ANESTHESIA
REVIEW

ANESTHESIA REVIEW

A Study Guide to
Anesthesia, Fifth Edition
and
Basics of Anesthesia, Fourth Edition

Lorraine M. Sdrales, M.D.
Assistant Clinical Professor
Department of Anesthesia and Perioperative Care
University of California, San Francisco, School of Medicine
San Francisco, California

Staff Anesthesiologist
Cedars-Sinai Medical Center
Los Angeles, California

Ronald D. Miller, M.D.
Professor and Chair
Department of Anesthesia and Perioperative Care
University of California, San Francisco, School of Medicine
San Francisco, California

Consulting Editor
Robert K. Stoelting, M.D.
Professor and Chair
Department of Anesthesia
Indiana University School of Medicine
Indianapolis, Indiana

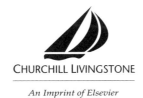

CHURCHILL LIVINGSTONE

An Imprint of Elsevier

CHURCHILL LIVINGSTONE
An Imprint of Elsevier

The Curtis Center
Independence Square West
Philadelphia, Pennsylvania 19106

Library of Congress Cataloging-in-Publication Data

Sdrales, Lorraine
Anesthesia review: a study guide to Anesthesia, 5th edition and Basics of Anesthesia, 4th edition / Lorraine Sdrales, Ronald D. Miller.

p.; cm.

ISBN 0–443–07978–1

1. Anesthesia—Examinations, questions, etc.   I. Miller, Ronald D., 1939-
  II. Stoelting, Robert K. Basics of anesthesia. III. Anesthesia. IV. Title.
  [DNLM: 1. Anesthesia—Examination Questions.   WO 218.2 S437a 2001]

RD82.3 .S385 2001   617.9′6′076—dc21   00–065746

Acquisitions Editor: Allan Ross
Project Manager: Agnes Hunt Byrne
Production Manager: Norman Stellander
Illustration Specialist: Robert Quinn
Book Designer: Steven Stave

ANESTHESIA REVIEW: A Study Guide to Anesthesia, Fifth Edition
and Basics of Anesthesia, Fourth Edition   ISBN 0–443–07978–1

Printed in the United States of America.

Last digit is the print number: 9   8   7   6   5   4

Preface

As with all medical disciplines, the practice of anesthesia requires a solid knowledge base as well as clinical competence. There are many textbooks that provide the student of anesthesiology with the information needed to practice anesthesia, although few have been updated. What was lacking was a book that allowed students at every level to actively participate in their learning. This study guide lets the reader evaluate his or her own knowledge and formulate answers alone or in groups, and it provides for an alternate means of study of the information.

The format of the book is question/answer. It is organized in a logical progression from basic anesthesia principles and concepts to more complex issues. These include the delivery of anesthesia in various settings, and the administration of anesthesia to patients with organ system dysfunction and disease states. All the answers are current, fully formed, and self-explanatory, and the page number references provided at the end of each question refer the reader to the *Basics of Anesthesia*, Fourth Edition, and *Anesthesia*, Fifth Edition, texts where further information on the given topic can be found.

There are several ways this study guide can be used. The first year anesthesia resident may use it to solidify information read. Anesthesia residents at every level may use it to prepare for specific clinical applications that they may be faced with on a subspecialty rotation or with given cases. Anesthesia residents can also use this study guide for group study in which they will be forced to verbalize answers to questions on given topics. Similarly, faculty may use the study guide to quiz residents orally in a coherent, progressive manner in formal or informal settings. Finally, anesthesiologists in practice may find the study guide useful to refresh their knowledge base and review old and new information that they may not have been taught during their residencies. The multiple uses of this study guide make it an appropriate choice for students and teachers of anesthesiology at every level.

Lorraine M. Sdrales
Ronald D. Miller

Contents

Chapter 1

Basic Pharmacologic Principles

1. What is pharmacokinetics?

2. What is pharmacodynamics?

3. What is the role of receptors in drug pharmacology?

4. What are three methods by which the effect of a drug is terminated?

STEREOCHEMISTRY

5. What is a racemic mixture? Give an example of a drug used in clinical anesthesia that is a racemic mixture.

6. What is the significance of the administration of racemic mixtures in clinical anesthesia?

TERMINOLOGY AND DEFINITIONS

7. What are agonist drugs?

8. What are antagonist drugs?

9. Define competitive and noncompetitive antagonism. Which of these is overcome by higher concentrations of the drug?

10. What does an additive drug effect mean? Give an example.

11. What does a synergistic drug effect mean? Give an example.

12. When an individual is described as hyporeactive to a drug, what does it refer to?

13. What is drug tolerance?

14. What is drug cross-tolerance?

15. What does tachyphylaxis to a drug refer to?

16. What does an idiosyncratic reaction to a drug refer to?

17. What does a dose-response curve illustrate? Draw and label one.

18. How is the potency of a drug depicted on a dose-response curve?

19. What does the effective dose 50 (ED_{50}) refer to?

20. How would an increased affinity of a drug for its receptor influence its dose-response curve?

21. What is reflected by the slope of a dose-response curve? What clinical problem may be associated with a steep dose-response curve?

22. What is a drug's efficacy? How is it depicted on the dose-response curve? What may limit a drug's efficacy clinically?

23. Can individual variability alter the dose-response curve?

PHARMACOKINETICS OF INTRAVENOUS DRUGS

24. What is the role of the volume of distribution and clearance of a drug in the evaluation of the pharmacokinetic properties of the drug?

25. Describe the two-compartment model used to describe the pharmacokinetic properties of a drug that has been administered as a bolus.

26. What is the volume of distribution of a drug?

27. What are three properties of a drug that will determine how much of the drug will pass from the plasma into the tissues after its intravenous administration?

28. How are drugs cleared from the body? How might the clearance rate of drugs be defined pharmacokinetically?

29. What is the role of the kidneys in the clearance of drugs from the plasma? How might the function of the kidneys in this regard be evaluated clinically?

30. What is the role of the liver in the clearance of drugs from the plasma? How is this accomplished by the liver?

31. Draw and label a typical curve illustrating the decrease in the plasma concentration of drug over time after its intravenous administration as a bolus. What are the two distinct phases that are represented on the curve?

32. What is the elimination half-time of a drug? What is the clinical relevance of a drug's elimination half-time?

33. What is the time necessary to achieve a steady-state plasma concentration of drug when it is administered as intermittent boluses? After a therapeutic concentration of drug is achieved in the plasma, how can a continued, unchanging plasma concentration be maintained?

34. Why might measured pharmacokinetic properties of drugs differ from what is observed clinically?

35. What is the context-sensitive half-time? What is its clinical usefulness?

36. What is the time to recovery from anesthesia dependent on? Why might a bispectral index monitor be useful in decreasing the time to recovery from anesthesia?

37. What does the effect-site equilibration time refer to? What is its clinical usefulness?

38. What is the pharmacokinetic relevance of the degree of ionization of a drug? What factors determine the degree of ionization of a drug?

39. What is the principal advantage of the intravenous administration of drugs?

40. What is the first-pass hepatic effect of drugs? When does it apply? What is its clinical effect?

41. What is the first-pass pulmonary effect of drugs? When does it apply? What is its clinical effect?

42. Describe the redistribution of a drug after its intravenous administration. What is the clinical relevance of redistribution?

PHARMACODYNAMICS OF INTRAVENOUS DRUGS

43. What are receptors? How are receptors identified and classified?

44. What are transmembrane signaling systems? What is their net effect?

45. Name an example of a receptor type that acts as a protein (ion) channel.

46. Name an example of a receptor type that opens an ion channel via membrane-bound G proteins when stimulated.

47. Name an example of a receptor type that acts via membrane-bound G proteins and an intracellular second messenger to exert its intracellular effects.

48. Name an example of a receptor type that acts through the activation of phospholipase C.

49. Why is the stereospecificity of drugs important with respect to their interaction with the receptor?

50. Are the number of receptors in lipid cell membranes static or dynamic? Give an example of down-regulation and up-regulation of a receptor.

51. How does aging change the responsiveness of receptors?

52. During steady-state conditions, what is the relationship between the concentration of drug at the receptors and the plasma concentration of drug?

PHARMACOKINETICS OF INHALED ANESTHETICS

53. What does the pharmacokinetics of inhaled anesthetics describe?

54. How does the inspired partial pressure (PI) of an inhaled anesthetic influence the onset of anesthesia?

55. How do the tissues of the body equilibrate with the inspired partial pressure (PI) of an inhaled anesthetic?

56. What is a clinical use of the alveolar partial pressure of an anesthetic?

57. What are some factors that act simultaneously to determine the alveolar partial pressure of an anesthetic?

58. What are some factors that act simultaneously to determine the partial pressure of an anesthetic in the brain?

59. How much does the metabolism and percutaneous loss of inhaled anesthetics influence the alveolar partial pressure of an anesthetic during the induction and maintenance of anesthesia?

60. What is the concentration effect? Clinically, with which inhaled anesthetic agent is the concentration effect solely possible? Why?

61. Why is the inspired partial pressure of an anesthetic often decreased after the induction of anesthesia?

62. What is the second gas effect? Does this depend on or occur independent of the concentration effect? Give an example of the second gas effect.

63. Is the second gas effect clinically significant?

64. What is alveolar hyperoxygenation? By what percent does the arterial partial pressure of oxygen increase during alveolar hyperoxygenation?

65. How does increasing alveolar ventilation affect the rate of the induction of anesthesia with an inhaled anesthetic?

66. How can controlled ventilation of the lungs affect the rate of increase of the alveolar partial pressure of an inhaled anesthetic during its initial administration?

67. How can switching from spontaneous to controlled ventilation of the lungs during the administration of an inhaled anesthetic affect the anesthetic depth?

68. Why might the brain be theoretically protected from a high inspired partial pressure of anesthetic with the institution of controlled ventilation? Why is the heart not similarly protected on a theoretical basis?

69. What are the three characteristics of the anesthetic breathing system that influence the rate of increase of the partial pressure of anesthetic in the alveoli?

70. How does an increased volume in the anesthetic breathing system affect the rate of increase of the alveolar partial pressure? How is this overcome?

71. How does the solubility of inhaled anesthetics in the components of the anesthetic breathing system affect the rate of increase of the alveolar partial pressure (P_A) of anesthetic on induction? How does the solubility of inhaled anesthetics in the components of the anesthetic breathing system affect the rate of decrease of the P_A of anesthetic upon the termination of anesthesia?

72. What does the partition coefficient define? What does a blood:gas partition coefficient of 10 mean? Does temperature influence a partition coefficient?

73. What is the single most important determinant of the rate at which the alveolar concentration (F_A) of an inhaled anesthetic increases toward the constant inspired concentration (F_I) of the anesthetic?

74. Why is the rate of increase of the alveolar partial pressure of an inhaled anesthetic, and therefore the rate of induction of anesthesia, influenced by the anesthetic's solubility in blood?

75. When an inhaled anesthetic has a low solubility in blood, is the rate of increase of the partial pressure of anesthetic in the alveoli rapid or slow?

76. How can the impact of a high blood:gas solubility on the rate of increase of alveolar partial pressure be offset clinically?

77. What are the three factors that influence the uptake of anesthetic at the tissues from the blood? What does a tissue:blood partition coefficient describe?

78. How can the time necessary for the equilibration of an inhaled anesthetic between a given tissue and the blood be predicted?

79. How does the time constant for isoflurane compare with the time constant for desflurane with respect to brain tissue?

80. Why does nitrous oxide transfer into air-filled cavities with its administration?

81. How does the transfer of nitrous oxide into air-filled cavities affect the cavity? What are some of the potential risks that can occur as a result?

82. What three factors will influence the net amount of gas that will transfer into an air-filled cavity during the administration of nitrous oxide?

83. By how much does the volume of an air-filled cavity expand secondary to the administration of nitrous oxide? Over what time period does this occur?

84. How does a patient's cardiac output influence the rate of induction of anesthesia? Why?

85. How do intracardiac shunts affect the rate of induction of anesthesia?

86. How does wasted ventilation influence the rate of induction of anesthesia?

87. Please complete the following table:

	PERCENT BODY MASS	PERCENT CARDIAC OUTPUT
Vessel-rich group		
Muscle group		
Fat group		
Vessel-poor group		

88. What does the alveolar-to-venous partial pressure difference (A-vD) reflect? How does the A-vD change over time with the induction of anesthesia?

89. How does the uptake of anesthetic in skeletal muscle and fat compare with the uptake of anesthetic in the vessel-rich organs? How does the uptake of anesthetic in skeletal muscle and fat influence the equilibration of the partial pressures of anesthetic between these tissues and the blood?

90. How might the recovery from anesthesia be defined?

91. What are three common factors that influence both the rate of induction of anesthesia and the rate of recovery from anesthesia? What are three factors that influence the rate of recovery from anesthesia that are unique to this phase, and do not influence the rate of induction of anesthesia?

92. How do tissue concentrations of inhaled anesthetics affect the alveolar partial pressure (PA) of anesthetic at the conclusion of anesthesia? What two factors will determine how much impact tissue concentrations will have on the rate of recovery of anesthesia?

93. Which volatile anesthetics undergo a significant amount of metabolism?

94. What is the clinical utility of the context-sensitive half-time in evaluating the time to recovery from an inhaled anesthetic?

95. What is diffusion hypoxia? When is diffusion hypoxia likely to occur? How can diffusion hypoxia be prevented?

PHARMACODYNAMICS OF INHALED ANESTHETICS

96. What is the minimum alveolar concentration (MAC) of an anesthetic? How does the MAC of an anesthetic relate to the anesthetic's dose-response curve?

97. How has the determination of the minimum alveolar concentration of various inhaled anesthetics enabled comparisons between the various anesthetics? How is the therapeutic index of an inhaled anesthetic derived?

98. What inhaled anesthetic is often administered concomitantly with volatile anesthetic agents to increase the potency of anesthesia? How is the combined minimum alveolar concentration calculated when two or more inhaled anesthetics are being administered?

99. Name some physiologic or pharmacologic factors that increase the minimum alveolar concentration for an individual patient.

100. Name some physiologic or pharmacologic factors that decrease the minimum alveolar concentration for an individual patient.

101. How do the duration of anesthesia, gender, anesthetic metabolism, and thyroid gland dysfunction each affect the minimum alveolar concentration of anesthesia for an individual patient?

102. What are some of the effects of inhaled anesthetics at the molecular level? Which of these is the mechanism by which inhaled anesthetics produce their depressant effects on the central nervous system?

103. Name some theories that have been proposed to explain the production of anesthesia by inhaled agents.

104. What is the protein (receptor) hypothesis? What is the evidence to support this theory?

105. Inhaled anesthetics may alter the availability of which neurotransmitter? How is this applied as a theory for the mechanism of action of inhaled anesthetics?

106. What is the Meyer-Overton theory? What is the evidence to support this theory? What is the basis for the opposition to the Meyer-Overton theory?

Answers*

1. Pharmacokinetics is the study of the absorption, distribution, metabolism, and elimination of inhaled or injected drugs and their metabolites. It is also the study of the time it takes for these processes to occur. It can be thought of as what the body does to the drug. (18; **15**)

2. Pharmacodynamics is the study of the responsiveness of receptors to drugs, the pharmacologic effects of the drugs, and the mechanism by which these effects occur. More simply put, it is the study of the relationship between a specific dose of drug and its effect on the body. It can be thought of as what the drug does to the body. (18; **34**)

3. Receptors are components of a cell, often lying within the cell membrane. Attachment of a drug to a receptor leads to a chain of events whose end result is the pharmacologic effects of the drug. Understanding receptors furthers the understanding of a drug's activity and effect, the selectivity of the receptor for a given drug, and the pharmacologic activity of receptor agonists and antagonists. (18; **34**)

4. The three methods by which a drug's effects are terminated are through its redistribution to inactive tissue sites, metabolism, and/or excretion. (18; **34**)

STEREOCHEMISTRY

5. A racemic mixture refers to a drug or compound that is made up of a 50:50 mixture of two enantiomers of a compound. Racemic mixtures of drugs actually represent two distinct drugs or compounds whose stereochemistries differ. Examples of drugs used in clinical anesthesia that are racemic mixtures include bupivacaine, ketamine, and volatile anesthetics. (18; **24–25**)

6. Because racemic mixtures of drugs actually represent two distinct drugs whose stereochemistry is different, the molecular interactions of each of these drugs with receptors results in different effects for each enantiomer. Each enantiomer may have different pharmacokinetic and pharmacodynamic properties, as well as different physiologic effects. For example, only one enantiomer may be responsible for the drug's desired result, whereas the other may be responsible for the drug's side effects. (18; **24–25**)

TERMINOLOGY AND DEFINITIONS

7. Agonist drugs are drugs that bind to and activate receptors. (18; **35**)

8. Antagonist drugs are drugs that bind to but do not activate receptors. Antagonists do not allow agonists to bind to the receptors while bound themselves, and therefore block the clinical response that would normally result from the binding of an agonist drug to the receptor. (18; **36**)

9. Antagonist drugs bind to but do not activate receptors. Once occupied by a receptor, an antagonist whose effect can be overcome by increasing the concentration of an agonist at the receptor is considered a competitive antagonist. With competitive antagonism, increasing concentrations of the agonist can progressively overcome, and thus "compete" with, the antagonist. An example of a competitive antagonist is a nondepolarizing neuromuscular blocking drug. Nondepolarizing neuromuscular blocking drugs bind to and occupy acetylcholine receptors in the neuromuscular junction, thereby

---

*Numbers in parentheses: lightface numbers refer to pages, figures, or tables in Stoelting RK, Miller RD: *Basics of Anesthesia*, 4th ed. Philadelphia, Churchill Livingstone, 2000; **boldface numbers** refer to pages, figures, or tables in Miller RD: *Anesthesia*, 5th ed. Philadelphia, Churchill Livingstone, 2000.

blocking the effect of acetylcholine at that receptor. The effects of nondepolarizing neuromuscular blocking drugs can be overcome by increasing the concentration of acetylcholine molecules at the receptor. This is the basis for the reversal of the effect of nondepolarizing neuromuscular blocking drugs by acetylcholine esterase inhibitors, such as neostigmine. Noncompetitive antagonism exists when increasing or even high concentrations of an agonist cannot overcome, or cannot "compete," with the antagonist. In these situations the receptor remains blocked despite the high concentration of agonist available at the receptor. (18; **36**)

10. An additive drug effect occurs when a second drug is administered with a first drug and then the first and second drug together produce an effect that is equal to the sum of their individual effects. An example of this is when the first and second drugs are inhaled anesthetics and their combined effect is equal to the sum of their respective minimum alveolar concentration values. (18; **44**)

11. A synergistic drug effect occurs when a second drug is administered with a first drug and the first and second drug together produce an effect that is greater than that expected from the sum of their individual effects (additive effect). An example of a synergistic drug effect is when the first and second drugs are aminoglycoside antibiotics and nondepolarizing neuromuscular blocking drugs. The resulting neuromuscular blockade produced is greater than the added effect of each individual drug. A synergistic drug effect occurs when nondepolarizing neuromuscular blocking drugs are administered in combination with aminoglycoside antibiotics despite the inability of aminoglycoside antibiotics to produce clinically significant neuromuscular blockade when administered alone. (18; **44, 463**)

12. An individual described as being hyporeactive to a drug has a decreased clinical effect from that expected from the administration of a particular dose of a drug. A hyperreactive individual responds in the opposite way, when a particular dose of a drug produces an increased clinical effect from that expected. (18; **44**)

13. When an individual is administered a drug on a chronic basis the receptors to which the drug binds can develop a decreased responsiveness to the drug. The patient thus develops an acquired hyporeactivity to the drug. This results in a decreased clinical response elicited by a particular dose of drug, such that the dose of drug that results in a particular effect must be increased from the dose that previously resulted in the effect. The patient under these circumstances is said to have developed a tolerance to the drug. (18; **45–46**)

14. When an individual is administered a drug on a chronic basis the patient may develop a *tolerance* to the drug. The administration of another drug that produces similar effects to the first drug may also result in a decreased clinical response. The patient thus also develops an acquired hyporeactivity to the second drug that is similar to the first drug. The patient under these circumstances is said to have developed a *cross-tolerance* to the second drug. (18; **45–46**)

15. *Tachyphylaxis* is a term used to describe tolerance to a drug that develops acutely after just a few doses of the drug have been administered. (18; **45–46**)

16. When an individual experiences an unusual effect of the drug it is termed an *idiosyncratic reaction*. Patients who are susceptible to an idiosyncratic reaction after the administration of a drug will demonstrate a reaction regardless of the dose of drug that is administered. It is believed that patients become susceptible to an idiosyncratic reaction of a drug secondary to hypersensitivity or genetic differences. (18; **46**)

17. A dose-response curve is a graph depicting the relationship between a dose of drug administered on the x-axis and the pharmacologic effect that results from its administration on the y-axis. (19, Fig. 2–1; **44–45, Fig. 2–34**)

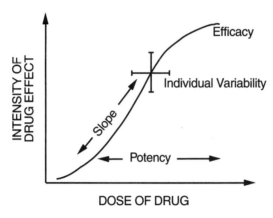

Figure 1–1. Dose-response curves are characterized by differences in potency, slope, efficacy, and individual responses. (From Stoelting RK, Miller RD: Basics of Anesthesia, 4th ed. Philadelphia, Churchill Livingstone, 2000, p 19.)

18. The potency of a drug is depicted by its location on the x-axis of the dose-response curve. Another method by which the potency of a drug can be quantified is by the dose of drug that is required to produce the maximal effect of the drug. (19, Fig. 2–1; **45**)

19. The effective dose 50 (ED_{50}) of a drug is the dose of the drug required to produce a given effect in 50% of the people to whom that dose of drug is administered. The ED_{50} of a drug only corresponds to one specific effect of that drug. (19; **45**)

20. An increased affinity of a drug for its receptor would move its dose-response curve to the left. This corresponds to an increased potency of the drug. A decreased affinity of a drug for its receptor would move its dose-response curve to the right, reflecting a decrease in drug potency. (19; **44**)

21. The slope of a dose-response curve reflects how much clinical effect results from the addition of drug. The number of receptors that must be occupied by a drug before a drug effect occurs will influence the slope of a dose-response curve. In the case in which a majority of the receptors must be occupied before seeing an effect of the drug, the slope of the dose-response curve would be steep. When a dose-response curve is steep, it indicates that small increases in the administered drug may result in large increases in the effect of the drug. Clinically, a small difference between a therapeutic and toxic concentration of drug may be associated with drugs whose dose-response curve is steep. (19; **44**)

22. The efficacy of a drug is the maximal clinical effect of the drug. An effect greater than the maximal one cannot be achieved even with the administration of more drug. The efficacy of a drug is depicted as the plateau on its dose-response curve. The maximal effect of a drug may not be possible to achieve clinically secondary to undesirable side effects of the drug that occur when maximal drug effects are approached. This may limit the efficacy of a drug clinically. (19, Fig. 2–1; **45**)

23. Individuals may vary with respect to the pharmacokinetics and/or the pharmacodynamics of a drug. Pharmacokinetics are affected by individual differences in renal function, liver function, cardiac function, and patient age. Pharmacodynamics are affected by individual differences in enzyme activity and genetic differences. This may be reflected as alterations in the position of the dose-response curve for the drug. (19; **46**)

PHARMACOKINETICS OF INTRAVENOUS DRUGS

24. The pharmacokinetics of administered drugs is the study of a drug's absorption, distribution, metabolism, and elimination. The volume of distribution of a drug reflects the apparent volume in which the drug will distribute itself. The clearance of the drug involves either its elimination via the kidneys or its metabolism by the liver. (19; **15–17**)

25. The two-compartment pharmacokinetic model is a conceptual model used to describe the biphasic manner in which the body appears to handle drugs administered as a bolus. The model describes two compartments in which the bolused drug will distribute itself. Initially, the drug will enter the central compartment. The central compartment, which is of a smaller volume, consists of the blood, plasma, and highly perfused organs such as the heart, lungs, kidneys, and liver. With time the drug will then transfer into the peripheral compartment. The peripheral compartment, which contains a large volume, consists of all other tissues or sites in which a drug may distribute itself. The transfer of drugs between these two compartments is depicted as rate constants. (19, Fig. 2–2; **26–29, Figs. 2–14, 2–15, 2–16**)

26. The volume of distribution of a drug is calculated as the dose of drug administered intravenously divided by the plasma concentration. Although the volume of distribution is a calculated number, it does not refer to absolute anatomic volumes but to a conceptual volume. The volume of distribution is used to conceptualize how much of the drug stays in the central compartment (plasma) after its intravenous injection. A volume of distribution for a given drug may be as small as the plasma volume of the patient, implying that nearly all the administered drug remains in the central compartment. Conversely, the volume of distribution of a drug may be large, implying the drug transfers quickly into the peripheral tissues. The volume of distribution is therefore a calculated number used to describe a specific drug's potential to transfer from the plasma to the tissues after its intravenous administration. (19–20; **16–17**)

27. Three properties of a drug that will determine how much of the drug will pass from the plasma into the tissues after its intravenous administration include its capacity to bind to plasma proteins, its degree of ionization, and its lipid solubility. Because these three factors will determine how much of the drug will stay in the central compartment after its intravenous administration, they also influence the drug's apparent volume of distribution. For example, drugs that are highly bound to protein, with a high degree of ionization, and a low lipid solubility will tend to remain in the plasma and have a high plasma concentration. These drugs will have a small calculated volume of distribution. (20; **17, 22**)

28. Drugs are cleared from the body through its elimination or metabolism. The clearance rate of a drug is defined as the volume of plasma that is cleared of drug per unit time. By knowing the clearance rate of a drug, the anesthesiologist is better able to administer a given drug at a rate in which inadequate levels of the drug in the plasma or the accumulation of drug levels in the plasma are minimized. (20; **17–22, 29–30, Fig. 2–3**)

29. The kidneys are primarily responsible for clearing drugs from the plasma through the excretion of drugs in the urine. Drugs that are water soluble and not bound to proteins are most efficiently excreted by the kidney. Clinical indicators of the capacity of the kidneys to eliminate drugs include the creatinine clearance or serum creatinine values. An abnormal laboratory value indicates that there is some degree of decreased kidney function, implying

that the clearance of drugs from the plasma may be prolonged. The degree of increase of the serum creatinine levels provides an indication of how much the drug dose should be decreased to prevent the accumulation of the drug in the plasma. (20; **17, 22**)

30. Although the kidneys, lungs, and gastrointestinal tract have limited potential for the metabolism of drugs, the liver is the organ primarily responsible for the metabolism of drugs, which facilitates their clearance from the plasma. Metabolism is the conversion of lipid-soluble drugs to water-soluble drugs, which allows for their excretion by the kidneys. Lipid-soluble drugs are poorly excreted by the kidneys because they are so easily reabsorbed by the renal tubules. Often the metabolism of drugs to a more water-soluble form converts the drug from a pharmacologically active to an inactive metabolite. The enzymes responsible for the metabolism of many drugs are located in the liver, specifically in the hepatic smooth endoplasmic reticulum, and are referred to as microsomal enzymes. The microsomal enzymes include the protein enzymes of the cytochrome P-450 system, which are believed to be responsible for the metabolism of many drugs. The principal determinant of microsomal enzyme activity is most likely genetic, accounting for the large variation among individuals with respect to the rate of drug metabolism. Microsomal enzymes may also be induced, increasing their activity and subsequently accelerating the rate of metabolism and clearance of some administered drugs. A drug that classically causes induction of the hepatic microsomal enzymes is phenobarbital. (20; **18–22, Figs. 2–7, 2–8**)

31. On the curve, the first phase of distribution, or the alpha phase, immediately follows the intravenous administration. It is characterized by a rapid decline in the plasma concentration of drug. The alpha phase represents the initial distribution of drug from the circulation to the tissues. The second phase, or beta phase, is clearly separate from the alpha phase. The beta phase is characterized by a slow decrease in the plasma concentration subsequent to the distribution phase. The beta phase represents the elimination of a drug from the central compartment by renal and hepatic clearance mechanisms. (20, Fig. 2–3; **30–33, Figs. 2–17, 2–18, 2–19**)

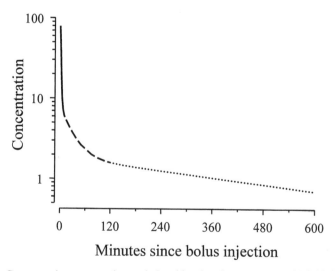

Figure 1–2. Concentration versus time relationship showing a very rapid initial decline after bolus injection. The terminal log-linear portion is only seen after most of the drug has left the plasma. This is characteristic of most anesthetic drugs. Different line types highlight the rapid, intermediate, and slow (log-linear) portions of the curve. (From Miller RD: Anesthesia, 5th ed. Philadelphia, Churchill Livingstone, 2000, p 31.)

32. The elimination half-time of a drug is the time necessary for the plasma concentration of a drug to decrease by 50% during the elimination phase. The drug is almost completely eliminated after five elimination half-times have passed. By knowing the elimination half-time of a drug, the anesthesiologist is theoretically better able to administer a given drug at a rate in which inadequate levels of the drug in the plasma are minimized. Repeated equal doses of a drug more frequently than five elimination half-times would result in the drug being administered at a rate greater than its clearance. The result would be an accumulation of the drug in the plasma. Drug accumulation does not occur when the rate of elimination of the drug is equal to the rate of drug administration. (21; **27–30, 33–34**)

33. The time necessary to achieve a steady-state plasma concentration of drug when it is administered as intermittent boluses is about five elimination half-times of the drug. In clinical practice this is often circumvented through the intravenous administration of a large initial dose of drug, or loading dose, to quickly achieve a therapeutic drug concentration. After a therapeutic concentration of the drug is achieved in the plasma, the clinician can give continuous or intermittent intravenous injections of the drug at a rate approximately equal to the rate of drug elimination to maintain an unchanging plasma concentration. (21; **27–30, 33–34, Fig. 2–4**)

34. Pharmacokinetic properties of drugs are measured in healthy, ambulatory adults. Observed pharmacokinetics of drugs may be very different in patients with chronic diseases, at the extremes of age, with abnormal hydration or nutritive status, or with decreased skeletal muscle mass. Patients with renal insufficiency or hepatic dysfunction are especially likely to have prolongation of the elimination half-time of an administered drug. In the presence of hepatic or renal dysfunction, the maintenance dose of a drug should be adjusted downward to prevent drug accumulation. (21; **17–22, 46–47**)

35. The context-sensitive half-time refers to the time required for the concentration of a particular drug to reach a specific percent after the discontinuation of its administration as a continuous intravenous infusion for a specific duration. The context-sensitive half-time of a drug depends mostly on the drug's lipid solubility and clearance mechanisms and is not directly related to its elimination half-time. Computer-simulated models of the context-sensitive half-time of a drug may be useful clinically in anesthesia to predict the duration of a particular drug's effects after its discontinuation. (21, Fig. 2–4; **391–392, Fig. 11–13**)

36. The time to recovery from anesthesia is dependent on multiple factors. In general, however, if the plasma concentration of a drug administered is just above that required for awakening, the time to recovery would be less than it otherwise would have been. For this reason, the use of a bispectral index monitor may be useful in allowing the anesthesiologist to better estimate the depth of anesthesia obtained with a given plasma concentration of drug for a given patient. That patient may then be maintained at a plasma concentration just greater than that required for awakening, thus decreasing the amount of plasma concentration of the drug that would be required before awakening. This, in turn, leads to a decrease in the time to recovery from anesthesia. (22, Fig. 2–5; **391–394**)

37. The effect-site equilibration time refers to the interval of time required between the time that a specific drug concentration is achieved in the plasma and a specific effect of the drug can be measured. The effect-site equilibration time reflects the time necessary for the circulation to deliver the drug to its site of action, such as the brain. Knowledge of the effect-site equilibration time for a particular drug may be clinically useful in determining dosing intervals or in the titration of particular drugs. (22; **391–395**)

38. The degree of ionization of a drug is a key factor in the pharmacokinetics of a drug with respect to its pharmacologic activity, solubility in lipids, transfer out of the central compartment, and clearance from the central compartment. Most drugs are weak acids or weak bases and, under physiologic conditions, exist in both ionized and nonionized forms. The pK of a drug is a constant that determines the degree of ionization of the drug at physiologic pH, or in solutions in which the pH deviates from physiologic pH. The pK_a of a drug is defined as the pH of the drug at which the drug will be 50% ionized. Therefore, when the pK_a of a drug and the pH of the surrounding fluid are identical, 50% percent of the drug exists in the ionized form. When the pK of a drug is close to the pH of the surrounding fluid, small changes in the pH of the surrounding fluid can result in large changes in the degree of ionization of the drug. Drugs that are weak acids tend to be highly ionized in a basic solution and nonionized in an acidic pH. The opposite is true for drugs that are weak bases, such that these drugs tend to be highly nonionized in a basic solution and ionized in an acidic pH. (22, Table 2–1; **17**)

39. The principal advantage of the intravenous administration of drugs is that the plasma concentration of drug that is achieved is more predictable than when drugs are administered orally or intramuscularly. After the intravenous administration of a drug, the highly perfused tissues will receive a proportionally larger amount of the total dose of drug than other tissues. The highly perfused tissues include the brain, heart, liver, and kidneys. Intravenously administered anesthetic drugs that are lipid soluble therefore reach the brain rapidly and cross the blood-brain barrier to exert their effects. (22; **30**)

40. The first-pass effect refers to the extensive metabolism of a drug before reaching the systemic circulation and exerting its pharmacologic effect. A drug administered orally becomes absorbed from the gastrointestinal tract, enters the portal venous blood, and then passes through the liver before entering the systemic circulation. This only applies to drugs administered orally and is referred to as the first-pass hepatic effect. The clinical effect is most significant when drugs are extensively metabolized by the liver. These drugs have large differences between the oral and intravenous doses that need to be administered for a similar pharmacologic effect. Examples of drugs that undergo extensive metabolism by the liver include lidocaine and propranolol. (23; **30**)

41. The first-pass pulmonary effect of drugs refers to the uptake of basic lipophilic amines by the lung. Examples of these drugs include lidocaine, propranolol, and fentanyl. Clinically, the first-pass pulmonary effect may influence the peak arterial concentration of these drugs. The lungs may also serve as a reservoir from which drug is released back into the systemic circulation. (23; **30**)

42. After the intravenous administration of a drug, highly perfused tissues rapidly take up drug from the plasma. Eventually the plasma concentration of drug will drop below the concentration of drug in the highly perfused tissues. The drug will then leave the highly perfused tissues, move into the plasma, and be delivered to less well-perfused tissue sites. This transfer of drug to inactive tissue sites, such as skeletal muscle and fat, is known as redistribution. A clinical example of redistribution can be seen after the administration of an intravenous bolus dose of thiopental for the induction of anesthesia. The transfer of drug to inactive tissue sites, or redistribution, is responsible for waning of the pharmacologic effect of the drug. Clinically, the redistribution of thiopental after the administration of an induction dose is reflected by patient awakening after the administration of the drug. Repeated doses or a continuous infusion of a drug such as thiopental can saturate the inactive tissue sites. As these sites become saturated, redistribution becomes a pro-

longed effect. The body tissues then depend on metabolism as the principal method of elimination of the drug. The result is a prolonged pharmacologic effect of the drug. In the case in which the drug is thiopental, the clinical effect may be delayed awakening. (23; **30–33, Fig. 2–13**)

PHARMACODYNAMICS OF INTRAVENOUS DRUGS

43. Receptors are components of a cell that selectively interact with compounds that are external to the cell. The interaction of the receptor with the compound results in the translation of the stimulus into a specific effect. Receptors are typically protein macromolecules present in the cell membrane, whereas the compounds with which they interact are frequently drugs in the plasma. Receptors are identified and classified on the basis of their effects after being stimulated by agonists or blocked by antagonists. Examples of classes of receptors include the alpha, beta, dopamine, histamine, and mu receptor types. These classifications are useful to summarize the pharmacologic effects of agonist and antagonist drugs. (23; **34–36, Figs. 2–24, 2–26**)

44. Transmembrane signaling systems describe the way in which receptors exert their effect after interacting with, or being activated by, a drug. The portion of the receptor that lies outside the cell membrane interacts with the drug, whereas the portion of the receptor that faces the inside of the cell exerts the cellular effect after activation. The collective end result of receptor activation most often is a change in transmembrane voltage and neuronal excitability. Receptors are therefore transmembrane signaling systems. (23; **38–39**)

45. Receptors for the neurotransmitter gamma-aminobutyric acid (GABA) are an example of protein (ion) channels. This type of receptor results in ion flow into or out of the cell when activated. In this example, after activation of the receptor by GABA, the ion channel changes configuration such that there is flow of chloride ions into the cell. (24; **40, Figs. 2–28, 2–31**)

46. An example of a receptor that opens an ion channel via membrane-bound G proteins when stimulated is the muscarinic receptor. The muscarinic receptor couples to the membrane bound guanine nucleotide binding protein (G protein) after its activation by an agonist. The result of this coupling is opening of the potassium ion channel and flow of potassium ions through the channel. (24; **38–39, 542–544, Figs. 2–28, 2–29, 2–30**)

47. Like the muscarinic receptor, other receptors act via binding of the receptor to a G protein. Unlike the muscarinic receptor, however, the coupling of the receptor with a G protein may result in activation of an intracellular second messenger to exert its intracellular effects. An example of a second messenger is cyclic adenosine monophosphate (cAMP), whose activity is regulated by adenylate cyclase. Adenylate cyclase can be stimulated through a stimulatory G protein, positively affecting its activity and resulting in an increase in the intracellular level of cAMP. An example of a receptor that acts this way is the beta-adrenergic receptor. Conversely, adenylate cyclase can be inhibited through an inhibitory G protein, negatively affecting its activity and resulting in a decrease in the intracellular level of cAMP. An example of a receptor that acts this way is the alpha-2 adrenergic receptor. (24; **38–42, 540–541, Figs. 2–28 through 2–32, 14–13**)

48. Alpha-1 receptors act by interacting with the membrane-bound enzyme phospholipase C once activated. Activation of phospholipase C catalyzes reactions, leading to second messengers that stimulate the release of calcium from intracellular stores. (24; **42, 540–541, Fig. 14–13**)

49. The stereospecificity of a drug is often important in how it configures with

the receptor to exert its pharmacologic response. Most drugs are synthesized as racemic mixtures containing about 50% each of the dextro (*d*) and levo (*l*) isomers. These stereoisomers of the same drug may have distinctly different biologic properties. The inactive isomer may be an impurity that does not contribute to its pharmacologic effect. The inactive isomer may, however, contribute to undesired drug effects. (24–25; **36–37**)

50. The number of receptors in lipid cell membranes is dynamic. Receptors increase in number (up-regulation) or decrease in number (down-regulation) in response to specific stimuli. Beta-adrenergic receptors are an example of a receptor that can behave this way. When beta-adrenergic receptors are chronically stimulated, down-regulation of the receptor can result. This can be seen to occur after chronic asthma treatment with beta agonists. The decrease in the number of beta receptors under these conditions explains the resulting tachyphylaxis. When beta receptors are chronically blocked, up-regulation of the receptor can result. The increased number of receptors can result in an exaggerated response if the blockade is discontinued. This explains the exaggerated hypertension that can result from discontinuation of a patient's beta-blockade therapy. (25; **45–46, 544**)

51. The mechanism by which the responsiveness of receptors changes is not well understood. The change in receptor responsiveness that occurs with age appears to occur independent from a change in the number of receptors. (25; **46**)

52. During steady-state conditions the concentration of a drug at the receptor is believed to be directly proportional to the plasma concentration of the drug. This allows for pharmacodynamic studies to be performed that evaluate the dose of drug required for specific responses. (25; **1092–1093**)

PHARMACOKINETICS OF INHALED ANESTHETICS

53. Pharmacokinetics is the study of the absorption, distribution, metabolism, and elimination of inhaled or injected drugs and their metabolites. The pharmacokinetics of inhaled anesthetics describes their absorption from the alveoli, distribution in the body, and metabolism via the liver or elimination via the lungs. (25; **15**)

54. The onset of anesthesia is dependent on achieving an appropriate partial pressure of anesthetic in the brain. The achievement of this relies on the concentration gradient of anesthetic from the anesthesia machine to the brain. By controlling the inspired partial pressure (PI) of an inhaled anesthetic the clinician is able to manipulate that concentration gradient. An increased PI will result in a greater concentration gradient, and a quicker achievement of the optimal partial pressure of anesthetic in the brain. This ultimately results in a more rapid onset of anesthesia. (25; **74, 77–78**)

55. The tissues of the body equilibrate with the inspired partial pressure of an inhaled anesthetic through the blood. The blood is responsible for the distribution of inhaled anesthetic to the various tissues of the body. The partial pressure of anesthetic in the arterial blood, or Pa, is thus an intermediary between the partial pressure of anesthetic in the alveoli (PA) and the partial pressure of anesthetic in the brain (Pbr). This is reflected in the equilibrium equation PA $\rightleftharpoons$ Pa $\rightleftharpoons$ Pbr. (25–26; **76–78**)

56. The alveolar partial pressure (PA) of an anesthetic is used clinically as a reflection of the partial pressure of anesthetic in the brain (Pbr). The PA of an anesthetic is therefore a useful clinical indicator of anesthetic depth. Maintaining a constant and optimal PA allows the anesthesiologist to achieve the same with the Pbr. It is also useful in monitoring the induction and

recovery of anesthesia when administering an inhaled anesthetic. Another clinical use of the PA of an anesthetic is that it provides a means by which inhaled anesthetics can be compared at equal potencies. (26)

57. In general terms the partial pressure of an anesthetic in the alveoli is a function of its input into the alveoli minus its uptake into the arterial blood. There are three things that influence the input of an anesthetic. These include the inspired partial pressure of the anesthetic, alveolar ventilation, and the characteristics of the anesthetic breathing system. There are also three things that influence the uptake of an anesthetic from the alveoli into the blood. These include the blood:gas partition coefficient of the anesthetic gas, the patient's cardiac output, and the alveolar-to-venous partial pressure difference. Together, these six factors determine the partial pressure of an anesthetic in the alveoli. (26; **74–82**)

58. The partial pressure of an anesthetic in the brain is determined by its brain:blood partition coefficient, cerebral blood flow, and the arterial-to-venous partial pressure difference. (26; **75–76**)

59. The metabolism and percutaneous loss of inhaled anesthetics do not significantly influence the alveolar partial pressure of an anesthetic during the induction and maintenance of anesthesia. (26; **79**)

60. With the administration of a given concentration of inhaled anesthetic, a certain amount of the anesthetic will be taken up by the blood. By administering a high inspired partial pressure (PI) of anesthetic initially, the impact of the uptake of anesthetic into the blood will be offset. The result is an accelerated rate of the induction of anesthesia. The rate of induction is reflected by the rate of increase in the alveolar partial pressure of the inhaled anesthetic. This effect of the high PI of anesthetic on the rate of rise of the alveolar concentration of the anesthetic is known as the *concentration effect*. The concentration effect occurs for two reasons. One is that the uptake of a large volume of anesthetic into the blood results in the remainder of the anesthetic gas being left in a smaller volume. The remainder of the gas is thus concentrated to a greater partial pressure than it otherwise would have been. The second reason why the concentration effect occurs is because of the augmentation of inspired ventilation. Augmentation of the inspired ventilation refers to the greater influence of the inspired gases when replacing larger volumes of lost gases in the alveoli. A high concentration of anesthetic must be given to produce the concentration effect. Clinically, this is only possible with nitrous oxide. (26, Fig. 2–10; **78, Figs. 4–3, 4–4**)

61. With the administration of a given concentration of inhaled anesthetic, a certain amount of the anesthetic will be taken up by the blood. The administration of a high inspired partial pressure (PI) of anesthetic initially offsets the impact of the uptake of anesthetic into the blood. The result is an accelerated rate of the induction of anesthesia. After the induction of anesthesia, the uptake of anesthetic into the blood will decrease. At this point the PI of anesthetic should be decreased from the high initial PI in order to maintain a constant and optimal partial pressure of anesthetic in the brain. If the PI of the anesthetic were maintained constant as the uptake of anesthetic into the blood decreased, the partial pressures of anesthetic in the alveoli and the brain would continue to increase. This could result in a greater than necessary, and even potentially toxic, partial pressure of anesthetic in the brain. (26; **76–78**)

62. When two gases exist in the alveoli, a large volume of uptake of the first gas from the alveoli results in an increase in the rate of rise of the partial pressure of the second gas in the alveoli. This is because the second gas remaining in

the alveoli is concentrated in a smaller total volume of gas in the alveoli. The uptake of the second gas into the blood is then increased as well. This is known as the second gas effect. The second gas effect occurs independent of the concentration effect. The classic example of the second gas effect is when the first and second gases are nitrous oxide and oxygen, respectively. The initial large volume of uptake of nitrous oxide into the blood accelerates the uptake of oxygen. (26–27; **78–79, Figs. 4–3 and 4–4**)

63. The second gas effect is not considered clinically significant. (27; **78–79**)

64. Alveolar hyperoxygenation refers to the increase in the uptake of oxygen when oxygen is administered with nitrous oxide due to the second gas effect. The increased uptake of oxygen in the blood results in a transient increase in the arterial partial pressure of oxygen by about 10% during the early phase of nitrous oxide administration. Although this phenomenon may be seen clinically, it is not considered to be clinically significant. (27; **78–79**)

65. An increase in alveolar ventilation helps to offset the impact of the uptake of anesthetic in the blood with its initial administration. The effect of increasing alveolar ventilation is a more rapid rate of increase in the partial pressure of an inhaled anesthetic in the alveoli and a more rapid rate of the induction of anesthesia. This is particularly true when the inhaled agent has a high blood:gas partition coefficient or is highly soluble in blood. Under these conditions there is a greater degree of uptake of anesthetic in the blood, and the more beneficial is the increase in alveolar ventilation in offsetting this. (27; **79–81, Fig. 4–5**)

66. Controlled ventilation of the lungs can cause an increase in the rate of the increase in the alveolar partial pressure of an inhaled anesthetic and a corresponding increase in the rate of induction of anesthesia. This may occur for two reasons. First, controlled ventilation of the lungs may result in an increase in alveolar ventilation, thereby increasing the input of anesthesia. Second, controlled ventilation of the lungs may decrease venous return. A corresponding decrease in cardiac output also results in a decrease in the uptake of an inhaled anesthetic into the blood. The net result of these is a more rapid rate of increase of the alveolar partial pressure of the inhaled anesthetic. (27; **80**)

67. Switching from spontaneous to controlled ventilation of the lungs during the initial administration of an inhaled anesthetic may result in an increase in the rate of induction of anesthesia through its potential combined effects of an increase in alveolar ventilation and a decrease in cardiac output. Also of note is the increased risk of anesthetic overdose with the switch from spontaneous to controlled ventilation of the lungs. This is particularly true with anesthetics with a high degree of solubility in blood. In a spontaneously ventilating patient, inhaled anesthetics affect alveolar ventilation such that they will cause respiratory depression, decreasing alveolar ventilation as alveolar partial pressures (PA) of the anesthetic increase. The resulting respiratory depression modulates the amount of anesthetic that is subsequently inspired. Respiratory depression progresses with increasing PA of the anesthetic until the patient becomes apneic, the ultimate prevention in further rises in the PA of the anesthetic. This intrinsic safety of limiting the maximal achievable PA of an anesthetic by the anesthetic itself is abolished by the institution of controlled ventilation of the lungs. For this reason it is recommended that the inspired partial pressure of an anesthetic be decreased when switching to controlled ventilation of the lungs to maintain the PA of the anesthetic that had been achieved. (27; **80**)

68. With the institution of controlled ventilation of the lungs there may be corresponding alveolar hyperventilation, as reflected by a decrease in the

arterial carbon dioxide partial pressure. This, in turn, results in a decrease in cerebral blood flow. Alveolar hyperventilation of the lungs increases the rate of increase of the alveolar partial pressure (PA) of the anesthetic with a potential increase in the delivery of anesthetic to the tissues. Because the brain relies on cerebral blood flow for the delivery of anesthetic, during hyperventilation the impact of the rate of increase of the PA of the anesthetic may be offset. Coronary blood flow is unlike cerebral blood flow in that coronary blood flow is not altered with hyperventilation. The myocardium is, therefore, not inherently protected from the possible increased input of anesthesia with the institution of controlled ventilation, and myocardial depression may result. (27; **642–643, 698**)

69. The three characteristics of the anesthetic breathing system that influence the rate of increase of the alveolar partial pressure of anesthetic are the volume of the system, the solubility of inhaled anesthetics in the components of the system, and gas inflow from the anesthetic machine. (27; **85–86**)

70. An increased volume in the anesthetic system slows the achievement of an optimal partial pressure of anesthetic in the brain by acting as a buffer. This can be overcome by using high gas inflows. (27; **85**)

71. The solubility of inhaled anesthetics in the plastic or rubber components of the anesthetic breathing system leads to absorption of anesthetic into the components. This results in slowing in the rate of increase in the alveolar partial pressure (PA) of anesthetic on the induction of anesthesia, as well as slowing in the rate of decrease in the PA of anesthetic upon the termination of anesthesia. Trace concentrations of anesthetic still remain in the components of the anesthetic breathing circuit at the conclusion of anesthesia. (27; **85, 91**)

72. The solubility of an inhaled anesthetic in blood and tissues is quantified as partition coefficients specific to the inhaled anesthetic. A partition coefficient describes how an inhaled agent will distribute itself between two phases when the partial pressures of the inhaled anesthetic in each phase are equal. For example, a blood:gas partition coefficient of 10 means that at equilibrium the ratio of the concentrations of anesthetic in blood:gas is 10:1. Therefore, the concentration of the anesthetic in the blood will be 10 times the concentration of the anesthetic in the gas. Partition coefficients are defined at a specific temperature, and are thus temperature dependent. Partition coefficients conventionally used in anesthesia have been defined at a temperature of 37°C. When temperatures are greater than this, the solubility of a gas in a liquid decreases. (27; **75–76, Table 4–1**)

73. The single most important determinant of how quickly the alveolar concentration (FA) of an anesthetic increases toward the constant inspired concentration (FI) of the anesthetic is the solubility of the inhaled anesthetic in blood. The solubility of the inhaled anesthetic in blood is defined by the anesthetic's blood:gas partition coefficient. Therefore, the rate of induction of anesthesia with an inhaled anesthetic is reflected by its blood:gas partition coefficient. The lower the blood:gas partition coefficient, the more quickly the FA of the anesthetic increases toward its FI, and the more rapidly the induction of anesthesia will be achieved. (27; **75–78**)

74. The rate of increase of the alveolar partial pressure (PA) of an inhaled anesthetic is influenced by the solubility of the anesthetic in blood. This is based on the premise that a gas that is highly soluble in blood will have a higher concentration of the gas taken up by the blood than a gas that is less soluble in blood. Likewise, an inhaled anesthetic with a high blood:gas partition coefficient will have a greater amount of anesthetic dissolved in the blood before reaching equilibrium. The inhaled anesthetic dissolved in blood does not quickly move to the tissues. The blood can therefore be considered

an inactive reservoir that takes up anesthetic but does not contribute to anesthesia. An anesthetic that is highly soluble in blood will have a slower rate of increase of its PA and a slower rate of induction of anesthesia, secondary to the greater amount of anesthetic that must dissolve in the blood before it can equilibrate with the tissues. (27; **75–78**)

75. When the blood solubility of an inhaled anesthetic is low, minimal amounts of anesthetic will have to be dissolved in the blood before the anesthetic can equilibrate with the tissues. For this reason, the rate of increase of the partial pressures of the anesthetic in the alveoli and brain are rapid. (27; **75**)

76. An anesthetic that is highly soluble in blood will have a slower rate of increase of its alveolar partial pressure (PA) and a slower rate of induction of anesthesia, secondary to the greater amount of anesthetic that must dissolve in the blood before it can equilibrate with the tissues. The impact of an anesthetic's high solubility in blood and its subsequent relatively slower rate of increase of its PA can be offset clinically to some extent by increasing the inspired concentration of the anesthetic. Increasing the inspired concentration of anesthetic will increase the amount of anesthetic delivered to the alveoli per unit of time, more rapidly fill the inactive blood reservoir with the soluble anesthetic, and decrease the amount of time required for equilibration with the tissues. (27; **75**)

77. The three factors that influence the uptake of anesthetic at the tissues from the blood include the blood flow to the given tissue, the arterial-to-tissue concentration gradient, and the tissue:blood partition coefficient of the anesthetic. The solubility of an inhaled anesthetic in blood and tissues is quantified as partition coefficients specific to the inhaled anesthetic. The tissue:blood partition coefficient describes how an inhaled agent will distribute itself between tissues and the blood when the partial pressures of the inhaled anesthetic in each phase are equal. The value of tissue:blood partition coefficients is that they are useful in predicting the time it will take for the anesthetic in the tissue to equilibrate with the anesthetic in the blood. (27; **76**)

78. The time necessary for the equilibration of an inhaled anesthetic between a tissue and the blood can be predicted by calculating a time constant for the anesthetic in the given tissue. The time constant is defined as the capacity of the system or tissue divided by the flow to the system. In the case of inhaled anesthetics and a specific tissue, the time constant is the amount of inhaled anesthetic that can be dissolved in a specific tissue divided by the blood flow to that tissue. Given this, tissues in which anesthetics do not dissolve well and tissues with a high volume of blood flow will have the shortest time constants and equilibrate most rapidly with the blood. For complete equilibration of anesthetic in the tissue and the blood, at least three time constants are required. (27; **76–77**)

79. The approximate time constant for isoflurane with respect to the brain is 3 to 4 minutes, whereas for desflurane it is about 2 minutes. Because cerebral blood flow in both cases is equal, the difference in the time constants for each of these agents is based solely on the difference in the solubility of the inhaled agents in the brain. The brain:blood partition coefficients are reflective of the solubility of these two agents. Three time constants, or the time required for almost complete equilibration of isoflurane with the tissue, results in equilibration of the partial pressures of anesthetic between the blood and the brain in 10 to 15 minutes. Inhaled anesthetics that are less soluble in blood, such as desflurane and nitrous oxide, require less time for the arterial partial pressure to equilibrate with the partial pressure of anesthetic in the brain. For this reason, desflurane and nitrous oxide require about 6 minutes for almost complete equilibration of their partial pressures in the blood and the brain. (27)

80. The transfer of nitrous oxide into air-filled cavities with its administration occurs as a result of the difference in solubility between nitrous oxide and nitrogen. The blood:gas partition coefficient of nitrous oxide is 0.46, and that of nitrogen is 0.014. Nitrous oxide is therefore 34 times more soluble in blood than nitrogen. Because nitrogen does not enter blood readily, nitrogen tends to remain in the air-filled cavity. Nitrous oxide is likely to enter the air-filled cavity until an equilibrium is established between the partial pressures of nitrous oxide in the air-filled cavity and the blood. Because of this preferential transfer of nitrous oxide, and the subsequent net transfer of gas into the air-filled cavity, the total amount of gas in the air-filled cavity increases. (28; **84–85**)

81. The air-filled cavity that is undergoing the net transfer of nitrous oxide may be surrounded by a compliant wall or a noncompliant wall. If the wall is compliant, as the gas enters the cavity the volume of the air-filled cavity will increase. Examples of potential compliant-walled, air-filled cavities include the intestines, pulmonary blebs, or blood vessels. If the wall is noncompliant, as the gas in the cavity increases the pressure in the air-filled cavity will increase. Examples of potential noncompliant-walled, air-filled cavities include the middle ear, cerebral ventricles, and supratentorial subdural space. The potential risk of the transfer of nitrous oxide into an air-filled cavity is that there may be expansion of the volume or an increase in the pressure of the cavity that can result in harm to the patient. For example, a contraindication to the administration of nitrous oxide is a closed pneumothorax or when an air embolus is suspected. When bowel gas volume is increased preoperatively, as in a small bowel obstruction, nitrous oxide administration is best limited to an inspired concentration of 50%. By following this guideline, bowel gas volume has been shown to double at most, even with prolonged operations. (28, Fig. 2–12; **84–85, Fig. 4–14**)

82. The three factors that will influence the net amount of gas that will transfer into an air-filled cavity during the administration of nitrous oxide include the alveolar partial pressure of nitrous oxide, the degree of blood flow to the air-filled cavity, and the duration of the administration of nitrous oxide. (28; **84–85**)

83. The degree of expansion of the volume of an air-filled cavity depends greatly on the concentration of nitrous oxide administered. When the concentration of inspired nitrous oxide is 50%, there may be a doubling of volume of an air-filled cavity. The volume of an air-filled cavity may quadruple in the presence of the administration of 75% nitrous oxide. The time course over which the expansion of the volume occurs is more variable. When nitrous oxide was administered to animals with a pneumothorax at an inhaled concentration of 75%, the volume of the pneumothorax doubled in 10 minutes and tripled in 30 minutes. The expansion of the volume of gas in the intestines secondary to the administration of nitrous oxide appears to be slower than this, but it may become significant during prolonged intra-abdominal surgical procedures. (28, Fig. 2–12; **84, Fig. 4–13**)

84. A patient's cardiac output influences the rate of induction of anesthesia by influencing how much anesthetic is carried away from the alveoli. For example, a high cardiac output will result in more rapid uptake of anesthetic by the blood. This is because more blood is exposed to the alveoli per unit time, and thus more of the anesthetic will be taken up by the blood. Less inhaled anesthetic remains in the alveolus under these conditions. Therefore, the rate of increase of the alveolar partial pressure (P_A) of anesthetic and the rate of induction of anesthesia are both slowed in patients with a high cardiac output. On the other hand, a low cardiac output, as in the shock state, results in less rapid uptake of anesthetic by the blood. This is because less blood is

exposed to the alveoli per unit time, and thus less of the anesthetic will be taken up by the blood. More inhaled anesthetic remains in the alveolus under these conditions. Therefore, the rate of increase of the P_A of anesthetic and the rate of induction of anesthesia are both rapid in patients with a low cardiac output. (28; **76, 81, Fig. 4–7**)

85. The effects of shunts on the rate of induction of anesthesia are intuitively obvious. A right-to-left shunt, whether intracardiac or intrapulmonary, results in blood from the venous system returning to the left ventricle of the heart without passing ventilated alveoli. This blood is not exposed to the anesthetic present in the alveoli. The partial pressure of anesthetic is decreased in the blood that will be delivered to the tissues because of the dilutional effect of the shunted blood, and the rate of induction of anesthesia is slowed in the presence of a right-to-left shunt. A left-to-right shunt, on the other hand, results in blood that has passed ventilated alveoli returning to the venous circulation without delivering the anesthetic. Examples of left-to-right shunts include an arteriovenous fistula and anesthetic-induced increases in cutaneous blood flow. Under these conditions the blood returning to the heart contains a higher partial pressure of anesthetic than blood that has passed through the tissues, increasing the partial pressure of anesthetic in the blood. Right-to-left or left-to-right cardiac shunts have little clinical impact, however. (28–29)

86. Wasted ventilation is the ventilation of alveoli that are not perfused. Under these conditions the rate of induction of anesthesia is not affected provided the minute ventilation remains the same. Wasted ventilation does increase the difference between the alveolar partial pressure of anesthetic and the partial pressure of anesthetic in the arterial blood. This effect is similar to the observed difference between the end-tidal partial pressure of carbon dioxide (P_{CO_2}) and partial pressure of arterial carbon dioxide (Pa_{CO_2}) seen in cases of wasted ventilation, such as in the case of a pulmonary embolus. (29; **593–594, 610–611**)

87. (29; **Table 4–2**)

	PERCENT BODY MASS	PERCENT CARDIAC OUTPUT
Vessel-rich group	10	75
Muscle group	50	19
Fat group	20	5
Vessel-poor group	20	1

88. The alveolar-to-venous partial pressure difference (A-vD) reflects the transfer of inhaled anesthetic from the blood to the tissues, or tissue uptake. Highly perfused tissues of the body include the brain, heart, kidneys, and liver. Although these tissues account for less than 10% of body mass, they receive 75% of the cardiac output. As a result, the equilibration of the partial pressures of anesthetic between the blood and these vessel-rich tissues is rapid. During times of greatest uptake by these vessel-rich tissues, or during the induction of anesthesia, the A-vD will be wide. After the vessel-rich group has taken up sufficient anesthetic to equilibrate with the blood, over 75% of the blood returning to the heart no longer delivers anesthetic to the tissues. This venous blood has a partial pressure of anesthetic that is similar to the alveolar partial pressure of anesthetic, and the A-vD becomes narrow. A narrow A-vD reflects a decrease in the amount of anesthetic that is taken up by the tissues. Furthermore, it reflects a near-equilibration of the inspired partial pressures with the partial pressures in alveoli, tissues, and venous blood. (29; **76**)

89. Skeletal muscle and fat together comprise about 70% of body mass but only receive less than 25% of cardiac output. As a result, these tissues act as reservoirs that slowly take up anesthetic for several hours after the induction of anesthesia. Because of the relatively low blood flow to these organs, equilibration of these organs with the partial pressure of anesthetic in the arterial blood is much slower than the equilibration of the tissues comprising the vessel-rich group. In fact, equilibration of the partial pressure of anesthetic in the blood with fat, which receives only 5% of the cardiac output, is probably not ever achieved. (29; **76**)

90. The recovery from anesthesia might be defined as the rate at which the alveolar partial pressure of anesthetic decreases with time. With the termination of the delivery of anesthetic, the partial pressure of the tissues will decrease as the anesthetic moves along its concentration gradient from tissues to the alveolus. The alveolar concentration is a reflection of the anesthetic that remains in the tissues. Initially, the partial pressure of anesthetic in the alveolus falls rapidly, followed by a slower rate of decline. (29, Fig. 2–13; **90**)

91. Three common factors that influence both the rate of induction of anesthesia and the rate of recovery from anesthesia include alveolar ventilation, the solubility of the anesthetic in blood, and the cardiac output. Three factors that influence the rate of recovery from anesthesia that are unique to this phase of anesthesia include the absence of a concentration effect on recovery, variable tissue concentrations of anesthetics at the start of recovery, and the potential importance of metabolism on the rate of decrease in the alveolar partial pressure of anesthetic. (29; **90–91**)

92. At the conclusion of anesthesia the variable tissue concentrations of anesthetic will serve as a source, or reservoir, that will maintain the alveolar partial pressure (PA) of anesthetic. The partial pressure gradient is reversed and anesthetic slowly comes off the tissues at varying rates, depending on the partial pressure of the anesthetic in the tissue. The PA of anesthetic during the recovery of anesthesia can never be zero. This is different than the induction of anesthesia, when all the tissues begin with a partial pressure of anesthetic of zero. The degree of impact that the partial pressures of anesthetic in tissues will have on the rate of recovery of anesthesia depends on the amount of anesthetic stored in the tissues during anesthesia. The amount of anesthetic stored in the tissues during anesthesia depends on the duration of anesthesia and the solubility of the anesthetic in the various tissue components. (29; **90–91**)

93. During the recovery phase of anesthesia metabolism may contribute to the removal of the volatile anesthetic from the tissues in addition to alveolar ventilation. The role of metabolism is only significant, however, with anesthetics that are highly lipid soluble. Of the volatile anesthetics in clinical use today, halothane alone undergoes a significant degree of metabolism such that the rate of decrease of the alveolar partial pressure (PA) of halothane at the conclusion of anesthesia is dependent on both metabolism and alveolar ventilation. For methoxyflurane, a highly lipid soluble volatile anesthetic that is not widely used clinically today, metabolism is a principal determinant in the rate of decrease of its PA. As opposed to methoxyflurane and halothane, the less lipid-soluble anesthetics isoflurane, desflurane, and sevoflurane principally rely on alveolar ventilation for recovery from anesthesia. (30, Fig. 2–14; **90–91**)

94. The context-sensitive half-time refers to the time required for the concentration of a particular drug to reach a specific percent after the discontinuation of its administration as a continuous intravenous infusion for a specific duration. For inhaled anesthetics the context-sensitive half-time depends on

the anesthetic's blood:gas solubility and the duration of its administration. As with intravenous drugs, computer-simulated models of the context-sensitive half-time of an anesthetic may be useful clinically in anesthesia to predict the duration of a particular drug's effects after its discontinuation. (31; **391–392, Fig. 11–13**)

95. Diffusion hypoxia refers to the hypoxemia that may occur at the conclusion of a nitrous oxide anesthetic in a patient breathing room air. Diffusion hypoxia may occur for two reasons. First, because the solubility of nitrous oxide in blood is so low, nitrous oxide will move quickly from the tissues to the alveoli down its concentration gradient when its administration is discontinued. Initially, the outpouring of nitrous oxide into the alveoli can displace the oxygen in the alveoli and dilute the alveolar partial pressure of oxygen (P_{AO_2}) so greatly that the arterial partial pressure of oxygen (PaO_2) decreases. The second reason why diffusion hypoxia may occur is because the dilution of carbon dioxide in the alveoli that can occur by the same mechanism may decrease the patient's respiratory drive. Diffusion hypoxia can be prevented by administering 100% oxygen to the patient at the conclusion of a nitrous oxide anesthetic. (31; **92–93**)

PHARMACODYNAMICS OF INHALED ANESTHETICS

96. A dose-response curve for an inhaled anesthetic is a graph of the alveolar concentration of an anesthetic and a pharmacologic response. The MAC of an anesthetic is defined as its *minimum alveolar concentration* at 1 atmosphere that prevents skeletal muscle movement in response to a noxious stimulus, such as surgical incision, in 50% of patients. The MAC of an inhaled anesthetic is one point on an inhaled anesthetic's dose-response curve for which the desired effect is no skeletal muscle movement on surgical incision. While a MAC of 1.0 prevents skeletal muscle movement in about 50% of patients undergoing surgery, the administration of approximately 1.3 MAC prevents skeletal muscle movement in nearly all patients undergoing surgery. (31; **50, 1095–1098**)

97. The MAC of an anesthetic is a reflection of the partial pressure of anesthetic required in the brain for a specific effect. The MAC can then be used as an index for comparing anesthetics for their potency by comparing the partial pressure of each anesthetic required at MAC. In addition, since a given MAC reflects a specific potency, inhaled anesthetics can be compared with regard to their other effects (e.g., decreases in blood pressure) at equal potency. This can be done by calculating the therapeutic index of the anesthetic for a given effect. The therapeutic index for an inhaled anesthetic is the alveolar concentration producing a given effect divided by its MAC. Through this use of MAC, comparisons of the effect of inhaled anesthetics on vital organs may facilitate the rational selection of a specific inhaled anesthetic for an individual patient. (31; **1095–1100**)

98. Because the MAC of nitrous oxide is 105%, it cannot be used as a sole anesthetic agent while allowing a sufficient alveolar oxygen concentration. Because nitrous oxide has minimal depressant cardiovascular and ventilation effects, it is often administered in combination with a volatile anesthetic to increase the MAC without increasing the negative effects of the volatile anesthetic. The effective MAC that is achieved when two or more inhaled anesthetics are being administered to a patient is the added MAC of each individual inhaled anesthetic agent. For example, the administration of 0.6 MAC of nitrous oxide and 0.5 MAC of isoflurane together produces an effect of 1.1 MAC. (31; **60, 1096**)

99. Physiologic or pharmacologic factors that increase the MAC for an individual patient include hyperthermia, infant age, hypernatremia, chronic ethanol abuse, and drugs that increase catecholamines in the central nervous system. Examples of drugs that increase central nervous system catecholamines include MAO inhibitors, cocaine, and amphetamines. (32; **Table 29–1**)

100. Physiologic or pharmacologic factors that decrease the MAC for an individual patient include hypothermia, preoperative medication, intravenous anesthetics, neonatal age, elderly age, pregnancy, alpha-2 agonists, acute ethanol ingestion, lithium, cardiopulmonary bypass, opioids, and an arterial partial pressure of oxygen <38 mm Hg. (32; **Table 29–1**)

101. The duration of anesthesia, gender, anesthetic metabolism, and thyroid gland dysfunction each have no effect on the minimum alveolar concentration of anesthesia for individual patients. (32; **Table 29–1**)

102. Some of the effects that anesthetics have at the molecular level include alterations in membrane properties, in the activity of neurotransmitters, in receptor responsiveness, and in chemical- and voltage-gated ion channels and enzymes. It has been difficult to generate a theory for the mechanism of action of general anesthetics that incorporates all these alterations. The precise mechanism by which inhaled anesthetics produce their depressant effects on the central nervous system is not known. (32; **52–58**)

103. Three theories that have been proposed to explain the production of anesthesia by inhaled agents include the Meyer-Overton theory (critical-volume hypothesis), the protein (receptor) hypothesis, and alterations in the availability of the neurotransmitter gamma-aminobutyric acid (GABA). (32; **58–67**)

104. The protein hypothesis proposes that inhaled anesthetics act on the hydrophobic regions of specific proteins in the central nervous system that serve as receptors. The evidence to support this theory comes from the steep dose-response curves of inhaled anesthetics. The curve changes quickly from 1 MAC to 1.3 MAC, suggesting that there may be a crucial receptor occupancy. Another supportive finding is that an anesthetic can lose its anesthetic properties by increasing its molecular weight, even while its lipid solubility increases. (32; **65–67**)

105. The inhibition of the metabolic breakdown of the inhibitory neurotransmitter gamma-aminobutyric acid (GABA) by inhaled anesthetics has led to speculation that anesthesia may result from enhanced inhibition of central nervous system activity by GABA. (32; **55–56, 65–66**)

106. The Meyer-Overton theory, or critical volume hypothesis, suggests that anesthesia occurs when a critical volume, or number, of anesthesia molecules dissolve in lipid cell membranes. The evidence for this theory is the close correlation between the lipid solubility of inhaled anesthetics and their MAC (potency). Lipid cell membrane expansion by a critical volume of 0.4% has been shown to result in anesthesia, lending further support to the Meyer-Overton theory. Subsequent exposure of these membranes to high pressures (40 to 100 atmospheres) partially reverses the action of inhaled anesthetics, presumably by externally forcing the lipid cell membranes to their previous contour. Sodium ion channels in lipid cell membranes could, in theory, be altered by the membrane expansion caused by the dissolving of anesthetic molecules into lipid cell membranes. The altered sodium channel may then prevent sodium flux, stopping flow of the ion that is necessary for the development of action potentials for synaptic transmission. The basis for the opposition to the Meyer-Overton theory is the observation that some lipid soluble compounds are not anesthetics. (33; **58–65**)

Chapter 2

Autonomic Nervous System

1. What is the most practical method to evaluate autonomic nervous system function at the bedside? What results would suggest autonomic nervous system dysfunction?

ANATOMY AND PHYSIOLOGY OF THE AUTONOMIC NERVOUS SYSTEM

2. What central nervous system structures make up the central autonomic nervous system? What functions do each of these structures control?

3. The peripheral autonomic nervous system is divided into what two systems? What is the path by which impulses are conducted in both these systems?

4. What is the function of autonomic ganglia? What neurotransmitter and receptor are involved in the autonomic ganglia?

5. For the parasympathetic nervous system, from where do the preganglionic fibers arise? What neurotransmitter is released by the postganglionic nerve fibers? What receptor type is found at the target organ? How are the postganglionic fibers distributed?

6. For the sympathetic nervous system, from where do the preganglionic fibers arise? What neurotransmitter is released by the postganglionic nerve fibers? What receptor type is found at the target organ? How are the postganglionic fibers distributed?

7. What are the three classes of adrenergic receptors? What endogenous neurotransmitter primarily stimulates each of these receptors?

8. How is the pharmacologic response of catecholamines altered by changes in the density and sensitivity of alpha and beta receptors?

9. How do alpha-2 receptors exert their physiologic effect when stimulated?

10. How is termination of the action of norepinephrine accomplished?

11. What are the two classes of cholinergic receptors? How is the action of acetylcholine terminated at these receptors?

12. Complete the following chart:

RECEPTOR	EFFECTOR ORGANS	RESPONSE TO STIMULATION	AGONIST DRUGS	ANTAGONIST DRUGS
Beta-1				
Beta-2				
Alpha-1				
Alpha-2				
Dopamine-1				
Dopamine-2				
Muscarinic				
Nicotinic				

CATECHOLAMINES

13. Name some examples of catecholamines that are and are not found endogenously. What is their basic chemical structure? Which receptors do they stimulate? What is their clinical use?

14. How does the dose of dopamine administered affect its clinical response? Why must dopamine be administered as a continuous intravenous infusion?

15. What clinical situation is dopamine most often used in?

16. What are the two methods by which dopamine exerts its myocardial inotropic effects?

17. What are the two methods by which dopamine increases urine output?

18. How does dopamine affect the ventilatory response to hypoxemia?

19. How does dopamine affect the release of insulin?

20. How should dopamine be prepared? What can result from the preparation of dopamine in alkaline solutions?

21. What does the local extravasation of dopamine result in? How can it be treated?

22. Which adrenergic effect of norepinephrine predominates, the alpha or the beta? How may norepinephrine be used clinically?

23. What are the two methods by which norepinephrine may decrease cardiac output?

24. Which adrenergic receptors are stimulated by epinephrine?

25. How does epinephrine affect systemic vascular resistance?

26. How does epinephrine affect renal blood flow?

27. How does epinephrine affect the myocardium and myocardial function?

28. What are the endocrine and metabolic effects of epinephrine?

29. What are some clinical uses of epinephrine?

30. Which adrenergic receptors are stimulated by isoproterenol?

31. How does isoproterenol affect the myocardium and myocardial function?

32. Why is isoproterenol of limited utility in patients with ischemic heart disease?

33. How does isoproterenol affect systemic vascular resistance and diastolic blood pressure?

34. How does isoproterenol affect the pulmonary bronchioles?

35. What are some clinical uses of isoproterenol?

36. Which adrenergic receptors are stimulated by dobutamine?

37. What are some of the clinical effects of dobutamine?

38. How does dobutamine affect systemic vascular resistance?

39. What are some clinical uses of dobutamine? Which patients may benefit from simultaneous infusions of dobutamine and dopamine?

40. How should dobutamine be prepared?

41. Complete the following chart indicating whether the administration of each catecholamine results in a mild, moderate, or marked decrease or mild, moderate, or marked increase in mean arterial pressure (MAP), heart rate (HR), cardiac output (CO), systemic vascular resistance (SVR), and renal blood flow (RBF).

CATECHOLAMINE	MAP	HR	CO	SVR	RBF
Dopamine					
Norepinephrine					
Epinephrine					
Isoproterenol					
Dobutamine					

SYMPATHOMIMETICS

42. What are sympathomimetics?

43. How are sympathomimetics classified?

44. What are some potential adverse cardiac effects that can result from the administration of sympathomimetics?

45. What can result from the administration of a direct-acting sympathomimetic or an indirect-acting sympathomimetic to a patient chronically treated with antihypertensives that decrease sympathetic nervous system activity?

46. What can result from the administration of a sympathomimetic to a patient on monoamine oxidase inhibitor or tricyclic antidepressant therapy? When are these patients at the greatest risk of this adverse reaction? How should the anesthetic technique be altered in these patients?

47. What is the current recommendation for the perioperative medical management of patients on monoamine oxidase inhibitors or tricyclic antidepressants?

48. What is the mechanism of action of ephedrine?

49. What are the cardiovascular effects of ephedrine?

50. Why does ephedrine have the potential to elicit cardiac dysrhythmias with its administration?

51. How are the clinical cardiovascular effects of ephedrine altered in patients with drug-induced beta-adrenergic blockade?

52. How is placental blood flow affected by the administration of ephedrine?

53. After how many doses of ephedrine does tachyphylaxis become apparent? What are two possible causes of this tachyphylaxis?

54. What is the mechanism of action for phenylephrine? What are its resultant clinical effects?

55. Does phenylephrine primarily stimulate alpha-1 receptors or alpha-2 receptors?

56. Why might the administration of phenylephrine result in a transient decrease in cardiac output?

57. Complete the following chart describing the stimulatory effect of each drug on the receptor by indicating no change or mild, moderate, or marked stimulation for each sympathomimetic at the given receptor.

SYMPATHOMIMETIC	ALPHA-1	ALPHA-2	BETA-1	BETA-2
Ephedrine				
Phenylephrine				
Metaraminol				
Mephentermine				
Methoxamine				

58. Of the five sympathomimetics—ephedrine, phenylephrine, metaraminol, mephent- ermine, and methoxamine, which act primarily directly and which act primarily indirectly at their given receptors?

ANTIHYPERTENSIVES

59. What is the mechanism by which antihypertensives decrease blood pressure by acting on the sympathetic nervous system?

60. How is the attenuation of sympathetic nervous system activity by antihypertensives reflected clinically?

61. What is the current recommendation for the perioperative medical management of patients on antihypertensive therapy?

62. What is the mechanism of action of angiotensin-converting enzyme inhibitors in the treatment of essential hypertension? Give some examples of this class of drugs.

63. What are some potential side effects of angiotensin-converting enzyme inhibitors?

64. What is the current recommendation for the perioperative medical management of patients on angiotensin-converting enzyme inhibitors?

65. What is potential problem during the induction of anesthesia that may be seen in patients who are taking an angiotensin-converting enzyme inhibitor for the treat- ment of essential hypertension?

66. Which adrenergic receptor does clonidine act on? How does the administration of clonidine result in a decrease in blood pressure?

67. How does the administration of clonidine affect the patient's anesthetic require- ments?

68. What are some of the potential negative effects associated with the initial and chronic administration of clonidine?

69. What is the duration of action of a single dose of clonidine?

70. What is the role of clonidine in opioid withdrawal?

71. How does clonidine affect the plasma catecholamine level of a patient with a pheochromocytoma?

72. What is the effect of clonidine injected into the epidural or intrathecal space? What are the benefits and drawbacks to this route of clonidine administration?

73. How does minoxidil act to decrease blood pressure?

74. What are some of the potential negative effects associated with the administration of minoxidil?

75. What is a topical minoxidil preparation used for?

76. What is the mechanism by which prazosin lowers blood pressure?

77. What are some potential uses of prazosin? What are two potential side effects associated with the administration of prazosin?

78. What is the mechanism by which verapamil lowers blood pressure? What are some potential intraoperative side effects of calcium channel blockers?

79. What is the mechanism by which labetalol lowers blood pressure?

80. What is a potential side effect that may be associated with the administration of labetalol?

BETA-ADRENERGIC AGONISTS

81. What is the primary clinical use of beta-1 agonists?

82. What is the primary clinical use of beta-2 agonists?

83. What are some potential adverse effects of the administration of beta-2 agonists?

84. What is tachyphylaxis to beta agonists attributed to?

BETA-ADRENERGIC ANTAGONISTS

85. What is the mechanism by which beta antagonists decrease blood pressure?

86. What are some clinical uses of beta antagonists?

87. What are some potential benefits of the administration of beta antagonists?

88. What are some potential adverse effects associated with beta-adrenergic blockade therapy?

89. What are some of the signs of excessive drug-induced beta blockade? What is the recommended treatment?

90. Which type of beta-adrenergic blocker is best selected for patients needing beta-blockade therapy who also have a history of bradycardia or depressed left ventricular function?

91. Which type of beta-adrenergic blocker is best selected for patients needing beta-blockade therapy who also have a history of asthma or chronic obstructive pulmonary disease?

92. What is the potential problem with the administration of beta-adrenergic blockers to patients with peripheral vascular disease?

93. What are two potential problems with the administration of beta blockers to patients with insulin-dependent diabetes mellitus?

94. What can result from the abrupt discontinuation of beta-adrenergic blockade?

PERIPHERAL VASODILATORS

95. Name two peripheral vasodilators commonly used as continuous intravenous infusions in clinical anesthesia practice to decrease systemic blood pressure. What is their mechanism of action?

96. What is a potential negative effect associated with the administration of nitroprusside?

97. What is the mechanism of action of adenosine? What is a clinical use of adenosine?

98. What is a clinical use of inhaled nitric oxide?

ANTICHOLINERGICS

99. What is the mechanism of action of anticholinergics?

100. Which of the anticholinergics has a quaternary ammonium structure? What is its major clinical use in clinical anesthesia?

101. Which of the anticholinergics are tertiary amines?

ANTICHOLINESTERASES

102. What is the mechanism of action of anticholinesterases?

103. Which of the anticholinesterases are quaternary ammonium structures? What is their major clinical use?

104. Which of the anticholinesterases are tertiary amine structures? What is their major clinical use in the perioperative period?

ANSWERS*

1. The most practical bedside evaluation of autonomic nervous system function preoperatively is a test for evidence of autonomic nervous system dysfunction. A test for autonomic nervous system dysfunction involves first measuring the blood pressure and heart rate while the patient is in the supine position. The patient then assumes an upright posture. After 5 minutes, blood pressure and heart rate measurements are again taken. A systolic blood pressure decrease of more than 30 mm Hg and the absence of an increase in heart rate indicates that the patient may have autonomic nervous system dysfunction. It implies that the autonomic nervous system does not respond to a decrease in blood pressure by increasing the heart rate, as would be expected from an intact autonomic nervous system. (34; **567**)

ANATOMY AND PHYSIOLOGY OF THE AUTONOMIC NERVOUS SYSTEM

2. The central autonomic nervous system is made up of the hypothalamus, medulla, and pons. The hypothalamus is responsible for the control of stress responses, blood pressure, and temperature regulation. The medulla and pons together provide for hemodynamic and ventilatory control. (34)

3. The peripheral autonomic nervous system is divided into the parasympathetic nervous system and the sympathetic nervous system. Both of these systems have myelinated, preganglionic fibers that arise from the central nervous system and synapse on postganglionic fibers. The unmyelinated, postganglionic fibers synapse on the target effector organs. (34, Fig. 3–1; **523–524, 526–529, Figs. 14–1, 14–5, 14–6**)

4. A number of cell bodies converge at the autonomic ganglia. This is where synapse between the preganglionic and postganglionic nerve fibers of the peripheral autonomic nervous system occurs. Autonomic ganglia may also serve integrative and processing functions that modulate the synapse. The neurotransmitter released at this site is acetylcholine, which acts on nicotinic cholinergic receptors. (34, Fig. 3–1; **549**)

5. Preganglionic nerve fibers of the parasympathetic nervous system arise from craniosacral nerves of the central nervous system. The neurotransmitter released by the postganglionic fibers is acetylcholine. Acetylcholine acts on muscarinic cholinergic receptors at the target, or effector, organ. The distribution of the postganglionic fibers of the parasympathetic nervous system is very selective and discrete. The terminal ganglia are near the innervated effector organs, resulting in the discrete discharge of impulses. (34, Fig. 3–1; **529, Fig. 14–5**)

6. Preganglionic nerve fibers of the sympathetic nervous system arise from the thoracolumbar nerves of the central nervous system. The neurotransmitter released by the postganglionic fibers is norepinephrine. Norepinephrine acts on adrenergic receptors at the target, or effector, organ. Postganglionic fibers of the sympathetic nervous system are widely distributed throughout the body. The discharge of impulses is generalized, such that a mass reflex

*Numbers in parentheses: lightface numbers refer to pages, figures, or tables in Stoelting RK, Miller RD: Basics of Anesthesia, 4th ed. Philadelphia, Churchill Livingstone, 2000; **boldface numbers** refer to pages, figures, or tables in Miller RD: Anesthesia, 5th ed. Philadelphia, Churchill Livingstone, 2000.

response results from stimulation of the sympathetic nervous system. (34, Fig. 3–1; **526–529, Fig. 14–5**)

7. The three classes of adrenergic receptors are the alpha, beta, and dopamine receptors. Alpha- and beta-adrenergic receptors are primarily stimulated by the endogenous neurotransmitter norepinephrine, whereas dopamine receptors are stimulated by the neurotransmitter dopamine. (34; **540–542, 550–553**)

8. The density and sensitivity of alpha and beta receptors play a role in the degree of pharmacologic response seen when these receptors are stimulated by a neurotransmitter. The number of receptors in lipid cell membranes is dynamic, such that receptors can increase in number (up-regulation) or decrease in number (down-regulation) in response to specific stimuli. For example, increased plasma concentrations of norepinephrine result in decreases in the density, or down-regulation, of beta receptors in cell membranes. This down-regulation of receptors decreases the sensitivity of the effector organ to the neurotransmitter. This response is known as tachyphylaxis and can be seen to occur after chronic asthma treatment with beta agonists. Conversely, when beta receptors are chronically blocked, up-regulation of the receptor can result. The increased number of receptors can result in an exaggerated response to minimal stimulation. This explains the rebound tachycardia that can result from discontinuation of a patient's beta-blockade therapy. (34; **544**)

9. Alpha-2 receptors are found presynaptically, or on the preganglionic cell that releases norepinephrine. When stimulated, the alpha-2 receptor functions to feedback negatively on the postganglionic cell, inhibiting the subsequent release of neurotransmitter from the cell. Postsynaptic alpha-2 receptors on platelets contribute to platelet aggregation when stimulated. (34, Fig. 3–2; **540–541, 556–557**)

10. Termination of the action of norepinephrine at its receptor is primarily by its reuptake into the postganglionic nerve ending. Monoamine oxidase is an enzyme in the cytoplasm of the postganglionic cell that acts to deaminate a small amount of the norepinephrine that has been taken up. Most of the norepinephrine, however, escapes deamination and is stored for re-release with subsequent stimulation. (34–35; **538–539**)

11. There are two classes of postsynaptic receptors in the parasympathetic nervous system; both cholinergic receptors are stimulated by acetylcholine. The nicotinic type of receptor lies in the autonomic ganglia between the preganglionic cell and the postganglionic cell. Nicotinic receptors are also subtypes of the cholinergic receptor that is found in the neuromuscular junction. The muscarinic type of receptor is found at the effector organ and is stimulated by the release of acetylcholine by the postganglionic cells. The action of acetylcholine is terminated at these receptors by its hydrolysis. The enzyme responsible for hydrolyzing acetylcholine at the receptor is acetylcholinesterase, or true cholinesterase. (35, Fig. 3–1; **547–548**)

12. (Table 3–1; **Tables 14–1, 14–3, 14–4, 14–6, 14–8**)

RECEPTOR	EFFECTOR ORGANS	RESPONSE TO STIMULATION	AGONIST DRUGS	ANTAGONIST DRUGS
Beta-1	Heart	Increased heart rate, contractility, and conduction velocity	Dobutamine Dopamine Isoproterenol	Metoprolol Esmolol Propranolol Timolol Labetalol
	Fat cells	Lipolysis		

RECEPTOR	EFFECTOR ORGANS	RESPONSE TO STIMULATION	AGONIST DRUGS	ANTAGONIST DRUGS
Beta-2	Blood vessels Bronchioles Uterus Kidney Liver Pancreas	Dilation Dilation Relaxation Renin secretion Gluconeogenesis Glycogenolysis Insulin secretion	Albuterol Ritodrine	Propranolol Timolol Labetalol

Alpha-1	Blood vessels
	Pancreas
	
	Intestine and
	  bladder
		Constriction
		Inhibited insulin
		  secretion
		Relaxation
		Constriction of
		  sphincters
			Phenylephrine	Prazosin
				Phentolamine
				Labetalol

Alpha-2	Postganglionic
	  central nervous
	  system
	Platelets
		Inihibition of
		  norepinephrine
		  release
		Aggregation
			Clonidine
			Dexmedetomidine
				Yohimbine
				Phentolamine

Dopamine-1	Blood vessels	Dilation	Dopamine	Droperidol

Dopamine-2	Postganglionic	Inhibition of
		  norepinephrine
		  release
			Dopamine	Domperidone

Muscarinic	Heart
	
	Bronchioles
	Salivary glands
	Intestine and
	  bladder
		Decreased heart rate,
		  contractility, and
		  conduction velocity
		Constriction
		Secretion
		Contraction and
		  relaxation of
		  sphincters
			Methacholine
			Carbachol
				Atropine
				Scopolamine
				Glycopyrrolate

Nicotinic	Neuromuscular
	  junction
	Autonomic
	  ganglia
		Skeletal muscle
		  contraction
		Sympathetic nervous
		  system stimulation
			Succinylcholine	Nondepolarizing
				  neuromuscular
				  blocking
				  drugs

CATECHOLAMINES

13. Examples of catecholamines found endogenously include dopamine, norepinephrine, and epinephrine. Isoproterenol and dobutamine are catecholamines that do not occur endogenously. The basic structure of catecholamines is a benzene ring of phenylethylamine, with hydroxyl groups on the 3 and 4 positions of the ring. Catecholamines stimulate the adrenergic receptors. Clinically, catecholamines are administered mostly for their cardiovascular effects, usually as intravenous infusions. (35, Fig. 3–3; **550–553, 992–994**)

14. Dopamine stimulates the adrenergic receptor subtypes (dopamine, beta, and alpha) depending on the dose of dopamine being administered. The clinical response to dopamine varies accordingly, depending on which subtype of receptor is primarily being stimulated. At doses between 0.5 and 3.0 μg/kg/min, dopamine receptors are stimulated. Dopamine infusions at a dose of 3 to 10 μg/kg/min result increasingly in beta-adrenergic receptor stimulation. Combined beta- and alpha-adrenergic receptor stimulation by dopamine occurs when it is administered at doses between 10 and 20 μg/kg/min. Alpha-adrenergic effects of dopamine predominate at doses greater than 20 μg/kg/min. Patients respond variably to dopamine, making it important to titrate its administration to a dose that yields the desired response. The rapid metabolism of dopamine requires that it be administered as a continuous intravenous infusion. (37; **553**)

15. Dopamine is most often used clinically in patients with symptoms of shock or severe congestive heart failure. Symptoms that are frequently treated with the administration of a dopamine infusion often include a decreased cardiac output, decreased blood pressure, increased left ventricular end-diastolic pressure, and oliguria. Inotropic effects of dopamine increase cardiac output, whereas its effect on redistributing blood flow to the kidneys helps to increase urine output. (37; **553**)

16. Dopamine exerts its myocardial inotropic effects through direct beta-adrenergic receptor stimulation, as well as indirectly by causing the release of endogenous stores of norepinephrine. Clinically, beta-adrenergic receptor stimulation by dopamine manifests as increased myocardial contractility without marked changes in heart rate or blood pressure. When cardiac catecholamine stores are depleted, as in chronic congestive heart failure, the indirect effect of dopamine on the heart is less reliable. (37; **553**)

17. Dopamine's ability to stimulate dopamine receptors and redistribute blood flow to the kidneys makes it unique among the catecholamines. There are two methods by which dopamine is able to increase urine output. First, dopamine administered in doses less than 3 μg/kg/min stimulates dopamine receptors, resulting in the redistribution of blood flow through the kidneys through renal vascular vasodilation. Second, dopamine administered at this dose inhibits the secretion of aldosterone. (37; **553, 683**)

18. Dopamine acts as an inhibitory neurotransmitter at the carotid bodies. This is in part reflected by its interference with the ventilatory response to hypoxemia. (37)

19. Insulin release is inhibited by dopamine administered at high doses as a result of the corresponding alpha-adrenergic receptor stimulation. Clinically, this may result in hyperglycemia. (37)

20. Dopamine should be prepared in a solution of 5% dextrose in water. Dopamine may be inactivated when prepared in solutions that are more alkaline than 5% dextrose in water. (37)

21. The local extravasation of dopamine causes an intense, painful, local vasoconstriction. This localized vasoconstriction can be treated with the local infiltration of phentolamine, an alpha-adrenergic receptor antagonist that opposes the vasoconstrictive action of alpha-1 adrenergic receptors. (37)

22. Norepinephrine is a neurotransmitter that stimulates both alpha- and beta-adrenergic receptors. Endogenously norepinephrine acts to maintain blood pressure by adjusting the systemic vascular resistance via its stimulation of these receptors. Its stimulatory effects on alpha-1 adrenergic receptors predominate over its beta-1 agonist effects, thereby explaining its primary effect of increasing the systemic vascular resistance. The increase in systemic vascular resistance resulting from its release is reflected by increases in systolic, diastolic, and mean arterial pressures. Norepinephrine may be used clinically to treat refractory hypotension. For example, it may be used intraoperatively to treat refractory hypotension that can occur immediately after ligation of the vascular supply to a pheochromocytoma. Prolonged intravenous infusions of norepinephrine can result in gangrene of the digits, owing to its profound peripheral vasoconstrictive properties. (38; **552–553**)

23. The administration of norepinephrine can result in a decrease in cardiac output by two methods. First, through increasing systemic vascular resistance, afterload is increased. This increases the pressure the heart must overcome to maintain its stroke volume. Second, baroreceptor-mediated reflex bradycardia in response to the increase in blood pressure may contribute to a decrease in cardiac output. (38; **552–553**)

24. Epinephrine stimulates alpha-1, beta-1, and beta-2 adrenergic receptors. (38; **550–552**)

25. Low dose infusions of epinephrine result in vasoconstriction of the skin, mucosa, hepatic, and renal vessels through its stimulation of alpha-1 receptors. Stimulation of beta-2 receptors during low-dose epinephrine infusions results in vasodilation of skeletal muscle vessels. The net effect is a decrease in systemic vasculature resistance and redistribution of blood flow to skeletal muscle. The administration of epinephrine at high doses results in marked alpha-adrenergic receptor stimulation and generalized potent vasoconstriction. (38; **550–552**)

26. Epinephrine is a potent renal vascular vasoconstrictor through its alpha-1 adrenergic effects. Even without changes in systemic blood pressure, renal blood flow is significantly decreased with the administration of epinephrine. (38; **551**)

27. The administration of epinephrine results in an increase in cardiac output through its beta-1 adrenergic effects. Stimulation of beta-1 adrenergic receptors by epinephrine increases heart rate, cardiac contractility, and cardiac automaticity. The increase in cardiac automaticity can manifest as cardiac irritability. Premature ventricular contractions are the most frequently seen clinical manifestations of cardiac irritability during epinephrine infusions. (38; **531, 550–552**)

28. Epinephrine increases metabolic activity through its beta-adrenergic effects and inhibits the release of insulin through its alpha-1 adrenergic effects. Together, the stimulation of these receptors by epinephrine results in adipose tissue lipolysis, liver glycogenolysis, and increased circulating levels of glucose, lactate, and free fatty acids. The endogenous release of epinephrine most likely accounts for the hyperglycemia often observed in patients in the perioperative period. (38; **532**)

29. There are several clinical uses of epinephrine. At low doses, epinephrine may be administered in situations of decreased cardiac contractility. The beta-1 effects of epinephrine directly increase contractility and cardiac output in those situations. The subcutaneous administration of epinephrine is commonly used in combination with local anesthetics to vasoconstrict the vasculature locally, improving operating conditions and prolonging the effect of the local anesthetic. The same mechanism accounts for the prolongation of the effect of local anesthetics by epinephrine in the epidural space. The subcutaneous administration of epinephrine may also be used to treat bronchospasm or to stabilize mast cells as in an allergic reaction. Inhaled racemic epinephrine may be administered to treat airway edema or bronchospasm. Finally, epinephrine may be administered as a bolus during times of life-threatening allergic reactions, refractory bradycardia, or cardiovascular collapse. (38; **550–552**)

30. Isoproterenol stimulates beta-1 and beta-2 adrenergic receptors. Isoproterenol does not have any apparent effect on alpha receptors. (38; **555**)

31. Isoproterenol exerts its myocardial effects through its stimulation of beta-adrenergic receptors. This is consistent with its observed cardiac effects of increased contractility, increased heart rate, increased cardiac output, increased automaticity, and an increase in systolic blood pressure. Isoproterenol may decrease coronary blood flow, which can have detrimental effects in patients with ischemic heart disease. This is secondary to its ability to cause an excessive tachycardia while decreasing diastolic blood pressure. This leads to an increase in myocardial oxygen demand while simultaneously decreasing its blood flow supply. (38; **555**)

32. Isoproterenol is of limited utility in patients with ischemic heart disease for several reasons. First, the administration of isoproterenol results in tachycardia combined with a decrease in diastolic blood pressure. This results in increases in myocardial oxygen demand while simultaneously decreasing myocardial oxygen delivery. Second, isoproterenol administration is associated with a high incidence of cardiac dysrhythmias due to increased cardiac automaticity. Finally, the beta-2 effects of isoproterenol result in the diversion of blood flow to skeletal muscles. These three events combined limit the utility of isoproterenol in patients with a history of ischemic heart disease. (38; **555**)

33. Isoproterenol decreases systemic vascular resistance and diastolic blood pressure. (38; **555–556**)

34. Isoproterenol, through its beta-2 stimulatory effects, dilates pulmonary bronchioles. (38; **556**)

35. Clinical uses of isoproterenol include its administration to increase the heart rate of a patient after heart transplantation and to decrease pulmonary vascular resistance in a patient with valvular heart disease. Isoproterenol has been used to act as a chemical pacemaker in patients with complete heart block but is now no longer included in the American Heart Association's Advanced Cardiac Life Support protocol. (38; **555**)

36. Dobutamine stimulates beta-1 adrenergic receptors without significant effects on beta-2 or alpha receptors. (38; **555**)

37. Dobutamine has similar clinical effects as isoproterenol with regard to increases in myocardial contractility and increases in cardiac conduction velocity. Dobutamine has minimal chronotropic or cardiac dysrhythmic effects, however. Clinically, the predominant effect of dobutamine is to increase cardiac output in a dose-dependent fashion. The dose for the infusion of dobutamine for this purpose is between 2 and 20 μg/kg/min. (38; **555**)

38. Dobutamine often decreases systemic vasculature resistance. (38; **555**)

39. Dobutamine may be useful clinically for patients with congestive heart failure or those who have a decreased cardiac output after a myocardial infarction. The direct-acting effects of dobutamine are effective in patients such as these who have depleted catecholamine stores, and dobutamine is less likely to cause tachycardia or extend the size of an infarct than other catecholamines. Dobutamine may be administered in combination with dopamine in patients who are hypotensive and oliguric, as can occur with cardiogenic shock. The combination of dobutamine and dopamine can increase cardiac output, augment blood pressure, and increase renal blood flow. Prolonged treatment with dobutamine can result in down-regulation of beta receptors, thereby decreasing the effectiveness of dobutamine. (39; **555**)

40. Dobutamine, like dopamine, may lose its clinical effects if it is not prepared in a solution of 5% dextrose in water. (39)

41. (36–38, Table 3–2)

CATECHOLAMINE	MAP	HR	CO	SVR	RBF
Dopamine	Mild increase	Mild increase	Marked increase	Mild increase	Marked increase
Norepinephrine	Marked increase	Mild decrease	Mild decrease	Marked increase	Marked decrease
Epinephrine	Mild increase	Moderate increase	Moderate increase	Moderate increase	Moderate decrease
Isoproterenol	Mild decrease	Marked increase	Marked increase	Moderate decrease	Mild decrease
Dobutamine	Mild increase	Mild increase	Marked increase	No change	Moderate increase

SYMPATHOMIMETICS

42. Sympathomimetics are synthetic drugs whose chemical structure resembles catecholamines. Sympathomimetics have actions at the adrenergic receptors that are similar to, but less potent than, those of catecholamines. They are often used clinically to reverse the hypotension that can accompany spinal, epidural, or general anesthesia. (39; **555**)

43. Sympathomimetics are classified according to the receptors that they selectively stimulate and by their mechanism of action. Sympathomimetics may act directly by binding to the receptor to mimic the effects of a catecholamine or indirectly by evoking the release of an endogenous catecholamine. (39; **553–555**)

44. The administration of a sympathomimetic may result in cardiac dysrhythmias or a decrease in cardiac output. Cardiac dysrhythmias may result from the administration of a sympathomimetic that has beta-1 adrenergic effects. A decrease in cardiac output may result from the administration of a sympathomimetic with alpha-adrenergic effects unopposed by beta-adrenergic effects. The mechanism by which the decrease in cardiac output may occur is primarily due to reflex-mediated bradycardia. A compensatory reflex-mediated bradycardia may accompany the peripheral vasoconstriction and increase in blood pressure caused by alpha-adrenergic receptor stimulation. (39; **553–555**)

45. Patients chronically treated with antihypertensives that decrease sympathetic nervous system activity, for example, beta-adrenergic receptor blockers, may have altered responses to sympathomimetics. When a direct-acting sympathomimetic is administered to these patients the pharmacologic response may be enhanced. This is because of the body's natural response to increase the number of receptors in response to the chronic blockade, so that a given amount of administered sympathomimetic will stimulate a greater number of receptors and exert a greater than normal response. Conversely, when an indirect-acting sympathomimetic is administered to these patients, the pharmacologic response may be decreased. While the sympathomimetic is attempting to elicit a response by endogenous catecholamine release, there is a direct antagonism of beta-adrenergic activity by the antihypertensive, thereby causing a lesser than normal response. (40; **993–994**)

46. Monoamine oxidase inhibitors and tricyclic antidepressants may increase the availability of endogenous norepinephrine. Monoamine oxidase is an enzyme found in the cytoplasm of postganglionic cells that deaminates norepinephrine such that it is unavailable for re-release. Inhibitors of monoamine oxidase prevent this deamination from occurring and increase the endogenous norepinephrine stores available for release from the nerve terminal. Ephedrine, an indirect-acting sympathomimetic, may cause exaggerated blood pressure responses with its administration to these patients. There is thus a potential danger with the administration of indirect-acting sympathomimetics. Patients being treated with monoamine oxidase inhibitors and tricyclic antidepressants are most at risk of an exaggerated response to sympathomimetics during the first 14 to 21 days of treatment. If the treatment of hypotension by a sympathomimetic is required during this time period, a direct-acting sympathomimetic such as phenylephrine should be administered in decreased doses. Hypertension in patients who take monoamine oxidase inhibitors or tricyclic antidepressants is effectively treated with a vasodilator. (40; **550, 561–562, 995–996**)

47. The current recommendation for the perioperative medical management of patients on monoamine oxidase inhibitors or tricyclic antidepressants is to

continue the medicines as prescribed throughout the perioperative period. The medicines are not believed to introduce an unacceptable anesthetic risk of an adverse drug reaction. (40; **562, 995–996**)

48. Ephedrine is primarily an indirect-acting sympathomimetic, with some direct-acting effects. It works to increase blood pressure principally by stimulating the release of endogenous norepinephrine. Ephedrine has stimulatory effects at alpha-1, beta-1, and beta-2 adrenergic receptors as well. (40; **553**)

49. Ephedrine, like epinephrine, increases systolic and diastolic blood pressures, heart rate, and cardiac output. These effects are primarily mediated through the beta-1 adrenergic receptor stimulation that results from the administration of ephedrine. The clinical cardiovascular effects of ephedrine are similar to those of epinephrine but are about 10 times less potent and persist about 10 times longer. Systemic vascular resistance is only minimally altered with ephedrine administration. This is because the effects of peripheral vasculature vasoconstriction due to alpha-adrenergic stimulation are counteracted by the vasodilation of the skeletal muscle vasculature due to beta-2 adrenergic stimulation. (40; **553**)

50. Ephedrine has the potential to elicit cardiac dysrhythmias with its administration secondary to its beta-adrenergic stimulatory effects. This potential for cardiac dysrhythmias increases in the presence of drugs or agents that sensitize the heart to the effects of catecholamines, such as halothane. (40)

51. The cardiovascular effects of ephedrine are primarily due to beta-1 receptor stimulation, although ephedrine does have stimulatory effects at alpha-1 adrenergic receptors. The administration of ephedrine typically manifests clinically as an increase in myocardial contractility and an increase in cardiac output. Patients on chronic beta-adrenergic blockade therapy, however, may clinically respond to the administration of ephedrine with effects resembling alpha-1 adrenergic stimulation. (40; **553**)

52. Placental blood flow is preserved with the administration of ephedrine. This makes ephedrine the treatment of choice for hypotension in parturients. (40; **553**)

53. Tachyphylaxis to ephedrine becomes apparent after the first dose. There are thought to be two reasons why the tachyphylaxis results. First, ephedrine may linger on the receptor for a longer period of time than indicated by its clinical effect. Then, when the second dose of ephedrine is administered, there are fewer receptors available to the newly administered ephedrine and the blood pressure response is less pronounced. The second way in which tachyphylaxis may result is by depletion of norepinephrine stores with the first dose, making less norepinephrine available for subsequent ephedrine doses. (40; **553, 988**)

54. Phenylephrine directly stimulates alpha-adrenergic receptors but lacks significant beta-adrenergic activity. Phenylephrine thus increases systemic vasculature resistance and blood pressure primarily through venoconstriction without significant constriction of arterial vessels. Clinically, phenylephrine mimics the effects of norepinephrine but is less potent and longer lasting. (40; **554, Table 14–8**)

55. Alpha-1 adrenergic receptors are stimulated at lower doses of phenylephrine than those required to stimulate alpha-2 receptors. (40)

56. The administration of phenylephrine might result in a transient decrease in cardiac output coincident with the increase in systemic blood pressure. This most likely occurs as a result of the reflex bradycardia that occurs in response to the increase in blood pressure. (40, Fig. 3–5; **554**)

57. (39–40, Table 3–3)

SYMPATHOMIMETIC	ALPHA-1	ALPHA-2	BETA-1	BETA-2
Ephedrine	Moderate	Unknown	Moderate	Mild
Phenylephrine	Marked	Unknown	None	None
Metaraminol	Marked	Unknown	Moderate	None
Mephentermine	Mild	Unknown	Moderate	Mild
Methoxamine	Marked	Unknown	None	None

58. Ephedrine, metaraminol, and mephentermine primarily act indirectly at their given receptors, whereas phenylephrine and methoxamine primarily act directly. (39, Table 3–3; **553–554**)

ANTIHYPERTENSIVES

59. Antihypertensives that act on the sympathetic nervous system to decrease blood pressure do so by affecting the heart, the peripheral vasculature, or both. When antihypertensives attenuate sympathetic nervous stimulation to the heart, parasympathetic nervous system activity at the heart predominates and bradycardia can result. (40; **557–559, 992–994**)

60. Clinically, attenuation of sympathetic nervous system activity by antihypertensives affects the patient's physiologic capacity to reflexively compensate for decreases in blood pressure. This may manifest as orthostatic hypotension. Intraoperatively, the inhibitory effects of antihypertensives may manifest as exaggerated decreases in blood pressure in response to hemorrhage, positive airway pressure, or sudden changes in body position. (40; **559, 992–994**)

61. The current recommendation for the perioperative medical management of patients on antihypertensive therapy is to continue the prescribed schedule of the antihypertensive throughout the operative period for the optimal control of blood pressure. This includes all types of antihypertensives, including calcium channel blockers, beta-adrenergic receptor blockade, and alpha-2 agonists. For those patients on chronic beta-adrenergic blockade therapy who are unable to receive oral medicines, the intravenous administration of a beta blocker, such as esmolol, can be administered. (41; **259–261, 560, 993–994**)

62. Angiotensin converting enzyme inhibitors act as antihypertensives by blocking the conversion of angiotensin I to angiotensin II. This prevents the vasoconstriction and sympathetic nervous system stimulation associated with angiotensin II. Examples of angiotensin converting enzyme inhibitors include captopril, enalapril, and lisinopril. (41; **562, 993**)

63. Overall there are very few side effects associated with angiotensin converting enzyme inhibitor therapy, making patient compliance high with this antihypertensive. Potential side effects include an increase in serum potassium levels, cough, upper respiratory congestion, and rhinorrhea. Patients who are especially at risk of elevated potassium levels are patients on potassium-sparing diuretics or patients with renal insufficiency. Patients with chronic obstructive pulmonary disease may experience an exacerbation of dyspnea and wheezing with angiotensin converting enzyme inhibitor therapy. There is some evidence to suggest that patients on angiotensin-converting enzyme inhibitors may have a more severe hypotension with the induction of anesthesia than the hypotension seen in patients on other antihypertensive agents. (41; **562, 993**)

64. The current recommendation for the perioperative management of patients on angiotensin converting enzyme inhibitor therapy is to continue these drugs

in the perioperative period. The rebound hypertension, bronchospasm, and metabolic changes that are frequently seen with the discontinuation of other antihypertensive agents have not been noted to occur with the discontinuation of angiotensin converting enzyme inhibitor agents, however. (41; **562, 993**)

65. There is some evidence to suggest that patients on angiotensin converting enzyme inhibitors may have a more severe hypotension with the induction of anesthesia than the hypotension seen in patients on other antihypertensive agents. In addition, prolonged hypotension intraoperatively during general anesthesia has been observed in these patients, particularly during operative procedures that involve large fluid shifts. For this reason, some anesthesiologists choose to discontinue angiotensin converting enzyme inhibitor therapy preoperatively. (41; **562, 993**)

66. Clonidine acts centrally by stimulating alpha-2 adrenergic receptors. Stimulation of alpha-2 adrenergic receptors causes a decrease in the outflow of sympathetic nervous system impulses to the periphery. Clinically, the effect of clonidine to decrease sympathetic nervous system activity results in decreases in cardiac output, systemic vascular resistance, and blood pressure. (41; **259–261, 554–555, 994**)

67. Small doses of clonidine administered preoperatively result in sedative and/or analgesic effects. This is reflected by a decrease in the minimum alveolar concentration (MAC) of anesthetic required. Sympathetic nervous system responses to direct laryngoscopy and surgical stimulation are attenuated with prior clonidine administration as well. (41; **259–261, 554–555**)

68. Negative side effects that may accompany the initial administration of clonidine include sedation, bradycardia, and dry mouth. The most significant adverse effect of chronic clonidine therapy is a rebound hypertensive crisis with abrupt discontinuation of the drug. Rebound hypertension is thought to result from an abrupt increase in systemic vascular resistance due to the release of catecholamines. During the perioperative period the rebound hypertension may be seen before the induction of anesthesia or in the early postoperative period. This rebound hypertension can usually be controlled by administering transdermal clonidine or an alternative antihypertensive. (41–42; **259–261, 554–555, 994**)

69. The duration of action of a single dose of clonidine is 6 to 24 hours. This explains why the administration of clonidine in the preoperative period may result in postoperative sedation. (41; **994**)

70. Clonidine has been used to suppress symptoms of opioid withdrawal. It is presumed to be effective secondary to its alpha-2 mediated inhibition of sympathetic nervous system activity. (42; **555, 994**)

71. Despite the ability of clonidine to lower plasma catecholamine levels in hypertensive patients, clonidine does not decrease the amount of circulating catecholamines in a patient with a pheochromocytoma. This reflects the ability of clonidine to block catecholamine release mediated by the central nervous system but not catecholamines released to the circulation from a source outside the central nervous system. The clonidine suppression test involves the administration of clonidine to patients with hypertension secondary to an unknown cause to distinguish between patients who have hypertension secondary to a pheochromocytoma or another cause. (42)

72. Clonidine injected into the epidural or intrathecal space has an analgesic effect. The benefit of this route of administration of clonidine is that, unlike opioids, it does not produce respiratory depression, pruritus, or nausea and vomiting. Bradycardia and sedation are the negative side effects of epidural or intrathecal clonidine administration. (42; **555**)

73. Minoxidil decreases blood pressure by directly relaxing arteriolar smooth muscle. (42)

74. Potential negative effects associated with the administration of minoxidil include reflex tachycardia, sodium retention, water retention, pulmonary hypertension, pericardial effusions, and cardiac tamponade. Minoxidil is presumed to cause a reflex tachycardia, sodium retention, and water retention secondary to its arterial vasodilatory effects. Because of this, minoxidil is often administered together with a beta-receptor antagonist and a diuretic. Minoxidil-induced pulmonary hypertension is most likely not a direct effect of the drug itself but rather a secondary effect because of fluid retention. Patients with a history of renal dysfunction are most at risk for pericardial effusions and cardiac tamponade, which can occur in a small number of patients on minoxidil therapy. (42)

75. Topical minoxidil administration is used to stimulate hair growth in patients with baldness. (42)

76. Prazosin is a selective alpha-1 receptor antagonist, with little alpha-2 receptor activity. Because it blocks the activity of norepinephrine at the alpha-1 receptor, it acts to lower blood pressure by decreasing systemic vascular resistance. (42; **557, 994**)

77. Potential uses of prazosin include the treatment of essential hypertension, decreasing afterload in patients with congestive heart failure, and as a preoperative medication in a patient with a pheochromocytoma. Two prominent side effects of prazosin therapy are fluid retention and orthostatic hypertension. (42, **557, 924, 994**)

78. Verapamil is a calcium channel blocker. Calcium channel blockers have several cardiovascular effects, including decreased heart rate, decreased cardiac contractility, decreased cardiac conduction velocity, and the dilation of cerebral, coronary, and systemic arterioles. Calcium channel blockers used intraoperatively may have exaggerated effects on blood pressure and myocardial depression when used in combination with inhaled anesthetics. Calcium channel blockers may potentiate the effects of neuromuscular blocking drugs, although this effect is not likely to be noted clinically. (42; **464, 994–995**)

79. Labetalol lowers blood pressure through its activity as an antagonist at alpha-1 and beta-adrenergic receptors. (42; **560–561**)

80. The administration of labetalol may be accompanied by prominent orthostatic hypotension, because both alpha and beta responses to decreases in blood pressure are blocked. Although potential bronchospasm is a concern for patients on beta-blocker therapy, bronchospasm appears to be less likely with labetalol than it is with other nonselective beta-adrenergic receptor antagonists. (42; **560–561**)

BETA-ADRENERGIC AGONISTS

81. The primary clinical use of beta-1 agonists is to increase heart rate and myocardial contractility. Isoproterenol is a primarily beta-1 selective agonist whose clinical uses include its administration to increase the heart rate in a patient after heart transplantation, to act as a chemical pacemaker in a patient with complete heart block, and to decrease pulmonary vascular resistance in a patient with valvular heart disease. The use of beta-1 agonists is limited by their potential to cause cardiac dysrhythmias and to increase myocardial oxygen requirements. (42–43; **555**)

82. The primary clinical use of beta-2 agonists is for the treatment of bronchial asthma and premature labor through their effects of bronchial and uterine

smooth muscle relaxation. Albuterol, a beta-2 agonist, is the current preferred treatment of bronchospasm in an anesthetized patient. The administration of albuterol under these conditions is best achieved through the use of a metered-dose inhaler during a mechanically produced inspiration. Each metered actuation of aerosol delivers about 90 μg to the patient. This method of delivery provides for rapid onset and minimizes systemic drug levels. Terbutaline is a beta-2 agonist that may be administered subcutaneously for the treatment of intraoperative bronchospasm. (42–43; **555–556**)

83. Although beta-2 agonists have fewer cardiac effects than beta-1 agonists, the administration of these drugs can lead to a reflex tachycardia either due to beta-2 mediated vasodilation and hypotension or by the direct stimulation of beta-1 receptors. A continuous intravenous infusion of a beta-2 agonist, as in the treatment of premature labor, may rarely result in pulmonary edema or cardiac dysrhythmias. A continuous infusion of a beta-2 agonist can also result in hypokalemia. The hypokalemia is thought to occur because of beta-2 mediated stimulation of insulin release and the subsequent intracellular transfer of potassium, and it may persist despite potassium supplementation. When this occurs, potassium levels are seen to return to pre-infusion levels about 30 minutes after discontinuing the infusion. The release of insulin may cause a reactive hypoglycemia in the fetus, particularly in parturients with diabetes mellitus. (43; **555–556**)

84. Chronic stimulation of beta-2 receptors leads to a tachyphylaxis, which is attributed to a decreased sensitivity or a decreased number of receptors. The number of receptors in lipid cell membranes is dynamic, such that the number of receptors can become down-regulated in response to specific stimuli. For example, increased plasma concentrations of norepinephrine result in decreases in the density, or down-regulation, of beta receptors in cell membranes. This down-regulation of receptors decreases the sensitivity of the effector organ to the neurotransmitter. This response is known as tachyphylaxis and can be seen to occur after chronic asthma treatment with beta agonists. (43; **544**)

BETA-ADRENERGIC ANTAGONISTS

85. Beta-adrenergic antagonists, or beta blockers, exert several effects. Most beta antagonists have antagonist effects at both beta-1 and beta-2 receptors, although with varying degrees of selectivity. Effects of beta-adrenergic antagonists include decreases in heart rate, cardiac contractility, and cardiac conduction velocity, renin release, lipolysis, bronchoconstriction, and peripheral vasoconstriction. Beta antagonists most likely decrease blood pressure by decreasing cardiac output. When a beta-adrenergic antagonist is administered, the beta-1 mediated effect of decreased heart rate lasts longer than the beta-1 mediated negative inotropic effects. This suggests that there is a possible subdivision of beta-1 receptors. (43; **541, 557–558**)

86. Beta antagonists are used clinically to decrease blood pressure, to decrease heart rate, for the treatment of myocardial ischemia, for postinfarction management, for the treatment of cardiac dysrhythmias, for thyrotoxicosis management, and as prophylaxis against migraine headaches. (43; **557–559**)

87. Beta antagonist therapy for the treatment of hypertension has several benefits that are exclusive to this class of drugs. Beta-adrenergic antagonists, through their ability to decrease heart rate and contractility, decrease myocardial oxygen requirements in addition to decreasing blood pressure. Clinically, in patients with ischemic heart disease, this may manifest as relief of angina pectoris. With regard to beta-adrenergic blockade therapy in the post–

myocardial infarction population, several studies have shown that the therapy results in a decrease in mortality and a decrease in the incidence of myocardial reinfarction. Orthostatic hypotension, which may accompany other methods of treating essential hypertension, does not occur with beta-adrenergic blockade therapy. Beta-blocker therapy in conjunction with vasodilator therapy may attenuate the baroreceptor-mediated reflex tachycardia that may accompany vasodilator therapy alone. (43; **558–559, 993**)

88. There are several potential adverse effects associated with beta-adrenergic blockade therapy. Two major adverse effects of this type of therapy are excessive myocardial depression and bronchoconstriction. Myocardial depression may precipitate congestive heart failure in some patients secondary to the decrease in myocardial contractility associated with beta-adrenergic blockade. Patients may also have life-threatening bradycardia or atrioventricular heart block associated with beta-blockade therapy. Bronchoconstriction associated with beta-blockade therapy is more commonly seen with medicines that have a high degree of beta-2-adrenergic receptor effects. The administration of beta-adrenergic antagonists may also accentuate increases in serum levels of potassium when potassium chloride is being infused. This is believed to be due to interference with the mechanism necessary for the movement of potassium ions across the cell membranes. Finally, beta-adrenergic blockade therapy is commonly associated with fatigue and lethargy, although the anesthetic requirements for individual patients have not been shown to be decreased when chronically on beta-adrenergic blockade therapy. (43, Fig. 3–6; **559–560**)

89. Signs of excessive drug-induced beta-adrenergic blockade include bradycardia and atrioventricular block. Atropine, a muscarinic antagonist, is the initial treatment of choice in these situations. If the beta blockade persists, the administration of a beta-specific agonist such as isoproterenol or dobutamine is indicated. Large doses of these drugs may be required to reverse the blockade. Another agent that may be useful for reversal of beta blockade is calcium chloride at conventional doses, although the mechanism by which this is effective is not known. (43–44; **559–560**)

90. In patients with bradycardia or depressed left ventricular function in whom beta-blockade therapy is indicated, drugs that have intrinsic sympathomimetic activity are the most appropriate treatment. Some myocardial depression with volatile anesthetics has been shown to occur, but the combined administration of volatile anesthetics with beta-adrenergic blockers has not been shown to have clinically significant additive effects. (43; **559, 993–994**)

91. The bronchoconstriction that may accompany beta-2 adrenergic blockade may be detrimental in patients who have a history of asthma or chronic obstructive pulmonary disease. Drugs that are selective for beta-1 adrenergic receptors are the most appropriate treatment for these patients when beta blockade therapy is indicated. Examples of beta-1 selective drugs include esmolol and metoprolol. (43; **560**)

92. The peripheral vasoconstriction associated with beta-2 adrenergic blockade may be detrimental in patients with peripheral vascular disease. For this patient population in whom beta blockade therapy is indicated, drugs that are selective for beta-1 adrenergic receptors are the most appropriate treatment. (43; **560**)

93. The administration of beta-adrenergic blockers to patients with insulin-dependent diabetes mellitus may have two detrimental effects. First, the warning signs and symptoms of hypoglycemia are blunted by beta blockade. The careful monitoring of blood sugar levels is therefore indicated for patients with diabetes mellitus who are also on beta-blockade therapy. Second, insulin

secretion is suppressed by beta-2 blockade, which may exacerbate diabetes in these patients. For insulin-dependent diabetic patients requiring beta-adrenergic blockade therapy, cardioselective beta-1 adrenergic blocker drugs are the most appropriate treatment. (43–44; **560**)

94. Chronic beta-adrenergic blockade therapy results in an up-regulation of the beta receptors. Abrupt discontinuation of beta-blockade therapy can be associated with excessive sympathetic nervous system activity from the increased amount of receptors activated with a single stimulus. The enhanced activity may manifest clinically as hypertension, tachycardia, and myocardial ischemia. (43; **559, 994**)

PERIPHERAL VASODILATORS

95. Two peripheral vasodilators commonly used as intravenous infusions in clinical anesthesia practice include nitroprusside and nitroglycerin. Nitroprusside is believed to act by both arteriolar and venous dilation, whereas nitroglycerin is believed to act primarily through venous dilation. The mechanism of action for both agents is believed to be through the generation of the intracellular endogenous vasodilator nitric oxide. (44; **643, 1474–1477**)

96. Two potential negative effects associated with the administration of nitroprusside include cyanide toxicity and methemoglobinemia. The breakdown of nitroprusside in the blood produces cyanide in a dose-dependent manner. (44; **1474**)

97. Adenosine is an endogenous compound that dilates coronary vessels through an as yet unknown mechanism. It has been postulated to work by increasing levels of cyclic adenosine monophosphate. It is used clinically to treat paroxysmal supraventricular tachycardia through its effect of producing a transient block of atrioventricular nodal conduction. (44; **643, 2539–2541**)

98. Inhaled nitric oxide has been used to manage patients with pulmonary hypertension. When used for this purpose it is administered at a dose of 5 to 40 ppm. It acts by vasodilating the pulmonary vasculature and improving arterial oxygenation. Nitric oxide is rapidly inactivated when bound to hemoglobin. Because of this, inhaled nitric oxide produces no systemic vasodilation. (44; **643, 1834**)

ANTICHOLINERGICS

99. Anticholinergics, including atropine, scopolamine, and glycopyrrolate, are muscarinic antagonists. The mechanism of action of these drugs is to competitively inhibit the action of acetylcholine at cholinergic receptors. (44; **564–565**)

100. Glycopyrrolate has a quaternary ammonium structure that prevents glycopyrrolate from crossing lipid membranes. The effects of glycopyrrolate are therefore limited to peripheral cholinergic receptors. In clinical anesthesia, glycopyrrolate is mostly used to block the muscarinic side effects of the anticholinesterase drugs that are being administered for the reversal of neuromuscular blockade. (44; **564–565, Table 14–13**)

101. Atropine and scopolamine are tertiary amines, making these drugs able to cross lipid membranes such as the blood-brain barrier and placenta. These drugs are therefore able to exert effects centrally and on the fetus of a parturient. (44; **564–565, Table 14–13**)

ANTICHOLINESTERASES

102. Anticholinesterases act by inhibiting the enzyme acetylcholinesterase, or true cholinesterase. Anticholinesterases inhibit the hydrolysis of acetylcholine at

cholinergic receptors after it has been released from the nerve terminal. Consequently, when an anticholinesterase has been administered, acetylcholine accumulates at nicotinic and muscarinic receptor sites and may compete more effectively for those receptors. (44; **565–566**)

103. Anticholinesterases that are quaternary ammonium structures and not able to cross lipid membranes such as the blood-brain barrier include neostigmine, pyridostigmine, and edrophonium. These anticholinesterases are used clinically in the reversal, or antagonism, of muscle relaxation produced by nondepolarizing neuromuscular blocking drugs. The quaternary ammonium structure limits the action of these drugs to peripheral cholinergic sites such as the neuromuscular junction. The accumulation of acetylcholine that results from the administration of these anticholinesterases allows acetylcholine to more effectively compete with nondepolarizing neuromuscular blocking drugs for sites on the nicotinic receptor. (44; **565–566**)

104. An anticholinesterase that is a tertiary amine structure and able to cross lipid membranes is physostigmine. The major clinical use of physostigmine in the perioperative period is the treatment of central anticholinergic syndrome. Central anticholinergic syndrome may manifest as emergence delirium in the postanesthesia care unit after the administration of atropine or scopolamine. Its method for the antagonism of atropine or scopolamine at cholinergic receptors is through the inhibition of the hydrolysis of acetylcholine at the receptor sites. (44; **565–566**)

Chapter 3

Effects of Inhaled Anesthetics on Ventilation and Circulation

1. What is the method by which the various pharmacologic effects of inhaled anesthetics have been studied?

2. In general, how similar are the properties and clinical effects of the two newer volatile anesthetic agents desflurane and sevoflurane when compared with the properties of the older volatile anesthetic agents isoflurane and halothane?

CIRCULATION

3. How do inhaled anesthetics affect arterial blood pressure? What is the mechanism by which this effect occurs?

4. How does the substitution of nitrous oxide for an equipotent dose of volatile anesthetic affect arterial blood pressure at a given anesthetic dose?

5. What are the cardiovascular effects of surgical stimulation? How do volatile anesthetics modify this response?

6. How do inhaled anesthetics affect heart rate? What is the mechanism by which this occurs?

7. How can the effect of inhaled anesthetics on heart rate during the induction of anesthesia be attenuated?

8. How do inhaled anesthetics affect cardiac output?

9. How is the cardiac stroke volume calculated? How do inhaled anesthetics affect the calculated cardiac stroke volume? What is the mechanism by which this occurs?

10. How do inhaled anesthetics affect myocardial contractility? What is the mechanism by which this occurs? Which patients may be at particular risk of the effects of inhaled anesthetics on myocardial contractility?

11. How do inhaled anesthetics affect right atrial pressure?

12. How is systemic vascular resistance calculated? How do inhaled anesthetics affect the calculated systemic vascular resistance?

13. How do inhaled anesthetics affect cerebral blood flow?

14. How do inhaled anesthetics affect skeletal muscle blood flow?

15. How do inhaled anesthetics affect coronary artery blood flow? What is coronary artery steal syndrome? What is its clinical relevance?

16. How do inhaled anesthetics affect pulmonary vascular resistance?

17. The administration of which inhaled anesthetic can lead to sympathetic nervous system stimulation?

18. How do inhaled anesthetics affect cardiac rhythm? What cardiac dysrhythmias are commonly seen? How should cardiac dysrhythmias in the presence of a volatile anesthetic be treated?

19. How do the circulatory effects of inhaled anesthetics change over time with the administration of the same, continuous dose of an inhaled anesthetic? What is the mechanism by which these changes occur?

20. How are the circulatory effects of volatile anesthetics altered during spontaneous ventilation versus mechanical ventilation?

21. What are some variables that may influence the cardiovascular effects produced intraoperatively by inhaled anesthetics?

22. Describe some of the clinical cardiovascular effects of isoflurane that support the belief that isoflurane may have mild beta-agonist properties.

23. What are some possible explanations for the less significant myocardial depressant effects associated with the administration of isoflurane than with the other volatile anesthetics?

24. What are some of the signs of mild sympathomimetic stimulation that are seen with the administration of nitrous oxide? What is the mechanism by which this occurs?

VENTILATION

25. How much influence does the choice of inhaled anesthetic have on the incidence of postoperative pulmonary complications?

26. How is the ventilatory drive affected by inhaled volatile anesthetics? What is the mechanism by which inhaled anesthetics are thought to affect the ventilatory drive?

27. How is the rate of breathing affected by inhaled volatile anesthetics? How does isoflurane differ from the other inhaled anesthetics with respect to how it influences the rate of breathing?

28. How is the tidal volume affected by inhaled volatile anesthetics?

29. How is the minute ventilation affected by inhaled volatile anesthetics?

30. What is the carbon dioxide response curve a plot of? What do the slope and the position on the x-axis of the carbon dioxide response curve represent?

31. What is the ventilatory response of an awake, healthy, spontaneously ventilating individual for every 1 mm Hg increase in the Pa_{CO_2}?

32. How do inhaled anesthetics affect the carbon dioxide response curve?

33. How does the presence of chronic obstructive pulmonary disease influence the Pa_{CO_2} of an individual being administered a volatile anesthetic?

34. How is the Pa_{CO_2} affected by the administration of nitrous oxide? How does the addition of nitrous oxide to a volatile anesthetic affect the Pa_{CO_2}?

35. How does surgical stimulation affect the ventilation of an anesthetized, spontaneously ventilating patient inhaling a volatile anesthetic?

36. How does the Pa_{CO_2} change over time with the administration of the same, continuous dose of a volatile anesthetic? How do inhaled anesthetics affect the carbon dioxide response curve with prolonged inhalation of the anesthetic?

37. How do inhaled anesthetics affect respiratory muscle function?

38. Define the apneic threshold. What is the approximate difference between the apneic threshold Pa_{CO_2} and the resting Pa_{CO_2}?

39. What is the most reliable method by which to decrease the Pa_{CO_2} of a spontaneously ventilating patient being administered a volatile anesthetic?

40. What is the ventilatory response to arterial hypoxemia in an awake, healthy, spontaneously ventilating individual?

41. How does the inhalation of an anesthetic at 0.1 minimun alveolar concentration (MAC) and at 1 MAC affect the ventilatory response to arterial hypoxemia?

42. How do subanesthetic doses of inhaled anesthetics affect the usual synergistic ventilatory response to arterial hypoxemia and hypercapnia? What is the clinical relevance of this?

43. How do volatile anesthetics affect bronchial tone? What is the mechanism by which this is thought to occur?

44. How beneficial is the administration of bronchodilating volatile anesthetics for the treatment of bronchospasm?

45. Which two volatile anesthetics are thought to be airway irritants? How is this manifest clinically? How does this limit their clinical utility?

46. How do inhaled anesthetics affect the hypoxic pulmonary vasoconstriction reflex?

Answers*

1. The pharmacologic effects of the inhaled anesthetics on ventilation and circulation have been studied in healthy volunteers. The comparative data were gathered from the volunteers while they were breathing equally potent concentrations of the anesthetics in the absence of extraneous influences. For example, the circulatory effects of inhaled anesthetics were studied in healthy volunteers who were administered the inhaled anesthetic during controlled ventilation to maintain normocarbia. Care should be taken when administering these agents clinically to take into account co-existing diseases present in the patient. (46)

2. The two newer volatile anesthetic agents, desflurane and sevoflurane, have lower blood and tissue solubilities than the older volatile anesthetic agents isoflurane and halothane. This property of desflurane and sevoflurane allows for greater control with its administration and potentially less time to recovery from anesthesia with its discontinuation. Other properties of these two agents, including their effects on circulation and ventilation, closely resemble the effects of the older volatile anesthetic agents. (46; **91–92**)

CIRCULATION

3. The volatile anesthetics all produce a dose-dependent decrease in mean arterial blood pressure, although the mechanism by which they exert their effects varies. Halothane primarily acts to decrease blood pressure by decreasing myocardial contractility and cardiac output. Isoflurane, desflurane, and sevoflurane primarily act to decrease blood pressure through their effects of peripheral vasodilation and an associated decrease in systemic vascular resistance. Nitrous oxide, when administered alone, does not alter blood pressure. (46, Fig. 4–1; **101–104, 114–115, Figs. 5–11, 5–12**)

4. Nitrous oxide, when administered alone, does not alter blood pressure. The substitution of nitrous oxide for an equipotent dose of a volatile anesthetic therefore results in less of a decrease in arterial blood pressure than would have otherwise occurred if the volatile anesthetic were administered alone. This is in part the basis for the administration of nitrous oxide in combination with a volatile anesthetic. The combination of nitrous oxide with a volatile anesthetic allows for an increase in the minimum alveolar concentration (MAC) of anesthesia delivered without the cardiovascular effects of the volatile anesthetic administered alone at the same MAC. (46, Fig. 4–2; **104, 114–115**)

5. Surgical stimulation results in sympathetic nervous system stimulation. This may manifest as an increase in heart rate and blood pressure, even while under

*Numbers in parentheses: lightface numbers refer to pages, figures, or tables in Stoelting RK, Miller RD: Basics of Anesthesia, 4th ed. Philadelphia, Churchill Livingstone, 2000; **boldface numbers** refer to pages, figures, or tables in Miller RD: Anesthesia, 5th ed. Philadelphia, Churchill Livingstone, 2000.

general anesthesia. Volatile anesthetics attenuate the sympathetic nervous system response in a dose-dependent manner. For example, 1.47 MAC halothane prevents the rise in blood pressure and heart rate in response to surgical incision in 50% of patients. Conversely, the sympathetic nervous system stimulation associated with surgical stimulation may attenuate the decrease in arterial blood pressure that is associated with a given dose of volatile anesthetic. (46; **104, 1095–1096, 1099, Fig. 29–8**)

6. The effect of the inhaled anesthetics on heart rate varies, but in general increases in heart rate are seen with the administration of all the volatile anesthetic agents except halothane. The administration of halothane does not result in any change in heart rate. The heart rate is unchanged by the administration of desflurane at doses up to 1 MAC. When higher levels of desflurane concentrations are achieved, desflurane increases heart rate in a dose-dependent manner. The administration of isoflurane increases heart rate, especially at doses less than 1 MAC. This effect of isoflurane on heart rate is more likely to occur in young patients than in elderly patients. Sevoflurane increases heart rate when it is administered at doses greater than 1.5 MAC. Heart rate is unchanged or minimally increased with the administration of nitrous oxide. The increase in heart rate that accompanies the administration of desflurane, isoflurane, and sevoflurane is thought to be mediated reflexively by the carotid sinus baroreceptors when decreases in arterial blood pressure are sensed. This reflex remains intact when these agents induce a decrease in blood pressure with their administration, although the resultant increase in heart rate varies. Halothane, however, inhibits the baroreceptor reflex response. The administration of halothane and the associated decrease in blood pressure are therefore not accompanied by an increase in heart rate. (47, Fig. 4–3; **104–105, 114–115**)

7. Opioids are useful in the attenuation of the volatile anesthetic-induced changes in heart rate during the induction of anesthesia. (47; **331–332**)

8. Halothane produces a dose-dependent decrease in cardiac output that parallels the decrease in blood pressure that is seen with the administration of these agents. It is believed that the reason for the decrease in cardiac output that is associated with halothane is the lack of a compensatory increase in heart rate. Neither desflurane, isoflurane, nor sevoflurane produces a dose-dependent decrease in cardiac output. This may be due in part to the increase in heart rate that accompanies the decrease in blood pressure when these agents are administered. Nitrous oxide is associated with a mild increase in cardiac output, possibly reflecting weak sympathomimetic effects of this drug. (48, Fig. 4–4; **96–99, 101–104, 112–115**)

9. Cardiac stroke volume is cardiac output divided by heart rate. Alterations in the cardiac stroke volume caused by the administration of volatile anesthetics can be calculated from the cardiac output and heart rate that results from the administration of each anesthetic. Because desflurane, isoflurane, and sevoflurane produce little change in cardiac output but increase heart rate, it follows that the stroke volume associated with the administration of each of these agents is decreased. Halothane causes myocardial depression, leading to decreases in cardiac output. Halothane inhibits the baroreceptor reflex, with a net result of a decrease in cardiac output, no change in the heart rate, and a decrease in stroke volume. Therefore, the calculated stroke volume is decreased by 15% to 30% by all these agents. Nitrous oxide administration has very little effect on the calculated stroke volume. (48; **96–99, 101–104, 112–113**)

10. The effects of inhaled anesthetics on myocardial contractility have been studied in vitro using isolated papillary muscle preparations. These studies have shown that the volatile anesthetics directly produce a dose-dependent decrease in myocardial contractility. This effect of myocardial depression was found to be

greatest with the administration of halothane, and less with isoflurane, sevoflurane, and desflurane. Nitrous oxide was also found to depress myocardial contractility, but to a lesser degree than that seen with the volatile anesthetics. The mechanism by which inhaled anesthetics depress myocardial contractility may be either due to decreasing free calcium concentrations or by altering the sensitivity of the contractile proteins to the available calcium. Despite the evidence found in vitro for myocardial depression and decreased contractility caused by the administration of inhaled anesthetics, in vivo cardiac depression is not consistently seen. This may be due to homeostatic mechanisms by the autonomic nervous system that obscures these direct effects. When comparisons were made between papillary muscles taken from animals in congestive heart failure and compared with papillary muscles of normal animals, it was found that the muscles from animals with congestive heart failure had a greater depression of myocardial contractility by the volatile anesthetics. This may imply that patients with congestive heart failure are at particular risk of the effects of inhaled anesthetics on myocardial contractility. (48; **96–99, 112–113, Figs. 5–3, 5–12**)

11. Right atrial pressure, or central venous pressure, is increased with the administration of halothane, isoflurane, desflurane, and nitrous oxide. These volatile agents probably produce an increase in right atrial pressure through direct negative inotropic effects on the myocardium. The increase in right atrial pressure associated with the administration of nitrous oxide is likely due to mild increases in pulmonary vascular resistance. The administration of sevoflurane does not appear to result in an increase in right atrial pressure. (48–49, Fig. 4–5; **104, 112–115**)

12. Systemic vascular resistance is calculated by the mean arterial pressure minus right atrial pressure divided by cardiac output. Alterations in systemic vascular resistance caused by the administration of volatile anesthetics can be calculated from the mean arterial pressure, right atrial pressure, and cardiac output that results from the administration of each anesthetic. Isoflurane, sevoflurane, and desflurane administration lead to dose-dependent decreases in systemic vascular resistance. The decrease in systemic vascular resistance produced by these agents parallels the decrease in blood pressure they produce. No significant change in systemic vascular resistance is noted with the administration of either halothane or nitrous oxide. (49, Fig. 4–6; **102–105, 114–115, Fig. 5–11**)

13. All the volatile anesthetics increase cerebral blood flow through vasodilation of the cerebral vasculature, although the anesthetics each affect the vasculature to varying degrees. The administration of halothane appears to increase cerebral blood flow the most, whereas the administration of isoflurane results in the least increase in cerebral blood flow. (49; **706–709, Fig. 19–7**)

14. The administration of isoflurane produces a twofold to threefold increase in skeletal muscle blood flow. The increase in skeletal muscle blood flow by isoflurane contributes to the associated decrease in systemic vascular resistance. No other volatile anesthetics increase skeletal muscle blood flow with their administration. Nitrous oxide does not result in any change in skeletal muscle blood flow, whereas the administration of halothane results in an indirect decrease in skeletal muscle blood flow through its effects of decreasing the perfusion pressure. (49)

15. Halothane, sevoflurane, and desflurane have been shown to cause mild coronary artery vasodilation. Isoflurane has been shown to selectively dilate small coronary arterioles in animal models. Coronary artery steal syndrome can occur when coronary arterioles undergo vasodilation and blood flow is diverted from narrowed arterioles that are already maximally dilated to healthy arterioles with less resistance. This theoretically could result in ischemia in the areas supplied

by the narrowed arterioles. Coronary artery steal syndrome is therefore a concern for individuals with ischemic heart disease who are being administered isoflurane. There is strong evidence against isoflurane-induced coronary artery steal syndrome, however. Most patients with ischemic heart disease do not develop myocardial ischemia during the administration of isoflurane. In addition, coronary artery autoregulation appears to be maintained during anesthesia produced by inhaled anesthetics. What is of greater importance is the avoidance of events such as tachycardia or hypotension that may result in myocardial ischemia. (49–50, Fig. 4–7; **105–111**)

16. Volatile anesthetics have minimal effect on the pulmonary vasculature in the absence of any underlying pulmonary disease. Nitrous oxide may increase pulmonary vascular resistance secondary to its mild sympathomimetic effects. This appears to be particularly true in patients with co-existing pulmonary hypertension. (50; **114–115**)

17. Sympathetic nervous system stimulation appears to accompany the administration of desflurane when an abrupt and large increase in the concentration of desflurane is delivered to the patient. This stimulation of the sympathetic nervous system is reflected as a transient increase in heart rate and systemic blood pressure. The plasma concentration of norepinephrine has been shown to be increased during this time of sympathetic nervous system stimulation. These transient responses to increased desflurane concentration delivery can be blunted by the prior administration of an opioid or by more gradually increasing the desflurane concentration. (50, Fig. 4–8; **112, Fig. 5–19**)

18. The only inhaled anesthetic that has any effect on cardiac rhythm is halothane. The administration of halothane may be accompanied by a junctional cardiac rhythm and a decrease in blood pressure. The junctional rhythm is likely due to the suppression of the activity of the sinus node by halothane. The administration of halothane also results in decreases in the amount of circulating epinephrine necessary to elicit premature ventricular contractions. Adults are more sensitive to this effect of halothane than children, such that children are able to tolerate higher doses of subcutaneous epinephrine injection during halothane anesthesia. Cardiac arrhythmias that occur in the presence of halothane should be treated directly, and not solely through the discontinuation of halothane. The basis for this comes from the study of the potential of halothane to cause cardiac dysrhythmias in animal models. These studies have shown that the risk of cardiac dysrhythmias when halothane is administered at a concentration of 0.5% is the same as the risk of cardiac dysrhythmias when halothane is administered at a concentration of 2%. (50–51, Fig. 4–9; **105, 552, 997**)

19. The inhalation of a volatile anesthetic for longer than 5 hours is associated with an increase in heart rate, cardiac output, and right atrial pressure when compared with the values of these after about 1 hour of anesthesia. The effects of increased cardiac output and decreased systemic vascular resistance together result in no change in blood pressure, or rather a recovery from the effects of the volatile anesthetic. The degree to which these changes occur vary with the inhaled anesthetic. The administration of halothane appears to have the greatest time-related changes in cardiovascular measurements after 5 hours of inhalation, whereas minimal changes occur over time with the administration of isoflurane and desflurane. Thus, the continued administration of halothane results in the greatest degree of recovery from its cardiovascular effects among the volatile anesthetics. The cardiovascular changes that are noted after 5 hours of volatile anesthetic inhalation are attenuated or completely prevented by the prior administration of propranolol. This suggests that the mechanism by which these cardiovascular time-related changes occur may be due to an increase in sympathetic nervous system activity. (51; **104**)

20. Circulatory effects of volatile anesthetics are altered during spontaneous ventilation versus mechanical stimulation mainly through associated differences in the Pa_{CO_2}. Carbon dioxide often accumulates when patients are spontaneously ventilating while an inhaled anesthetic is being administered. The accumulation of carbon dioxide may stimulate the sympathetic nervous system, leading to an increase in heart rate, an increase in myocardial contractility, an increase in cardiac output, peripheral vasodilation, and a decrease in systemic vascular resistance. A patient who is being administered a volatile anesthetic does not exhibit any significant alterations in blood pressure when switched from controlled ventilation to spontaneous ventilation. This may be due to the increase in venous return that also accompanies spontaneous ventilation, thereby opposing the effects that may otherwise have been noted by the accumulation of carbon dioxide. (51–52; **613–614, Table 15–5**)

21. There are several variables that may influence the cardiovascular effects produced intraoperatively by inhaled anesthetics. First, the patient's co-existing diseases may contribute to the cardiovascular response to inhaled anesthetics, particularly if the disease is cardiac in nature. Some cardiac disease states that may influence the patient's cardiovascular response include congestive heart failure, ischemic heart disease, and stenotic valvular lesions. Second, a patient's regularly prescribed drug therapy may influence the cardiovascular effects of inhaled anesthetics. For example, beta-adrenergic antagonists or calcium channel blockers may lead to an exaggeration in the magnitude of cardiac depression produced by some volatile anesthetics. In addition, angiotensin-converting enzyme inhibitor therapy that is continued through the morning of surgery may exaggerate decreases in blood pressure seen intraoperatively. Finally, the degree of surgical stimulation may influence the cardiovascular effects produced by the inhaled anesthetics intraoperatively. The MAC of anesthesia required to prevent a sympathetic nervous system response to surgical incision is greater than that required to prevent movement with skin incision. (52, Fig. 4–10; **97–101, 992–995**)

22. Isoflurane is alone among the volatile anesthetics with regard to its mild beta-adrenergic agonist property. This property of isoflurane is consistent with many of the clinical cardiovascular effects that are associated with the administration of isoflurane. Some of these clinical cardiovascular effects include a maintenance of cardiac output, an increase in heart rate, an increase in skeletal muscle blood flow, dilation of the coronary arterioles, and a decrease in systemic vascular resistance. (53)

23. There are several possible explanations for the less significant myocardial depressant effects associated with the administration of isoflurane than with the other volatile anesthetics. First, isoflurane may have mild beta-agonist properties. Second, the administration of isoflurane reduces myocardial intracellular calcium less than the other agents. Third, isoflurane is less likely than halothane to depress the baroreceptor reflex. Finally, isoflurane may have a greater anesthetic potency. That is, isoflurane may depress the brain more readily than the other agents, and thus spare the heart at a given MAC value. Evidence that this may be true is by comparison of the ratio of the fatal anesthetic concentration to MAC in animals for the various anesthetics. For isoflurane it is 3.0, compared with 2.5 for desflurane and 2.0 for halothane. (53; **96–99**)

24. The administration of nitrous oxide produces several effects that are signs of its ability to mildly stimulate the sympathetic nervous system. Examples of these effects include an increase in plasma concentrations of circulating catecholamines, mydriasis, and an increase in systemic and pulmonary vascular resistance. These effects of nitrous oxide are seen whether nitrous oxide is administered alone or in combination with a volatile anesthetic. Nitrous oxide is

thought to stimulate the sympathetic nervous system by directly acting on the suprapontine areas of the brain. (53; **112–115**)

VENTILATION

25. The choice of inhaled anesthetics administered to maintain anesthesia has not been shown to influence the incidence of postoperative pulmonary complications. (53)

26. Inhaled volatile anesthetics produce a dose-dependent depression of the ventilatory drive. The mechanism by which this occurs is thought to be primarily through the direct depression of the medullary ventilatory centers, with some contribution from depressant effects on intercostal muscle function. Each inhaled anesthetic depresses ventilation to a different degree. For example, the resting $PaCO_2$ was found to be increased more by the administration of desflurane and isoflurane than with sevoflurane and halothane when equipotent doses of each volatile anesthetic was administered to healthy volunteers. (53, Fig. 4–11; **135–140, Figs. 5–28, 5–29**)

27. Inhaled volatile anesthetics produce a dose-dependent increase in the rate of breathing. Although the exact mechanism for this effect of inhaled anesthetics is unclear, it is believed to result from central nervous system stimulation by the anesthetic. Isoflurane differs from the other anesthetics with regard to its effects on the rate of breathing in that it only increases the rate of breathing when administered at doses of up to 1 MAC. The administration of isoflurane at doses above 1 MAC does not further increase the rate of breathing. (53; **136–137, Fig. 5–29**)

28. Inhaled volatile anesthetics decrease the tidal volume of individuals breathing the inhaled anesthetic. The mechanism by which this occurs is unclear. (53; **136–137, Fig. 5–29**)

29. Overall, the breathing pattern of patients who are being administered an inhaled volatile anesthetic is regular, rhythmic, rapid, and shallow. The decrease in tidal volume is not sufficiently compensated by the increase in respiratory rate, however. This results in a decrease in the minute ventilation of individuals breathing an inhaled anesthetic. The resting $PaCO_2$ of these patients is increased as a result. The resting $PaCO_2$ is used as an index to evaluate the degree of respiratory depression that is produced by inhaled anesthetics. (53; **136–137, Fig. 5–29**)

30. The carbon dioxide response curve is a plot of the volume of ventilation at increasing levels of $PaCO_2$. The slope of the carbon dioxide response curve represents the sensitivity to the ventilatory stimulant effects of carbon dioxide. The placement of the carbon dioxide response curve along the x-axis represents the ventilatory responsiveness to carbon dioxide. (54; **140–141**)

31. The minute ventilation increases by 1 to 3 L/min in an awake, healthy, spontaneously ventilating individual for every 1 mm Hg increase in the $PaCO_2$. (54; **140**)

32. The carbon dioxide response curve gives useful information about the effects of drugs on ventilation. Inhaled anesthetics, including nitrous oxide, produce both a dose-dependent depression of the slope and a rightward shift of the carbon dioxide response curve. The decreased slope of the carbon dioxide response curve represents a decreased sensitivity to the ventilatory stimulant effects of carbon dioxide. The rightward displacement of the carbon dioxide response curve represents an attenuation of the response to carbon dioxide. (54–55; **140–141, Fig. 5–36**)

33. Patients with chronic obstructive pulmonary disease appear to have an obtunded ventilatory response to an increased $PaCO_2$ that is proportional to the degree of

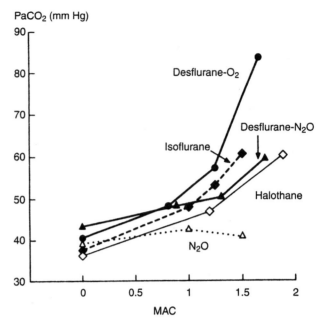

Figure 3–1. Inhaled anesthetics produce drug-specific and dose-dependent increases in $Paco_2$ (From Eger EI. Desflurane (Suprane®): A Compendium and Reference. Nutley, NJ. Anaquest 1993, pp 1–119.)

obstruction of the airways. These patients may therefore have an accentuated increase in $Paco_2$ when administered a volatile anesthetic. (55; **139, 141, 143, Fig. 5–35**)

34. The administration of 1.5 MAC nitrous oxide to patients in a hyperbaric chamber decreases the patient's ventilatory response to carbon dioxide by 15%. Clinically, however, the administration of nitrous oxide to patients does not change their $Paco_2$ levels from awake levels. Although there is an increase in the anesthetic depth when nitrous oxide is added to a volatile anesthetic, the patient's $Paco_2$ does not change with the addition of nitrous oxide to the volatile anesthetic. Similarly, the substitution of nitrous oxide for an equivalent dose of a volatile anesthetic results in less of an increase in the $Paco_2$ than that which would have otherwise occurred with the volatile anesthetic alone. Desflurane may be an exception to this, however. (55, Fig. 4–11; **140–141, Fig. 5–30**)

35. Surgical stimulation leads to an increase in both a patient's respiratory rate and tidal volume. The minute ventilation may increase by as much as 40% with surgical stimulation, and the $Paco_2$ subsequently decreases. The decrease in $Paco_2$ is partially offset secondary to an increase in the production of carbon dioxide during surgical stimulation, such that the decrease in the $Paco_2$ is only by 4 to 6 mm Hg. (55, Fig. 4–13; **142–143, Fig. 5–30**)

36. The increase in $Paco_2$ lessens with time during the administration of the same, continuous dose of a volatile anesthetic. This results in a $Paco_2$ closer to the patient's baseline after prolonged exposure to a volatile anesthetic than it was during the initial administration of the volatile anesthetic. This is reflected in the carbon dioxide response curve, which returns to baseline after more than 5 hours of continuous inhalation of a volatile anesthetic. The mechanism by which this occurs is unknown. (55; **136, 139–140**)

37. Normal breathing relies on proper functioning of the intercostal muscles and the diaphragm. Expansion of the rib cage is produced by contraction of the intercostal muscles, which is coupled with descent of the diaphragm for optimal respiratory function. The administration of inhaled anesthetics, and in particular halothane, suppresses intercostal muscle function while sparing the diaphragm.

This depression of intercostal muscle function results in an impairment of rib cage expansion and has several effects. First, there is impairment of rib cage expansion in response to chemical stimuli such as arterial hypoxemia and hypercapnia. Second, the impairment of rib cage expansion results in inward chest collapse on inspiration, decreasing lung volume. This, in turn, leads to a decrease in the patient's functional residual capacity. (55; **138–139, Figs. 5–31, 5–32, 5–33**)

38. The apneic threshold is defined as the maximum $PaCO_2$ level that a patient can have that will not initiate spontaneous ventilation. The difference between the apneic threshold $PaCO_2$ and the resting $PaCO_2$ is about 5 mm Hg. This appears to be true regardless of the resting $PaCO_2$ of a patient. (55; **140, Fig. 5–36**)

39. The most reliable method by which to decrease the $PaCO_2$ of a spontaneously ventilating patient being administered a volatile anesthetic is through the initiation of mechanical ventilation of the lungs. Assisted ventilation of the lungs is not reliable, given that a spontaneously ventilating individual will become apneic when the $PaCO_2$ has decreased by about 5 mm Hg below the resting $PaCO_2$. (55–56; **140**)

40. In an awake, healthy, spontaneously ventilating individual there is an increase in the minute ventilation in response to a decrease of PaO_2 below 60 mm Hg. This response is mediated by the carotid bodies. (56; **141–142**)

41. The inhalation of a volatile anesthetic at 0.1 MAC significantly obtunds the ventilatory response to arterial hypoxemia, whereas the inhalation of a volatile anesthetic at 1 MAC obliterates the ventilatory response to arterial hypoxemia. (56; **142–143, Figs. 5–37, 5–38**)

42. Subanesthetic doses of inhaled anesthetics have a greater effect on the ventilatory response to hypoxemia than on the ventilatory response to hypercapnia. The synergistic effect to stimulate ventilation that occurs when arterial hypoxemia and hypercapnia are both present in healthy, awake individuals is also attenuated by inhaled anesthetics. Clinically, this effect of subanesthetic doses of inhaled anesthetics becomes relevant in patients recovering from anesthesia. Patients in the postanesthesia care unit may not respond appropriately to arterial hypoxemia by increasing ventilation secondary to the residual effects of the inhaled anesthetic. (56; **142–143, Figs. 5–37, 5–38**)

43. Volatile anesthetics have all been shown to be bronchodilators and exert some attenuation of bronchospasm with their administration. The exact mechanism by which these bronchodilating effects occur is not known. They may exert this effect primarily by decreasing efferent vagal tone from the central nervous system. The additive effects of halothane and a beta-2 agonist on bronchial tone lends further evidence that this may be the case. It is believed that they also directly relax bronchial smooth muscle. (56, Figs. 4–14, 4–15; **125–129, Figs. 5–22, 5–23**)

44. There may be some benefit to the administration of the volatile anesthetics for the treatment of bronchospasm because the bronchodilating effects of halothane in combination with albuterol have been shown to be additive. There is, however, no evidence to show that the bronchodilating effects of volatile anesthetics are an effective method for treating status asthmaticus. (57; **128**)

45. Isoflurane and desflurane are both considered to be modestly irritating to the airways when administered to awake patients. Clinically, the administration of these volatile anesthetics to awake patients may result in coughing, breath holding, and the production of secretions. This effect of isoflurane and desflurane is not attenuated by the prior administration of nitrous oxide or an opioid. Isoflurane and desflurane are thus limited in their clinical utility for an inhalation induction of anesthesia. (57; **128–129**)

46. Hypoxic pulmonary vasoconstriction is a reflex response of pulmonary arterioles to vasoconstrict in areas of low alveolar Pa_{O_2} in an attempt to decrease perfusion to underventilated alveoli, as in atelectasis. Inhaled anesthetics directly inhibit the hypoxic pulmonary vasoconstriction reflex in models studied to evaluate this effect. The mechanism for the effect is unknown, but it is believed to be multifactorial. (57, Fig. 20–5; **131–135, Figs. 5–26, 5–27**)

Chapter 4

Intravenous Anesthetics

1. Name some examples of intravenous anesthetics. What are the potential clinical uses of intravenous anesthetics?

PROPOFOL

2. What type of chemical structure is propofol?

3. What is the mechanism of action of propofol?

4. How is propofol cleared from the plasma?

5. What degree of metabolism does propofol undergo? How should the dose of propofol be altered when administered to patients with liver dysfunction?

6. What is the context-sensitive half-time of propofol relative to other intravenous anesthetics? What is the effect-site equilibration time of propofol relative to other intravenous anesthetics?

7. How does the emergence from a propofol anesthetic or propofol induction differ from the emergence seen with the other induction agents?

8. How readily does propofol cross the placenta? What effects does it have on the neonate when administered to a parturient?

9. How does propofol affect the cardiovascular system?

10. How does propofol affect ventilation?

11. How does propofol affect the central nervous system?

12. How does propofol affect the seizure threshold?

13. What is the relationship between propofol and nausea and vomiting?

14. How is propofol administered for sedation?

15. How is propofol administered for maintenance anesthesia?

16. How can the pain associated with the intravenous injection of propofol be attenuated?

17. Why is asepsis important when handling propofol?

18. Which patients may be at risk for a life-threatening allergic reaction to propofol?

BARBITURATES

19. Name some of the barbiturates. From what chemical compound are they derived?

20. What is the mechanism of action of barbiturates?

21. How are barbiturates cleared from the plasma?

22. What degree of metabolism do barbiturates undergo?

23. What is the context-sensitive half-time of barbiturates relative to other intravenous anesthetics? What is the effect-site equilibration time of barbiturates relative to other intravenous anesthetics?

24. How do methohexital and thiopental compare with regard to induction doses, duration of action, and clinical utility?

25. How do barbiturates affect the arterial blood pressure?

26. How do barbiturates affect the heart rate?

27. How do barbiturates affect ventilation?

28. How do barbiturates affect laryngeal and cough reflexes?

29. How do barbiturates affect the central nervous system? How do barbiturates affect an electroencephalogram?

30. How should thiopental be administered and dosed for cerebral protection in patients with persistently elevated intracranial pressures?

31. What are the various routes and methods for the administration of barbiturates in clinical anesthesia practice?

32. What are some potential adverse complications of the injection of thiopental?

33. What is the risk of a life-threatening allergic reaction to barbiturates?

ETOMIDATE

34. What type of structure is etomidate? What is its mechanism of action?

35. How is etomidate cleared from the plasma?

36. What degree of metabolism does etomidate undergo?

37. What is the context-sensitive half-time of etomidate relative to other intravenous anesthetics? What is the effect-site equilibration time of etomidate relative to other intravenous anesthetics?

38. How does etomidate affect the cardiovascular system?

39. How does etomidate affect ventilation?

40. How does etomidate affect the central nervous system?

41. How does etomidate affect the seizure threshold?

42. What are the endocrine effects of etomidate?

43. What are some potential negative effects associated with the administration of etomidate?

KETAMINE

44. What chemical compound is ketamine a derivative of? What is its mechanism of action?

45. How do patients appear clinically after an induction dose of ketamine?

46. What is the mechanism by which the effects of ketamine are terminated?

47. What are the induction doses for intravenous and intramuscular routes of administration of ketamine? What is the time of onset for the effect of ketamine subsequent to its administration?

48. How does ketamine affect the cardiovascular system?

49. How does ketamine affect ventilation?

50. How does ketamine affect skeletal muscle tone? How does this affect the upper airway?

51. How does ketamine affect the central nervous system?

52. What does the emergence delirium associated with ketamine refer to? What is the incidence? How can it be prevented?

53. What are some common clinical uses of ketamine?

54. What can the repeated administration of ketamine lead to? How is it manifest clinically?

55. How common are allergic reactions to ketamine?

BENZODIAZEPINES

56. Name some of the commonly used benzodiazepines. What are some of the clinical effects and properties of benzodiazepines that make them useful in anesthesia practice?

57. What is the mechanism of action of benzodiazepines?

58. Where are benzodiazepine receptors located?

59. How does midazolam compare with diazepam with regard to its affinity for the benzodiazepine receptor?

60. How does water-soluble midazolam cross the blood-brain barrier to gain access to the central nervous system?

61. What is the effect-site equilibration time of benzodiazepines relative to other intravenous anesthetics? How do the context-sensitive half-times of the benzodiazepines compare?

62. How do benzodiazepines affect the cardiovascular system?

63. How do benzodiazepines affect ventilation?

64. How do benzodiazepines affect the central nervous system?

65. What are some clinical uses of benzodiazepines in anesthesia practice?

66. How do midazolam and diazepam compare with regard to time of onset and degree of amnesia when administered for sedation?

67. What are some advantages and disadvantages of benzodiazepines for use as induction agents?

68. How can the effects of benzodiazepines be reversed?

69. What organic solvent is used to dissolve diazepam into solution? What are some of the effects of this solvent?

70. How common are allergic reactions to benzodiazepines?

ANSWERS*

1. Examples of intravenous anesthetics include the barbiturates, benzodiazepines, opioids, etomidate, propofol, and ketamine. These drugs can be used as induction agents or, in combination with other anesthetics, for the maintenance of anesthesia. (58)

PROPOFOL

2. Propofol is a lipid-soluble isopropyl phenol formulated as an emulsion. The current formulation consists of 1% propofol, soybean oil, glycerol, and purified egg phosphatide. (58, Fig. 5–1; **249–250, Fig. 9–17**)

3. The mechanism by which propofol exerts its effects is not fully understood, but it appears to be in part via the gamma-aminobutyric acid (GABA) activated chloride ion channel. Evidence suggests that propofol may interact with the

*Numbers in parentheses: lightface numbers refer to pages, figures, or tables in Stoelting RK, Miller RD: Basics of Anesthesia, 4th ed. Philadelphia, Churchill Livingstone, 2000; **boldface numbers** refer to pages, figures, or tables in Miller RD: Anesthesia, 5th ed. Philadelphia, Churchill Livingstone, 2000.

GABA receptor and maintain it in an activated state for a prolonged period, thereby resulting in greater inhibitory effects on synaptic transmission. Propofol may also inhibit the NMDA subtype of the glutamate receptor. (58; **251**)

4. Propofol is cleared rapidly from the plasma through both redistribution to inactive tissue sites and rapid metabolism by the liver. (58; **250**)

5. Propofol is extensively metabolized by the liver to inactive, water-soluble metabolites, which are then excreted in the urine. Less than 1% of propofol administered is excreted unchanged in the urine. The metabolism of propofol is extremely rapid. Patients with liver dysfunction appear to rapidly metabolize propofol as well, lending some proof that extrahepatic sites of metabolism exist. This has been further supported by evidence of metabolism during the anhepatic phase of liver transplantation. (58; **250, Fig. 9–18**)

6. The context-sensitive half-time refers to the time required to pass for the concentration of a particular drug to reach 50% of its peak plasma concentration after the discontinuation of its administration as a continuous intravenous infusion for a given duration. The context-sensitive half-time of a drug depends mostly on the drug's lipid solubility and clearance mechanisms. The continuous infusion of propofol rarely results in cumulative drug effects. After the continuous administration of propofol for several days for sedation in the intensive care unit the discontinuation of the infusion resulted in the rapid recovery to consciousness. The lack of cumulative effects of propofol illustrates that the context-sensitive half-time of propofol is short. The effect-site equilibration time refers to the interval of time required between the time that a specific plasma concentration of the drug is achieved and a specific effect of the drug can be measured. The effect-site equilibration time reflects the time necessary for the circulation to deliver the drug to its site of action, such as the brain. The rapid administration of an induction dose of propofol results in unconsciousness in less than 30 seconds, illustrating its rapid effect-site equilibration time. (60; **250**)

7. After the administration of propofol, patients experience a rapid return to consciousness with minimal residual central nervous system effects. Patients who are to undergo brief procedures or outpatient surgical patients may especially benefit from the rapid wake-up associated with propofol anesthesia. Propofol also tends to result in the patient awakening with a general state of well-being and mild euphoria. Patient excitement has also been observed. Hallucinations and sexual fantasies have been reported to have occurred in association with the administration of propofol. (58; **250–251**)

8. Propofol readily crosses the placenta, but it has minimal effects on the neonate because it is rapidly cleared from the neonatal circulation. (60)

9. The administration of an induction dose of propofol results in a decrease in systolic blood pressure by 25% to 40% and a decrease in cardiac output by about 15%. These effects of propofol appear to be due to both direct myocardial depression and vasodilation, which are dose dependent. The cardiovascular effects produced by propofol are similar to, but more pronounced than, those produced by barbiturates. Unlike the barbiturates, the heart rate is usually unchanged with the administration of propofol. Propofol may selectively decrease sympathetic nervous system activity more than parasympathetic nervous system activity. (60; **253**)

10. The administration of an induction dose of propofol (1.5 to 2.5 mg/kg) almost always results in apnea through a dose-dependent depression of ventilation in a manner similar to, but more prolonged than, that of thiopental. The apnea that results appears to last for 30 seconds or greater and is followed by a return of

ventilation that is characterized by rapid, shallow breathing such that the minute ventilation is significantly decreased for up to 4 minutes. (60; **252–253**)

11. The administration of propofol results in decreases in intracranial pressure, cerebral blood flow, and cerebral metabolic oxygen requirements in a dose-dependent manner. In patients with an elevated intracranial pressure the administration of propofol may be accompanied by undesirable decreases in the cerebral perfusion pressure, however. (60; **251–252, 720**)

12. The effects of propofol on the seizure threshold are controversial. The administration of propofol has resulted in seizures and opisthotonos and has been used to facilitate the mapping of seizure foci. Propofol has also been used to treat seizures. High doses of propofol can result in burst suppression on the electroencephalogram. (60, 61; **251–252**)

13. Propofol appears to have a significant antiemetic effect, given the low incidence of nausea and vomiting in patients who have received a propofol anesthetic. In addition, propofol administered in subhypnotic doses of 10 to 15 mg has successfully treated both postoperative nausea and vomiting and nausea in patients receiving chemotherapy. (61; **254**)

14. Propofol may be administered for sedation through a continuous intravenous infusion at a rate of 25 to 100 µg/kg/min. At these doses propofol will provide sedation and amnesia without hypnosis. (60; **255–256**)

15. Propofol may be administered for maintenance anesthesia through a continuous intravenous infusion at a rate of 100 to 200 µg/kg/min. The clinician may use signs of light anesthesia such as hypertension, tachycardia, diaphoresis, or skeletal muscle movement as indicators for the need to increase the infusion rate of propofol. For procedures lasting more than 2 hours, the use of propofol for maintenance anesthesia may not be cost effective. (61; **254–255**)

16. The injection of propofol intravenously can cause pain in awake patients. The pain can be attenuated by using large veins for its administration, or with the prior administration of lidocaine at the injection site. Alternatively, lidocaine may be mixed with the propofol for simultaneous infusion. (58; **256**)

17. Asepsis is important when handling propofol because the solvent for propofol, Intralipid, provides for a favorable culture medium for bacterial growth. Ethylenediaminetetraacetic acid has been added to the propofol formulation in the United States in an attempt to suppress bacterial growth. (61; **254**)

18. Patients at risk for a life-threatening allergic reaction to propofol are those with a history of atopy or allergy to other drugs that also contain a phenyl nucleus or isopropyl group. Anaphylactoid reactions to the propofol itself and separate from the lipid emulsion have been reported. (61; **253**)

BARBITURATES

19. Thiopental is the most commonly used barbiturate in the practice of anesthesia. Other barbiturates include secobarbital, pentobarbital, thiamylal, and methohexital. The barbiturate compounds are a derivative of barbituric acid. Structural alterations of two of the carbon atoms of barbituric acid result in the barbiturates used in clinical practice. Historically, the barbiturates had been classified as short-acting or long-acting agents. This method of classification is no longer used because of the erroneous implication that the duration of action is predictable for a given agent. (61; **209–210, Figs. 8–1, 8–2**)

20. The mechanism of action of barbiturates is based on their ability to enhance and mimic the action of the neurotransmitter gamma-aminobutyric acid (GABA) in the central nervous system. GABA is the main inhibitory neurotransmitter in the central nervous system. Barbiturates bind to the GABA receptor and increase

the duration of activity of the GABA receptor, such that the chloride ion influx into the cells is prolonged. The chloride ion hyperpolarizes the cell and inhibits postsynaptic neurons. At higher concentrations the chloride ion channel may be stimulated by the barbiturate alone even in the absence of GABA. (61; **209–211, Fig. 8–3**)

21. Barbiturates are cleared from the plasma primarily through its rapid redistribution to inactive tissue sites after its administration as a bolus. (61–62; **211–214, Figs. 8–4, 8–5, 8–6**)

22. Barbiturates are eliminated from the body through hepatic metabolism. Less than 1% of the drug is excreted unchanged by the kidneys. (62; **211–212**)

23. Barbiturates are most often used for the intravenous induction of general anesthesia. Maximal brain uptake and onset of effect takes place within 30 seconds after the rapid intravenous injection of a barbiturate. Rapid awakening follows the administration of an induction dose of a barbiturate secondary to the rapid redistribution of these drugs. This accounts for the short effect-site equilibration time for these agents. The duration of action of barbiturates after its intravenous injection is dictated by its redistribution from the plasma to inactive sites. Large or repeated doses of the lipid-soluble barbiturates can result in saturation of the inactive sites. This may lead to the accumulation of drug and to prolonged effects of the usually short-acting drugs. The context-sensitive half-time of barbiturates is thus prolonged. (61, Fig. 5–3; **211–214, Figs. 8–4 through 8–6, 8–17**)

24. The induction dose of methohexital is 1 to 1.5 mg/kg intravenously, whereas the induction dose of thiopental is 3 to 5 mg/kg IV. Methohexital undergoes greater hepatic metabolism than thiopental, resulting in a shorter duration of action and more rapid awakening. Based on the shorter duration of action of methohexital, it is sometimes chosen over thiopental for the induction of anesthesia for patients undergoing outpatient procedures when rapid awakening is desired. An example of a procedure in which methohexital is frequently chosen for the induction of anesthesia is electroconvulsive shock therapy. This is not only due to the short duration of action of methohexital, but also to its epileptogenic property. (62; **211–214, 216, 224, Table 8–6**)

25. The administration of barbiturates typically results in a decrease in blood pressure by 10 to 20 mm Hg. This decrease in blood pressure primarily results from peripheral vasodilation. The vasodilation that accompanies the administration of barbiturates is due to a combination of depression of the vasomotor center in the medulla and a decrease in sympathetic nervous system outflow from the central nervous system. Exaggerated blood pressure decreases may be seen in patients who are hypertensive, whether or not they are being treated by antihypertensives. The administration of barbiturates should also be undertaken with caution in patients who are dependent on the preload to the heart to maintain cardiac output, as in patients with ischemic heart disease, pericardial tamponade, congestive heart failure, heart block, or hypovolemia. (62, Fig. 5–4; **219**)

26. The administration of barbiturates results in an increase in heart rate. This increase in heart rate is thought to be due to a baroreceptor-mediated reflex response to the decrease in blood pressure caused by the administration of the barbiturate. The increase in heart rate may increase myocardial oxygen requirements during a time when significant decreases in blood pressure may decrease coronary artery blood flow as well. Given this, the administration of a barbiturate to patients with ischemic heart disease must be done with extreme caution. Although the administration of barbiturates typically results in an increase in heart rate, the cardiac output may be decreased. This is in part due to the direct myocardial contractile depression that results from the administration of barbiturates. The effect of a decrease in cardiac output by barbiturates

is not of such significance that it is frequently seen clinically, however. (62, Fig. 5–4; **219**)

27. Barbiturates depress ventilation centrally by depressing the medullary ventilatory centers. This is manifest clinically as a decreased responsiveness to the ventilatory stimulatory effects of carbon dioxide. Depending on the dose administered, the patient will have a slow breathing rate and small tidal volumes to the extent that apnea follows. Typically, after an induction dose of barbiturate transient apnea will result and require controlled ventilation of the lungs. When spontaneous ventilation is resumed, it is again characterized by a slow breathing rate and small tidal volumes. (62–63; **218, Fig. 8–12**)

28. Induction doses of thiopental alone do not reliably depress laryngeal and cough reflexes. Stimulation of the upper airway, as with the placement of an oral airway or an endotracheal tube, can result in laryngospasm or bronchospasm. It is therefore recommended that adequate suppression of these reflexes be obtained before instrumenting the airway. This can be accomplished with increased doses of a barbiturate, by the administration of a neuromuscular blocking drug, or by the addition of another preoperative medicine, such as opioids, to augment the anesthetic effects of thiopental during stimulation of the upper airway. (63; **218**)

29. Barbiturates are potent cerebral vasoconstrictors. This results in a decrease in cerebral blood flow, a decrease in cerebral blood volume, a decrease in intracranial pressure, and a decrease in cerebral metabolic oxygen requirements. Barbiturates are also thought to depress the reticular activating system, which is believed to be important in maintaining wakefulness. Thiopental produces a dose-dependent depression of the electroencephalogram. A flat electroencephalogram may be maintained with a continuous infusion of thiopental. Methohexital is the only barbiturate that does not decrease electrical activity on an electroencephalogram. In fact, methohexital activates epileptic foci and is often used intraoperatively to identify epileptic foci during the surgical ablation of these foci. The effects of barbiturates on the central nervous system indicate that barbiturates are useful for patients in whom elevated intracranial pressures are a concern. Examples of patients who may benefit from the administration of a barbiturate as an induction agent or as maintenance anesthesia include patients with space-occupying lesions or patients who have suffered head trauma. (63; **217–218, 223, Fig. 8–11**)

30. In patients with persistently elevated intracranial pressures, barbiturates may be administered intravenously in high doses to decrease the intracranial pressure. Care must be taken to avoid decreases in mean arterial pressure that would compromise the cerebral perfusion pressure under these conditions. To ascertain the optimal dose of barbiturate administered for these patients an electroencephalogram can be obtained. The dose of barbiturate can be titrated to a flat-line electroencephalogram. When the electroencephalogram is isoelectric there is no further depression of cerebral metabolism or of cerebral metabolic oxygen requirements with increasing doses of barbiturate. This allows the clinician to administer the dose of barbiturate that provides the maximal benefit with minimal adverse effects. Barbiturates may offer some cerebral protection for patients with regional cerebral ischemia. Patients with global cerebral ischemia, such as from cardiac arrest, are not thought to derive any protection from the administration of barbiturates. (63; **223, 719–720, Fig. 8–18**)

31. There are various routes and methods for the administration of barbiturates in clinical anesthesia practice. For instance, the rapid intravenous administration of a bolus of barbiturate is indicated for a rapid sequence induction of anesthesia. The bolus of barbiturate should be immediately followed by the administration of succinylcholine or a nondepolarizing neuromuscular blocking drug to produce

skeletal muscle paralysis and facilitate tracheal intubation under these conditions. Alternatively, small doses of intravenous thiopental, in the range of 0. 5 to 1 mg/kg, may be administered to adult patients who have difficulty accepting the application of an anesthesia mask and/or the inhalation of a volatile anesthetic. The rectal administration of the barbiturate methohexital can be used to facilitate the induction of anesthesia in young or uncooperative patients. (63; **215, 2102**)

32. Potential adverse complications of the injection of thiopental may result from accidental intra-arterial, subcutaneous, and even appropriate venous administration of thiopental. The accidental intra-arterial injection of barbiturates results in excruciating pain and intense vasoconstriction that can last for hours. It is believed that barbiturate crystal formation in the blood causes the occlusion of distant small diameter arteries and arterioles. There are several treatment modalities for this potential problem, including the intra-arterial injection of papaverine and/or lidocaine, sympathetic nervous system blockade by stellate ganglion block of the involved upper extremity, and the administration of heparin to prevent thrombosis. Despite aggressive therapy, gangrene of the extremity often results. The accidental subcutaneous injection of barbiturates results in local tissue irritation. The irritation may proceed to pain, edema, erythema, or even tissue necrosis, depending on the volume and concentration injected. It has been recommended that 5 to 10 ml of 0.5% lidocaine be injected locally when the subcutaneous injection of thiopental occurs in an attempt to dilute the barbiturate. Venous thrombosis has been seen after the intravenous administration of thiopental. It is presumed that the thrombosis results from the deposition of barbiturate crystals in the vein. The crystallization of barbiturates is more likely to occur when the pH of the blood is too low to keep the alkaline barbiturate in solution. (63–64; **217, 221**)

33. Life-threatening allergic reactions to barbiturates are rare. The risk has been estimated to be 1 in 30,000. (64; **217**)

ETOMIDATE

34. Etomidate is an imidazole derivative. The mechanism by which etomidate exerts its effects is not completely understood. It appears that etomidate acts in part through agonist effects at the GABA receptor. (64; **245, Fig. 9–14**)

35. The induction dose of etomidate is 0.3 mg/kg. The administration of etomidate in induction doses results in unconsciousness in less than 30 seconds. The duration of action of etomidate after an induction dose is very short, owing to its rapid clearance from the plasma through redistribution to inactive tissue sites. (64; **245–246, Fig. 9–15**)

36. Etomidate rapidly undergoes nearly complete ester hydrolysis to pharmacologically inactive metabolites by the liver, with less than 3% of the drug being excreted in the urine unchanged. (64; **245–246**)

37. Like thiopental and propofol, etomidate is highly lipid soluble, which allows it to quickly cross the blood-brain barrier to exert its effects. This accounts for the short effect-site equilibration time for these agents. The context-sensitive half-time of etomidate may be prolonged if repeated or continuous doses of the drug result in saturation of the inactive sites. It is less likely than thiopental to accumulate and have prolonged effects, however. (64; **245–246**)

38. The administration of etomidate provides cardiovascular stability in that induction doses of etomidate result in minimal changes in heart rate, mean arterial pressure, central venous pressure, stroke volume, or cardiac index. Minimal decreases in blood pressure may result from the administration of etomidate to hypovolemic patients. The cardiovascular stability associated with etomidate

sets it apart from the other induction agents and is the basis for its usefulness as an induction agent in patients with limited cardiac reserve. When etomidate is administered to these patients it is important to realize that it does not have any analgesic effects. Supplemental agents need to be administered in conjunction with etomidate to blunt the stimulatory effects of direct laryngoscopy. (64, Fig. 5–5; **247**)

39. The administration of etomidate alone appears to result in less depressant effects on ventilation than propofol or thiopental. The effects of etomidate on ventilation may be augmented when administered in combination with other anesthetics or opioids. (64; **247**)

40. The administration of etomidate results in decreases in cerebral blood flow, intracranial pressure, and cerebral metabolic oxygen requirements. Etomidate has similar effects as barbiturates on the electroencephalogram as well, such that etomidate may be titrated to an isoelectric electroencephalogram to maximally decrease cerebral metabolic oxygen requirements. (64; **246, 720**)

41. The administration of etomidate has been shown to increase the activity of seizure foci on an electroencephalogram. Etomidate is similar to methohexital in this regard. Its effects can be used intraoperatively to facilitate intraoperative mapping of seizure foci for surgical ablation. (64; **246**)

42. The administration of etomidate is associated with the suppression of adrenocortical function. The suppression of adrenocortical function may last for up to 8 to 20 hours after the induction dose of etomidate has been administered. The concern regarding this suppression of adrenocortical function is the potential for the adrenal cortex to be unresponsive to adrenocorticotropic hormone. Should the adrenal cortex be unresponsive to adrenocorticotropic hormone, desirable protective responses against the stresses that accompany the perioperative period may be prevented. No adverse outcomes have been shown to have occurred secondary to short-term adrenocortical suppression associated with the administration of etomidate, however. (64, Fig. 5–6; **247–248, Fig. 9–16**)

43. Potential negative effects associated with the administration of etomidate include pain during intravenous injection, superficial thrombophlebitis, involuntary myoclonic movements, and an increased incidence of postoperative nausea and vomiting. (65; **249–250**)

KETAMINE

44. Ketamine is a derivative of phencyclidine. The administration of ketamine produces unconsciousness and analgesia that is dose related. The exact mechanism by which ketamine exerts its effects is unknown. Ketamine occupies some mu opioid receptors in the brain and spinal cord, which may partially explain its analgesic effects. Ketamine also binds to the NMDA receptor, which is believed to mediate the general anesthetic actions of ketamine. Other receptors that ketamine interacts with include monoaminergic receptors, muscarinic receptors, and calcium ion channels. Functionally, ketamine is believed to cause selective depression of the projections from the thalamus to the limbic system and cortex. The anesthesia derived from the administration of ketamine has thus been termed a *dissociative anesthesia*. There have not been any drugs isolated that are able to antagonize the effects of ketamine. (65; **240, Fig. 9–12**)

45. After an induction dose of ketamine the patient appears to be in a cataleptic state. The appearance of the patient may be characterized as eyes remaining open with a slow nystagmic gaze; the maintenance of cough, swallow, and corneal reflexes; moderate dilation of the pupils; lacrimation; salivation; and an increase in skeletal muscle tone with apparently coordinated but purposeless movements of the extremities. Induction doses of ketamine provide an intense

analgesia and amnesia in patients despite the patient appearing as if he or she may be awake. (65; **241**)

46. The redistribution of highly lipid-soluble ketamine to inactive tissue sites allows for rapid awakening after the administration of a bolus of ketamine. Ketamine undergoes extensive hepatic metabolism to norketamine for its elimination. Norketamine has between 20% and 30% the potency of ketamine and may contribute to some of the delayed effects of ketamine when administered as a continuous infusion. (65; **240, Fig. 9–13**)

47. For the induction of anesthesia, the intravenous dose of ketamine is 1 to 2 mg/kg, whereas the intramuscular dose is 5 to 10 mg/kg. The induction of anesthesia after intravenous administration is achieved within 60 seconds. The induction of anesthesia after intramuscular administration is achieved within 2 to 4 minutes. Return of consciousness after an intravenous induction dose of ketamine usually requires 10 to 20 minutes, whereas full orientation may take 60 to 90 minutes. Ketamine may also be administered orally or rectally. (66; **244, Table 9–7**)

48. The administration of ketamine results in an increase in systemic blood pressure, pulmonary artery blood pressure, heart rate, and cardiac output. The systemic blood pressure may increase by 20 to 40 mm Hg over the first 5 minutes after induction doses of ketamine are administered. The rise in blood pressure is often sustained for over 10 minutes. The degree of hemodynamic change elicited by the administration of ketamine is not influenced by the dose of ketamine that is administered, but it can be blunted by the prior administration of barbiturates, benzodiazepines, opioids, or droperidol. These cardiovascular effects of ketamine are most likely mediated centrally through the activation of the sympathetic nervous system and the direct stimulation of sympathetic nervous system outflow. Endogenous norepinephrine release has been found to accompany the administration of ketamine. This property of ketamine may make it useful as an induction agent in hypovolemic patients in whom hemodynamic support is beneficial. Conversely, patients with a history of myocardial ischemia may be adversely affected by the increases in myocardial oxygen demand induced by the administration of ketamine, making ketamine a poor choice as an induction agent in this patient population. Of note, the cardiovascular stimulatory effects of ketamine may not be as pronounced and may even be absent in patients who are catecholamine depleted. In catecholamine-depleted patients, such as the trauma patient, the administration of ketamine may actually lead to myocardial depression and a decrease in systemic blood pressure. (65–66; **242–243**)

49. The administration of ketamine can result in a transient depression of ventilation, even apnea with large doses, but the resting $PaCO_2$ is typically unaltered in these patients. Ketamine is a bronchial smooth neuromuscular blocking drug. This effect of ketamine is most likely mediated by its sympathomimetic effects and may make it useful as an induction agent in patients with bronchial asthma. The administration of ketamine also induces an increase in airway secretions. When ketamine is used as an induction agent, the administration of an antisialagogue preoperatively may be useful in decreasing the amount of airway secretions. (66; **243**)

50. Ketamine preserves and may even increase skeletal muscle tone. Patients have varying degrees of purposeful skeletal muscle movement and hypertonus after an induction dose of ketamine. The preservation of skeletal muscle tone results in maintenance of a patent upper airway and the preservation of cough and swallow reflexes. Despite this, airway protection by these reflexes against regurgitation or vomiting cannot be assumed. (66; **243**)

51. Ketamine has excitatory effects on the central nervous system such that there are increases in cerebral metabolism, cerebral blood flow, intracranial pressure,

and cerebral metabolic oxygen requirements associated with its administration. These excitatory effects of ketamine are reflected by the development of theta wave activity on the electroencephalogram when ketamine is administered. Because of the central nervous system excitatory effects of ketamine, it is not recommended as an induction agent in patients with space-occupying intracranial lesions or after head trauma in whom increases in the intracranial pressure can be detrimental. (66; **241–242**)

52. The emergence after the administration of ketamine has been associated with a delirium, often referred to as an emergence delirium. The severity of the emergence delirium varies. The emergence delirium manifests as vivid dreaming, visual and auditory illusions, and a sense of floating outside the body. These sensations are often associated with confusion, excitement, and fear, and are unpleasant to the patient. The emergence delirium typically occurs in the first hour after emergence and persists for 1 to 3 hours. The incidence of emergence delirium with ketamine administration has been estimated to be up to 30%, and it is more likely to occur when ketamine is used as the sole anesthetic agent. The risk of emergence delirium can be decreased with the preoperative or postinduction administration of benzodiazepines. (66; **241–242**)

53. Some common clinical uses of ketamine include its administration for the induction of anesthesia in hypovolemic patients, its intramuscular injection for the induction of anesthesia in children or in developmentally disabled patients who are difficult to manage, and for dressing changes and debridement procedures in burn patients. Small doses of ketamine may be titrated for its analgesic effects. (66; **243–244**)

54. The repeated administration of ketamine may result in the development of a tolerance to the analgesic effects of ketamine. Clinically, this would manifest as an increase in the dose of ketamine required with each subsequent anesthetic to provide sufficient analgesic effects. An example in which this situation may arise is in burn patients who are being administered ketamine while undergoing recurrent dressing changes. (66; **244**)

55. Allergic reactions to ketamine are uncommon. (66)

BENZODIAZEPINES

56. Benzodiazepines that are commonly used in the perioperative period include midazolam, diazepam, and lorazepam. The most common effects of benzodiazepines are their anxiolytic and sedative effects. When administered at higher doses, benzodiazepines may also produce unconsciousness. Other properties of benzodiazepines include anterograde amnesia, a lack of retrograde amnesia, minimal cardiopulmonary depression, anticonvulsant activity, and relative safety when taken in overdose. Clinical uses of benzodiazepines include their use for preoperative medication, for intravenous sedation, for the intravenous induction of anesthesia, and for the suppression of seizure activity. (66–67; **229**)

57. Benzodiazepines exert their effects through their actions on the gamma-aminobutyric acid (GABA) receptor. When GABA receptors are stimulated by the inhibitory neurotransmitter GABA, a chloride ion channel opens, allowing chloride ions to flow into the cell. This results in hyperpolarization of the neuron and a resistance of the neuron to subsequent depolarization. Benzodiazepines enhance the effect of GABA by binding to subunits of the GABA receptor and maintaining the chloride channel open for a longer period of time. (67, Fig. 5–7; **231–232, Fig. 9–6**)

58. Benzodiazepine receptors are located primarily on postsynaptic nerve endings in the central nervous system. The greatest density of benzodiazepine receptors

is in the cerebral cortex. The distribution of benzodiazepine receptors is consistent with the minimal cardiopulmonary effects of these drugs. (67; **231–232**)

59. Midazolam has almost two times the affinity for benzodiazepine receptors than diazepam, which is consistent with its greater potency. (67; **232–233**)

60. Midazolam is a hydrophilic drug. When midazolam is exposed to the pH of the blood it undergoes a change in its structure and becomes highly lipid soluble. This change in structure allows it to cross the blood-brain barrier and gain access to the central nervous system. (67; **232–233**)

61. Benzodiazepines are highly lipid-soluble drugs. This allows them to gain rapid entrance into the central nervous system by crossing the blood-brain barrier, where they are able to exert their effects. Thus the effect-site equilibration time of benzodiazepines is short, although it is slower than propofol or thiopental. The duration of action of benzodiazepines is dependent on the redistribution of the drug from the brain to inactive tissue sites. A continuous infusion or repeated boluses can result in saturation of the inactive tissue sites and a prolongation of the drug effect, particularly for the benzodiazepines that have active metabolites. For instance, diazepam undergoes hepatic metabolism to active metabolites, whereas midazolam has no active metabolites. The context-sensitive half-times for diazepam and lorazepam are prolonged when compared with that of midazolam. (67; **230, Table 9–2**)

62. Induction doses of midazolam may lead to decreases in systemic blood pressure that are greater than those seen with the induction dose of diazepam. This effect of midazolam may be particularly pronounced in patients who are hypovolemic. The decrease in systemic blood pressure is believed to be due to decreases in systemic vascular resistance. (67–68; **234–235**)

63. In general, benzodiazepines alone produce dose-dependent ventilatory depressant effects. Apnea may occur with the rapid administration of induction doses of midazolam, particularly if an opioid has been used for premedication. (68; **233–234, Fig. 9–8**)

64. Benzodiazepines decrease cerebral blood flow and cerebral metabolic oxygen requirements in a dose-dependent manner. This makes benzodiazepines safe for use in patients with space-occupying lesions, although the administration of benzodiazepines to patients with intracerebral pathologic processes may make subsequent neurologic evaluation of the patient difficult secondary to the potentially prolonged effects of these drugs. Benzodiazepines also have anticonvulsant effects that are thought to occur through the enhancement of the inhibitory effects of the neurotransmitter gamma-aminobutyric acid in the central nervous system. Benzodiazepines have been shown to increase the seizure threshold or treat seizures due to local anesthetic toxicity, alcohol withdrawal, and epilepsy. The dose of diazepam used to treat seizures is 0.1 mg/kg intravenously. An isoelectric electroencephalogram is not able to be achieved with the administration of benzodiazepines. (68; **233**)

65. Clinical uses of benzodiazepines in anesthesia practice include preoperative medication, intravenous sedation, the intravenous induction of anesthesia, and the suppression of seizure activity. (68; **235–236**)

66. When administered for sedation, midazolam has a more rapid onset and produces a greater degree of amnesia than diazepam. The slow onset and greater duration of action of lorazepam limits its usefulness as a preoperative medication. All benzodiazepines may have prolonged and more pronounced sedative effects in the elderly. (68; **235**)

67. The intravenous induction doses of midazolam and diazepam are 0.1 to 0.2 mg/kg and 0.2 to 0.3 mg/kg, respectively. The time of onset of midazolam is

anywhere between 30 and 80 seconds, depending on the dose and premedication. The time of onset of midazolam is more rapid than the time of onset of diazepam, making it the benzodiazepine of choice for the induction of anesthesia. The speed of onset of both these agents can be facilitated by the prior administration of opioids. Benzodiazepines are advantageous over barbiturates for the induction of anesthesia only because of its potentially lesser circulatory effects and greater reliability for the production of amnesia. A disadvantage of benzodiazepines for the induction of anesthesia is their lack of analgesic properties. Additional medicines would need to be administered to blunt the cardiovascular and laryngeal responses to direct laryngoscopy. The major disadvantage of benzodiazepines for the induction of anesthesia is delayed awakening, which limits the usefulness of benzodiazepines for this purpose. Midazolam is the shortest-acting of the benzodiazepines and therefore the most appropriate choice of benzodiazepine for the induction of anesthesia. Even so, awakening after a single induction dose of midazolam in healthy volunteers takes more than 15 minutes. The benzodiazepines, diazepam and lorazepam, require even greater periods of time before awakening after an induction dose, precluding their use as anesthesia induction agents. (68; **236**)

68. The effects of benzodiazepines can be reversed by a specific antagonist drug, flumazenil. Flumazenil is a competitive antagonist that binds to the benzodiazepine receptor but has little intrinsic activity. Flumazenil should be titrated to effect by administering 0.2 mg intravenously every 60 seconds up to a total dose of 1 to 3 mg. Flumazenil binds tightly to the benzodiazepine receptor but is cleared rapidly from the plasma. This results in a short duration of action of only about 20 minutes. The short duration of action of flumazenil requires that the patient be closely monitored for re-sedation after a dose of flumazenil is administered to reverse the effects of a benzodiazepine. Alternatively, an infusion of flumazenil may be started and titrated to the desired effect to maintain a constant plasma level of this reversal agent. (68; **237–240, Fig. 9–11**)

69. Propylene glycol is an organic solvent used to dissolve lipid soluble diazepam into solution. Propylene glycol is likely responsible for the unpredictable absorption of diazepam when administered intramuscularly. It is also responsible for the pain and possible subsequent thrombophlebitis experienced by patients on the intravenous injection of diazepam. (68; **229**)

70. Allergic reactions to benzodiazepines are extremely rare. (68)

Chapter 5

Opioids

STRUCTURE ACTIVITY RELATIONSHIPS

1. Name some of the commonly used opioids in anesthesia practice. Which opioids occur naturally and are obtained from the poppy plant?

MECHANISM OF ACTION

2. What is the mechanism of action of opioids?

3. Describe the location, subtypes, and pharmacologic responses of the opioid receptors. What are the primary receptor subtypes for supraspinal and spinal analgesia?

4. What endogenous ligands normally bind to and activate opioid receptors?

5. How does the affinity of the opioid for the receptor correlate with its potency?

6. Where are the opioid receptors located in the spinal cord?

7. How do differences in lipid solubility influence the action of epidural opioids?

8. How significant is the systemic absorption of opioid after its administration into the intrathecal or epidural space?

9. What are some potential side effects of neuraxially administered opioids?

10. What is the time course of respiratory depression that may be seen after the administration of neuraxial opioids? How can it be treated?

11. What are some risk factors for respiratory depression after the administration of neuraxial opioids?

OPIOID AGONISTS

12. How effective is morphine for the relief of pain? What are some other clinical effects of morphine?

13. What is the benefit derived from the administration of opioids minutes before the induction of anesthesia?

14. What is preemptive analgesia?

15. What are the potency, time of onset, and duration of action of opioids dependent on? How rapid is the effect-site equilibration time of morphine relative to the other opioids?

16. How are opioids cleared from the plasma? Which opioids have active metabolites?

17. What are the effects of opioids on the cardiovascular system?

18. What are the effects of opioids on ventilation?

19. What are the effects of opioids on the central nervous system?

20. What are the effects of opioids on the thoracoabdominal muscles? How can it be treated?

21. What are the effects of opioids on the gastrointestinal system?

22. What are the effects of opioids on the genitourinary system?

23. What is the mechanism by which opioids are thought to cause nausea and vomiting?

24. Over what time course does acute tolerance to the analgesic effects of morphine develop? What are some of the characteristics of the opioid withdrawal syndrome in opioid-dependent patients?

25. How do opioids modulate immune function?

26. What is the potency of meperidine relative to morphine?

27. What are some clinical effects of meperidine that are unique to this opioid?

28. What is the potency of fentanyl relative to morphine?

29. How does fentanyl compare with morphine with regard to its effect-site equilibration time?

30. How are the effects of fentanyl terminated? How does the context-sensitive half-time of fentanyl compare with other opioids?

31. What are some systemic clinical effects associated with the administration of fentanyl?

32. What are some clinical uses of fentanyl in anesthesia practice? What are some alternative routes for the administration of fentanyl?

33. What is the potency of sufentanil relative to morphine?

34. How does sufentanil compare with the other opioids with respect to its effect-site equilibration time and its context-sensitive half-time?

35. What are some systemic clinical effects associated with the administration of sufentanil?

36. What is the potency of alfentanil relative to morphine?

37. How does alfentanil compare with the other opioids with respect to its effect-site equilibration time and its context-sensitive half-time?

38. What are some clinical uses of alfentanil?

39. What is the potency of remifentanil relative to morphine?

40. How does remifentanil compare with the other opioids with respect to its effect-site equilibration time and its context-sensitive half-time?

41. What are some clinical uses of remifentanil?

OPIOID AGONIST-ANTAGONISTS

42. Name some of the agonist-antagonist opioids. What opioid receptors do these drugs often have strong and weak agonist affinities for?

43. What are some advantages and disadvantages to the administration of agonist-antagonist opioids?

OPIOID ANTAGONISTS

44. Name some of the opioid antagonist drugs. What is the mechanism of action of opioid antagonists?

45. What is the dose of naloxone for the reversal of undesirable effects of opioids? How should it be administered?

46. What are some of the systemic clinical effects that may be associated with the administration of naloxone?

ANSWERS*

STRUCTURE ACTIVITY RELATIONSHIPS

1. Opioids that are commonly used in anesthesia practice include morphine, meperidine, fentanyl, sufentanil, alfentanil, and remifentanil. The only clinically significant opioids that occur naturally and are derived from the poppy plant are papaverine, codeine, and morphine. Papaverine lacks any opioid activity. Morphine is considered the prototype opioid with which all other opioids are compared. (70, Table 6–1; **275–276**)

MECHANISM OF ACTION

2. Opioids exert their effects through their agonist actions at the opioid receptor. Opioids bind to the opioid receptor in the ionized state. After an opioid binds to a receptor, there are at least two mechanisms by which opioids alter the activity of the cell. The main action of opioids appears to be through the interaction with G proteins, resulting in inhibition of the activity of adenylate cyclase and increasing potassium conductance. This ultimately results in hyperpolarization of the cell and leads to a suppression of synaptic transmission. The second mechanism by which opioids may produce their effect is through the interference of calcium ion intracellular transport in the presynaptic cell. This results in interference with the release of neurotransmitter from the presynaptic cell and again suppresses synaptic transmission. Neurotransmitters that are affected by this mechanism of action of opioids include acetylcholine, dopamine, norepinephrine, and substance P. (70; **279–280**)

3. Opioid receptors are located in various tissues throughout the central nervous system, including the cerebral cortex, medial thalamus, periaqueductal gray matter, substantia gelatinosa, and sympathetic preganglionic neurons. The five subtypes of opioid receptors are the mu-1, mu-2, delta, kappa, and sigma receptors. The responses evoked by agonists at the mu-1 receptor include supraspinal analgesia, euphoria, miosis, nausea and vomiting, urinary retention, and pruritus. The responses evoked by agonists at the mu-2 receptor include respiratory depression, sedation, bradycardia, and ileus. The responses evoked by agonists at the delta receptor include the modulation of mu receptor activity and physical dependence. The responses evoked by agonists at the kappa receptor include spinal analgesia, sedation, and miosis. The responses evoked by agonists at the sigma receptor include dysphoria, hypertonia, and mydriasis. Supraspinal analgesia is mediated primarily by the mu receptors, whereas spinal analgesia is mediated primarily by the delta and kappa receptors. (70, Table 6–2; **278–279, Table 10–4**)

4. Endorphins and enkephalins are endogenous ligands that normally bind to and activate opioid receptors. (70; **278, 283–284**)

5. The greater the affinity of the opioid for its receptor, the smaller the dose of opioid required to exert a given effect. Therefore, the affinity with which an opioid binds to the opioid receptor directly correlates with its analgesic potency. It also correlates with the opioid molecule's stereochemistry. (70; **278–279**)

6. Opioid receptors of the mu, kappa, and delta type are located in the substantia gelatinosa in the spinal cord. (70; **281–282**)

7. Opioids administered in the epidural space must diffuse across the dura to bind

*Numbers in parentheses: lightface numbers refer to pages, figures, or tables in Stoelting RK, Miller RD: Basics of Anesthesia, 4th ed. Philadelphia, Churchill Livingstone, 2000; **boldface numbers** refer to pages, figures, or tables in Miller RD: Anesthesia, 5th ed. Philadelphia, Churchill Livingstone, 2000.

to opioid receptors on the spinal cord. The more lipid soluble the opioid, the more rapid the diffusion across the dura at the sight of injection. In contrast, the less lipid-soluble agents diffuse slowly and have more potential to migrate cephalad in the cerebrospinal fluid. For this reason, epidurally administered fentanyl and sufentanil, which are more lipid soluble than morphine, will tend to have a quicker onset and shorter duration of action and will exert their effects more locally than epidurally administered morphine. (70; **311–312, 2330**)

8. The systemic absorption of intrathecal opioid is minimal. Opioids administered in the epidural space are significantly absorbed systemically, however, such that the plasma concentration of the opioid is similar to what it would have been if the same dose had been intramuscularly administered. (71; **2330**)

9. Side effects associated with the neuraxial administration of opioids appear to occur in a dose-dependent manner. The side effects are likely due to both the systemic absorption of opioid as well as the effects of opioid in the cerebrospinal fluid. Therefore, some of the potential side effects of neuraxially administered opioids that can potentially occur are similar to those that can occur with the intravenous administration of opioids. These include sedation, nausea and vomiting, and, most importantly, respiratory depression. Side effects that are more specific to neuraxially administered opioids include pruritus and urinary retention. (71–72, Table 6–3; **2330–2333**)

10. Clearly the most concerning side effect that may accompany the epidural or spinal administration of opioids is respiratory depression. The patient must be in an environment where he or she can be assessed for at least 24 hours after the administration of the opioid. The assessment must be global, because the patient's ventilatory status is not adequately assessed by respiratory rate alone. In fact, a decrease in the patient's level of consciousness is also an indicator of hypercarbia and respiratory depression. Respiratory depression after the administration of epidural opioids can occur early or be delayed. Early respiratory depression, occurring in the first 2 hours after injection, is thought to be due to vascular uptake and redistribution. Delayed respiratory depression can occur between 6 and 12 hours after injection and is believed to be due to the rostral spread of opioid in the cerebrospinal fluid to the ventilatory centers located in the floor of the fourth ventricle. Respiratory depression should be treated immediately with the support of ventilation by the administration of oxygen and positive-pressure ventilation if necessary. Naloxone, an opioid antagonist, administered in small doses and titrated to effect, may reverse the respiratory depression without reversing the analgesia provided by the opioid. The patient should be closely observed, because the duration of action of naloxone is much shorter than that of the opioid. Naloxone should be immediately available for patients who have been administered neuraxial opioids should respiratory depression occur. (71–72; **348–349, 2330–2333**)

11. Risk factors for respiratory depression after the administration of neuraxial opioids include high administered opioid doses, the administration of an opioid with a low lipid solubility, the administration of concurrent intravenous opioids or other intravenous sedatives, the administration of opioids to a patient who lacks tolerance to opioids, and advanced age. (72, Table 6–4; **295–296, 351–352, 2330–2331**)

OPIOID AGONISTS

12. Morphine appears to be highly effective for the relief of pain that arises from the viscera, skeletal muscles, and joints. Other clinical effects of morphine include euphoria, sedation, and altered mentation. (72)

13. The administration of opioids minutes before the induction of anesthesia may be beneficial in that it may attenuate the blood pressure and heart rate responses

to direct laryngoscopy and intubation of the trachea. It may also contribute to preemptive analgesia. (72; **302, 331–332, 2325**)

14. Preemptive analgesia has been defined as "antinociceptive treatment that prevents the establishment of altered central processing, which amplifies postoperative pain." Some studies have suggested that an intensely noxious stimulus can result in sensitization of the central nervous system to subsequent painful stimuli, resulting in a level of pain that is subsequently perceived to be higher than it otherwise would have been. Given this, preemptive analgesia describes the phenomenon in which the injection of an opioid before a noxious stimulus results in decreases in the amount of narcotic required after the pain-inducing stimulus for the subsequent control of the pain. For example, the injection of an opioid before painful surgical stimulation may decrease the amount of narcotic needed in the postoperative period for analgesia. (72; **2325**)

15. The potency of an opioid is related to its affinity for the opioid receptor. The time of onset, or effect-site equilibration time, and duration of action of an opioid are related to its lipid solubility and degree of ionization at physiologic pH. A greater lipid solubility and greater nonionization allow for quicker crossing of the blood-brain barrier, quicker access to the central nervous system to exert its effects, and quicker redistribution to inactive tissue sites. For example, morphine has a relatively low lipid solubility and is only 10% to 20% nonionized at physiologic pH, accounting for its relatively prolonged effect-site equilibration time. In fact, less than 0.1% of intravenously administered morphine has reached the blood-brain barrier at the time of peak plasma concentration, which takes 15 to 30 minutes to occur. The intramuscular injection of morphine exerts its peak effect in 45 to 90 minutes. (72; **310–312, 318–320, Figs. 10–27, 10–28, Table 10–12**)

16. Opioids are cleared principally by hepatic metabolism. Morphine is the only opioid that possesses an active metabolite. About 10% of the metabolism of morphine is to the active metabolite morphine-6-glucuronide. Morphine-6-glucuronide has analgesic and ventilatory depressant effects and is eliminated by renal excretion. It is more potent at the mu receptor than morphine and has a similar duration of action. Care must be taken when administering morphine to patients with renal failure because the elimination of the active metabolite of morphine may be prolonged. Morphine's principal metabolite, morphine-3-glucuronide, is inactive. (72; **313**)

17. There are several mechanisms by which the administration of opioids may result in hypotension. These include histamine release, centrally mediated decreases in sympathetic tone, vagal-induced bradycardia, and direct and indirect venous and arterial vasodilation. For example, morphine may result in hypotension primarily due to histamine release or through centrally mediated decreases in sympathetic tone. The release of histamine is most likely to accompany the administration of morphine when high doses of morphine are administered rapidly. The effects of morphine on blood pressure may manifest clinically only as orthostatic hypotension in the supine, normovolemic patient. The hypotension associated with the administration of morphine may also occur due to vagal stimulation. Hypertension may accompany the administration of opioids secondary to inadequate dosing of the opioid or to the ill-timed administration of the opioid relative to the stimulus inducing the increase in blood pressure. (72–73, Fig. 6–2; **298–302**)

18. All the mu-receptor agonist opioids produce a dose-dependent depression of ventilation. This is reflected by an increase in the resting $Paco_2$, an increase in the apneic threshold, a decrease in the responsiveness to the ventilatory stimulant effects of carbon dioxide, and a decrease in the hypoxic ventilatory drive. The administration of opioids also affects the rate of breathing and the tidal volume.

The respiratory rate is typically slowed and insufficiently compensated by an increase in the tidal volume. Consequently, the minute ventilation is decreased. The mechanism by which these effects of opioids on ventilation occurs is thought to be through the direct depression of the medullary ventilatory centers. Opioids may cause a decrease in the release of acetylcholine neurotransmitter at these centers. When apnea occurs as a result of opioid administration, the patient may spontaneously breathe if directed to do so. (73; **293–297, Fig. 10–12**)

19. The administration of opioids results in several central nervous system effects. First, the administration of opioids has been shown to cause modest cerebral vascular vasoconstriction when the Pa_{CO_2} has been maintained normal under controlled ventilation. This may also result in modest decreases in cerebral blood flow and intracranial pressure. Opioids are unable to produce a dose-related general depression of the central nervous system typical of other general anesthetics. This is reflected by their inability to produce an isoelectric electroencephalogram. Instead, opioids have a ceiling effect that is not overcome by increasing the administered dose of opioids. Opioids do contribute to the MAC of anesthesia delivered and decrease the amount of volatile agent required to achieve a given anesthetic depth. Opioids are not considered to be true anesthetics, however, because of their inability to reliably produce unconsciousness even in high doses. Finally, the administration of opioids causes miosis through its cortical inhibition of the Edinger-Westphal nucleus. (73; **284–292, Figs. 10–8, 10–9, 10–10, 10–11, Tables 10–5, 10–7**)

20. The administration of opioids can result in increased thoracoabdominal muscle tone, which may result in chest wall stiffness. This "stiff-chest" syndrome can be so severe that the muscle rigidity interferes with ventilation. The impairment of ventilation in these patients has been shown to be primarily due to closure of the vocal cords and not just the rigid chest wall. This syndrome can also result in increases in pulmonary artery pressure and central venous pressure. Although the exact mechanism for this muscle rigidity is not known, it appears to occur most frequently when rapid, large boluses of an opioid are initially administered. Termination of the rigidity to allow for ventilation can be accomplished through the administration of a neuromuscular blocking drug or an opioid antagonist such as naloxone. Prophylaxis against this muscle rigidity can be achieved through the administration of a priming dose of a nondepolarizing neuromuscular blocking drug and the slow, intermittent administration of opioid. (73; **291–292, Tables 10–8, 10–9**)

21. Among the several effects opioids have on the gastrointestinal system are effects on gastrointestinal motility, gastric emptying, and biliary smooth muscle tone. Opioids increase tone and decrease propulsive motility in both the small and large intestines. Opioids also increase the gastric emptying time through both central and peripheral effects of the opioid. Centrally, this effect is mediated by the vagus nerve. Peripherally, binding of an opioid to the opioid receptors in the myenteric plexus and cholinergic nerve terminals inhibits the release of acetylcholine at these nerve terminals. Opioids also increase pyloric sphincter tone, further contributing to a delay in gastric emptying. Opioids can cause spasm of biliary smooth muscle, increasing biliary duct pressure. Opioids also increase the tone of the sphincter of Oddi. In patients receiving intraoperative cholangiograms, approximately 3% of patients who have been administered opioids have opioid-induced spasm of the sphincter of Oddi. Together these can result in an increase in intrabiliary pressure that may manifest as biliary colic or mimic angina pectoris in the awake patient. The clinician can distinguish between opioid-induced biliary colic pain and myocardial ischemia through the administration of naloxone. Naloxone can relieve the pain of biliary colic, but it has no effect on the pain caused by myocardial ischemia. Glucagon also

reverses biliary spasm due to opioids. Nitroglycerin has resulted in pain relief in both circumstances, making diagnosis difficult. (73; **306–307, Fig. 10–17**)

22. Opioids can enhance detrusor and ureteral sphincter tone, leading to urinary retention in some patients. When this occurs there may be the need to catheterize the patient's bladder to drain it. (73; **2333**)

23. There are several mechanisms by which opioids are thought to cause nausea and vomiting. The primary mechanism appears to be through the direct stimulation of dopamine receptors in the chemoreceptor trigger zone in the area postrema of the medulla. In addition to this, opioids also increase gastrointestinal secretions, decrease gastrointestinal tract motility, and prolong gastric emptying time. Other influences of the incidence of nausea and vomiting elicited by the administration of opioids are the age of the patient, female gender, obesity, type of surgery, duration of surgery, a history of gastroparesis, and the administration of nitrous oxide or etomidate. (73–74; **307–308, Fig. 10–18**)

24. Tolerance is the need over time to increase the dose of an agent to achieve a given effect. With analgesic doses of morphine, for instance, after 2 to 3 weeks of administration acute tolerance to its analgesic effects begins to develop. Tolerance to the respiratory depressant effects of opioids may take months to develop. When patients are opioid dependent, the withdrawal of opioids can lead to a typical withdrawal abstinence syndrome within 15 to 20 hours. The syndrome is characterized by diaphoresis, muscle spasms, vomiting, diarrhea, fever, chills, hypertension, tachycardia, and behavioral disturbances. The withdrawal syndrome peaks in 2 to 3 days. (74; **304–305**)

25. Opioids have been shown to modulate immune function through the modulation of neutrophil chemotaxis, phagocytic activity, and the secretion of cytokines. The clinical significance of this is under investigation. (74; **310**)

26. Meperidine is about one tenth as potent as morphine. (74, Table 6–1)

27. Meperidine is unique among the opioids due to its chemical structure, effects on the heart, effects on shivering, and central nervous stimulatory effects of its metabolite. The chemical structure of meperidine resembles atropine, which may account for its atropine-like effects on the heart. The administration of meperidine may lead to an increase in heart rate and a decrease in myocardial contractility. Meperidine may also lead to mydriasis rather than miosis, again likely due to its atropine-like structure. Meperidine uniquely is effective in treating postoperative shivering. The mechanism for this is believed to be through stimulation of the kappa receptors. The metabolite of meperidine, normeperidine, can produce central nervous stimulation resulting in seizures with its administration. Caution must be taken with the administration of meperidine to patients with renal failure because normeperidine is cleared renally. (74; **293, 298–299, 313–314**)

28. Fentanyl is 75 to 125 times more potent than morphine. (74, Table 6–1)

29. Fentanyl administered intravenously has a more rapid onset and shorter duration of action than morphine. This reflects its greater lipid solubility. The effect-site equilibration time of fentanyl is about 6.5 minutes. Its shorter duration of action is also reflective of its rapid redistribution to inactive tissue sites, leading to a rapid decrease in the plasma concentration of fentanyl. (74; **311–314**)

30. The effects of fentanyl are terminated through its redistribution to inactive tissue sites followed by its metabolism by the liver. High intravenous doses of fentanyl or a continuous intravenous infusion can lead to saturation of the inactive tissue sites. This may result in prolonged redistribution, prolonged elimination, and prolonged pharmacologic effects of the drug. The cumulative drug effects during continuous intravenous infusions of fentanyl, sufentanil, alfentanil, and

remifentanil have been compared. Alfentanil and remifentanil do not seem to produce clinically significant cumulative drug effects, and awakening appears to be prompt with minimal lingering side effects when compared with fentanyl. The context-sensitive half-time of fentanyl is therefore greater than for these other opioids, particularly for continuous infusions of greater than 2 hours' duration. (74; **317–318, Fig. 10–26**)

31. The administration of fentanyl is associated with a decrease in heart rate. The administration of fentanyl alone leads to little change in systemic blood pressure, whereas its administration after a benzodiazepine may lead to decreases in blood pressure. There are also synergistic effects between fentanyl and benzodiazepines on ventilatory depression and sedation. (74–75, Fig. 6–3; **293–296, 298–299**)

32. Clinical uses of fentanyl in anesthesia practice include perioperative analgesia, the induction and maintenance of anesthesia, the inhibition of the sympathetic nervous system response to direct laryngoscopy or surgical stimulation, and preemptive analgesia. Opioids are most commonly used during the maintenance of anesthesia as a supplement to inhaled anesthetics. Opioids used in this manner are often administered in small intravenous boluses or as a continuous infusion. High doses of a narcotic, especially fentanyl or sufentanil, may be used as the sole anesthetic agent in patients who are unable to tolerate any effects of cardiac depression that inhaled anesthetics may produce. A disadvantage of an opioid-based anesthetic is the potential for patient awareness. Transmucosal, transdermal, and oral preparations provide alternative routes for the administration of fentanyl. (75; **330–332, 338–343**)

33. Sufentanil is 500 to 1000 times more potent than morphine. (75, Table 6–1)

34. Sufentanil has an effect-site equilibration time similar to fentanyl. Its context-sensitive half-time is less than that of alfentanil for infusions lasting less than 8 hours, but it is greater than that of remifentanil. (75; **315, 317–318, Figs. 10–26, 10–40**)

35. Systemic clinical effects associated with the administration of sufentanil include depression of ventilation and bradycardia that appears to be greater than that produced by fentanyl. Sufentanil in large doses may result in thoracoabdominal muscle rigidity as well. (75–76; **291–292, 299**)

36. Alfentanil is 10 to 25 times more potent than morphine. (76, Table 6–1)

37. Alfentanil has an effect-site equilibration time that is shorter than that of fentanyl and sufentanil, about 1.4 minutes. This is as a result of its low pK, which allows for about 90% of the drug to be nonionized and lipid soluble at physiologic pH. The context-sensitive half-time of alfentanil varies by as much as 10 times among individuals. This is believed to be due to individual variations in its metabolism. Even so, the context-sensitive half-time of alfentanil is considered to be short when compared with other opioids, particularly with continuous infusions greater than 8 hours. (76, Fig. 6–5; **314–315, 317–318, Figs. 10–26, 10–40**)

38. The rapid, short-acting effect of alfentanil makes it useful for situations in which the response to a single, brief, intense, noxious stimulus requires blunting. Examples include the response to direct laryngoscopy and tracheal intubation or the performance of a retrobulbar block. (76, Fig. 6–5; **314–315, 333**)

39. Remifentanil is 250 times more potent than morphine. (76, Table 6–1)

40. Remifentanil has an effect-site equilibration time of about 1.4 minutes, which is shorter than that of fentanyl and sufentanil and about equal to that of alfentanil. The context-sensitive half-time of remifentanil is much shorter than that of the other opioids, about 4 minutes. It is also independent of the duration

of the continuous infusion, which is unique to remifentanil among the opioids. The basis for this is its structure, which has an ester link. The ester link allows for hydrolysis in the plasma to inactive metabolites. This accounts for its rapid titratability, noncumulative effects, and rapid recovery. (76–77, Figs. 6–4, 6–6; **315–318, Figs. 10–29, 10–40**)

41. Like alfentanil, the unique pharmacokinetic profile of remifentanil makes it desirable in cases where the response to a brief, intense stimulus requires blunting. It can also be used as maintenance anesthesia when rapid recovery might be desired, as during an intraoperative wake-up test for the evaluation of motor nerve integrity during spine surgery. When remifentanil is used as maintenance anesthesia, a longer-acting opioid may need to be administered before patient arousal for analgesia. (77; **315–318, 334–335**)

OPIOID AGONIST-ANTAGONISTS

42. Some of the agonist-antagonist opioids include pentazocaine, butorphanol, nalbuphine, buprenorphine, and dezocine. These agonist-antagonist opioids often have strong affinities for the kappa and delta receptors and only weakly bind the mu receptor. (77, Fig. 6–8; **345–348**)

43. The advantage of the administration of agonist-antagonist opioids is that they may only minimally depress ventilation. In addition, they are less prone to being abused secondary to their minimal euphoric effects. Unfortunately, agonist-antagonist opioids have limited analgesic properties. These drugs have a ceiling effect, or a maximal dose above which increasing doses of drug do not provide additional analgesia. This limits their usefulness for the control of pain, making them infrequently used in the perioperative period. (77; **345–348, Table 10–20**)

OPIOID ANTAGONISTS

44. Opioid antagonist drugs include naloxone, naltrexone, and nalmefene. These drugs exert their effects by binding to the mu opioid receptor, thereby displacing opioids from the receptor. (77–78, Fig. 6–9; **348–350**)

45. In clinical anesthesia practice the administration of naloxone is best achieved with intermittent low doses until the opioid-induced depression of ventilation or pruritus is reversed while leaving a sufficient amount of analgesia for patient comfort. The administration of naloxone for the reversal of undesirable effects of opioids should be done in doses of 1 to 4 μcg/kg. The rapid onset of naloxone allows for rapid, easy titration of the drug to the desired effect. The duration of action of naloxone is brief, about 30 minutes. It is possible that the previously reversed effects of the opioid may recur when the effects of naloxone pass. For this reason it is important to observe the patient for the recurrence of the opioid-induced effects that may necessitate a repeated administration of naloxone. Alternatively, a continuous infusion of naloxone may be administered. (78; **348–349**)

46. High doses of naloxone administered rapidly can result in rapid awakening with intense pain. Even in the absence of pain the administration of naloxone may result in intense sympathetic nervous system activity with tachycardia, hypertension, pulmonary edema, and cardiac dysrhythmias, including ventricular fibrillation. Caution should be used when administering naloxone for opioid reversal to patients who are at risk of myocardial ischemia. (77; **348–349**)

Chapter 6

Local Anesthetics

HISTORY

1. What was the first local anesthetic introduced into clinical practice? What was its clinical use?

STRUCTURE ACTIVITY RELATIONSHIPS

2. What is the basic structure of local anesthetics?

3. Why are local anesthetics marketed as hydrochloride salts?

4. What are two differences between ester and amide local anesthetics that make classifying local anesthetics important?

5. Name four ester local anesthetics.

6. Name six amide local anesthetics.

MECHANISM OF ACTION

7. What is the mechanism of action of local anesthetics?

8. Do local anesthetics most likely exert their action by working inside or outside the nerve membrane?

9. How is the effect of a local anesthetic on the nerve terminated?

10. How is the resting membrane potential and the threshold potential altered in nerves that have been infiltrated by local anesthetic?

11. What is the temporal progression of the interruption of the transmission of neural impulses between the autonomic nervous system, motor system, and sensory system after the infiltration of a mixed nerve with local anesthetic?

12. What is frequency-dependent blockade? How does frequency-dependent blockade relate to the activity of local anesthetics?

CLASSIFICATION OF NERVES AND SENSITIVITY TO LOCAL ANESTHETICS

13. What three characteristics are nerve fibers classified by? What are the three main nerve fiber types?

14. Which types of nerve fibers are myelinated? What is the function of myelin and how does it affect the action of local anesthetics?

15. How many consecutive nodes of Ranvier must be blocked for the effective blockade of the nerve impulse by local anesthetic?

16. Which two nerve fiber types primarily function to conduct sharp and dull pain impulses? Which of these two nerve fibers is more readily blocked by local anesthetic?

17. Which two nerve fiber types primarily function to conduct impulses that result in large motor and small motor activity?

18. Which nerve fibers are more readily blocked by local anesthetics than any other nerve fiber?

19. How do local anesthetics diffuse through nerve fibers when deposited around a nerve? Which nerve fibers are blocked first as a result?

SPREAD OF ANESTHESIA AND PERIPHERAL NERVE BLOCKADE

20. How are the nerve fibers arranged from the mantle to the core in the dorsal nerve roots with respect to nerve diameter? How does this correlate with the apparent sensitivity to the effects of intrathecal local anesthetics between the small diameter and large diameter nerves of the dorsal nerve root?

21. How are the nerve fibers arranged from the mantle to the core in a peripheral nerve with respect to the innervation of proximal and distal structures? How does this correlate with the temporal progression of local anesthetic-induced blockade of proximal and distal structures?

PHARMACOKINETICS

22. Is the pKa of local anesthetics more than or less than 7.4?

23. At physiologic pH does most local anesthetic exist in the ionized or nonionized form? What form must the local anesthetic be in to cross nerve cell membranes?

24. Does local tissue acidosis create an environment for higher or lower quality local anesthesia? Why?

25. What is the primary determinant of local anesthetic potency?

26. After a local anesthetic has been absorbed from the tissues, what are the primary determinants of local anesthetic peak plasma concentrations?

27. How are ester local anesthetics cleared?

28. How are amide local anesthetics cleared?

29. What percent of local anesthetic undergoes renal excretion unchanged?

30. What are two organs that influence the potential for local anesthetic systemic toxicity?

31. Which type of local anesthetic, the esters or the amides, is more likely to result in systemic toxicity? Why?

32. Patients with atypical plasma cholinesterase are at an increased risk for what complication with regard to local anesthetics?

33. What disease states may influence the rate of clearance of lidocaine from the plasma?

34. Does lidocaine or its metabolites produce cardiac antidysrhythmic effects?

35. How does the addition of epinephrine or phenylephrine to a local anesthetic solution prepared for injection affect its systemic absorption?

36. How does the addition of epinephrine or phenylephrine to a local anesthetic solution prepared for injection affect its duration of action?

37. How does the addition of epinephrine or phenylephrine to a local anesthetic solution prepared for injection affect its potential for systemic toxicity?

38. How does the addition of epinephrine or phenylephrine to a local anesthetic solution prepared for injection affect the rate of onset of anesthesia?

39. How does the addition of epinephrine or phenylephrine to a local anesthetic solution prepared for injection affect local bleeding?

40. What are some potential negative effects of the addition of epinephrine to a local anesthetic solution prepared for injection?

41. Name some situations in which the addition of epinephrine to a local anesthetic solution prepared for injection may not be recommended.

SIDE EFFECTS

42. What are some potential negative side effects associated with the administration of local anesthetics?

43. What is the most common cause of local anesthetic systemic toxicity?

44. What are the factors that influence the magnitude of the systemic absorption of local anesthetic from the tissue injection site?

45. From highest to lowest, what is the relative order of peak plasma concentrations of local anesthetic associated with the following regional anesthetic procedures: brachial plexus, caudal, intercostal, epidural, sciatic/femoral?

46. Which two organ systems are most likely to be affected by excessive plasma concentrations of local anesthetic?

47. What are the initial and subsequent manifestations of central nervous system toxicity due to increasingly excessive plasma concentrations of local anesthetic?

48. What is a possible pathophysiologic mechanism for seizures that result from excessive plasma concentrations of local anesthetic?

49. What are some potential adverse effects of local anesthetic-induced seizures? What is the treatment of local anesthetic-induced seizures?

50. What is the indication for and disadvantage of the administration of neuromuscular blocking drugs for the treatment of seizures?

51. Is the cardiovascular system more or less susceptible to local anesthetic toxicity than the central nervous system?

52. What are two mechanisms by which local anesthetics produce hypotension?

53. What is the mechanism by which local anesthetics exert their cardiotoxic effects? How is this manifested on the electrocardiogram?

54. How is the relative cardiotoxicity between local anesthetic agents compared? What is the relative cardiotoxicity between lidocaine, bupivacaine, and ropivacaine?

55. How does bupivacaine differ from lidocaine with respect to their cardiotoxic effects? What is a potential explanation for the differing effects of bupivacaine and lidocaine on the heart?

56. What is the maximum recommended concentration of bupivacaine to be administered for obstetric epidural anesthesia? Why?

57. Why is ropivacaine unique among local anesthetics?

58. The administration of which local anesthetic has been associated with methemoglobinemia? What is the mechanism by which this occurs? How can it be treated?

59. What is the nature of the neurotoxicity produced by chloroprocaine? What is the mechanism by which this occurs?

60. What is transient radicular irritation? What is the mechanism by which it occurs?

61. What is the mechanism by which local anesthetics have resulted in cauda equina syndrome?

62. What is the allergenic potential of local anesthetics? What are the potential causes of an allergic reaction to local anesthetics?

63. Does cross-sensitivity exist between the classes of local anesthetics?

CLINICAL USES

64. What regional anesthetic procedures are local anesthetics commonly used for?

65. What are some clinical uses of lidocaine that make it unique among the local anesthetics?

66. What is unique to cocaine with respect to its use as a local anesthetic?

67. Name some possible manifestations of cocaine-induced cardiovascular effects. How should these effects be treated?

For questions 68 through 74 please select from the following local anesthetics: procaine, chloroprocaine, tetracaine, lidocaine, mepivacaine, bupivacaine, etidocaine, prilocaine, and ropivacaine.

68. Which two local anesthetics may be used for topical anesthesia?

69. What is eutectic mixture of local anesthetics (EMLA)?

70. Which eight local anesthetics may be used for local infiltration?

71. Which two local anesthetics may be used for intravenous regional anesthesia?

72. Which eight local anesthetics may be used for peripheral nerve block anesthesia?

73. Which seven local anesthetics may be used for epidural anesthesia?

74. Which five local anesthetics may be used for spinal anesthesia?

ANSWERS*

HISTORY

1. The first local anesthetic introduced into clinical practice was cocaine. It was introduced by Koller in 1884 as a topical anesthetic for the cornea. Its use was limited by its propensity toward causing a psychological dependence and for its irritant properties when placed topically or near nerves. (80; **5**)

STRUCTURE ACTIVITY RELATIONSHIPS

2. Local anesthetics consist of a lipophilic end and a hydrophilic end connected by a hydrocarbon chain. The lipophilic end is an unsaturated benzene ring, and the hydrophilic end is a tertiary amine and proton acceptor. The bond that links the hydrocarbon chain to the lipophilic end of the structure is either an ester (—CO—) bond or an amide (—HNC—) bond. The local anesthetic is thus classified as either an ester or an amide local anesthetic. (80, Table 7–2; **491–493, Table 13–1**)

3. Local anesthetics are bases that are poorly water soluble. For this reason they are marketed as hydrochloride salts. The resulting solution is slightly acidic with a pH of about 6. (80; **497**)

4. The site of metabolism and the potential to produce allergic reactions differ

*Numbers in parentheses: lightface numbers refer to pages, figures, or tables in Stoelting RK, Miller RD: Basics of Anesthesia, 4th ed. Philadelphia, Churchill Livingstone, 2000; **boldface numbers** refer to pages, figures, or tables in Miller RD: Anesthesia, 5th ed. Philadelphia, Churchill Livingstone, 2000.

between ester and amide local anesthetics, making this classification of local anesthetics important. (80; **510, 516**)

5. The ester local anesthetics include procaine, chloroprocaine, cocaine, and tetracaine. (80, Fig. 7–1, Table 7–2; **501**)

6. The amide local anesthetics include lidocaine, mepivacaine, bupivacaine, etidocaine, prilocaine, and ropivacaine. (80, Fig. 7–1, Table 7–2; **501**)

MECHANISM OF ACTION

7. Local anesthetics act by producing a conduction blockade of neural impulses in the affected nerve. This is accomplished through the prevention of the passage of sodium ions through ion selective sodium channels in the nerve membranes. The sodium channels are functionally inactivated by being maintained in the closed conformation. The inability of sodium ions to pass through their ion selective channels results in slowing of the rate of depolarization. As a result, the threshold potential is not reached and an action potential is not propagated in these nerves. (80; **497–501**)

8. Local anesthetics are thought to exert their action on the nerve by binding to a specific receptor on the sodium ion channel. The location of the binding site appears to be on the inner portion of the sodium channel. They may also alter sodium permeability by blocking sodium channels near their external openings. This may explain why local anesthetics bind more rapidly and with a greater affinity to the receptors while the nerve is in the activated state. Regardless of the exact location of the binding site for the local anesthetic, the binding of local anesthetic to the receptor inactivates the sodium ion channel by preventing the flow of sodium ions through the channel. (80; **498–501**)

9. The conduction blockade produced by a local anesthetic is completely reversible. Reversal of the blockade is spontaneous. (80; **499**)

10. Neither the resting membrane potential nor the threshold potential is altered by local anesthetics. (80; **498**)

11. The temporal progression of the interruption of the transmission of impulses is autonomic, sensory, and then motor nerve blockade. This yields a temporal progression of autonomic nervous system blockade, then sensory nervous system blockade, followed by skeletal muscle paralysis. (80; **501**)

12. Local anesthetics induce conduction blockade in nerves during action potentials when the sodium channel is in the activated, open state. In between action potentials there is recovery of blockade. However, during the subsequent action potential the sodium channel is accessed and again blocked by the local anesthetic. This is referred to as frequency-dependent blockade. This reflects the finding that local anesthetics gain access to receptors when the sodium channels are in the activated, open state. For this reason, local anesthetics may selectively block nerves that fire more frequently. This may mean that the greater the frequency of firing of the nerve, the greater the subsequent inhibition of the nerve produced by the local anesthetic. (81; **499–500**)

CLASSIFICATION OF NERVES AND SENSITIVITY TO LOCAL ANESTHETICS

13. Fiber diameter, the presence or absence of myelin, and function are the three characteristics by which nerve fibers are classified. A, B, and C are the three main types of nerve fibers. (81, Table 7–1; **494, Table 13–3**)

14. The A and B nerve fiber types are myelinated. Myelin is composed of plasma membranes of specialized Schwann cells that wrap around the axon during

axonal growth. Myelin functions to insulate the axolemma, or nerve cell membrane, from the surrounding conducting media. It also forces the depolarizing current to flow through periodic interruptions in the myelin sheath called the nodes of Ranvier. The sodium channels that are instrumental in nerve pulse propagation and conduction are concentrated at these nodes of Ranvier. Myelin increases the speed of nerve conduction and makes the nerve membrane more susceptible to local anesthetic-induced conduction blockade. (81; **494, 496, Figs. 13–3, 13–4**)

15. At least three consecutive nodes of Ranvier must be exposed to adequate concentrations of local anesthetic for the effective blockade of nerve impulses to occur. (82; **496**)

16. The nerve fiber type A delta, which is myelinated, conducts sharp pain impulses. The nerve fiber type C, which is unmyelinated, conducts dull pain impulses. The large-diameter A delta type fiber appears to be more sensitive to blockade by local anesthetics than the smaller diameter C type fiber. This lends support to the theory that myelination of nerves has a greater influence than nerve fiber diameter on the conduction blockade produced by local anesthetics. (80–81, Table 7–1; **501–503, Table 13–3**)

17. The nerve fiber types A alpha and A beta, which are both myelinated, conduct motor nerve impulses. The nerve fiber type A alpha conducts large motor nerve impulses, and the nerve fiber type A beta conducts small motor nerve impulses. (80–81, Table 7–1; **501, Table 13–3**)

18. Preganglionic type B fibers are more readily blocked by local anesthetics than any other nerve fiber. This is presumed to be due to a combination of its relatively small diameter and the presence of myelin. (81, Table 7–1; **501, Table 13–3**)

19. Local anesthetics diffuse along a concentration gradient from the outer surface, or mantle, of the nerve toward the center, or core, of the nerve. As a result, the nerve fibers located in the mantle of the nerve are blocked before those in the core of the nerve. (81; **494**)

SPREAD OF ANESTHESIA AND PERIPHERAL NERVE BLOCKADE

20. Small-diameter nerve fibers are closer to the mantle, or nerve root surface, in dorsal nerve roots. Large-diameter nerves, conversely, are situated deep in the core of the dorsal nerve root. The diffusion path for local anesthetics is shorter to the mantle of the dorsal nerve root. In the case of dorsal nerve roots, this correlates to a shorter diffusion distance to the small diameter nerve fibers when local anesthetics are placed in the intrathecal space. The small diameter nerve fibers therefore appear to be more sensitive to local anesthetic blockade as a result of dorsal nerve root anatomy. This may explain the clinical finding of sensory nerve blockade occurring before motor nerve blockade with the onset of spinal anesthesia. In fact, the minimum concentration of local anesthetic (Cm) necessary for motor nerve blockade is twice that of sensory nerves. (82; **500–501**)

21. In a peripheral nerve the nerve fibers in the mantle most often innervate more proximal anatomic structures. The distal anatomic structures are more frequently innervated by nerve fibers near the core of the nerve. This physiologic orientation of nerve fibers in a peripheral nerve explains the observed initial proximal analgesia with subsequent progressive distal spread as local anesthetics diffuse to reach more central core nerve fibers. (82, Fig. 7–4; **500–501**)

PHARMACOKINETICS

22. The pKa of local anesthetics is more than 7.4. This means that the pH at which local anesthetics will exist divided equally between the ionized, cationic form, and nonionized form is greater than 7.4. (82–83, Table 7–2; **493–494, 497–499, Table 13–2**)

23. Most local anesthetic exists in the ionized, hydrophilic form at physiologic pH. Local anesthetics must be in the nonionized, lipid-soluble form to cross the lipophilic nerve cell membranes. (82–83; **493–494, 497–499, Fig. 13–2**)

24. Local tissue acidosis is thought to be associated with a lower quality of local anesthesia. This is presumed to be due to an increase in the ionized fraction of the drug in an acidotic environment. Because the pKa of local anesthetics is greater than 7.4, it follows that when the pH is less than 7.4 a greater fraction of the local anesthetic will exist in the ionized form. This results in a decrease in the amount of local anesthetic available to cross nerve cell membranes. (83; **497, 502**)

25. The primary determinant of the potency of a local anesthetic is its lipid solubility. (83; **502**)

26. The rate of tissue distribution and the rate of clearance of the drug are the two primary determinants of peak plasma concentrations of a local anesthetic after its absorption from tissue sites. (83; **510**)

27. Ester local anesthetics are cleared by hydrolysis by pseudocholinesterase enzymes in the plasma. (83; **510**)

28. Amide local anesthetics undergo degradation in the liver by hepatic microsomal enzymes. The metabolites are then excreted by the kidneys. (83; **510**)

29. Less than 5% of the injected dose of local anesthetic undergoes renal excretion unchanged. The low water solubility of local anesthetics limits their renal excretion. (84; **509**)

30. The lungs and the liver both influence the potential for local anesthetic systemic toxicity. The ability of the lungs to extract local anesthetics from the circulation, or the first-pass pulmonary extraction of local anesthetic, influences systemic toxicity by preventing the accumulation of local anesthetics in the plasma. The liver also influences local anesthetic systemic toxicity, especially the amide local anesthetics that are metabolized by the liver. (83; **510**)

31. The administration of amide local anesthetics is more likely to result in systemic toxicity than the administration of ester local anesthetics secondary to the mechanisms by which they are cleared. Amide local anesthetics are more slowly metabolized than the hydrolysis responsible for the clearance of ester local anesthetics. The slower metabolism of amide local anesthetics creates the potential for more sustained plasma concentrations, and thus the greater potential for systemic toxicity. (83; **510**)

32. Patients with atypical plasma cholinesterase enzyme may be at an increased risk for developing excessive plasma concentrations of ester local anesthetics. Ester local anesthetics rely on plasma hydrolysis for their metabolism, which may be limited or absent in these patients. (83–84)

33. Lidocaine, an amide local anesthetic, is cleared by hepatic metabolism. The clearance of lidocaine from the plasma parallels hepatic blood flow. Liver disease or decreases in hepatic blood flow as can occur with congestive heart failure or general anesthesia can decrease the rate of metabolism of lidocaine. Likewise, neonates with immature liver enzyme function are likely to have a prolonged elimination time for lidocaine. (83–84; **510**)

34. Both lidocaine and its metabolites possess cardiac antidysrhythmic effects. (84, Fig. 7–5)

35. The addition of epinephrine or phenylephrine to a local anesthetic solution prepared for injection produces a local tissue vasoconstriction. This results in a slowing of the rate of systemic absorption of the local anesthetic. (84; **503, 509**)

36. The addition of epinephrine or phenylephrine to a local anesthetic solution prepared for injection produces a local tissue vasoconstriction. This results in a prolonged duration of action of the local anesthetic by keeping the anesthetic solution in contact with the nerve fibers for a longer period of time. (84; **503**)

37. The addition of epinephrine or phenylephrine to a local anesthetic solution prepared for injection causes a slower rate of systemic absorption and a prolonged duration of action. This increases the likelihood that the rate of metabolism will match the rate of absorption, resulting in a decrease in the possibility of systemic toxicity. (84; **503, 509**)

38. The addition of epinephrine or phenylephrine to a local anesthetic solution has little effect on the rate of onset of anesthesia. (84; **502**)

39. The addition of epinephrine or phenylephrine to a local anesthetic solution decreases bleeding in the area infiltrated due to its vasoconstrictive properties. (84; **503**)

40. The systemic absorption of epinephrine in the local anesthetic solution may contribute to cardiac dysrhythmias or accentuate hypertension in vulnerable patients. (84)

41. The addition of epinephrine to a local anesthetic solution may not be recommended in patients with unstable angina pectoris, cardiac dysrhythmias, uncontrolled hypertension, or uteroplacental insufficiency. The addition of epinephrine to a local anesthetic solution is not recommended for intravenous anesthesia or for peripheral nerve block anesthesia in areas that may lack collateral blood flow, such as the digits or the penis. (84)

SIDE EFFECTS

42. Potential negative side effects associated with the administration of local anesthetics include systemic toxicity, neurotoxicity, and allergic reactions. (84)

43. Local anesthetic systemic toxicity occurs as a result of excessive plasma concentrations of a local anesthetic drug. The most common cause of local anesthetic systemic toxicity is accidental intravascular injection of local anesthetic solution during the performance of a nerve block. (84; **510–511**)

44. The magnitude of the systemic absorption of local anesthetic from the tissue injection site is influenced by the pharmacologic profile of the local anesthetic, the total dose injected, the vascularity of the injection site, and the inclusion of a vasoconstrictor in the local anesthetic solution. (84; **509**)

45. The relative order from highest to lowest of peak plasma concentrations of local anesthetic associated with regional anesthesia is intercostal nerve block, caudal block, epidural, brachial plexus, and sciatic/femoral. (84, Fig. 7–6; **509, Fig. 13–13**)

46. The central nervous system and cardiovascular system are most likely to be affected by excessive plasma concentrations of local anesthetic. (84–85; **511**)

47. The initial manifestations of central nervous system toxicity due to excessive plasma concentrations of local anesthetic include lightheadedness and dizziness. These symptoms are then followed by alterations in visual and auditory sensations, such as difficulty focusing, vertigo, and tinnitus, and may proceed to

symptoms of disorientation, restlessness, and slurred speech. With progressively increasing concentrations of local anesthetic in the plasma, symptoms may progress to manifestations of central nervous system excitation, such as facial and extremity muscular twitching and tremors. Finally, tonic-clonic seizures, apnea, and death can follow. (84; **511**)

48. Local anesthetic drugs in excessive plasma concentrations sufficient to cause seizures are believed to initially depress inhibitory pathways in the cerebral cortex. This allows for the unopposed action of excitatory pathways in the central nervous system, which manifests as seizures. As the concentration of local anesthetic in the plasma increases, there is subsequent inhibition of both excitatory and inhibitory pathways in the brain. Ultimately this leads to generalized global central nervous system depression. (84; **511**)

49. Potential adverse effects of local anesthetic-induced seizures are arterial hypoxemia, metabolic acidosis, and the pulmonary aspiration of gastric contents. The mainstay of the treatment of local anesthetic-induced seizures, as with all seizures, is aimed toward supporting the patient while attempting to abort the seizure with anticonvulsant drugs. Supplemental oxygen should be administered. The patient's airway may need to be secured with a cuffed endotracheal tube if there is a need to facilitate the delivery of oxygen to the lungs, to protect the airway from the aspiration of gastric contents, or to facilitate hyperventilation of the lungs. Hyperventilation of the lungs has two additional benefits with respect to local anesthetic-induced seizures. First, hyperventilation of the lungs decreases additional local anesthetic delivery to the brain through its effects of cerebral vasoconstriction. Second, the respiratory alkalosis and hypokalemia that result from hyperventilation of the lungs offsets the metabolic acidosis and hyperpolarizes nerve cell membranes, decreasing the central nervous system excitatory effect of local anesthetics. Anticonvulsant drugs that can be used to stop local anesthetic-induced seizures include diazepam and thiopental. Diazepam should be administered at a dose of 0.1 mg/kg intravenously. Thiopental should be administered in small doses of 0.5 to 2 mg/kg intravenously as well, typically as a temporizing measure until the onset of action of diazepam. The short duration of action of thiopental limits its usefulness for the treatment of seizures. (84–85; **511, 515, 722**)

50. The administration of paralyzing doses of a rapidly acting neuromuscular blocking drug may be necessary to facilitate intubation of the trachea during a seizure. The administration of a neuromuscular blocking drug with prolonged paralytic effects during a seizure may be indicated when benzodiazepines and barbiturates have not been effective in stopping the seizure activity. The advantage of neuromuscular blocking drugs for this purpose is twofold. First, it decreases the contribution of motor activity to the formation of lactic acid and metabolic acidosis. Second, it facilitates controlled hyperventilation of the lungs to offset potentially life-threatening metabolic acidosis and to facilitate the delivery of oxygen to the lungs. The disadvantage of neuromuscular blockade is that, although it aborts the peripheral seizure activity, it does not alter the abnormal cerebral electrical activity. The cerebral electrical activity should therefore be monitored by an electroencephalogram in patients who have had neuromuscular blocking drugs administered during seizure activity. (85; **722**)

51. The cardiovascular system is less susceptible to local anesthetic toxicity than the central nervous system. That is, the dose of local anesthetic required to result in central nervous system toxicity is less than the dose of local anesthetic required to result in cardiotoxicity. (85; **511**)

52. Two mechanisms by which local anesthetics produce hypotension include the direct relaxation of peripheral vascular smooth muscle and direct myocardial depression. (85; **512–513**)

53. Local anesthetics exert their cardiotoxic effect directly through the blockade of sodium ion channels in the myocardium. This blockade of sodium channels results in an increase in the conduction time throughout the heart. Local anesthetics also produce a dose-dependent negative inotropic effect. Clinically, these may result in a decreased cardiac output. With extremely elevated levels of local anesthetic in the serum, bradycardia and sinus arrest can result. Manifestations of local anesthetic-induced cardiotoxicity on an electrocardiogram include a prolongation of the PR interval and widening of the QRS complex. (85; **512, Table 13–11**)

54. The relative cardiotoxicity between local anesthetic agents is made through a comparison of the cardiovascular collapse to central nervous system toxicity ratio. This ratio compares the concentration of drug required to produce cardiovascular collapse relative to the dose required to produce central nervous toxicity. Through the evaluation of these ratios, it has been determined that bupivacaine is twice as cardiotoxic as lidocaine and that ropivacaine is intermediate between the two. (85; **513, Fig. 13–16, Table 13–12**)

55. Bupivacaine is more cardiotoxic than lidocaine per dose administered to achieve a given anesthetic effect. The injection of an accidental intravenous bolus of bupivacaine can result in precipitous hypotension, cardiac dysrhythmias, and atrioventricular heart block. The risk of cardiotoxicity from bupivacaine appears to be greater than it otherwise would have been if epinephrine had been added or if the patient was on beta-adrenergic blockade therapy. The toxicity to the heart caused by bupivacaine is also qualitatively different than that caused by lidocaine in several ways. First, bupivacaine may induce ventricular arrhythmias and ventricular fibrillation with its rapid intravenous administration, whereas lidocaine is unlikely to. Second, cardiovascular resuscitation after cardiovascular collapse induced by bupivacaine is more difficult to achieve than after cardiovascular collapse induced by lidocaine. Finally, acidosis and hypoxia markedly potentiate the cardiotoxicity induced by bupivacaine. The exact reasons why bupivacaine has greater and differing cardiotoxic effects than lidocaine is mostly unknown, although bupivacaine is known to differ in its effects on the myocardium. The rapid phase of depolarization of the cardiac Purkinje fibers and ventricular muscle is more greatly depressed by bupivacaine than lidocaine. In addition, bupivacaine is highly lipid soluble, making its dissociation from cardiac sodium channels slower. This accounts for the fast-in, slow-out characteristic of the binding to cardiac sodium channels that is associated with bupivacaine. These may account at least in part for the greater and more persistent cardiac effects of bupivacaine. (85–86; **512–514, Table 13–12**)

56. The maximum recommended concentration of bupivacaine to be administered for epidural anesthesia in obstetrics is 0.5%. This recommendation comes as a result of numerous cardiotoxic reactions that have occurred with the administration of 0.75% bupivacaine to this patient population. It is possible that elevated levels of progesterone associated with pregnancy increase the sensitivity of the myocardium to the cardiotoxic effects of bupivacaine as well. (Fig. 7–7; **505, 513–514**)

57. Ropivacaine is unique from all other local anesthetics because it is prepared as a levoisomer rather than a racemic mixture. Ropivacaine was developed in response to the cardiotoxic effects of bupivacaine. Ropivacaine appears to cause less persistent myocardial depression than bupivacaine. In addition, the reversal of cardiotoxicity with aggressive cardiopulmonary resuscitation appears to result in more favorable outcomes with ropivacaine than bupivacaine in animal studies. (86; **514–515**)

58. The administration of prilocaine has been associated with methemoglobinemia in a dose-dependent manner. It appears that this effect specific to prilocaine

among the local anesthetics occurs when administered in doses higher than 600 mg. Methemoglobinemia results from the accumulation of *ortho*-toluidine, a metabolite of prilocaine. Ortho-toluidine is an oxidizing compound that oxidizes hemoglobin to methemoglobin, creating methemoglobinemia. Patients with sufficient levels of methemoglobinemia may appear cyanotic, and their blood may appear chocolate colored. Methemoglobinemia that occurs through the administration of prilocaine is spontaneously reversible. Alternatively, methylene blue may be administered intravenously to treat this condition. (86; **515–516**)

59. The administration of chloroprocaine has been associated with neurotoxicity when administered at recommended doses. Its administration in the subarachnoid space has resulted in prolonged motor and sensory deficits. Chloroprocaine is the only local anesthetic that has been shown to have this effect, and it is not recommended for administration in the subarachnoid space or for intravenous regional anesthesia as a result. The mechanism by which these effects have occurred appears to be due to a combination of the low pH of 3.0 of the local anesthetic solution and to sodium bisulfite, an antioxidant included in the preparation of chloroprocaine. Newer preparations of chloroprocaine do not contain sodium bisulfite. (86; **516, Table 13–13**)

60. Transient radicular irritation, also called transient neurologic symptoms, is a finding that occurs within 24 hours of the recovery from a spinal anesthetic in which the patient complains of pain in the lower back, posterior thighs, or buttocks. It appears to be due to a direct neural inflammatory reaction caused by the local anesthetic. Full recovery from the symptoms usually occurs within 1 week. Risk factors for transient radicular irritation include the use of lidocaine for spinal anesthesia, lithotomy position during surgery, and outpatient status. Indeed, when these three risk factors are combined the incidence has been found to be 24%. Age, gender, history of back pain, needle type, and lidocaine concentration do not appear to have any influence over the risk of transient radicular irritation, whereas obesity may have some minor influence. To minimize the risk, alternative local anesthetics may be chosen, particularly for patients who will be placed in the lithotomy position and will be discharged to home after the procedure. (86; **516–517**)

61. Cauda equina syndrome occurs after the lumbosacral plexus sustains diffuse injury. Symptoms may include sensory anesthesia, bowel and bladder sphincter dysfunction, and paraplegia. In the past, microbore spinal catheters were associated with cauda equina syndrome. This risk of cauda equina syndrome was greatest for patients receiving 5% lidocaine via the catheter. It is believed that the pooling of local anesthetic in the most dependent portion of the subarachnoid space led to high concentrations of local anesthetic at those spinal nerves and subsequent irreversible neurotoxicity. Although small microbore catheters for continuous spinal anesthesia are no longer used, caution must be taken with the administration of a continuous spinal anesthetic. Because cauda equina syndrome is still a potential complication, alternatives to 5% lidocaine should be considered for the spinal local anesthetic. (86; **516–517**)

62. Less than 1% of all adverse reactions to local anesthetics are believed to be true allergic reactions. When a true allergic reaction to a local anesthetic is suspected to have occurred, full documentation should be made in the chart regarding the dose and route of local anesthetic administered and the reaction that occurred. A true allergic reaction might yield a rash, laryngeal edema, hypotension, and/or bronchospasm. In contrast to this, the accidental intravenous injection of an epinephrine-containing local anesthetic solution may result in a vasovagal response manifested by hypotension, syncope, tachycardia, or bradycardia. There are two potential causes of an allergic reaction due to local anesthetics. First, a metabolite of the ester local anesthetics, *para*-aminobenzoic

acid, may induce an allergic reaction. Esters are more likely than amides to cause allergic reactions on this basis. Second, the preservative methylparaben used in some commercial preparations of both amides and esters may also have antigenic potential. (86–87; **516**)

63. Cross-sensitivity has not been found to exist between the classes of local anesthetics. A patient found to be allergic to ester local anesthetics has not been shown to have an allergy to amide local anesthetics when intradermal tests have been performed. (87; **516**)

CLINICAL USES

64. Local anesthetics are most often used to produce regional anesthesia. Regional anesthesia is typically classified by the site of injection. Four sites of injection for local anesthetics include topical or surface anesthesia, local or subcutaneous infiltration anesthesia, intravenous regional anesthesia, and nerve block anesthesia. Nerve block anesthesia includes spinal, epidural, and peripheral nerve anesthesia. (87, Table 7–3; **505**)

65. Clinical uses of lidocaine that make it unique among the local anesthetics include its use intravenously to prevent or treat cardiac ventricular dysrhythmias, to attenuate pressor responses associated with intubation of the trachea, to prevent or treat increases in the intracranial pressure, and to minimize coughing during intubation or extubation of the trachea. Lidocaine, as well as tetracaine, may be used topically on the mucous membranes of areas such as the nose, mouth, or tracheobronchial tree. (87)

66. Cocaine is unique to all other local anesthetics by producing topical anesthesia and vasoconstriction. The mechanism for this is the inhibition of norepinephrine reuptake into postganglionic nerve endings. This property of cocaine is useful when topically preparing the nasal mucosa for a nasal intubation, which has the potential of nasal hemorrhage. Vasoconstriction of the coronary arteries is a risk of the topical administration of cocaine. The abuse potential of cocaine is also a disadvantage of this drug. (88; **509, 2192–2193**)

67. Manifestations of cocaine-induced cardiovascular effects may include coronary artery vasoconstriction, myocardial ischemia, cardiac dysrhythmias, or hypertension. The hypertension induced by cocaine has resulted in cerebral vascular accidents. The administration of cocaine with epinephrine, or in the presence of volatile anesthetics that sensitize the myocardium to catecholamines, may augment these potential effects of cocaine. The cardiovascular effects of cocaine may be treated by titrating esmolol to the desired heart rate, typically less than 100 beats per minute. A concern with the administration of beta-adrenergic blockers to these patients is the possible exacerbation of coronary artery vasospasm. Nitroglycerin may be administered to treat myocardial ischemia. (88; **2192–2193**)

68. Tetracaine and lidocaine may be used as topical anesthetics. (87–88, Table 7–3; **507–509, Table 13–9**)

69. Eutectic mixture of local anesthetics (EMLA) is a topical anesthetic cream that consists of lidocaine 2.5% and prilocaine. EMLA cream requires 45 to 60 minutes to exert its peak effect. (88, Table 7–3; **508, Table 13–9**)

70. Procaine, chloroprocaine, lidocaine, mepivacaine, bupivacaine, ropivacaine, etidocaine, and prilocaine may be used for local infiltration anesthesia. (88, Table 7–3; **505, Table 13–4**)

71. Lidocaine and prilocaine may be used for intravenous regional anesthesia. (87, Table 7–3; **505–506**)

72. Procaine, chloroprocaine, lidocaine, mepivacaine, bupivacaine, etidocaine, prilo-

caine, and ropivacaine may be used for peripheral nerve block anesthesia. (87, Table 7–3; **506, Table 13–6**)

73. Chloroprocaine, lidocaine, mepivacaine, bupivacaine, etidocaine, prilocaine, and ropivacaine may be used for epidural anesthesia. (87, Table 7–3; **507, Table 13–7**)

74. Procaine, tetracaine, lidocaine, ropivacaine, and bupivacaine may be used for spinal anesthesia. (87, Table 7–3; **507, Table 13–8**)

Chapter 7

Neuromuscular Blocking Drugs

1. What are some clinical situations in which skeletal muscle relaxation is desired?

2. What are some methods by which skeletal muscle relaxation can be achieved without the administration of neuromuscular blocking drugs?

3. What analgesic effects do neuromuscular blocking drugs have?

4. What are some characteristics of neuromuscular blocking drugs that may influence the choice of which drug is administered for clinical use for a given patient?

NEUROMUSCULAR JUNCTION

5. What is the neuromuscular junction?

6. What events lead to the release of neurotransmitter at the neuromuscular junction? What is the neurotransmitter that is released?

7. What class of receptors are located on postjunctional membranes? What clinical effect results from the stimulation of these receptors?

8. How and in what time course is the action of acetylcholine terminated in the synaptic cleft? What is the clinical relevance of this?

9. With respect to the neuromuscular junction, what are the three sites at which nicotinic cholinergic receptors are located?

10. What is the role of prejunctional receptors?

11. What is the role of extrajunctional receptors? What is their effect when stimulated?

12. What is the structure of nicotinic cholinergic receptors? How is the junction of the cholinergic receptor related to its structure?

13. What is the binding site for an agonist at the nicotinic cholinergic receptor?

14. When an overdose of a nondepolarizing neuromuscular blocking drug is given, how is the neuromuscular blocking drug thought to exert its effect such that the blockade it causes is irreversible?

15. How may the properties of the nicotinic cholinergic receptor and ion channel be altered by volatile anesthetics?

STRUCTURE ACTIVITY RELATIONSHIPS

16. How does the chemical structure of neuromuscular blocking drugs relate to their pharmacologic action?

17. What portion of the chemical structure of neuromuscular blocking drugs allows them to be attracted to a portion of the cholinergic receptor?

DEPOLARIZING NEUROMUSCULAR BLOCKING DRUGS

18. What is the intubating dose of succinylcholine? What are its approximate time of onset and duration of action when administered at this dose?

19. What is the mechanism of action of succinylcholine?

20. What is phase I neuromuscular blockade?

21. What is phase II neuromuscular blockade? What is the mechanism by which it occurs? When is phase II neuromuscular blockade most likely to occur clinically?

22. What occurs clinically as a result of the opening of the nicotinic cholinergic receptor ion channel that occurs with the administration of succinylcholine?

23. How efficiently does plasma cholinesterase hydrolyze succinylcholine? Where is plasma cholinesterase produced?

24. How is the effect of succinylcholine at the cholinergic receptor terminated?

25. How is the duration of action of succinylcholine influenced by plasma cholinesterase?

26. What are some drugs, chemicals, or clinical diseases that may affect the activity of plasma cholinesterase?

27. What is atypical plasma cholinesterase? What is its clinical significance?

28. What is dibucaine? What is its clinical use?

29. What is the normal dibucaine number? For heterozygous and homozygous atypical cholinesterase patients, what is their associated dibucaine number, duration of action of an intubating dose of succinylcholine, and incidence in the population?

30. Why is succinylcholine usually not administered to children under nonemergent conditions?

31. What are some adverse cardiac rhythms that may result from the administration of succinylcholine? When and why are they likely to occur?

32. How can the potential risk of adverse cardiac rhythms associated with the administration of succinylcholine be minimized?

33. What is the mechanism by which the administration of succinylcholine may be associated with increases in heart rate and arterial blood pressure?

34. What is the mechanism by which succinylcholine may induce a hyperkalemic response with its administration? Which patients are especially at risk for this effect of succinylcholine?

35. How effective is pretreatment with a nondepolarizing neuromuscular blocking drug for decreasing the magnitude of a hyperkalemic response to the administration of succinylcholine in susceptible patients?

36. Are renal failure patients at greater risk for a hyperkalemic response to the administration of succinylcholine?

37. What is the mechanism by which succinylcholine may induce postoperative myalgias with its administration? Which muscles are typically affected? Which patients are especially at risk for this effect of succinylcholine?

38. How might the fasciculations associated with the administration of succinylcholine be blunted?

39. What effect does the administration of succinylcholine have on intraocular pressure? What is the clinical significance of this?

40. What effect does the administration of succinylcholine have on intragastric pressure? What is the clinical significance of this?

41. What effect does the administration of succinylcholine have on intracranial pressure? What is the clinical significance of this?

42. What effect does the administration of succinylcholine have on masseter muscle tension? What is the clinical significance of this?

NONDEPOLARIZING NEUROMUSCULAR BLOCKING DRUGS

43. What are some characteristics of nondepolarizing neuromuscular blocking drugs that influence the clinician's choice of drug?

44. What is the mechanism of action of nondepolarizing neuromuscular blocking drugs?

45. What are two methods by which the onset time of nondepolarizing neuromuscular blocking drugs may be decreased? What is the mechanism by which these are thought to produce their effect?

46. Describe the lipid solubility of nondepolarizing neuromuscular blocking drugs. How does this influence its volume of distribution and clinical effect?

47. What are some of the methods by which nondepolarizing neuromuscular blocking drugs are cleared? How does this influence its duration of action?

48. What are some drugs and physiologic states that may enhance the neuromuscular blockade produced by nondepolarizing neuromuscular blocking drugs?

49. What is the mechanism by which volatile anesthetics are believed to enhance the neuromuscular blockade produced by nondepolarizing neuromuscular blocking drugs?

50. What is the mechanism by which antibiotics and magnesium are believed to enhance the neuromuscular blockade produced by nondepolarizing neuromuscular blocking drugs? What type of antibiotic exerts this effect? How might this effect be reversed?

51. Which two cardiac antidysrhythmic agents are thought to enhance the neuromuscular blockade produced by nondepolarizing neuromuscular blocking drugs? What is the mechanism by which this occurs?

52. What type of injury has been associated with resistance to the effects of nondepolarizing neuromuscular blocking drugs? What is the time course after injury in which this effect peaks and subsides?

53. What are some of the methods by which nondepolarizing neuromuscular blocking drugs are able to exert cardiovascular effects?

54. What is a concern regarding patients receiving long-term nondepolarizing neuromuscular blocking drugs in the intensive care unit?

55. Which patients are at risk for developing a myopathy after the administration of nondepolarizing neuromuscular blocking drugs in the intensive care unit? How might they present clinically?

56. How common are allergic reactions to nondepolarizing neuromuscular blocking drugs?

LONG-ACTING NONDEPOLARIZING NEUROMUSCULAR BLOCKING DRUGS

57. Name some long-acting nondepolarizing neuromuscular blocking drugs. What is their approximate time of onset and duration of action?

58. How is the clearance of pancuronium affected by renal or liver disease?

59. What are the cardiovascular effects associated with the administration of pancuronium? What is the mechanism by which these effects occur?

INTERMEDIATE-ACTING NONDEPOLARIZING NEUROMUSCULAR BLOCKING DRUGS

60. Name some intermediate-acting nondepolarizing neuromuscular blocking drugs. What is their approximate time of onset and duration of action?

61. What are some advantages and disadvantages of intermediate-acting nondepolarizing neuromuscular blocking drugs when compared with long-acting nondepolarizing neuromuscular blocking drugs?

62. How is vecuronium excreted from the body? How does renal failure affect the clearance of vecuronium?

63. How does the time of onset of rocuronium compare with the time of onset of succinylcholine?

64. How is rocuronium excreted from the body? How does renal failure affect the clearance of rocuronium?

65. How are cisatracurium and atracurium structurally related?

66. How are atracurium and cisatracurium cleared from the plasma? How does renal failure affect the clearance of these drugs?

67. What is the principal metabolite of atracurium and its potential adverse physiologic effect? Which patients are especially at risk for this adverse effect?

68. What are some of the cardiovascular effects of atracurium?

69. What are some differences between cisatracurium and atracurium that make cisatracurium more desirable for clinical use?

SHORT-ACTING NONDEPOLARIZING NEUROMUSCULAR BLOCKING DRUGS

70. Name a short-acting nondepolarizing neuromuscular blocking drug. What is its approximate time of onset and duration of action?

71. How is mivacurium cleared from the plasma? How is the duration of action of mivacurium altered in patients who have deficiencies in plasma cholinesterase enzyme, liver disease, or renal disease?

72. Does the administration of neostigmine reverse the neuromuscular blockade produced by mivacurium?

73. What are some of the cardiovascular effects of mivacurium?

RAPID-ONSET AND SHORT-ACTING NONDEPOLARIZING NEUROMUSCULAR BLOCKING DRUGS

74. Name a rapid-onset and short-acting nondepolarizing neuromuscular blocking drug. What is its approximate time of onset and duration of action?

75. How is rapacuronium cleared from the plasma?

76. What are some other clinical effects of rapacuronium?

MONITORING THE EFFECTS OF NONDEPOLARIZING NEUROMUSCULAR BLOCKING DRUGS

77. What is the most common method for monitoring the effects of neuromuscular blocking drugs during general anesthesia?

78. What are two ways in which a peripheral nerve stimulator may be useful during the administration of neuromuscular blocking drugs during general anesthesia?

79. Which nerve and muscle are most commonly used to evaluate the neuromuscular blockade produced by neuromuscular blocking drugs?

80. Which nerves may be used for the evaluation of the neuromuscular blockade produced by neuromuscular blocking drugs through the use of a peripheral nerve stimulator when the arm is not available to the anesthesiologist?

81. How do the neuromuscular blocking drugs vary with regard to their time of onset at the adductor pollicis muscle, orbicularis oculi muscle, laryngeal muscles, and diaphragm?

82. What are some of the mechanical responses evoked by a peripheral nerve stimulator that are used to monitor the effects of neuromuscular blocking drugs? What are some methods by which to evaluate the mechanically evoked response?

83. How may the duration of neuromuscular blockade be defined using a single muscle twitch as the mechanically evoked response?

84. How may the depth of neuromuscular blockade be defined using a single muscle twitch as the mechanically evoked response?

85. What percent of depression of a mechanically evoked single twitch response from its control height correlates with adequate neuromuscular blockade for intubation of the trachea or for the performance of intra-abdominal surgery? What approximate percent of nicotinic cholinergic receptors must be occupied by a nondepolarizing neuromuscular blocking drug to achieve this effect?

86. What is the train-of-four stimulus delivered by a peripheral nerve stimulator? What is its clinical use?

87. What is the train-of-four ratio? What is its clinical use?

88. What train-of-four ratio correlates with the complete return to control height of a single twitch response?

89. What is the train-of-four ratio during phase I neuromuscular blockade resulting from the administration of a depolarizing neuromuscular blocking drug such as succinylcholine?

90. What is the train-of-four ratio during phase II neuromuscular blockade resulting from the administration of a depolarizing neuromuscular blocking drug such as succinylcholine?

91. How accurate is the estimation of the train-of-four ratio by clinicians evaluating the response visually and manually? What percent of the first twitch control height must be present before the fourth twitch is detectable?

92. What is the double burst suppression stimulus delivered by a peripheral nerve stimulator? What is its clinical use?

93. What is tetany? How might it be mechanically produced by a peripheral nerve stimulator?

94. How is the normal response to tetany altered by the administration of depolarizing and nondepolarizing neuromuscular blocking drugs?

95. What must the train-of-four ratio be to have a sustained response to a tetanic stimulus?

96. What is post-tetanic stimulation? What is its clinical use?

DRUG-ASSISTED ANTAGONISM OF NONDEPOLARIZING NEUROMUSCULAR BLOCKING DRUGS

97. What is the mechanism by which the neuromuscular blockade produced by nondepolarizing neuromuscular blocking drugs is antagonized?

98. How are the cardiac muscarinic effects of anticholinesterases attenuated?

99. Which class of anticholinesterase is used for the antagonism of the neuromuscular blockade produced by neuromuscular blocking drugs?

100. Name two factors that influence the choice of anticholinesterase drug to be administered to antagonize the neuromuscular blockade produced by nondepolarizing neuromuscular blocking drugs.

101. When might neostigmine or edrophonium be an appropriate choice of anticholinesterase drug to be administered to antagonize neuromuscular blockade? What anticholinergic drug is often paired with each?

102. When is the antagonism of the neuromuscular blockade produced by neuromuscular blocking drugs not recommended?

103. What are some tests that can be done to evaluate the adequacy of the recovery from the effects of neuromuscular blockade?

104. Which type of neuromuscular blocking drug is most commonly associated with postoperative weakness?

105. How might the residual effects of neuromuscular blockers be manifest clinically in the awake patient?

106. What are some pharmacologic or physiologic factors that may interfere with the antagonism of the neuromuscular blockade produced by neuromuscular blocking drugs?

ANSWERS*

1. Skeletal muscle relaxation is desired most frequently to facilitate intubation of the trachea. Other clinical situations in which skeletal muscle relaxation is desired include to facilitate mechanical ventilation of the lungs either intraoperatively or in the intensive care unit and to optimize surgical working conditions. (89; **413–414, 472**)

2. Skeletal muscle relaxation can be achieved without the administration of neuromuscular blocking drugs through the administration of high doses of volatile anesthetics, by the administration of regional anesthesia, and by proper patient positioning on the operating table. (89; **432–33, 445–446, 462**)

3. Neuromuscular blocking drugs do not have any anesthetic or analgesic effects.

*Numbers in parentheses: lightface numbers refer to pages, figures, or tables in Stoelting RK, Miller RD: Basics of Anesthesia, 4th ed. Philadelphia, Churchill Livingstone, 2000; **boldface numbers** refer to pages, figures, or tables in Miller RD: Anesthesia, 5th ed. Philadelphia, Churchill Livingstone, 2000.

The potential therefore exists for the patient to be rendered paralyzed without adequate anesthesia. (89; **413**)

4. Neuromuscular blocking drugs vary in their mechanism of action, speed of onset, duration of action, route of elimination, and associated side effects. These characteristics of a neuromuscular blocking drug may influence whether a specific neuromuscular blocking drug is chosen for administration to a given patient. (89; **417–418, 426**)

NEUROMUSCULAR JUNCTION

5. The neuromuscular junction is the location where the transmission of neural impulses at the nerve terminal becomes translated into skeletal muscle contraction at the motor endplate. The highly specialized neuromuscular junction consists of the prejunctional motor nerve ending, a highly folded postjunctional skeletal muscle membrane, and the synaptic cleft in between. (89, Fig. 8–1; **735–739, Figs. 20–1, 20–2**)

6. A nerve impulse conducted down the motor nerve fiber, or axon, ends in the prejunctional motor nerve ending. The resulting stimulation of the motor nerve terminal causes an influx of calcium into the nerve terminal. The influx of calcium results in a release of the neurotransmitter acetylcholine into the synaptic cleft. The nerve synthesizes and stores acetylcholine in vesicles in the motor nerve terminals, which is available for release with the influx of calcium. Acetylcholine released into the synaptic cleft binds to receptors in the postjunctional skeletal muscle membrane, leading to skeletal muscle contraction. (89–90; **738–739, Fig. 20–2**)

7. Nicotinic cholinergic receptors are located on the skeletal muscle membrane, or postjunctional membrane. When acetylcholine binds to the nicotinic cholinergic receptor there is a change in the permeability of the skeletal muscle membrane to sodium and potassium ions. The resultant movement of these ions down their concentration gradients causes a decrease in the membrane potential of the skeletal muscle cell from the resting membrane potential to the threshold potential. The resting membrane potential is the electrical potential of the skeletal muscle cell at rest, usually about -90 mV. The threshold potential is about -45 mV. When the threshold potential is reached, an action potential becomes propagated over the surfaces of skeletal muscle fibers. This leads to the contraction of these skeletal muscle fibers. (90; **732, 739–741, Fig. 20–3**)

8. Acetylcholine is hydrolyzed in the synaptic cleft by the enzyme acetylcholinesterase, or true cholinesterase. This occurs rapidly, within 15 msec. Clinically, this allows for the restoration of the membrane to its resting membrane potential. The metabolism of acetylcholine also prevents sustained depolarization of the skeletal muscle cells, and thus prevents tetany from occurring. (90; **739**)

9. Nicotinic cholinergic receptors are located in three separate sites relative to the neuromuscular junction and are referred to by their varied locations. Each of these receptors also has a different functional capacity with regard to its role in skeletal muscle contraction. The three types of nicotinic cholinergic receptors are prejunctional, postjunctional, and extrajunctional receptors. Prejunctional receptors are located at the motor nerve terminal. Postjunctional receptors are located just opposite the prejunctional receptors in the endplate and are the most important receptors for the action of neuromuscular blocking drugs. Extrajunctional receptors are immature in form and are located throughout the skeletal muscle membrane. They are located in areas other than the endplate region of the muscle membrane as well as at the motor endplate region. (90; **745–748**)

10. Prejunctional receptors are located on the motor nerve terminal. The exact role of prejunctional receptors remains under investigation, but it is believed that prejunctional receptors serve two functions. Prejunctional nicotinic cholinergic receptors are believed to influence the release of acetylcholine from the nerve terminal and to regulate the replenishment of acetylcholine in the nerve terminal. (90; **747–748**)

11. Extrajunctional receptors are located throughout the skeletal muscle membrane. They differ from the other two types of nicotinic cholinergic receptors both in their location as well as by their molecular structure. Under normal circumstances the synthesis of extrajunctional receptors is suppressed by neural activity and has minimal contribution to skeletal muscle action. Extrajunctional receptors may proliferate under conditions of denervation, trauma, strokes, or burn injury. The proliferation of extrajunctional receptors appears to occur within 24 hours of the injury. Conversely, when neuromuscular activity returns to normal, extrajunctional receptors quickly lose their activity. Extrajunctional receptors are stimulated by lower concentrations of agonists and depolarizing neuromuscular blocking drugs than are prejunctional or postjunctional receptors. In addition, extrajunctional receptors remain open longer and permit more ions to flow across the skeletal muscle cell membrane once activated. Clinically, this may manifest as an exaggerated hyperkalemic response when succinylcholine is administered to patients with denervation injuries. Extrajunctional receptors are less sensitive to nondepolarizing neuromuscular blocking drugs than are the other nicotinic cholinergic receptors. This makes the potential hyperkalemic clinical response of extrajunctional receptors associated with the administration of depolarizing neuromuscular blocking drugs difficult to block by pretreatment with nondepolarizing neuromuscular blocking drugs. (90; **745–748**)

12. Nicotinic cholinergic receptors are made up of glycoproteins divided into five subunits. There are two alpha subunits and one each of beta, gamma, and delta subunits. The subunits are arranged in such a way that they form a channel in the membrane, with the binding site for the agonist being the alpha subunits. When the receptor becomes stimulated by the binding of an agonist or acetylcholine, the channel changes conformation such that it allows the flow of ions through the cell membrane along their concentration gradient. Extrajunctional receptors differ slightly from postjunctional nicotinic cholinergic receptors in that the gamma and delta subunits of these receptors are altered from those of the postjunctional receptors. The two alpha subunits, however, are identical. (90, Fig. 8–2; **739–741, 745–747, Figs. 20–3, 20–4**)

13. The binding site for agonists at the nicotinic cholinergic receptor is the alpha subunit. Acetylcholine must bind to both of the two alpha subunits of the receptor to stimulate the receptor to change conformation and allow the flow of ions through the resulting ion channel. Nondepolarizing neuromuscular blocking drugs also bind to the alpha subunits of the receptor but only require that one alpha subunit be bound to exert their pharmacologic effect. With the binding of a nondepolarizing neuromuscular blocking drug to an alpha subunit on the receptor, acetylcholine is unable to bind to the receptor, the flow of ions across the channel does not occur, and the physiologic effect of skeletal muscle contraction becomes blocked. The binding of a depolarizing neuromuscular blocking drug, like acetylcholine, requires that both alpha subunits be bound before stimulating the receptor to change conformation and the resulting skeletal muscle contraction. Succinylcholine, a depolarizing neuromuscular blocking drug, exerts its effect in this manner. The elimination of succinylcholine is through its clearance from the plasma and requires a few minutes to occur. This accounts for its prolonged binding period on the nicotinic cholinergic receptor and subsequent skeletal muscle paralysis for the minutes after its administration. (90, Fig. 8–2; **741–742, Figs. 20–3, 20–4**)

14. Conventional doses of nondepolarizing neuromuscular blocking drugs may be reversed with the administration of an acetylcholinesterase inhibitor. The administration of the acetylcholinesterase inhibitor results in a greater concentration of acetylcholine available at the receptor to compete with the nondepolarizing neuromuscular blocking drug for the alpha subunit on the nicotinic cholinergic receptor. The administration of an overdose of a nondepolarizing neuromuscular blocking drug results in skeletal muscle relaxation that is not reversible. This is believed to be due to the physical obstruction of the ion channel caused by the large molecules of neuromuscular blocking drug, which results in a physical obstruction to the normal flow of ions across the channel. This prevents depolarization of the skeletal muscle membrane and inhibits skeletal muscle contraction. (90; **741–742, 748**)

15. The properties of the nicotinic cholinergic receptor and ion channels may be altered by drugs that alter the lipid membrane environment around the receptor. Examples of such drugs are the volatile anesthetics. (90–91; **741**)

STRUCTURE ACTIVITY RELATIONSHIPS

16. Both depolarizing and nondepolarizing neuromuscular blocking drugs have a chemical structure similar to that of acetylcholine, which explains its pharmacologic activity at the nicotinic cholinergic receptor. Succinylcholine is two acetylcholine molecules linked together by methyl groups. The nondepolarizing neuromuscular blocking drugs are much larger and bulkier than acetylcholine but have an internal structure that is chemically related to acetylcholine and allows for interaction with the nicotinic cholinergic receptor. (91, Fig. 8–3; **418–419, Fig. 12–4**)

17. Both depolarizing and nondepolarizing neuromuscular blocking drugs, like acetylcholine, are quaternary ammonium structures. Each of the neuromuscular blocking drugs contains at least one positively charged quaternary ammonium group, which allows for its attraction to the negatively charged cholinergic receptor. (91; **418–419**)

DEPOLARIZING NEUROMUSCULAR BLOCKING DRUGS

18. The only depolarizing neuromuscular blocking drug in use clinically is succinylcholine. Succinylcholine is most often used to facilitate intubation of the trachea through its effects of skeletal muscle relaxation, particularly with regard to relaxation of the laryngeal muscles and diaphragm. The usual intubating dose of succinylcholine when administered intravenously is 1 to 1.5 mg/kg. The onset of muscle paralysis after the administration of succinylcholine is typically within 30 to 60 seconds. The duration of action, or duration of skeletal muscle paralysis, after the administration of an intubating dose of succinylcholine is usually 5 to 10 minutes. (91; **419–420**)

19. Succinylcholine acts at the nicotinic cholinergic receptor through a similar mechanism as acetylcholine. Succinylcholine attaches to the two alpha subunits on the nicotinic cholinergic receptor and causes the ion channel in the muscle cell to open. This results in depolarization of the skeletal muscle cell. Unlike acetylcholine, succinylcholine is not hydrolyzed at the motor endplate but continues to attach to the cholinergic receptors until it is cleared from the plasma. The administration of succinylcholine therefore results in sustained depolarization of the motor endplate. The skeletal muscle paralysis associated with the administration of succinylcholine is due to the inability of the

depolarized postjunctional membrane to respond to a subsequent release of acetylcholine. (91; **742–743**)

20. Phase I neuromuscular blockade refers to the blockade of the transmission of neuromuscular impulses caused by succinylcholine with its initial administration. This neuromuscular blockade is due to succinylcholine remaining on the receptor and the sustained depolarization of skeletal muscle cells that results. The sustained depolarization prevents the muscle cell from being able to respond to a subsequent release of acetylcholine. (91; **425–426, 742–743, Table 12–5**)

21. Phase II neuromuscular blockade refers to the blockade of the transmission of neuromuscular impulses produced by succinylcholine after repolarization of the cell membrane has taken place, but while the cell membrane does not yet respond normally to the release of acetylcholine. Phase II neuromuscular blockade resembles the blockade produced by nondepolarizing neuromuscular blocking drugs. The mechanism of phase II neuromuscular blockade is not completely understood, but it is believed to result from the development of a nonexcitable area around the motor endplate that interferes with the spread of subsequent impulses that have been initiated by the release of acetylcholine. Phase II neuromuscular blockade is most likely to occur when the neuromuscular junction is continuously exposed to a depolarizing neuromuscular blocking drug. This may occur with a succinylcholine infusion, with the administration of a second dose of succinylcholine after the first, or when the intravenous dose of succinylcholine administered exceeds 3 to 5 mg/kg. (91–93, Table 8–1; **422–426, 742–745, Table 12–5**)

22. The sustained depolarization, and subsequent sustained opening of the cholinergic receptor ion channel, that results from the administration of succinylcholine clinically manifests as skeletal muscle fasciculations. Sustained opening of the nicotinic cholinergic receptor ion channel is also associated with leakage of potassium from the interior of cells into the plasma. The leakage of potassium ions associated with the administration of an intubating dose of succinylcholine is sufficient to increase the serum potassium level by about 0.5 mEq/L. (93; **424, 742–743**)

23. The enzyme responsible for the hydrolysis of succinylcholine is plasma cholinesterase, or pseudocholinesterase. This is in contrast to acetylcholinesterase, or true cholinesterase, the enzyme responsible for the hydrolysis of acetylcholine. Plasma cholinesterase hydrolyzes succinylcholine at a rapid rate and extremely efficiently, such that only a small fraction of succinylcholine reaches the receptor after its intravenous administration. Plasma cholinesterase is produced in the liver. (93, Fig. 8–4; **419–420, Fig. 12–5**)

24. The effect of succinylcholine at the cholinergic receptor is terminated by the diffusion of succinylcholine away from the neuromuscular junction and into the extracellular fluid. In the extracellular fluid succinylcholine is rapidly hydrolyzed by plasma cholinesterase. (93; **419–420, 742–743**)

25. Plasma cholinesterase influences the duration of action of succinylcholine by limiting the amount of succinylcholine that reaches the receptor for its initial action and by hydrolyzing succinylcholine on its diffusion away from the receptor. (93; **419–420, 742–743, Fig. 12–5**)

26. Potent anticholinesterases often used in insecticides or for the treatment of myasthenia gravis, and certain chemotherapeutic drugs such as nitrogen mustard and cyclophosphamide, can significantly decrease plasma cholinesterase activity. Prolonged effects of succinylcholine manifested as prolonged skeletal muscle paralysis may be clinically apparent with the administration of these drugs. Liver disease may also result in a decrease in the amount of

circulating plasma cholinesterase and a subsequent prolonged clinical effect of succinylcholine. The degree of liver disease must be severe before the synthesis of plasma cholinesterase is sufficiently decreased to result in prolonged muscle paralysis after the administration of succinylcholine, however. (93; **424–425**)

27. Atypical plasma cholinesterase is an abnormal genetic variant of the plasma cholinesterase enzyme that lacks the ability to hydrolyze ester bonds in drugs such as succinylcholine and mivacurium. Patients who are otherwise healthy may have atypical plasma cholinesterase enzyme. Clinically, the presence of this enzyme manifests as prolonged skeletal muscle paralysis after the administration of a conventional dose of succinylcholine. These patients may have skeletal muscle paralysis that persists for over an hour after the administration of succinylcholine. (93; **419–421**)

28. Dibucaine is an amide local anesthetic that greatly inhibits normal plasma cholinesterase activity, but it has limited inhibition of the activity of atypical plasma cholinesterase. This characteristic of dibucaine has led to an evaluation of the percent of inhibition of plasma cholinesterase activity by dibucaine, the result of which is referred to as the dibucaine number. By determining the dibucaine number for a given patient the diagnosis of the presence of atypical plasma cholinesterase may be established. It is important to realize that the dibucaine number reflects the quality, and not the quantity, of the circulating plasma cholinesterase enzyme in the plasma. For instance, patients with liver disease severe enough to decrease the number of circulating plasma cholinesterase enzymes would still have a normal dibucaine number. (93–94; **419–421, Table 12–3**)

29. The normal dibucaine number is 80. That is, normal plasma cholinesterase enzyme is inhibited by 80% in the presence of dibucaine. An individual heterozygous for atypical plasma cholinesterase would have a dibucaine number between 40 and 60. In these individuals a conventional dose of succinylcholine would lead to neuromuscular blockade that persisted for approximately 20 minutes. The incidence of individuals heterozygous for atypical plasma cholinesterase is about 1 in 480. An individual homozygous for atypical plasma cholinesterase would have a dibucaine number of about 20. In these individuals a conventional dose of succinylcholine would lead to neuromuscular blockade persisting for 60 to 180 minutes. The incidence of individuals homozygous for atypical plasma cholinesterase is about 1 in 3200. (94, Table 8–2; **419–421, Table 12–3**)

30. Succinylcholine is usually not administered to children under nonemergent conditions. This is mostly secondary to a number of case reports of cardiac arrest in children and adolescents who were otherwise apparently healthy and had been administered succinylcholine. Hyperkalemia, rhabdomyolysis, and acidosis were frequently documented in these cases. It is believed that many of these children had undiagnosed myopathies. (94; **422, 456**)

31. Succinylcholine may induce a wide variety of cardiac dysrhythmias with its administration. Among the most likely adverse cardiac rhythms to result from the administration of succinylcholine are sinus bradycardia, junctional rhythms, and ventricular arrhythmias. This is likely due to the similarity of the chemical structures of succinylcholine and acetylcholine. In addition to stimulating nicotinic receptors, succinylcholine may stimulate cardiac postganglionic muscarinic receptors in the sinus node of the heart and mimic the normal effect of acetylcholine at these receptors. This potential adverse effect of the administration of succinylcholine is most likely to occur when a second intravenous dose of succinylcholine is administered about 5 minutes after the first. (94; **421–422**)

32. The potential risk of adverse cardiac rhythms associated with the administration of succinylcholine may be minimized by pretreating patients before the administration of succinylcholine. The most effective pretreatment regimens include the intravenous administration of atropine or subparalyzing doses of nondepolarizing neuromuscular blocking drugs 1 to 3 minutes before administration of succinylcholine. (94–95; **421–422**)

33. Succinylcholine, because of its similar structure to acetylcholine, may mimic the effects of acetylcholine at the autonomic nervous system ganglia. Stimulation of the nicotinic receptors of the autonomic ganglia may be associated with increases in arterial blood pressure and heart rate when succinylcholine is administered. (95, Table 8–3; **421, 440**)

34. The administration of succinylcholine in healthy patients often results in an increase in serum levels of potassium by about 0.5 mEq/L. This increase in serum potassium levels associated with the administration of succinylcholine may be exaggerated in some patients. A hyperkalemic response to succinylcholine in susceptible patients is thought to occur secondary to a proliferation of extrajunctional receptors in the area of skeletal muscle after a denervation injury. These extrajunctional receptors are especially sensitive to succinylcholine. With the administration of succinylcholine to patients with a history of denervation injury there are more ion channels being opened, and more sites for the leakage of potassium out of cells during depolarization. In fact, patients with a history of denervation injury may be placed at risk of hyperkalemia sufficient to cause cardiac arrest when administered succinylcholine. Patients especially at risk are those with disease leading to skeletal muscle atrophy and those with unhealed skeletal muscle injury as produced by third-degree burns, upper motor neuron injury, and multiple trauma. Patients who have had denervation injuries are at risk of a hyperkalemic response to the administration of succinylcholine from 4 days to up to 3 to 6 months after the injury. Susceptibility to the hyperkalemic response peaks 7 to 10 days after the injury. The current recommendation is the avoidance of the administration of succinylcholine to the patient more than 24 hours after the denervation injury has occurred. (95; **422–423, 472, 746**)

35. Patients susceptible to a hyperkalemic response with the administration of succinylcholine do not benefit from pretreatment with nondepolarizing neuromuscular blocking drugs. In theory, the binding of extrajunctional receptor sites with a nondepolarizing neuromuscular blocking drug before the administration of succinylcholine may prevent the sustained depolarization and opening of the ion channels associated with the administration of succinylcholine. Extrajunctional receptors are not very sensitive to nondepolarizing neuromuscular blocking drugs, however. Therefore, there is minimal benefit of pretreatment with nondepolarizing neuromuscular blocking drugs for decreasing the magnitude of potassium release that results from the administration of succinylcholine in patients susceptible to a hyperkalemic response. (95; **746**)

36. Renal failure patients who are normokalemic can safely receive succinylcholine without being placed at risk for an exaggerated hyperkalemic response. This excludes patients with renal failure who have neuropathy secondary to uremia. (95; **423**)

37. Transient, generalized, unsynchronized skeletal muscle contractions referred to as fasciculations often accompany the administration of succinylcholine. This occurs secondary to the depolarization of the skeletal muscle membrane that occurs with the administration of succinylcholine. It is believed that these fasciculations can result in skeletal muscle damage and myalgias postoperatively. The presence of myoglobinuria may be a clinical sign of skeletal muscle damage in these patients. Postoperative myalgias associated with the

administration of succinylcholine most often occur in the muscles of the neck, back, and abdomen. Myalgias localized to the neck may be described as a sore throat by the patient and may be incorrectly attributed to tracheal intubation as the cause of the pain. Young, muscular adults undergoing minor surgical procedures that allow for early ambulation are most likely to complain about myalgias after the administration of succinylcholine. (95; **424**)

38. The cause of postoperative myalgias after the administration of succinylcholine has been speculated to be due to the fasciculations associated with the administration of this drug. A nondepolarizing neuromuscular blocking drug can be administered at a dose of 5% to 10% of its ED$_{95}$ dose 2 to 4 minutes before the administration of succinylcholine to blunt the fasciculations. When pretreatment with a nondepolarizing neuromuscular blocking drug has been given to block fasciculations, the subsequent dose of succinylcholine should be increased by 50% to 70%. Pretreatment with a defasciculating dose of a nondepolarizing neuromuscular blocking drug has been shown to decrease the incidence of postoperative myalgias but not abolish them completely. (95; **424**)

39. The administration of succinylcholine is associated with transient increases in intraocular pressure. The mechanism by which this occurs is not clearly understood, but it may be due to the contraction of extraocular muscles. The increase in intraocular pressure peaks 2 to 4 minutes after the administration of succinylcholine. The clinical concern regarding this effect of succinylcholine is that of the possibility of the extrusion of global contents when succinylcholine is administered to patients with open-eye injuries. Clinical experience with succinylcholine in these patients, however, has not shown this to be the case. This is in part due to the multitude of other factors that may also influence the intraocular pressure. For example, the administration of thiopental results in a decrease in intraocular pressure. When thiopental is administered before succinylcholine, the potential increase in intraocular pressure associated with succinylcholine may be attenuated. The prior administration of subparalyzing doses of nondepolarizing neuromuscular blocking drugs may also prevent succinylcholine-induced increases in intraocular pressure. In addition, the benefit of skeletal muscle paralysis associated with the administration of succinylcholine to patients with open eye injuries far outweighs the risk of the markedly elevated intraocular pressures that are associated with bucking on an endotracheal tube. (95; **423**)

40. The administration of succinylcholine produces increases in intragastric pressure that are unpredictable. Increases in intragastric pressure with succinylcholine administration, when they do occur, appear to correlate with the magnitude and the intensity of fasciculations. The increase in intragastric pressure is assumed to be due to fasciculation of the abdominal skeletal muscles. There is a theoretical risk of the aspiration of gastric fluid and contents with the increased intragastric pressure associated with the administration of succinylcholine. This risk appears to be increased in patients with ascites, obesity, a hiatal hernia, or an intrauterine pregnancy secondary to the altered angle of entry of the esophagus into the stomach in these patients. Because the magnitude of increase of intragastric pressure appears to be related to the intensity of fasciculations, the prior administration of subparalyzing doses of nondepolarizing neuromuscular blocking drugs may prevent the increase in intragastric pressure from occurring and decrease the theoretical risk of aspiration. (95; **423–424**)

41. The administration of succinylcholine results in transient and modest increases in intracranial pressure. This may be of concern in patients with intracranial lesions or after head injury in which increases in intracranial pressure may be hazardous. For these patients, the increase in intracranial

pressure associated with the administration of succinylcholine may be attenuated or prevented by the prior administration of thiopental or propofol, or by pretreatment with subparalyzing doses of nondepolarizing neuromuscular blocking drugs. (96; **424**)

42. The administration of succinylcholine can result in varying degrees of increased masseter muscle tension. In extreme cases this can result in trismus and in difficulty opening the mouth for direct laryngoscopy and intubation of the trachea. Pediatric patients are especially at risk for this complication of succinylcholine administration. Patients who develop trismus in association with the administration of succinylcholine may be susceptible to the subsequent development of malignant hyperthermia. (96; **424**)

NONDEPOLARIZING NEUROMUSCULAR BLOCKING DRUGS

43. Characteristics of nondepolarizing neuromuscular blocking drugs that influence the clinician's choice of drug include their time of onset, duration of action, rate of recovery, metabolism, clearance mechanism, and cost. (96, Table 8–4; **426, 431–432, Table 12–7**)

44. Nondepolarizing neuromuscular blocking drugs compete with acetylcholine for the binding sites on the alpha subunit of the nicotinic cholinergic receptor. With the binding of a nondepolarizing neuromuscular blocking drug to one or both alpha subunits on the receptor there are no two alpha subunits available for acetylcholine to bind. Subsequent depolarization in the postjunctional membrane through the actions of acetylcholine cannot occur, and skeletal muscle paralysis results. Fasciculations do not accompany the administration of nondepolarizing neuromuscular blocking drugs. (96; **426, 741–742**)

45. The onset time of a nondepolarizing neuromuscular blocking drug may be decreased by at least two methods. First, an extremely large dose of the drug can be given. The dose may be six to eight times the ED_{95} of the nondepolarizing neuromuscular blocking drug. The second method of decreasing the onset time of a nondepolarizing neuromuscular blocking drug is via the priming principle. The priming principle is the administration of a dose of neuromuscular blocking drug at 10% to 20% of the ED_{95} of the drug. This is followed in 2 to 5 minutes by two to three times the ED_{95} of the same nondepolarizing neuromuscular blocking drug. The concept underlying this method is that the initial small dose of neuromuscular blocking drug binds a certain number of "spare" receptors without exerting any significant clinical effect on the awake patient. The second, much larger dose is then administered and the speed of onset decreased secondary to the "spare" receptors already being bound. (**465**)

46. Nondepolarizing neuromuscular blocking drugs have very limited lipid solubility. This is due to the highly ionized state of nondepolarizing neuromuscular blocking drugs at physiologic pH. This limits their accessibility to the various tissues and results in a small volume of distribution. The small volume of distribution implies that neuromuscular blocking drugs are limited primarily to the extracellular fluid. Physiologically, the highly ionized state of nondepolarizing neuromuscular blocking drugs minimizes their transfer across lipid membrane barriers. This includes lipid membranes such as the blood-brain barrier, renal tubular epithelium, gastrointestinal epithelium, and placenta. Clinically, nondepolarizing neuromuscular blocking drugs therefore produce minimal central nervous system effects, undergo minimal renal

tubular absorption, are ineffective when administered orally, and do not affect the fetus when administered to a parturient. (96; **429–431**)

47. Because of the hydrophilic nature of nondepolarizing neuromuscular blocking drugs, all these neuromuscular blocking drugs may be eliminated by glomerular filtration via the kidneys. When additional methods of clearance of the drugs are possible, the duration of action of the drug shortens. This is the basis for the intermediate-acting and short-acting nondepolarizing neuromuscular blocking drugs. For example, the long-acting neuromuscular blocking drugs, such as pancuronium, undergo little or no metabolism and are primarily cleared by the kidneys. Several other pathways exist for the clearance of nondepolarizing neuromuscular blocking drugs in addition to glomerular filtration, such that intermediate-acting and short-acting nondepolarizing neuromuscular blocking drugs are relatively independent of renal function for their clearance from the plasma. For example, vecuronium and rocuronium are cleared primarily through biodegradation in the liver, cisatracurium undergoes chemodegradation by Hoffman elimination and ester hydrolysis, and mivacurium is cleared principally by ester hydrolysis by the enzyme plasma cholinesterase. (96; **428–431, 435–439, Fig. 12–8, Table 12–10**)

48. There are several drugs that are often administered in the perioperative period that may enhance the neuromuscular blockade produced by nondepolarizing neuromuscular blocking drugs. These drugs include volatile anesthetics, local anesthetics, cardiac antidysrhythmic agents, and calcium channel blockers. Hypothermia, hypokalemia, and decreases in pH may also prolong the action of nondepolarizing neuromuscular blocking drugs. (97; **461–465**)

49. Volatile anesthetics produce an enhancement of the magnitude and duration of neuromuscular blockade that is dose dependent and drug specific. Volatile anesthetics are thought to enhance the effects of nondepolarizing neuromuscular blocking drugs by directly inducing central nervous system depression and causing a corresponding decrease in skeletal muscle tone. In addition, nondepolarizing neuromuscular blocking drugs may alter the lipid membrane around the nicotinic cholinergic receptors, changing the properties of the ion channel. In this respect, volatile anesthetics may alter the sensitivity of postjunctional membranes to depolarization. (97; **461–462, Figs. 12–40, 12–41, 12–42**)

50. Aminoglycoside antibiotics enhance the neuromuscular blockade produced by nondepolarizing neuromuscular blocking drugs. Aminoglycoside antibiotics and magnesium are thought to enhance the effects of nondepolarizing neuromuscular blocking drugs through several mechanisms. The enhanced blockade results from a combination of a decrease in the release of acetylcholine from the nerve terminal, from reduced sensitivity of the postjunctional membrane, and by stabilization of the postjunctional membrane. It is postulated that the decreased release of acetylcholine from the nerve terminal reflects a competition of the antibiotic or magnesium with calcium for entry into the terminal. For this reason the enhancement of neuromuscular blockade associated with both aminoglycoside antibiotics and magnesium may be reversed through the administration of calcium. The response to the administration of calcium under these conditions, however, has been shown to be unpredictable. (97; **463–464**)

51. The cardiac antidysrhythmic agents lidocaine and quinidine, as administered to treat cardiac dysrhythmias, are believed to enhance the neuromuscular blockade produced by nondepolarizing neuromuscular blocking drugs. In addition to lidocaine, nearly all the local anesthetics have been shown to have this effect on neuromuscular blockade. These agents are thought to exert their effect by decreasing the amount of acetylcholine released from the nerve

terminal, through the stabilization of postjunctional membranes, and by directly depressing skeletal muscle fibers. (97; **464**)

52. Third-degree burn injuries involving more than 30% of the body have been associated with resistance to the effects of nondepolarizing neuromuscular blocking drugs. This resistance appears to be due to an increase in the number of acetylcholine receptors in the neuromuscular junction that are required to be blocked to achieve skeletal muscle relaxation. The patient's hypermetabolic state may also contribute by increasing the rate of hepatic and renal clearance of the nondepolarizing neuromuscular blocking drug. This resistance seems to peak about 40 days after injury and usually declines after 60 days after injury but has been documented to exist for more than a year. The relative resistance to the effects of nondepolarizing neuromuscular blocking drugs in patients with a burn injury may be overcome by increasing the dose of nondepolarizing neuromuscular blocking drug administered to these patients to achieve a given effect. (97; **472**)

53. Nondepolarizing neuromuscular blocking drugs may exert cardiovascular effects through several methods. First, they may induce the release of histamine. Second, nondepolarizing neuromuscular blocking drugs may have some direct action at cardiac postganglionic muscarinic receptors. Finally, nondepolarizing neuromuscular blocking drugs may have some direct effects on nicotinic receptors at the autonomic ganglia. The clinical significance of the cardiovascular effects produced by neuromuscular blocking drugs is minimal, however. (97, Table 8–3; **439–444**)

54. Most patients receiving neuromuscular blocking drugs for a prolonged period of time in the intensive care unit recover full muscle strength within a few hours of discontinuation of the drug. There have been reports of a subset of patients who, after receiving neuromuscular blocking drugs for several days or weeks, have had persistent skeletal muscle weakness after the discontinuation of the neuromuscular blocking drug. In some cases the skeletal muscle weakness has persisted for months. Weaning the patient from mechanical ventilation of the lungs is therefore delayed. (97; **472–474, Tables 12–17, 12–18**)

55. Risk factors for developing a myopathy secondary to the administration of nondepolarizing neuromuscular blocking drugs in the intensive care unit include patients with asthma, female patients with renal failure receiving vecuronium, the concurrent administration of high doses of corticosteroids, and the administration of large doses of neuromuscular blocking drugs for prolonged periods. Clinically, these patients may present with flaccid quadriplegia and increased creatine kinase concentrations. The pathophysiology of the myopathy is not known. (97–98; **472–474**)

56. Allergic reactions to neuromuscular blocking drugs are rare. When an allergy does exist, the antigenic group is believed to be the quaternary ammonium nitrogen molecule. Because the quaternary ammonium nitrogen molecule is common to all the neuromuscular blocking drugs, including succinylcholine, there is likely to be a cross-sensitivity among all the neuromuscular blocking drugs when an allergy is present. (98)

LONG-ACTING NONDEPOLARIZING NEUROMUSCULAR BLOCKING DRUGS

57. The long-acting nondepolarizing neuromuscular blocking drugs include *d*-tubocurarine, gallamine, and pancuronium. Their approximate time of onset

is 3 to 5 minutes. Their approximate duration of action is 60 to 90 minutes. (98, Table 8–4; **432**)

58. The principal route of clearance of pancuronium, like the other long-acting nondepolarizing neuromuscular blocking drugs, is by glomerular filtration. The clearance of all these long-acting nondepolarizing neuromuscular blocking drugs is greatly affected by renal disease, such that the plasma clearance of pancuronium in patients with renal failure is decreased by 30% to 50%. Patients with renal disease are therefore likely to exhibit prolonged neuromuscular blockade with the administration of conventional doses of pancuronium. Pancuronium is also metabolized by the liver to a limited degree. A metabolite of pancuronium, 3-desacetylpancuronium, possesses limited muscle relaxant properties. Patients with biliary obstruction or cirrhosis of the liver may also manifest decreased plasma clearance and prolonged elimination half-times of pancuronium, although not to as great an extent as that seen with renal disease. (98; **428, 435–437, 446–447, Table 12–10**)

59. The administration of pancuronium results in a modest increase in heart rate and arterial blood pressure by 10% to 15%. This effect of pancuronium is primarily due to muscarinic receptor blockade at the sinus node of the heart exerted directly by pancuronium. This selective vagal blockade of the heart is similar to the mechanism by which atropine increases heart rate. The increase in heart rate associated with the administration of pancuronium is dose-related and additive, such that subsequent doses of pancuronium will result in similar, additional increases in heart rate as previous doses. This increase in heart rate cannot be blunted or avoided through the slower injection of the drug. A minimal contributor to the increases in heart rate and blood pressure associated with the administration of pancuronium is activation of the sympathetic nervous system. Patients with altered atrioventricular conduction of cardiac impulses, such as patients with atrial fibrillation, appear to be the most likely to have marked increases in heart rate associated with the administration of pancuronium. (98; **441, 443, 447, Fig. 12–16**)

INTERMEDIATE-ACTING NONDEPOLARIZING NEUROMUSCULAR BLOCKING DRUGS

60. The intermediate-acting nondepolarizing neuromuscular blocking drugs include atracurium, cisatracurium, vecuronium, and rocuronium. Their approximate time of onset is 3 to 5 minutes. Their approximate duration of action is 20 to 35 minutes, or 33% to 50% shorter than that of long-acting neuromuscular blocking drugs. The intermediate-acting neuromuscular blocking drug rocuronium stands apart from all the other agents with respect to its time of onset, which is 1 to 2 minutes. (98, Table 8–4; **434–439, 448–449**)

61. There are two advantages of the intermediate-acting nondepolarizing neuromuscular blocking drugs when compared with the long-acting nondepolarizing neuromuscular blocking drugs. First, intermediate-acting nondepolarizing neuromuscular blocking drugs have minimal cumulative effects when administered as a continuous intravenous infusion. This is as a result of their rapid, efficient clearance from the plasma. Second, these drugs possess a relative lack of cardiovascular effects. One disadvantage of the intermediate-acting nondepolarizing neuromuscular blocking drugs when compared with the long-acting nondepolarizing neuromuscular blocking drugs is their relatively higher cost. (98; **435–439, 448–449, Table 12–10**)

62. Vecuronium is metabolized by deacetylation in the liver to 3-, 17-, and 3,17-hydroxy metabolites. Only the 3-hydroxy metabolite has any significant

neuromuscular blocking properties. Up to 60% of the injected dose of vecuronium, whether metabolized or unchanged, is excreted in the bile. Vecuronium is also partially cleared by the kidneys. Patients with renal failure may have impaired excretion of the unchanged form of vecuronium as well as the active 3-hydroxy metabolite of vecuronium. This may result in cumulative effects of vecuronium with the administration of large or repeated doses of vecuronium in renal failure patients. There are reports of prolonged neuromuscular blockade in renal failure patients in the intensive care unit being administered continuous infusions of vecuronium. (99; **436–437, 448–449, 472–474**)

63. Rocuronium has an onset time of 1 to 2 minutes at its ED_{95} dose, which makes it unique among the intermediate-acting nondepolarizing neuromuscular blocking drugs. In the event that a more rapid onset time is desired, rocuronium may be administered at a dose of three to four times its ED_{95} dose. This increased dose results in an onset time similar to that of succinylcholine. Because of the relative decreased potency of rocuronium when compared with the other intermediate-acting nondepolarizing neuromuscular blocking drugs, the duration of action of rocuronium at this increased dose remains intermediate. (99, Fig. 8–8; **449**)

64. Rocuronium is mostly cleared from the plasma through the bile largely unchanged. About 30% of rocuronium administered is excreted renally. Large or repeated doses of rocuronium in patients with renal failure may theoretically produce prolonged effects of the drug, although this has not been seen clinically. (99; **449**)

65. Cisatracurium is an isolated form of a stereoisomer of atracurium. (99; **451**)

66. The clearance of atracurium and cisatracurium from the plasma is completely independent of the kidneys. Two thirds of administered atracurium or cisatracurium undergoes ester hydrolysis, whereas the remaining third undergoes nonenzymatic spontaneous degradation by Hofmann elimination. Hofmann elimination is dependent on the pH and temperature of the plasma. The metabolism of these drugs is also independent of plasma cholinesterase since nonspecific plasma esterases are responsible for the ester hydrolysis. Both of the routes of metabolism for these drugs are independent of the kidneys or liver, making the duration of action of atracurium or cisatracurium unaltered in patients with hepatic or renal failure. (99; **450–452**)

67. The principal metabolite of atracurium is laudanosine, which has no neuromuscular blocking effects. Laudanosine freely crosses the blood-brain barrier and, in high concentrations, can act as a central nervous system stimulant. Patients who have been administered continuous infusions of atracurium for several days, as in an intensive care unit setting, are especially at risk for the accumulation of the metabolite laudanosine and its central nervous system stimulatory effects. Laudanosine is primarily cleared through the liver. Patients with impaired hepatic function further increase their risk of the adverse effects of laudanosine. (99; **437–438, 450–452**)

68. The administration of atracurium can result in a transient decrease in systolic blood pressure by as much as 20%, along with facial erythema. These effects of atracurium are related to histamine release and only occur when doses of three times ED_{95} of atracurium are administered rapidly. (100; **451**)

69. Cisatracurium undergoes primarily Hofmann elimination to laudanosine and does not seem to undergo ester hydrolysis. In contrast to atracurium, the plasma concentrations of laudanosine after the administration of cisatracurium are very small, making it less likely to exert any central nervous system–stimulating effects. In addition, cisatracurium has minimal cardiovascular

effects and does not invoke the release of histamine with its administration. (100; **437–438, 451–452**)

SHORT-ACTING NONDEPOLARIZING NEUROMUSCULAR BLOCKING DRUGS

70. A short-acting nondepolarizing neuromuscular blocking drug is mivacurium. Its approximate time of onset is 3 to 5 minutes. Its approximate duration of action is 10 to 20 minutes, or 30% to 40% shorter than intermediate-acting neuromuscular blocking drugs. (100, Table 8–4; **452–454**)

71. Mivacurium is dependent on the enzyme plasma cholinesterase for its clearance. Patients who have either atypical plasma cholinesterase or a decreased concentration of plasma cholinesterase will have a prolonged duration of action of mivacurium in a similar manner as succinylcholine. For instance, the administration of an intubating dose of mivacurium in patients who are heterozygous for atypical plasma cholinesterase will result in a prolonged duration of effect by 30% to 50%, whereas patients who are homozygous for atypical plasma cholinesterase will have a prolonged effect to 3 to 4 hours. Although the metabolism of mivacurium is completely independent of the kidneys and liver, patients with liver failure may have a prolonged effect of mivacurium secondary to decreases in the concentration of plasma cholinesterase and a subsequent slower rate of clearance. Patients with renal failure who have been on continuous intravenous infusions of mivacurium may also have a mildly prolonged duration of action of mivacurium to 10 to 15 minutes. This is thought to be due to modest decreases in the plasma cholinesterase enzyme concentration in these patients as well. (100; **438–439, 452–454**)

72. Neostigmine is an anticholinesterase that inhibits the activity of both plasma cholinesterase and true cholinesterase. The reversal of the neuromuscular blockade produced by mivacurium may be accomplished with the administration of neostigmine. The benefits of increasing the concentration of acetylcholine available to compete for binding sites on the nicotinic cholinergic receptor in the neuromuscular junction outweigh the inhibition of the activity of plasma cholinesterase in this circumstance, and the actions of mivacurium may be reversed. (100; **452–454**)

73. The administration of mivacurium rapidly and at doses of three times ED_{95} may result in histamine release and associated transient decreases in systemic blood pressure. (100; **452–454**)

RAPID-ONSET AND SHORT-ACTING NONDEPOLARIZING NEUROMUSCULAR BLOCKING DRUGS

74. A rapid-onset, short-acting nondepolarizing neuromuscular blocking drug is rapacuronium. Its approximate time of onset is 1 to 2 minutes when administered at two times ED_{95}. Its approximate duration of action is 15 minutes. Alternatively, if a dose of three times ED_{95} is administered to shorten the onset time of rapacuronium, its duration of action can be shortened by the administration of neostigmine 2 to 5 minutes after its injection. This quicker onset time may be useful in situations in which the rapid onset of neuromuscular blockade is desirable, such as for the emergent intubation of the trachea. Repeated doses of rapacuronium can lead to the prolongation of neuromuscular blockade such that its duration of action resembles the inter-

mediate-acting nondepolarizing neuromuscular blocking drugs. (100, Table 8–4; **434, 452–454**)

75. Rapacuronium is cleared from the plasma through ester hydrolysis. The principal metabolite of rapacuronium is pharmacologically active and renally cleared. Patients with renal failure may have prolonged effects of rapacuronium if the drug is administered in repeated doses or in a very large dose. (101; **438–439, 449–450**)

76. Rapacuronium administration has been associated with histamine release and bronchospasm, particularly when administered at large doses. (101; **449–450**)

MONITORING THE EFFECTS OF NONDEPOLARIZING NEUROMUSCULAR BLOCKING DRUGS

77. The most common method for monitoring the effects of neuromuscular blocking drugs during general anesthesia is through the use of a peripheral nerve stimulator. The peripheral nerve stimulator works by stimulating a motor nerve to conduct an impulse. A mechanically evoked muscle response is then evaluated by the clinician. The mechanical motor response of the muscle reflects the number of muscle fibers that are blocked and provides an indication to the clinician of the degree of neuromuscular blockade. (101; **414–418, 1351–1352**)

78. A peripheral nerve stimulator may be useful during the administration of neuromuscular blocking drugs during general anesthesia in at least two ways. First, a peripheral nerve stimulator allows the clinician to titrate the neuromuscular blocking drug to optimize skeletal muscle relaxation for surgery without unnecessarily overdosing the patient. Second, a peripheral nerve stimulator may be used as an objective means with which to judge the recovery from neuromuscular blockade at the conclusion of surgery either before or after the antagonism of a nondepolarizing neuromuscular blocking drug with an anticholinesterase drug. (101; **414–418, 1351–1352**)

79. The ulnar nerve and adductor pollicis muscle are the nerve and muscle most commonly used for the evaluation of the neuromuscular blockade produced by neuromuscular blocking drugs through the use of a peripheral nerve stimulator. The adductor pollicis muscle is solely innervated by the ulnar nerve. This means that the only source for motor stimulation of the adductor pollicis muscle is through the mechanical stimulation of the ulnar nerve. Different muscle groups differ in their sensitivities to neuromuscular blocking drugs. The adductor pollicis muscle is more sensitive to the effects of neuromuscular blockers than are the diaphragm or upper airway muscles. (101; **414, 1351–1352, Fig. 36–9**)

80. When the arm is not available to the anesthesiologist, the facial nerve and orbicularis oculi muscle are often used for the evaluation of the neuromuscular blockade produced by neuromuscular blocking drugs through the use of a peripheral nerve stimulator. Other nerves that may be used include the median, posterior tibial, and common peroneal nerves. (101; **414, 1357–1358**)

81. In general, the administration of nondepolarizing neuromuscular blocking drugs produces laryngeal muscle relaxation and conditions favorable for intubation of the trachea more rapidly than relaxation of the adductor pollicis muscle as measured by ulnar nerve stimulation. Facial nerve stimulation and measurement of neuromuscular blockade of the orbicularis oculi muscle more closely correlate laryngeal muscle relaxation and vocal cord paralysis than ulnar nerve stimulation. An exception to the pattern of neuromuscular block-

ade onset in the various muscles is with the administration of succinylcholine and rapacuronium. The administration of both of these neuromuscular blocking drugs results in neuromuscular blockade at the adductor pollicis muscle and the laryngeal muscles at approximately the same time. Thus the measurement of neuromuscular blockade at the ulnar nerve provides a better indication of vocal cord paralysis when these agents are administered. The diaphragm muscle appears to be resistant to the effects of neuromuscular blocking drugs, such that greater doses of drug are required to produce relaxation of the diaphragm than doses required for relaxation of either the laryngeal muscles, orbicularis oculi, or adductor pollicis muscles. (101, Figs. 8–9, 8–10; **416–417, 1357–1358, Figs. 12–2, 12–3, 36–10, 36–11, Table 12–2**)

82. Some of the mechanical responses evoked by a peripheral nerve stimulator and used to monitor the effects of neuromuscular blocking drugs include a single twitch response, a train-of-four ratio, double burst suppression, tetanus, and post-tetanic stimulation. The various methods of evaluation of the mechanically evoked response vary with regard to ease and accuracy. The mechanically evoked response can be evaluated visually, manually by touch, or by recording. (101–102; **415–416, 1352–1356**)

83. The duration of neuromuscular blockade may be defined as the time difference between the time of drug administration and the time a mechanically evoked single twitch recovers to a certain percentage of its control height. (102)

84. The depth of neuromuscular blockade may be defined as the percent inhibition of a mechanically evoked single twitch from its control height. (102)

85. Depression by 90% or more of a mechanically evoked single twitch response from its control height correlates with adequate neuromuscular blockade for the performance of intra-abdominal surgery or tracheal intubation. Greater than 70% of nicotinic cholinergic receptors must be occupied by a nondepolarizing neuromuscular blocking drug to achieve this. (102, Figs. 8–10, 8–15; **1352, 1361, Fig. 36–1**)

86. The train-of-four (TOF) stimulus delivered by a peripheral nerve stimulator is four electrical stimuli at 2 Hz each delivered every 0.5 second. The TOF stimulus is useful for the evaluation of the degree of neuromuscular blockade based on the premise that each successive electrical stimulus will further deplete stores of acetylcholine in the nerve terminal. In the presence of neuromuscular blockade produced by nondepolarizing neuromuscular blocking drugs, there will be a resultant decrease in the mechanically evoked muscle response with each stimulus. The amount of decrease in the mechanical muscle response correlates with the degree of neuromuscular blockade. Only four twitches are used in the TOF stimulus because any further stimulation of the nerve after the fourth does not result in any further depletion of acetylcholine stores at the nerve terminal. (102, Fig. 8–12; **1346–1347, Fig. 36–2**)

87. The train-of-four (TOF) ratio is a calculation of the height of the fourth evoked twitch response divided by the height of the first evoked twitch response of a TOF stimulus. For example, if the height of the fourth twitch is one half the height of the first twitch, the TOF ratio would be 0.5. The TOF ratio reflects how much fade has occurred, which correlates with the degree of neuromuscular blockade. The control, or baseline, TOF ratio should be 1.0 before the administration of neuromuscular blocking drugs. This corresponds to a height of the fourth mechanically evoked twitch response being equal to the height of the first evoked twitch response. (102–103; **1352–1353**)

88. A train-of-four (TOF) ratio of 0.7 or greater correlates with the complete return to control height of a single twitch response. That is, when the height of the fourth mechanically evoked twitch response is 70% of the height of the first evoked twitch response in a TOF stimulus, a single twitch response will have returned to its control height. (103; **1361**)

89. After the administration of succinylcholine for neuromuscular blockade, phase I neuromuscular blockade is reflected in the train-of-four (TOF) as a TOF ratio near 1.0. This means that the decrease in height of the first twitch is the same as the decrease in height of the fourth twitch, and there is no fade in the mechanically evoked muscle response. (103, Fig. 8–12; **1362–1363, Figs. 36–2, 36–17**)

90. After the administration of succinylcholine for neuromuscular blockade, phase II neuromuscular blockade may be reflected in the train-of-four (TOF) response as a TOF ratio less than 0.3. The TOF response thus shows some fade of the fourth twitch when compared with the first twitch of the TOF stimulus when phase II neuromuscular blockade is present. (103; **1362–1363**)

91. Estimation of the train-of-four (TOF) response by clinicians evaluating the response visually and manually is not very accurate. Although clinicians have difficulty assessing the TOF ratio, the assessment of the absolute number of twitches evoked by the TOF stimulus is much more reliable. When the first twitch is approximately 35% of the control twitch height, the fourth twitch is able to be detected. This corresponds to a TOF ratio of about 0.35. (103; **414–416, 1363–1364**)

92. The double burst suppression stimulus delivered by a peripheral nerve stimulator is two bursts of three 50 Hz electrical stimuli separated by 750 milliseconds between each, but it is perceived by the clinician as two separate twitches. The use of the double burst suppression stimulus appears to make the estimation of the fade response easier for clinicians. It is thought that the estimation of the ratio between the two twitches is easier for clinicians because the middle two twitches of the train-of-four (TOF) response are eliminated. A TOF ratio of 0.3 or less is most accurately detected by clinicians when using the double burst suppression stimulus. Accuracy of the estimation of a TOF ratio greater than 0.7 is still poor, however. (103, Fig. 8–13; **414–416, 1355–1356, Fig. 36–7**)

93. Tetany is a continuous skeletal muscle contraction that occurs secondary to continuous stimulation of the postjunctional receptors. Tetany can be mechanically produced through the use of a peripheral nerve stimulator. The delivery of a continuous electrical stimulus of about 50 Hz for 5 seconds is frequently used in clinical anesthesia practice to induce tetany for the evaluation of neuromuscular blockade. (103; **1353–1354**)

94. The normal response to tetany is a sustained muscular contraction. This response is altered by the administration of neuromuscular blocking drugs. Phase I neuromuscular blockade subsequent to the administration of depolarizing neuromuscular blocking drugs, such as succinylcholine, induces a mechanical muscle contraction in response to a tetanic stimulus that is greatly decreased from the control response and does not undergo fade over time. The administration of nondepolarizing neuromuscular blocking drugs induces a mechanical muscular contraction in response to a tetanic stimulus that fades over time. (103; **1353–1354, Fig. 36–3**)

95. A sustained response to a tetanic stimulus correlates to a train-of-four ratio greater than 0.7. (103–104; **1353–1354, 1361**)

96. Post-tetanic stimulation refers to the evaluation of a train-of-four (TOF) response after a tetanic stimulus has been delivered. The mechanical muscle

response to a TOF stimulus after the delivery of a tetanic stimulus is useful during intense neuromuscular blockade when there is no evoked mechanical response to either a single twitch or a TOF stimulus. The clinical use of post-tetanic stimulation is derived from the transient enhancement of the mechanical muscle response obtained when a TOF stimulus is delivered immediately after a tetanic stimulus. This enhancement is due to an increase in the available stores of acetylcholine in the nerve terminals after a tetanic stimulus and is termed post-tetanic facilitation. (104, Fig. 8–14; **1354–1355, Fig. 36–4**)

DRUG-ASSISTED ANTAGONISM OF NONDEPOLARIZING NEUROMUSCULAR BLOCKING DRUGS

97. The antagonism of the neuromuscular blockade produced by nondepolarizing neuromuscular blocking drugs is achieved through the intravenous administration of anticholinesterases. The anticholinesterases most often used for this purpose are neostigmine and edrophonium. These drugs exert their effect by inhibiting the activity of acetylcholinesterase, the enzyme that hydrolyzes acetylcholine in the neuromuscular junction. As a result of the inhibition of the hydrolysis of acetylcholine, acetylcholine accumulates in the neuromuscular junction. With more acetylcholine available at the neuromuscular junction the competition between acetylcholine and the nondepolarizing neuromuscular blocking drug is altered such that it is more likely that acetylcholine will bind to the postjunctional receptor. In addition to increasing the amount of acetylcholine available in the neuromuscular junction to compete for sites on the nicotinic cholinergic receptors, acetylcholine also accumulates at the muscarinic cholinergic receptor sites through the same mechanism. (104; **466–467, 748–749**)

98. Anticholinesterases increase the concentration of acetylcholine available at the muscarinic cholinergic receptors as well as the nicotinic cholinergic receptors. This may result in profound bradycardia through the stimulation of muscarinic cholinergic receptors in the heart. To attenuate the cardiac muscarinic effects of anticholinesterases, a peripheral-acting anticholinergic such as atropine or glycopyrrolate is administered intravenously before or simultaneous with the intravenous administration of the anticholinesterase. (104; **466–467, 748–749**)

99. Anticholinesterases that have a quaternary ammonium structure are used for the antagonism of the neuromuscular blockade produced by nondepolarizing neuromuscular blocking drugs. In contrast to the tertiary amine-structured anticholinesterases, the quaternary ammonium structure makes these agents less lipid soluble and prevents them from easily crossing lipid membranes. This restricts their ability to gain access to the central nervous system by crossing the blood-brain barrier, thereby minimizing their central nervous system effects. (104; **748–749**)

100. Two factors that influence the choice of anticholinesterase drug to be administered to antagonize neuromuscular blockade include the approximate duration of action of the nondepolarizing neuromuscular blocking drug that had been administered and the intensity of the neuromuscular blockade that exists at the conclusion of surgery. (104–105; **466–467, Fig. 12–45**)

101. Neostigmine and edrophonium are the quaternary ammonium-structured anticholinesterases that are most frequently administered for the antagonism of the effects of nondepolarizing muscle relaxants. Neostigmine should be administered for the antagonism of the effects of nondepolarizing neuromuscular blocking drugs when the neuromuscular blockade is intense and/or

when the neuromuscular blocking drug that had been administered is long acting. This is primarily due to the prolonged duration of effect of neostigmine when compared with the duration of effect of edrophonium. Glycopyrrolate is often paired with neostigmine as the anticholinergic of choice because its delayed cardiac anticholinergic effects more closely parallel the time of onset of the muscarinic effects produced by neostigmine. Conversely, edrophonium has a shorter time of onset and shorter duration of action than neostigmine. Edrophonium should be administered for the antagonism of the effects of nondepolarizing neuromuscular blocking drugs when there has been adequate spontaneous recovery from the effects of these drugs and/or when the nondepolarizing neuromuscular blocking drug that had been administered was short or intermediate acting. Atropine is often paired with edrophonium as the anticholinergic of choice because its shorter time of onset is similar to the short onset time of edrophonium. (104–105; **466–467, 748–749**)

102. Antagonism of the neuromuscular blockade produced through the administration of anticholinesterases is not recommended when a mechanical muscle twitch response to an electrical stimulus is unable to be evoked. The degree of neuromuscular blockade in these patients is believed to be so intense that its antagonism by an anticholinesterase is not possible. Instead, these patients should be maintained on mechanical ventilation of the lungs until a twitch response can be evoked. (104; **1364**)

103. Confirmation of the recovery from the effects of neuromuscular blockade that have occurred either spontaneously or through the administration of anticholinesterases should be obtained before extubation of the patient's trachea at the conclusion of general anesthesia. Often the mechanical muscle response to a train-of-four (TOF) stimulus is difficult for the clinician to evaluate manually or visually. When this is the case, the evaluation of the muscular response to a continuous tetanic stimulation may be useful. A sustained muscular contraction to a continuous tetanic stimulus usually indicates a TOF ratio greater than 0.7 and is an indication of adequate recovery from neuromuscular blockade. Alternatively, a double burst suppression stimulus may be delivered by the peripheral nerve stimulator to facilitate the clinician's ability to evaluate the degree of fade. Clinical tests that may also be used to evaluate the adequacy of the reversal of neuromuscular blockade include the patient's ability to open the eyes, cough, stick out the tongue, and sustain a head lift for 5 to 10 seconds; grip strength; vital capacity; and maximal inspiratory force. Of these clinical tests, a sustained head lift is considered to be the most sensitive test to evaluate the adequacy of the recovery from neuromuscular blockade. (105; **466–467, 1361, Table 14–1**)

104. Long-acting neuromuscular blocking drugs such as pancuronium are most commonly associated with postoperative weakness. (104; **417, 422, Figs. 12–46, 12–47**)

105. Residual effects of neuromuscular blockers may manifest clinically in awake patients as diplopia, decreased hand grip strength, difficulty swallowing, and difficulty speaking. Patients may also have difficulty sustaining their minute ventilation without assistance. (105; **1361, Table 36–1**)

106. There are several pharmacologic and physiologic factors that may interfere with the antagonism of the neuromuscular blockade produced by neuromuscular blocking drugs. Physiologic factors include abnormalities in the patient's temperature, acid-base status, electrolytes, or metabolism pathways. These may all interfere with the metabolism and clearance of the neuromuscular blocking drug. In particular, renal or liver disease may result in markedly prolonged elimination times and prolonged clinical effects of certain nondepolarizing neuromuscular blocking drugs. Pharmacologic factors include the

concurrent administration of aminoglycoside antibiotics, local anesthetics, volatile anesthetics, magnesium, dantrolene, and cardiac antidysrhythmic agents. Another cause of an apparent inability to antagonize the effects of neuromuscular blocking drugs is not allowing sufficient time to pass for an anticholinesterase to begin exerting its effect. Finally, the lack of a mechanically evoked muscular response to a train-of-four stimulus is an indication that the antagonism of the neuromuscular blockade is not possible. (105; **460–467**)

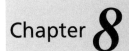

Chapter 8

Preoperative Evaluation and Choice of Anesthetic Technique

1. What should be accomplished in the preoperative evaluation and visit by the anesthesiologist according to the standard adopted by the American Society of Anesthesiologists?

2. What are some important aspects that should be included in the preoperative medical evaluation of the surgical patient?

3. What should be included in the discussion of informed consent for anesthesia by the anesthesiologist? Is it required that the anesthesiologist discuss with the patient all the remote risks of anesthesia, including death?

4. What situations may justify the anesthesiologist to delay the surgical procedure?

HISTORY

5. What are some important aspects of a patient's history that are obtained by the anesthesiologist preoperatively?

CURRENT DRUG THERAPY

6. Why is a patient's current drug therapy important information for the anesthesiologist to obtain preoperatively? How might the gathering of this information be expedited?

7. What is the general recommendation regarding the maintenance of a patient's current drug regimen perioperatively?

8. What is the general recommendation regarding the maintenance of a patient's current monoamine oxidase inhibitor or tricyclic antidepressant drug therapy perioperatively?

PHYSICAL EXAMINATION

9. What are some important aspects of a patient's physical examination that should be evaluated by the anesthesiologist preoperatively?

LABORATORY DATA

10. What patient laboratory data should be obtained preoperatively?

11. Which patients should receive a routine preoperative electrocardiogram?

12. Which patients should receive a routine preoperative chest radiograph?

13. Which patients should receive a routine preoperative pulmonary function test?

PHYSICAL STATUS CLASSIFICATION

14. What is the physical status classification of the American Society of Anesthesiologists based on? What is its use?

15. Describe what qualifies a surgical patient for each of the physical status classifications defined by the American Society of Anesthesiologists.

ANESTHETIC TECHNIQUE

16. Name some considerations that influence the choice of anesthetic technique.

17. How is the induction of general anesthesia often achieved?

18. What is the purpose of preoxygenation? How is it achieved?

19. Describe a rapid sequence induction.

20. When is a rapid sequence induction indicated?

21. Describe an inhalation induction.

22. When is an inhalation induction indicated?

23. What are some objectives of maintenance anesthesia?

24. What are some advantages of nitrous oxide for general anesthesia? What are some advantages of volatile anesthetics for general anesthesia? Why are the two often administered in combination?

25. Why might neuromuscular blocking drugs be used intraoperatively?

26. What are some of the advantages of injected opioids for general anesthesia? What is a disadvantage of injected opioids for general anesthesia?

27. What are some regional anesthetic techniques?

28. What surgical procedures are regional anesthetics often administered for?

29. What are some advantages of peripheral nerve blocks for surgical anesthesia?

30. What are some disadvantages of peripheral nerve blocks for surgical anesthesia?

PREPARATION FOR ANESTHESIA

31. What are some advantages and disadvantages to having a separate room from the operating room for the induction of anesthesia?

32. Regardless of the anesthetic technique, what are some routine preparations the anesthesiologist should make before anesthetizing a patient?

ANSWERS*

1. According to the standard adopted by the American Society of Anesthesiologists, preoperatively the anesthesiologist is responsible for determining the medical status of the patient, obtaining and reviewing tests and consultations necessary for the conduct of anesthesia, developing a plan of anesthesia care, and reviewing with the patient or a responsible adult the proposed anesthesia care plan. (108; **824**)

2. Important aspects that should be included in the preoperative medical evaluation of the surgical patient include data gathering and the imparting of information to the patient. The anesthesiologist needs to gather information regarding the patient's history and physical examination, current drug therapy regimen, and the ordering or interpretation of laboratory data. In turn, he or she must provide the patient and the patient's family with information regarding the events of the day of surgery, preoperative instructions regarding medicines and fasting, the anesthetic, and the potential risks of anesthesia. In addition, informed consent

---

*Numbers in parentheses: lightface numbers refer to pages, figures, or tables in Stoelting RK, Miller RD: *Basics of Anesthesia,* 4th ed. Philadelphia, Churchill Livingstone, 2000; **boldface numbers** refer to pages, figures, or tables in Miller RD: *Anesthesia,* 5th ed. Philadelphia, Churchill Livingstone, 2000.

for the procedure must be obtained. The overriding goal of the preoperative medical evaluation of the surgical patient is to decrease perioperative morbidity and mortality. (108, Table 9–1; **824–828**)

3. The discussion of informed consent for anesthesia should include a discussion of the planned method of anesthesia and specific potential complications relative to the patient, anesthetic technique, and the surgical case. Informed consent does not require that the anesthesiologist discuss with the patient all the remote risks of anesthesia. The patient or responsible adult should sign an informed consent statement before surgery. (108)

4. The anesthesiologist may be justified to delay the surgical procedure if the patient is not found to be in optimal medical condition or if consultation for further evaluation of a particular medical condition is desired. This would need to be discussed with both the patient's primary care physician and surgeon. In cases of urgent or emergent surgical indications, the risk of delaying surgery may be greater than the risk of proceeding. (108–109; **828, Table 23–3**)

HISTORY

5. Important aspects of a patient's history that are obtained by the anesthesiologist preoperatively include previous anesthetics and any anesthesia-related adverse events, any current medical problems or symptoms, the current medical drug therapy regimen, any history of allergies (including an allergy to latex), and any history of smoking tobacco, use of illicit drugs, or excessive alcohol intake. (109–110, Table 9–2; **829–833**)

CURRENT DRUG THERAPY

6. A patient's current drug therapy is important information for the anesthesiologist to obtain preoperatively for several reasons. It may provide information with respect to the patient's co-existing disease and its severity. It may influence the choice of intraoperative medicines or technique, and potential adverse drug interactions may be avoided. Asking the patient to bring his or her medicines to the preoperative visit expedites the retrieval of that information. (110, Table 9–3; **829–833**)

7. The general recommendation is for patients to maintain their current drug regimen perioperatively. One possible exception to this applies to patients taking angiotensin converting enzyme inhibitors for the treatment of hypertension. Some anesthesiologists may prefer that this drug be discontinued preoperatively because it has been shown to cause the patient to be at an increased risk for hypotension after the induction of anesthesia and intraoperatively. (110; **992–994**)

8. The general recommendation is for patients to continue their current monoamine oxidase inhibitor or tricyclic antidepressant drug therapy perioperatively. (110; **995–996**)

PHYSICAL EXAMINATION

9. Important aspects of a patient's physical examination that should be evaluated by the anesthesiologist preoperatively include the patient's cardiovascular, pulmonary, neurologic, and upper airway examinations. Additional evaluation by physical examination should be guided by the patient's medical history and the surgical procedure. For instance, if the procedure involves placing the patient in an abnormal position, demonstration of the patient's ability to comfortably achieve that position while awake may be indicated. (110, Table 9–4; **832**)

LABORATORY DATA

10. Laboratory data that are ordered by the anesthesiologist preoperatively should be based on the age of the patient, co-existing medical problems, the current drug therapy regimen, the possibility that a patient may be pregnant, and the nature of the surgical procedure. Routine ordering of preoperative laboratory data and diagnostic studies without indication is considered inappropriate and is costly. Abnormal hemoglobin levels may be an indication for the need for further medical evaluation before elective surgery. For instance, patients with polycythemia may be at an increased risk for hemorrhage and thrombosis. Causes of polycythemia such as chronic obstructive pulmonary disease and diuretic therapy should be considered. For patients receiving routine blood chemistries in the absence of indications, up to 7.5% of the results may be abnormal. Elderly patients are most likely to have incidental abnormal findings. A preoperative potassium level might be ordered in patients at risk for abnormal potassium levels, such as those on diuretic therapy or with renal disease. (111–112, Table 9–5; **838–842, 846–852**)

11. A routine preoperative electrocardiogram may be recommended in men and women older than the age of 40 or for any patient whose history indicates there may be cardiac compromise. The electrocardiogram in the operating room should be evaluated before the induction of anesthesia for every patient. (113; **843–846**)

12. A routine preoperative chest radiograph should not be obtained unless indicated by the patient's history or physical examination. (113; **843**)

13. Routine preoperative pulmonary function testing should not be obtained unless indicated by the patient's history, physical examination, chest radiograph, or the surgical procedure. (113; **899–902**)

PHYSICAL STATUS CLASSIFICATION

14. The physical status classification of the American Society of Anesthesiologists is based on a patient's severity of illness and physical condition independent of the surgical procedure. It is intended to standardize terminology for use as a common language among anesthesiologists at various institutions and not as a predictor of operative risk. (113, Table 9–6; **807–808, 2216**)

15. The physical status classifications as defined by the American Society of Anesthesiologists has six classifications, followed by an "E" to denote that the surgery the patient is scheduled to undergo is emergent. Physical status class I denotes a normal, healthy patient. Physical status class II denotes a patient with mild systemic disease that does not cause functional limitations. Physical status class III denotes a patient with severe systemic disease that causes the patient functional limitations. Physical status class IV denotes a patient with severe systemic disease that is a constant threat to life. Physical status class V denotes a moribund patient not expected to survive without the operation. Physical status class VI denotes a patient declared brain dead whose organs are being harvested for donation. (113, Table 9–6; **2216, Table 65–3**)

ANESTHETIC TECHNIQUE

16. Considerations that influence the choice of anesthetic technique include the patient's history of medical problems and diseases, site of surgery, body position of patient during surgery, whether the surgery is elective or emergent, the likelihood of the aspiration of gastric contents, the age of the patient, and patient preference. (114; **823–828**)

17. The induction of general anesthesia is often achieved with the administration of

an intravenous anesthetic, typically thiopental, propofol, etomidate, or ketamine. These medicines are all beneficial in that they rapidly produce unconsciousness. The induction of anesthesia is often followed with the administration of a neuromuscular blocking drug to facilitate intubation of the trachea. (114; **1430**)

18. The purpose of preoxygenation, or denitrogenation, is to replace the air in the patient's functional residual capacity with 100% oxygen. This allows for a greater amount of time to pass before the onset of arterial hypoxemia after the patient becomes apneic. Preoxygenation is therefore done as a safety measure. Preoxygenation can be achieved with the administration of 100% oxygen for 3 full minutes while the patient is spontaneously ventilating with normal tidal volumes. Alternatively, preoxygenation can be achieved by asking the patient to take eight maximal inspiratory and expiratory, or vital capacity, breaths of 100% oxygen over 60 seconds. Both these methods result in similar times to arterial hypoxemia with apnea. In contrast, the patient may be asked to take four vital capacity breaths of 100% oxygen over 30 seconds, which also increases arterial oxygenation but results in shorter times to arterial hypoxemia than the other two methods. (114; **434–435, 1432**)

19. A rapid sequence induction should be preceded with preparations such as the placement of routine monitors, confirmation of a functioning suction catheter, positioning the patient in an advantageous position to achieve intubation of the trachea by direct laryngoscopy, premedication with an antacid to neutralize the acidity of gastric contents, preoxygenation, and cricoid pressure. An induction dose of intravenous anesthetic agent, typically thiopental or propofol, followed by a dose of 1 to 2 mg/kg succinylcholine are then administered together in rapid sequence. After approximately 30 seconds, which corresponds to the onset of muscle relaxation, direct laryngoscopy should be instituted with the anesthesiologist's laryngoscope blade of choice. Only after successful intubation of the trachea has been confirmed by at least two methods should cricoid pressure be released. Alternatives to succinylcholine for neuromuscular blockade for a rapid sequence induction include rapacuronium at two times ED_{95} or rocuronium at two to three times ED_{95}. (114–115; **434–435, 1429–1430, 1432**)

20. A rapid sequence induction is indicated when patients are at an increased risk of the aspiration of gastric contents with the induction of anesthesia and the corresponding loss of protective laryngeal reflexes. These patients should also have an airway examination that does not indicate that visualization of the glottis via direct laryngoscopy, and therefore intubation of the trachea, may be difficult. Among the patients at an increased risk of the aspiration of gastric contents are patients with neurologic compromise, intoxicated patients, patients in cardiopulmonary arrest, patients with a hiatal hernia or history of gastroesoph-ageal reflux, patients with a history of gastroparesis, patients with an obstructed bowel, obese patients, pregnant patients, and those undergoing emergency sur-gery. (115; **1432, Table 39–6**)

21. An inhalation induction is the induction of anesthesia with the patient spontane-ously breathing nitrous oxide in conjunction with a volatile anesthetic by mask. Because of their relative lack of pungency, the volatile anesthetics most accepted by awake patients are halothane and sevoflurane. In some cases, the prior administration of a premedicant may be indicated. (115; **2100–2102**)

22. An inhalation induction is frequently used as the induction method of choice in pediatric patients in whom intravenous access is difficult to achieve while awake. Another benefit of an inhalation induction is the maintenance of the capacity to breathe spontaneously, which may be beneficial in patients in whom the administration of neuromuscular blocking drugs may place the patient at some risk. (115; **2100–2102**)

23. Objectives of maintenance anesthesia are to maintain amnesia, analgesia, and

skeletal muscle relaxation and to control sympathetic nervous system stimulation. These objectives are often achieved through combining drugs to optimize their effects. (115)

24. Advantages of nitrous oxide for general anesthesia include its relative lack of significant cardiovascular effects and its low blood-gas solubility. Advantages of volatile anesthetics for general anesthesia include their high potency, their ability to attenuate sympathetic nervous system responses, and their ease of administration. Nitrous oxide and volatile anesthetics are often administered in combination to decrease the concentration of the volatile anesthetic necessary for a given anesthetic effect. This also decreases the cardiovascular depression that may result from the administration of volatile anesthetics alone. (116; **112–115**)

25. Neuromuscular blocking drugs are used intraoperatively to ensure lack of patient movement during certain operative procedures, as in neurosurgery. With the administration of neuromuscular blocking drugs during general anesthesia there is the inherent risk of paralysis with an inadequate depth of anesthesia and resultant patient awareness. Therefore, neuromuscular blockade must be accompanied with adequate levels of anesthesia. (116; **413–414**)

26. Advantages of injected opioids for general anesthesia are the increased depth of anesthesia and analgesia produced with its administration in the absence of significant cardiovascular depression. A disadvantage of injected opioids when compared with inhaled anesthetics for general anesthesia is an inability to easily titrate opioids intraoperatively. (116; **284–285, 297**)

27. Regional anesthetic techniques include spinal, epidural, and caudal anesthetics. (116; **1491–1492**)

28. Regional anesthetics are often administered for procedures involving the lower abdomen or lower extremities. (116; **1492**)

29. Peripheral nerve blocks for surgical anesthesia provide an isolated anesthetic effect without manipulation of the airway or prolonged systemic effects. They typically do not cause any cardiopulmonary impairment, nor are protective airway reflexes compromised. (116)

30. One disadvantage of peripheral nerve blocks for anesthesia is the unpredictability of the adequacy of the block for surgery. Other disadvantages of peripheral nerve blocks are related to the potential complications of the peripheral nerve block itself, such as nerve injury and systemic local anesthetic toxicity. (116)

PREPARATION FOR ANESTHESIA

31. An advantage to having a separate room from the operating room for the induction of anesthesia is that peripheral nerve blocks or epidural catheter placement can be achieved before the availability of the operating room. The distinct disadvantage to having an induction room is that the practice of moving anesthetized patients may be unsafe. (117)

32. Regardless of the anesthetic technique, some routine preparations the anesthesiologist should make before anesthetizing a patient include evaluation of the anesthesia machine and monitors and confirmation of the availability of emergency drugs, anesthetic drugs, and equipment that might be necessary for controlled ventilation or the emergent intubation of the trachea. (117, Table 9–7)

Chapter 9

Preoperative Medication

PSYCHOLOGICAL PREMEDICATION

1. How is psychological premedication for the patient and their family best provided?

PHARMACOLOGIC PREMEDICATION

2. Name some goals of pharmacologic premedication.

3. When is pharmacologic premedication most often administered?

4. What are some factors that influence the choice of pharmacologic premedicant drug and dose that is administered to the preoperative patient?

DRUGS ADMINISTERED FOR PHARMACOLOGIC PREMEDICATION

5. Name some classes of drugs that can be used for pharmacologic premedication for the preoperative patient.

6. What are some advantages of benzodiazepines for use as pharmacologic premedicants?

7. What are some disadvantages of benzodiazepines for use as pharmacologic premedicants?

8. What are some advantages of opioids for use as pharmacologic premedicants?

9. What are some disadvantages of opioids for use as pharmacologic premedicants?

10. What are some advantages of antihistamines for use as pharmacologic premedicants?

11. What are some disadvantages of antihistamines for use as pharmacologic premedicants?

12. What are some advantages of alpha-2 agonists for use as pharmacologic premedicants?

13. What are some disadvantages of alpha-2 agonists for use as pharmacologic premedicants?

14. What are some advantages of antiemetics for use as pharmacologic premedicants?

15. What are some disadvantages of antiemetics for use as pharmacologic premedicants?

16. What are some advantages of anticholinergics for use as pharmacologic premedicants?

17. What are some disadvantages of anticholinergics for use as pharmacologic premedicants?

18. What are some advantages of histamine-2 antagonists for use as pharmacologic premedicants?

19. What are some disadvantages of histamine-2 antagonists for use as pharmacologic premedicants?

20. What are some advantages of antacids for use as pharmacologic premedicants?

21. What are some disadvantages of antacids for use as pharmacologic premedicants?

22. What are some advantages of metoclopramide for use as a pharmacologic premedicant?

23. What are some disadvantages of metoclopramide for use as a pharmacologic premedicant?

OUTPATIENTS

24. What additional objective of pharmacologic premedicants applies to patients undergoing outpatient surgical procedures?

PEDIATRIC PATIENTS

25. What age of pediatric patients typically do not require pharmacologic premedication?

26. What age of pediatric patients typically benefit from pharmacologic premedication?

27. What are some pharmacologic premedicants that can be used in the pediatric patient population?

EVALUATION OF DEPRESSANT DRUGS USED FOR PHARMACOLOGIC PREMEDICATION

28. How did pharmacologic premedicants compare to placebo in a well-controlled trial comparing their respective effects on plasma concentrations of beta endorphins preoperatively?

FASTING BEFORE ELECTIVE SURGERY

29. What is the basis for the recommendation that patients fast the night before surgery?

30. After the ingestion of solid food, what is its passage time through the stomach?

31. After the ingestion of clear liquid, what is its passage time through the stomach?

32. Who are some patients who are at increased risk for a delayed gastric emptying time?

33. What are the current recommendations for fasting preoperatively for healthy patients exclusive of parturients advocated by the American Society of Anesthesiologists?

RECOMMENDED PREOPERATIVE MEDICATION FOR ADULT PATIENTS UNDERGOING ELECTIVE SURGERY

34. How should preoperative medications be selected for patients undergoing elective surgery?

ANSWERS*

PSYCHOLOGICAL PREMEDICATION

1. Psychological premedication for the patient and their family is best provided by the anesthesiologist. The anesthesiologist is able to provide the patient with information regarding the future perioperative events, the planned anesthetic, and postoperative pain. Quality contact with an anesthesiologist preoperatively has been shown to be more effective in decreasing the patient's preoperative anxiety than premedication with barbiturates. In addition, postoperative analgesic requirements have been shown to be decreased when the preoperative interaction with the anesthesiologist provided the patient with information, allayed anxiety, and answered questions. (119, Table 10–1; **824–825, 2217–2218, Fig. 65–2**)

PHARMACOLOGIC PREMEDICATION

2. Goals of pharmacologic premedication may include the relief of anxiety, sedation, analgesia, amnesia, a decrease in oral secretions, an increase in gastric fluid pH, a decrease in gastric fluid volume, an attenuation of sympathetic nervous system stimulation, a decrease in anesthetic requirements, and prophylaxis against allergic reactions. (119; **1015–1016, 2218**)

3. Pharmacologic premedication is most often administered intravenously within the hour before the induction of anesthesia. Patients are often premedicated in a holding area before entering the operating room. (120; **2218**)

4. Factors that influence the pharmacologic premedicant drug and dose that is administered to the preoperative patient include the desired effect of the premedicant, patient age and weight, physical status, level of anxiety, level of consciousness, tolerance for depressant drugs, previous preoperative experience, allergies, whether the surgery is elective or emergent, and whether the surgery is being performed on an inpatient or outpatient basis. (120, Table 10–2; **2218**)

DRUGS ADMINISTERED FOR PHARMACOLOGIC PREMEDICATION

5. Classes of drugs that can be used for premedication for the preoperative patient include benzodiazepines, opioids, antihistamines, alpha-2 agonists, anticholinergics, histamine-2 antagonists, metoclopramide, and antacids. (120, Table 10–3)

6. Advantages of benzodiazepines for use as pharmacologic premedicants include their ability to produce sedation and anxiolysis in the absence of significant cardiovascular or respiratory depression, the production of amnesia, and the ability to antagonize their effects with flumazenil. (120–121, Fig. 10–1; **235, 2219, Table 65–5**)

7. Disadvantages of benzodiazepines for use as pharmacologic premedicants include their potential for prolonged sedation in some patients, particularly the elderly. This can lead to postoperative confusion and disorientation and may prolong the recovery of patients undergoing outpatient surgical procedures. (121; **235, 2219**)

---

*Numbers in parentheses: lightface numbers refer to pages, figures, or tables in Stoelting RK, Miller RD: Basics of Anesthesia, 4th ed. Philadelphia, Churchill Livingstone, 2000; **boldface numbers** refer to pages, figures, or tables in Miller RD: Anesthesia, 5th ed. Philadelphia, Churchill Livingstone, 2000.

8. Advantages of opioids for use as pharmacologic premedicants include their minimal cardiovascular effects, the provision of analgesia, and the ability to antagonize their effects with naloxone. Opioids are useful preoperatively in patients who are undergoing preoperative procedures, such as the placement of intra-arterial or central venous catheters, or for regional anesthesia. Furthermore, there is evidence that the preoperative administration of opioids may decrease the need for postoperative analgesia in the early postoperative period. This is termed *preemptive analgesia.* The mechanism for preemptive analgesia is believed to be due to the inhibition of changes in the central nervous system that occur as a result of painful stimulation. These changes in the central nervous system are believed to act to amplify postoperative pain. (121–123, Figs. 10–2, 10–3; **330, 2219**)

9. Disadvantages of opioids for use as pharmacologic premedicants include their effects of nausea and vomiting, pruritus, medullary ventilatory center depression, biliary tract smooth muscle spasm, decreased gastric emptying time, and increased gastric volume. (123; **220, 2219**)

10. Advantages of antihistamines, such as diphenhydramine, for use as pharmacologic premedicants include sedation without respiratory depression and prophylaxis against allergic reactions. (123; **2221**)

11. Disadvantages of antihistamines for use as pharmacologic premedicants include their potential for disorientation and prolonged recovery postoperatively. (123)

12. Advantages of alpha-2 agonists, such as clonidine and dexmedetomidine, for use as a pharmacologic premedicant include sedation, a decrease in the subsequent minimum alveolar concentration (MAC) of anesthesia required, the attenuation of sympathetic nervous system stimulation with minimal respiratory depression, and the ability to antagonize their effects with atipamezole. (123; **554–555, 2219**)

13. Disadvantages of alpha-2 agonists for use as pharmacologic premedicants include sedation that may be prolonged, dry mouth, and bradycardia. (123; **554–555, 2219**)

14. Advantages of antiemetics for use as pharmacologic premedicants include the potential to decrease postoperative nausea and vomiting and, with some agents, sedation and hypnosis in the absence of respiratory depression. Antiemetics that may be administered preoperatively include ondansetron, droperidol, metoclopramide, and perphenazine. (123–124, Fig. 10–4; **2220–2221**)

15. Disadvantages of antiemetics for use as pharmacologic premedicants include the high cost of some antiemetics, the variability in their efficacy, and the risk of dysphoria and rare extrapyramidal reactions. Extrapyramidal reactions may occur secondary to the central dopaminergic actions associated with butyrophenones, such as droperidol. Extrapyramidal reactions may include dyskinesias of the face, trouble speaking or swallowing, trismus, oculogyric spasms, and torticollis; they may be treated with diphenhydramine (Benadryl). The dysphoria that frequently accompanies the administration of droperidol is associated with a fear of death, hallucinations, distorted images, and the refusal of surgery after being administered droperidol as a premedicant. Droperidol may also result in delayed postoperative recovery and postoperative vertigo and restlessness. (124; **2220**)

16. Advantages of anticholinergics for use as pharmacologic premedicants include a decrease in oral secretions, sedation, amnesia, and the prevention of reflex bradycardia. When chosen for its antisialagogue effect, glycopyrrolate has twice the potency and a longer duration of action than atropine. Scopolamine has three times the potency of atropine with regard to its antisialagogue effect.

Because of their tertiary amine structure and ability to cross blood-brain barriers, atropine and scopolamine both have central effects of sedation and amnesia. Scopolamine is 8 to 10 times more sedating than atropine. Glycopyrrolate does not cross the blood-brain barrier and therefore does not produce central effects. The use of these drugs for the prevention of reflex bradycardia may be useful in pediatric anesthesia practice. (124, Table 10–4; **565–566, 1438–1439, 2221**)

17. Disadvantages of anticholinergics for use as pharmacologic premedicants include disorientation, tachycardia, relaxation of the lower esophageal sphincter, the potential for the suppression of sweat gland activity and subsequent increased body temperature, and mydriasis and cycloplegia, which may lead to impaired visual ability postoperatively. Scopolamine and glycopyrrolate have fewer cardioaccelerator effects than atropine. Atropine and scopolamine are tertiary amines that can cross blood-brain barriers and produce central anticholinergic syndrome. This syndrome is characterized by prolonged somnolence and delirium after anesthesia. This occurs secondary to muscarinic cholinergic receptor blockade in the central nervous system produced by the tertiary amines, particularly scopolamine. Central anticholinergic syndrome may be treated with physostigmine, a tertiary amine anticholinesterase. (125–126; **565–566, 2221**)

18. Advantages of histamine-2 antagonists for use as pharmacologic premedicants include their effectiveness at increasing gastric fluid pH and decreasing gastric fluid volume. (126; **968, 2222**)

19. Disadvantages of histamine-2 antagonists for use as pharmacologic premedicants include possible mental confusion in the elderly and the potential of some histamine-2 antagonists to alter the metabolism and elimination of numerous drugs. Most significantly, cimetidine, a histamine-2 antagonist, inhibits the metabolism of drugs that are metabolized by the cytochrome P-450 system in the liver. (126; **968, 2222**)

20. An advantage of antacids for use as pharmacologic premedicants includes their reliable increase in the gastric fluid pH within 15 to 30 minutes of administration. Antacids are, therefore, especially useful for patients at risk for the pulmonary aspiration of gastric contents. (126–127; **2222**)

21. Disadvantages of antacids for use as pharmacologic premedicants include their effects of an increase in the gastric fluid volume and the potential for the inhalation of particulate matter, initiating a pulmonary inflammatory reaction. Only antacids that are nonparticulate, such as sodium citrate, should be used for premedication. (126–127, Table 10–6; **2222**)

22. An advantage of metoclopramide for use as a pharmacologic premedicant is its ability to rapidly decrease the gastric emptying time by increasing gastric motility and decreasing pyloric sphincter tone. Other gastrointestinal prokinetic agents include cisapride and erythromycin. (127; **2222**)

23. Disadvantages of metoclopramide for use as a pharmacologic premedicant include its lack of effect on the gastric fluid pH, the capacity for it to be counteracted by other administered drugs, the potential for abdominal cramping with its administration, and, rarely, central nervous system effects. (127, Table 9–4; **2222**)

OUTPATIENTS

24. An additional objective of pharmacologic premedicants for patients undergoing outpatient surgical procedures is the avoidance of drugs that may result in prolongation of the recovery from anesthesia and a delay in being discharged to home. (127–128; **2218**)

PEDIATRIC PATIENTS

25. Pediatric patients younger than 1 year of age typically do not require pharmacologic premedication. (128; **2098–2099**)

26. Pediatric patients older than 1 year of age may benefit from pharmacologic premedication. After about 5 years of age communication with the preoperative pediatric patient becomes easier, although these patients may still benefit from pharmacologic premedicants for anxiolysis. The primary purpose of premedicants in the preschool age group is to facilitate separation from the parents. (128; **2098–2099**)

27. Among the pharmacologic premedicants that can be used preoperatively in the pediatric patient population are oral, intranasal, or intravenous midazolam, rectal methohexital, and oral or intravenous fentanyl. (128; **2098–2099**)

EVALUATION OF DEPRESSANT DRUGS USED FOR PHARMACOLOGIC PREMEDICATION

28. Preoperative plasma concentrations of beta endorphins in patients who have been administered pharmacologic premedicants are decreased when compared with preoperative plasma concentrations of beta endorphins in patients who have been administered a placebo. Nevertheless, because anxiety is a subjective response to surgery, it is difficult to evaluate the effectiveness of premedicants for anxiolysis. (128, Fig. 10–5)

FASTING BEFORE ELECTIVE SURGERY

29. It is recommended that patients fast the night before surgery to decrease the risk of the pulmonary aspiration of gastric contents during anesthesia when protective laryngeal reflexes will be impaired. (128; **2222–2223, 2852–2861**)

30. The passage time of solid food through the stomach is usually 4 to 6 hours after its ingestion, but it may take up to 12 hours. (128)

31. The passage time of clear liquid through the stomach is 12 to 20 minutes after its ingestion. (129)

32. Patients at an increased risk for a delayed gastric emptying time include patients in pain, patients who have been administered narcotics, patients who are pregnant or in labor, obese patients, intoxicated patients, trauma patients, patients undergoing emergency surgery, and patients with diabetes, myxedema, peptic ulcer disease, inflammatory bowel disease, and electrolyte abnormalities. (129)

33. Healthy patients should fast from clear liquids for 2 hours and from milk and solids 6 hours before an elective surgical procedure. Clear liquids include water, pulp-free juices, carbonated beverages, clear tea, and black coffee. The solids consumed 6 hours before should consist of a light, non-fatty meal. Infants consuming breast milk should fast from breast milk for 4 hours preoperatively. Patients may take their medicines with up to 150 ml of water in the hour before the induction of anesthesia. These recommendations do not apply to parturients. (129, Table 10–7; **2852–2861**)

NOTES

RECOMMENDED PREOPERATIVE MEDICATION FOR ADULT PATIENTS UNDERGOING ELECTIVE SURGERY

34. Preoperative medications for a patient undergoing elective surgery should be chosen based on the effects desired specific to that patient. Frequently a short-acting benzodiazepine such as midazolam is administered to the patient to produce anxiolysis, mild sedation, and amnesia. Patients at an increased risk for the pulmonary aspiration of gastric contents may benefit from an agent that will decrease the gastric fluid volume or increase the gastric pH, or both. Alternatively, if a patient is to have his or her trachea intubated under fiberoptic guidance, a medication that will decrease oral secretions may be useful. The premedicant drugs selected, timing of administration, and dose administered should be tailored to the individual patient. (129; **2218**)

Chapter 10

Anesthesia Systems

1. An anesthesia system is composed of what two components?

ANESTHESIA MACHINE

2. What are some components of an anesthesia machine?

3. What is the purpose of the fail-safe valve? What triggers the fail-safe valve on the anesthesia machine?

4. Can a hypoxic mixture be delivered from the anesthesia machine with an intact fail-safe valve? Explain.

5. How are the air, oxygen, and nitrous oxide gases that are used in anesthesia typically delivered to the anesthesia machine? At what pressure must these gases be delivered for proper function of the anesthesia machine?

6. How is the delivery of erroneous gases to the anesthesia machine minimized?

7. What is the purpose of the cylinders of air, oxygen, and nitrous oxide that are found on the back of the anesthesia machine?

8. How is an erroneous hook-up of a gas cylinder to the anesthesia machine minimized?

9. Please complete the following table illustrating the characteristics of compressed gases stored in E sized cylinders:

CHARACTERISTICS	OXYGEN	NITROUS OXIDE	CARBON DIOXIDE	AIR
Cylinder color				
Physical state in cylinder (gas or liquid)				
Cylinder contents (liters)				
Cylinder pressure full (psi)				

10. How is the pressure of oxygen related to the volume of oxygen in an oxygen gas cylinder?

11. How is the pressure of nitrous oxide related to the volume of nitrous oxide in a cylinder containing nitrous oxide gas?

12. Why does atmospheric water vapor accumulate as frost on the outside surface of oxygen tanks and nitrous oxide tanks in use?

FLOWMETERS

13. What is the purpose of flowmeters on an anesthesia machine?

14. How do flowmeters on an anesthesia machine work?

15. Are flowmeters for various gases interchangeable?

16. Why is the oxygen flowmeter the last flowmeter in series on the anesthesia machine with respect to the direction in which the gas flows?

17. What is the purpose of the oxygen flush valve?

18. What is the flow of oxygen delivered to the patient when the oxygen flush valve is depressed?

19. What is the pressure of oxygen delivered to the patient via the oxygen flush valve? What is the risk of this?

VAPORIZERS

20. Why do volatile anesthetics require placement in a vaporizer for their inhaled delivery to patients via the anesthesia machine?

21. What is vapor pressure? What influence does temperature have on vapor pressure?

22. What is the heat of vaporization?

23. Describe how a vaporizer for a volatile anesthetic works.

24. Contemporary vaporizers are classified as agent-specific, variable-bypass, flow-over, temperature-compensated, out-of-circuit vaporizers. What does the term *flow-over* refer to?

25. What does the term *variable-bypass* refer to?

26. What does the term *temperature-compensated* refer to? Between what temperatures is vaporizer output reliably constant?

27. What does the term *agent-specific* refer to?

28. What does the term *out-of-circuit* refer to?

29. How can intermittent backpressure that transmits pressure back into the vaporizer affect vaporizer output?

30. How does the composition of the gases that flow through a vaporizer affect the concentration of the anesthetic delivered by the vaporizer?

31. Over what range of fresh gas flows delivered to a vaporizer is the concentration of the anesthetic delivered by the vaporizer accurate?

32. How does tipping of a vaporizer affect vaporizer output?

33. What is the most common cause of a vaporizer leak?

34. How is the delivery of two different volatile anesthetics to the same patient via the same anesthesia machine prevented?

35. How is the potential risk of filling the agent-specific vaporizer with the erroneous volatile anesthetic minimized?

36. Why are contemporary vaporizers unsuitable for desflurane?

37. How frequently do manufacturers recommend vaporizer maintenance?

ANESTHETIC BREATHING SYSTEMS

38. What composes an anesthetic breathing system? How do anesthetic breathing systems impart resistance to the spontaneously ventilating patient?

39. What are some features of an anesthetic breathing system that enable them to be classified as either open, semi-open, closed, or semi-closed?

40. Describe the Mapleson F anesthetic breathing system. What is another name for this anesthetic breathing system?

41. What are some advantages of the Mapleson F anesthetic breathing system?

42. What are some disadvantages of the Mapleson F anesthetic breathing system?

43. When is the Mapleson F anesthetic breathing system commonly used?

44. Describe the Bain circuit anesthetic breathing system.

45. What are some advantages of the Bain circuit anesthetic breathing system?

46. What are some disadvantages of the Bain circuit anesthetic breathing system?

47. Is a circle anesthetic breathing system a semi-open, semi-closed, or closed system? What are the components that make up a circle anesthetic breathing system?

48. What are some advantages of the circle anesthetic breathing system?

49. What are some disadvantages of the circle anesthetic breathing system?

50. What is the purpose of unidirectional valves in the circle system? What would occur if one of the unidirectional valves should become incompetent?

51. What is the most advantageous arrangement of the unidirectional valves in a circle system?

52. What is advantageous about the large-diameter, corrugated tubing that delivers gases to the patient?

53. What inhaled gas flow rates can be supplied by the circle system? How does this compare with the gas flow rates that are conventionally supplied by the anesthesia machine?

54. What is the purpose of the adjustable pressure limiting valve, or pop-off, on the circle system?

55. What are two different ways in which anesthesia machine ventilators are powered?

56. What is the purpose of the bellows on the anesthesia machine ventilator? What is the advantage to bellows that ascend during exhalation instead of inhalation?

57. Are most anesthesia ventilator machines time cycled or volume cycled?

58. Does the degree of rebreathing of exhaled gases influence the inhaled concentration of the gases in a semi-closed circle anesthetic breathing system? How?

59. What constitutes a closed anesthetic breathing system?

60. What is the inflow of fresh gases in a closed anesthetic breathing system?

61. What are some advantages to the closed circle anesthetic breathing system?

62. What are some disadvantages to the closed circle anesthetic breathing system?

63. Are inspired concentrations of oxygen more or less predictable when nitrous oxide is also being delivered in a closed circle anesthetic breathing system? Why?

64. How can the potential problem of the inadequate delivery of oxygen using a closed circle anesthetic breathing system be minimized?

65. In a closed circle anesthetic breathing system, to what extent is the inhaled concentration of anesthetic dependent on the exhaled concentration of anesthetic? What is the potential problem with this?

CHECKING THE ANESTHESIA MACHINE AND CIRCLE SYSTEM FUNCTION

66. How should the anesthesia machine be checked each day before the administration of an anesthetic? What are the most important checks of the anesthesia machine?

67. What anesthesia machine checks should be made before the delivery of each anesthetic during the course of the day?

ELIMINATION OF CARBON DIOXIDE

68. How can carbon dioxide be eliminated in an open anesthetic breathing system?

69. How can carbon dioxide be eliminated in a semi-closed or closed anesthetic breathing system?

70. What are two types of chemicals that are used to neutralize carbon dioxide? What products are formed? Are the neutralization reactions endothermic or exothermic?

71. What does soda lime consist of?

72. Why is silica added to soda lime?

73. What is the pH of the water that is formed from the reaction of soda lime with carbon dioxide?

74. What does baralyme consist of?

75. How does the size of the carbon dioxide absorbent granules affect the efficiency of carbon dioxide neutralization?

76. What is the optimal carbon dioxide absorbent granule size?

77. For optimal carbon dioxide neutralization, what amount of a patient's tidal volume should be accommodated within the canister containing the carbon dioxide absorbent?

78. What makes the carbon dioxide absorbent granules change color with use?

79. What is the maximum volume of carbon dioxide that can be absorbed per 100 g of absorbent granules?

80. What does channeling in the carbon dioxide absorbent granule-containing canister refer to? How does channeling in the canister affect the efficiency of carbon dioxide neutralization?

81. What is the most frequent cause of channeling in the carbon dioxide absorbent granule-containing canister? How can it be minimized?

82. What is a potentially toxic interaction between the carbon dioxide absorbent and sevoflurane?

83. What is a potentially toxic interaction between the carbon dioxide absorbent and desflurane?

HUMIDIFICATION

84. How can inhaled gases delivered to the patient be humidified?

85. How are inhaled gases normally humidified in awake patients breathing through their native airway?

86. How is the humidification of gases delivered to a patient from an anesthesia machine accomplished?

87. What are some of the benefits of the humidification of inspired gases?

BACTERIAL CONTAMINATION OF ANESTHESIA EQUIPMENT

88. What are some reasons why anesthesia equipment is rarely implicated as a cause for respiratory infection?

89. How frequently do airborne bacteria from patients with known respiratory infections become transmitted to the anesthesia machine?

90. What is the recommendation regarding maintenance of the anesthesia machine after its use for a patient with suspected or known tuberculosis?

POLLUTION OF THE ATMOSPHERE WITH ANESTHETIC GASES

91. What is the recommendation by the National Institute of Occupational Safety and Health for the maximum atmospheric concentrations of nitrous oxide and volatile anesthetics in parts per million?

92. What concentration of nitrous oxide in parts per million should alert personnel to examine the anesthesia machine for leaks?

93. Where might be the source of a high pressure leak of nitrous oxide?

94. Where might be the source of a low pressure leak of nitrous oxide?

95. What are some ways in which the control of spillage of anesthetic gases might be achieved?

96. From which part of the anesthesia breathing system are gases scavenged?

ANSWERS*

1. The anesthesia system is composed of the anesthesia machine and the anesthesia breathing system. The anesthesia breathing system is commonly referred to as the circuit. (131; **174**)

ANESTHESIA MACHINE

2. Components of an anesthesia machine include the compressed gas source, flowmeters, and vaporizers. The anesthesia machine may also be equipped with a mechanical ventilator. (131, Figs. 11–1, 11–2; **174–175, Figs. 7–1, 7–2, 7–3**)

3. The purpose of the fail-safe valve on the anesthesia machine is to prevent the continued delivery of gases when the oxygen supply to the machine has malfunctioned. The fail-safe valve on the anesthesia machine is triggered when the pressure of oxygen in the delivery line falls to 28 psi. When the fail-safe valve is triggered, it either shuts off or proportionally decreases the flow of all other supply gases, depending on the anesthesia machine. Note, it is only the pressure of oxygen that the fail-safe valve responds to. (131; **177–178, Figs. 7–4, 7–5**)

4. An intact fail-safe valve is actually a pressure-sensor valve. The oxygen pressure needs only to be present to hold open the pressure-sensor valve. The valve does not respond to the flow, volume, delivery, or composition of the gas it is responding to. Presumably, it shuts off or proportionally decreases the flows of all other gases when the oxygen supply pressure is less than 28 psi. It does not, however, prevent hypoxic mixtures from being delivered from the anesthesia machine. A hypoxic mixture may still be delivered to the patient if the valve is sensing an adequate pressure in the circuit with no flow of oxygen. This confirms the importance of the oxygen analyzer on the anesthesia machine. (131; **177–178, Figs. 7–4, 7–5**)

5. The air, oxygen, and nitrous oxide gases that are used in anesthesia are typically delivered to the anesthesia machine as compressed gases from a central supply source. The central supply source is frequently located in the hospital. The

*Numbers in parentheses: lightface numbers refer to pages, figures, or tables in Stoelting RK, Miller RD: Basics of Anesthesia, 4th ed. Philadelphia, Churchill Livingstone, 2000; **boldface numbers** refer to pages, figures, or tables in Miller RD: Anesthesia, 5th ed. Philadelphia, Churchill Livingstone, 2000.

gases enter the anesthesia machine through pipeline inlet connections. These gases must be delivered at a pressure of about 50 psi for the anesthesia machine to function properly. (131; **176**)

6. The delivery of erroneous gases from the central supply source to the pipeline inlet connections on the anesthesia machine is minimized in two ways. First, the hoses are color-coded. Second, and more importantly, the connection of the hoses to the pipeline inlet connections are gas-specific Diameter Index Safety System threaded fittings. The Diameter Index Safety System threaded fittings are not interchangeable, thereby minimizing the risk of misconnections. (131; **176**)

7. The purpose of the cylinders of air, oxygen, and nitrous oxide that are found on the back of the anesthesia machine is for the delivery of those gases if the pipeline supply source is not available or fails. (131; **176–177**)

8. An erroneous hook-up of a gas cylinder to the anesthesia machine is minimized in two ways. First, the cylinders are color-coded. Second, and more importantly, the connections of the cylinders to the anesthesia machine are via hanger yoke assemblies. The hanger yoke assembly functions to support and orient the cylinder, provide a gas-tight seal, and provide for the unidirectional flow of gases into the machine. The hanger yoke assembly connections are made gas-specific by the Pin Index Safety System. The Pin Index Safety System consists of two metal pins that fit with two corresponding holes in the gas cylinder. Thus the connection is said to be *pin-indexed*. Each gas has its own specific pin arrangement, thereby minimizing the risk of misconnections. (131; **176–177**)

9. (131, Table 11–1)

CHARACTERISTICS	OXYGEN	NITROUS OXIDE	CARBON DIOXIDE	AIR
Cylinder color	Green	Blue	Gray	Yellow
Physical state in cylinder (gas or liquid)	Gas	Liquid and gas	Liquid and gas	Gas
Cylinder contents (liters)	625	1590	1590	625
Cylinder pressure full (psi)	2200	750	838	1800

10. The pressure of oxygen is directly proportional to the volume of oxygen in an oxygen gas cylinder, allowing the volume of gas in an oxygen cylinder to be estimated based on the oxygen pressure. For example, a full oxygen cylinder is evidenced by a pressure of approximately 2000 psi. If the pressure gauge on an oxygen cylinder were to read 500 psi, one fourth of the initial pressure, it can be estimated that only one fourth of the volume remains in the oxygen cylinder. The volume in the cylinder could be estimated to be 625/4, or about 155 L. (131–132)

11. The pressure of nitrous oxide is unrelated to the volume of nitrous oxide in the cylinder. The pressure gauge on a nitrous oxide cylinder will continue to read about 750 psi despite what the volume of nitrous oxide is in the cylinder. This is because nitrous oxide exists partially as a gas and partially as a liquid in the cylinder. The vapor pressure of the liquid is 750 psi, so as long as there is any liquid left in the cylinder the pressure will remain the same. When the stores of nitrous oxide become so depleted that there is no liquid left, the pressure in the cylinder will start to decrease in proportion to the volume of gas. The nitrous oxide in a cylinder becomes fully vaporized to gas when it is approximately 75% depleted. Therefore, when a decrease in pressure is noted in a cylinder of nitrous oxide, the cylinder must be near empty. (132)

12. Atmospheric water vapor accumulates as frost on the outside surface of oxygen tanks in use because the expansion of the compressed oxygen in the tank absorbs heat from the metal cylinder and the surrounding atmosphere. Atmospheric water vapor accumulates as frost on the outside surface of nitrous oxide tanks in use because the vaporization of the liquefied gas in the tank absorbs heat from the metal cylinder and the surrounding atmosphere. (132)

FLOWMETERS

13. Flowmeters on an anesthesia machine are constructed to accurately measure gas flow, allowing the anesthesiologist the control of flow of gases to the common gas outlet. (132; **178–180**)

14. Flowmeters on an anesthesia machine consist of a tapered glass tube, a float, and a scale. When the knob on the flowmeter is turned, gas flows through the vertical tube from the bottom upward in the space between the wall of the tapered tube, which confers resistance, and the float, which is balanced by gravity. The upper end of the round portion of the float provides the measurement for the flow on the corresponding scale. Flowmeters are individually calibrated by hand, because flow tubes and floats from the manufacturer may differ. The scale on the flowmeter is specific only to that flow tube and float. (132; **178–180, Figs. 7–6, 7–7, 7–8**)

15. Flowmeters for various gases are not interchangeable. The flowmeters are individually calibrated for a specific gas. The physical properties of the gas that influence its flow through a constricted orifice are its density and its viscosity. Because the density and viscosity of no two gases are the same, the flowmeters are not interchangeable. (132–133; **179–180**)

16. The oxygen flowmeter is the last flowmeter in series on the anesthesia machine with respect to the direction in which the gas flows to minimize the risk of the delivery of hypoxic mixtures secondary to a leak in a flowmeter. By placing the oxygen flowmeter last in the series of flowmeters, any leaks upstream from the flowmeter would result only in the delivery of decreased concentrations of the gases upstream, not of oxygen. A crack in the oxygen flowmeter would lead to a loss of volume of the gases being delivered, but the relative concentrations of each gas would likely remain the same. A leak in the oxygen flowmeter may still lead to the delivery of a hypoxic mixture, however. (133–134; **180, 182, Figs. 7–9, 7–10**)

17. The purpose of the oxygen flush valve is to provide large volumes of oxygen to the patient quickly. Oxygen delivered to the patient when the oxygen flush valve is depressed bypasses pressure regulators, the flowmeters, and the manifold. (134; **183**)

18. The flow of oxygen that is delivered to the patient via the oxygen flush valve is 35 to 75 L/min. (134; **183**)

19. The pressure of oxygen delivered to the patient via the oxygen flush valve is the pressure at which oxygen is supplied to the anesthesia machine from the central supply source, about 50 psi. Some anesthesia machine models deliver oxygen at reduced pressures when the oxygen flush valve is depressed. A risk of barotrauma exists when the oxygen flush valve is depressed during an inspiratory breath delivered by the mechanical ventilator. (134; **183**)

VAPORIZERS

20. Volatile anesthetics exist as liquids at room temperature and at atmospheric pressure. The inhaled delivery of anesthetics requires that the anesthetics be vaporized. Vaporizers allow not only the vaporization of liquid anesthetics, but

they also reliably and accurately deliver the specified concentration of anesthetic to the common gas outlet and ultimately to the patient. (134; **183–184**)

21. Placement of a volatile liquid in a closed container will result in liquid molecules reaching a steady-state equilibrium with gas molecules in the container over time. The vapor pressure is the pressure exerted by the gas on the walls of the container at equilibrium. An increase in temperature increases the amount of liquid molecules that become gas molecules, thus increasing the pressure exerted by the gas on the container. An increase in temperature therefore results in an increase in the vapor pressure. (134; **183–184, Fig. 7–13**)

22. The heat of vaporization is the heat required to convert 1 g of a liquid to a gas at a given temperature. (134; **184, Fig. 7–13**)

23. Volatile anesthetic vaporizers are classified as agent-specific, variable-bypass, flow-over, temperature-compensated, out-of-circuit vaporizers. After passing through the flowmeters, gases mix in the common manifold, then enter the vaporizers. Once in the vaporizer there are three different streams of flow that the gases can take. The gases may be diverted by a temperature-compensating bypass valve, they may enter the mixing bypass chamber, or they may enter the vaporizing chamber

 The temperature-compensating bypass valve adjusts the amount of gas that enters the other two chambers. When the temperature of the vapor is warm, more gas is directed to the vaporizer outlet than when the temperature is relatively cooler. The opposite occurs when the temperature of the vapor is cool. That is, more of the gas is directed toward the other two chambers. The temperature-compensating valve allows the vaporizer to compensate for changes in temperature so the desired concentration of volatile anesthetic is maintained.

 The flow of gases not diverted by the temperature-compensating bypass valve is divided between the mixing bypass chamber and vaporizing chamber, depending on the dialed concentration. Typically about 20% of the gas flows through the vaporizing chamber. A higher-dialed concentration will result in more gas going to the vaporizing chamber than otherwise. In the vaporizing chamber, there are a series of wicks that have been saturated with the liquid anesthetic. As the gas passes over the series of wicks, the gas becomes saturated with the anesthetic vapor. The gas, now saturated with anesthetic vapor, enters the mixing bypass chamber. In the mixing bypass chamber, the saturated gas mixes with the unsaturated gas that has been diverted there. Together the gases pass through the vaporizer outlet toward the common gas outlet at the desired concentration of volatile anesthetic. (134–135, Figs. 11–3, 11–4; **184–187, Figs. 7–14, 7–15, 7–16**)

24. The term *flow-over* refers to the method by which gases become saturated by volatile anesthetic in the vaporizer. Saturation of the gases occurs because the gases flow over wicks that are saturated with liquid anesthetic. (134–135; **185–186**)

25. The term *variable-bypass* refers to the division of gas into either the mixing bypass chamber or the vaporizing chamber based on the dialed concentration. (134–135; **184–185**)

26. The term *temperature-compensated* refers to the compensation of the vaporizer for changes in temperature to maintain the dialed concentration of volatile anesthetics. Vaporizer output is maintained nearly equivalent between the temperatures of 20° C and 35° C. (135; **186–187**)

27. The term *agent-specific* refers to the vaporizer being calibrated for a single, specific anesthetic agent. Vaporizers for different anesthetics are not interchangeable. (135–136; **184–188**)

28. The term *out-of-circuit* refers to the vaporizer being separate from the anesthetic breathing circuit. (135; **185**)

29. Any backward transmission of pressure downstream from the vaporizer could conceivably lead to the delivery of a concentration of vapor anesthetic that is higher than the dialed concentration. Pressure downstream can be pressure anywhere between the vaporizer and the patient, including pressure from positive-pressure ventilation. Such pressure could result in the backward flow of gases into the vaporizer that had already passed through the vaporizer. These gases would become even more saturated with volatile anesthetic. Newer vaporizers are now equipped with an outlet check valve designed to protect against reverse flow into the vaporizer. (135; **187**)

30. The composition of the gases that flow through vaporizers does not affect the concentration of volatile anesthetic delivered to the patient. (135; **187**)

31. Vaporizers are able to deliver accurate concentrations of volatile anesthetics to the patient when fresh gas flows are between 250 mL/min and 15 L/min. Gas flows less than 250 mL/min and greater than 15 L/min can result in the delivery of volatile anesthetic whose concentration is less than the intended dialed concentration. Gas flows less than 250 mL/min result in an inadequate delivered pressure and inadequate turbulence of gas in the vaporizer to vaporize to gas the liquid anesthetic saturating the wicks. Gas flows greater than 15 L/min result in incomplete mixing in the vaporizing chamber. (135; **186**)

32. Tipping a vaporizer can result in an increase in the delivered concentration of volatile anesthetic. With tipping, liquid anesthetic enters the mixing bypass chamber of the vaporizer. This results in an increase in the amount of gas that is exposed to liquid anesthetic. Gases that were not intended to flow over liquid anesthetic become saturated with anesthetic gas, making the concentration of volatile anesthetic delivered to the patient higher than the intended dialed concentration. (135; **188**)

33. The most common cause of a vaporizer leak is a loosely fitted cap on the volatile anesthetic filling chamber. (135; **188**)

34. The simultaneous delivery of two different volatile anesthetics to the same patient via the same anesthesia machine is prevented by a safety interlock system. The interlock system ensures that only one vaporizer may be turned on at a time. (135–136; **188**)

35. The potential risk of filling the agent-specific vaporizer with the erroneous volatile anesthetic is minimized by the use of agent-specific, color-coded, and keyed filler devices. These devices minimize the risk of filling the vaporizer with a liquid anesthetic that is different than the one for which the vaporizer was calibrated. There are vaporizers that do not have keyed filler devices, however, and errors in filling have resulted. (136; **188**)

36. Contemporary vaporizers are unsuitable for desflurane because the vapor pressure of desflurane is three to four times higher than that of the other volatile anesthetics. In addition, the boiling point of desflurane is near room temperature. If desflurane were to be placed in a contemporary vaporizer, many more volumes of desflurane would be delivered to the patient than intended. Desflurane vaporization requires a vaporizer that is electrically heated and pressurized for these reasons. (134; **188, Fig. 7–18**)

37. Manufacturers recommend that vaporizers undergo maintenance about one time a year. (136)

ANESTHETIC BREATHING SYSTEMS

38. An anesthetic breathing system is composed of the components that are necessary for the delivery of oxygen and anesthetic gases from the anesthesia machine

to the patient. Anesthetic breathing systems impart resistance to spontaneously ventilating patients due to the unidirectional valves, connectors, and tubing through which gas flows in the system to the patient. The resistance to breathing can be minimized by increasing the lumen of the tubing. Alternatively, controlled ventilation can be instituted. (136; **191–192, Fig. 7–19**)

39. Features of an anesthetic breathing system that enable them to be classified as open, semi-open, closed, or semi-closed include the presence or absence of a gas reservoir bag in the circuit, rebreathing of exhaled gases, neutralization of exhaled carbon dioxide, and/or unidirectional valves. Further descriptions of anesthetic breathing systems may include the fresh gas inflow rate, the composition of gases inhaled, and whether the system is preferred for spontaneous or controlled ventilation. (136, Table 11–2; **191–192**)

40. The Mapleson F anesthetic breathing system has a T-piece, at the end of which is a gas reservoir bag. The adjustable pressure limiting valve, or pop-off valve, is located at the end of the gas reservoir bag. The T-piece is on an L-connector. On the other leg of the L-connector can be connected either a face mask or an endotracheal tube. Fresh gas flows into the Mapleson F anesthetic breathing system opposite the mask on the L-connector. Another name for this anesthetic breathing system is the Jackson-Rees circuit. (136–138, Fig. 11–6; **191–192, Fig. 7–19**)

41. Advantages of the Mapleson F anesthetic breathing system include its low resistance to breathing and minimal deadspace, the ability to be used with either a mask or endotracheal tube, the ability to visualize a patient's respiratory efforts by the excursion on the gas reservoir bag, the ability to deliver controlled ventilation of the lungs, and the potential for adding a scavenging system. (136–137, Fig. 11–6; **191–192, Fig. 7–19**)

42. Disadvantages of the Mapleson F anesthetic breathing system include its lack of humidification, the need for high fresh gas flows to prevent rebreathing, and the possibility of high pressures delivered to the lungs and resultant barotrauma if the adjustable pressure-limiting valve is not appropriately set or malfunctions. To minimize the risk of rebreathing with this anesthetic breathing system it is recommended that fresh gas flows are delivered at a rate three times the patient's minute ventilation. Fresh gas flows may be delivered through a humidifier as well. (137–138, Fig. 11–6; **191–192, Fig. 7–19**)

43. The Mapleson F anesthetic breathing system is commonly used while transporting patients after an anesthetic procedure and during pediatric anesthesia. This anesthetic breathing system is advantageous for pediatric anesthesia because of its light weight, low resistance to breathing, and minimal deadspace. (136–137, Fig. 11–6; **191–192, Fig. 7–19**)

44. The Bain circuit anesthetic breathing system is similar to the Mapleson D circuit. The Bain circuit is a coaxial circuit, in which fresh gas flows through a narrow inner tube that lies within a wider corrugated tube. The wider corrugated tube is used for the exhaled gases. At the end of the tubes is a gas reservoir bag with the adjustable pressure limiting valve at the point where the gas reservoir bag joins the tubing. Fresh gas flows enter the circuit, the narrow inner tubing, just proximal to the gas reservoir bag and adjustable pressure limiting valve. (138, Fig. 11–7; **192, Fig. 7–20**)

45. Advantages of the Bain circuit anesthetic breathing system include its light weight, the fact that it is easily sterilized and reusable, the warming of the fresh gases in the inner tube by the exhaled gases in the outer tube, the improved humidification of inspired gases by partial rebreathing, the easily scavenged waste from the adjustable pressure limiting valve, and the ability to deliver controlled ventilation of the lungs. (138, Fig. 11–7; **192, Fig. 7–20**)

46. Disadvantages of the Bain circuit anesthetic breathing system include the requirement for high fresh gas flows to prevent the rebreathing of gases and the potential for unrecognized disconnection, kinking, or cracking of the inner tube that provides the patient with the fresh gas flows for inhalation. The outer, corrugated tube for exhalation is transparent to enable the anesthesiologist to visually assess the patency of the inner tube. (138, Fig. 11–7; **192, Fig. 7–20**)

47. A circle anesthetic breathing system can be a semi-open, semi-closed, or closed system depending on the amount of fresh gas flow versus the amount of rebreathing that occurs in the circuit. The components of a circle anesthetic breathing system include a reservoir bag, an adjustable pressure limiting valve, an inspiration limb and an expiration limb connected to a Y-piece, unidirectional valves, a fresh gas flow inlet, a carbon dioxide neutralization canister, and a selector switch that allows the anesthesiologist to select either the reservoir bag or the mechanical ventilator. These components are all arranged in a circular manner. (139, Fig. 11–8; **192–193, Fig. 7–21**)

48. Advantages of the circle anesthetic breathing system include the ability to conserve airway humidification and warmth through the partial rebreathing of gases, the relative consistency in the inspired concentrations of gases, the ability to allow spontaneous ventilation with minimal fresh gas flow rates through the partial rebreathing of gases and the neutralization of carbon dioxide, the potential to decrease the use of anesthetic gases, the ability to switch from spontaneous to controlled ventilation of the lungs, the ability to convert to a closed anesthetic breathing system, and the ability to scavenge waste gases. (139; **192–193**)

49. Disadvantages of the circle anesthetic breathing system include its bulkiness, lack of portability, and the increased potential for malfunction associated with its complexity. For instance, there are at least 10 connections in the circle system. Disconnections may occur at any one of these. (139; **192–193**)

50. The purpose of unidirectional valves in the circle system is to prevent the patient from rebreathing carbon dioxide or from breathing gases that have not been supplemented with more oxygen. Incompetence of one of the unidirectional valves can result in hypercarbia or, if the valves were to become stuck, occlusion of the entire circuit. (139; **192–193**)

51. The most advantageous arrangement of the unidirectional valves in a circle system is to place them close to the patient. To prevent the rebreathing of carbon dioxide, the valves must be placed between the patient and the reservoir bag on both the inspiratory and expiratory limbs of the circuit. In addition, the fresh gas flow cannot enter the circuit between the patient and the expiratory valve. Finally, the adjustable pressure limiting valve cannot be located between the patient and the inspiratory valve. (139; **193**)

52. The large-diameter tubing that delivers gases to the patient is corrugated to prevent kinking and is of a large diameter to minimize the resistance to breathing. (139)

53. Inhaled gas flow rates of up to 60 L/min can be supplied by the circle system secondary to the gas reserve in the gas reservoir bag. Conventional gas flow rates supplied by the anesthesia machine are 3 to 5 L/min. (139; **192–193**)

54. The adjustable pressure limiting valve, or pop-off valve, on the circle system allows the anesthesiologist to increase the pressure in the circuit to assist or control ventilation of the lungs. (139; **193**)

55. The power source for anesthesia machine ventilators is either compressed air or electricity. When powered by compressed air they are said to be a pneumatic

ventilator, and when powered by electricity they are said to be an electric ventilator. (139; **195**)

56. Bellows on the anesthesia machine ventilator deliver the anesthetic gases to the patient when compressed by air or driven by electricity. An advantage to bellows that ascend during exhalation instead of inhalation is that the bellows fill with gas during expiration. If there is a leak in the circuit, there will not be a sufficient amount of gas to fill the bellows and the bellows will not ascend. This gives the anesthesiologist a signal that there is a leak or a disconnection in the anesthetic breathing system. In contrast, bellows that descend during exhalation may descend by the entrainment of room air by gravity during exhalation when there is a leak in the circuit. Therefore, bellows that descend during exhalation continue to cycle up and down even with a leak in the circuit. Most contemporary ventilators have ascending bellows. (139–140; **195–196**)

57. Most anesthesia ventilator machines are time-cycled. (140; **195**)

58. The degree of rebreathing of exhaled gases influences the inhaled concentration of the gases in a semi-closed circle anesthetic breathing system. When rebreathing exhaled gases, the inhaled concentration of the gases then becomes dependent on the amount of tissue uptake of anesthetic gases that is occurring in the patient. For example, when the uptake of inhaled anesthetics is high, as during the induction of anesthesia, the concentration of anesthetic gases that is exhaled by the patient is low. The greater the degree of rebreathing of those gases, the lower the inhaled concentration of gases that will be delivered to the patient with the next breath. Given this rationale, the greater the degree of rebreathing, the greater the influence of exhaled gases on the inhaled concentration of gases. It then follows that during times of induction when the uptake of inhaled anesthetics is high, fresh gas flows may be increased to offset the greater uptake of anesthetic. Once tissue uptake decreases, fresh gas flows can be decreased. (140–141, Figs. 11–8, 11–9; **86–88, 193**)

59. A closed anesthetic breathing system is one in which the fresh gas inflow into the system is only sufficient to replace the anesthetic gases and oxygen used by the patient. The neutralization of carbon dioxide allows for the system to be completely closed, including the adjustable pressure limiting valve, such that no gases are lost to the outside. In reality, there are often leaks in closed systems that are difficult to control. In addition, anesthesiologists often create a leak by sampling gases from the circuit for analysis. (140; **86–88, 192–193**)

60. The fresh gas inflow in a closed anesthetic breathing system is typically between 150 to 500 mL/min. (140; **86–88**)

61. Advantages to the closed circle anesthetic breathing system include the maximal degree of warming and humidifying of inhaled gases, a decrease in the amount of potential pollution of the environment by waste gases, and the economical use of anesthetics. (140; **86–88**)

62. Disadvantages to the closed circle anesthetic breathing system include the inability to make rapid adjustments in the concentration of inhaled anesthetics and oxygen, the risk of delivering insufficient concentrations of oxygen, and the unknown concentration of anesthetic gases being delivered to the patient. (140; **86–88**)

63. Inspired concentrations of oxygen are less predictable when nitrous oxide is also being delivered in a closed circle anesthetic breathing system because the degree of uptake of nitrous oxide decreases with time. This results in an increase in the exhaled concentration of nitrous oxide, and a concomitant decrease in the inhaled concentration of oxygen if the dialed concentration of oxygen for delivery is unchanged. Over time this results in a decrease in the proportional

concentration of oxygen that is being inhaled by the patient. (140, Table 11–3; **86–88**)

64. The potential problem of the inadequate delivery of oxygen using a closed circle anesthetic breathing system can be minimized through the proper calibration and use of the oxygen analyzer on the anesthesia machine, and through the use of continuous pulse oximetry. (140; **86–88**)

65. In a closed circle anesthetic breathing system, the inhaled concentration of anesthetic is greatly influenced by the exhaled concentration of anesthetic, and therefore the amount of uptake that has occurred in the patient. The potential problem with this is that during periods of high uptake of anesthetic gases by the patient, as during the induction of anesthesia, there must be a high concentration of anesthetic delivered to the patient. Once the patient uptake of anesthetic diminishes, the exhaled concentration of anesthetic increases, and the dialed concentration of anesthetic for administration to the patient must be decreased to avoid an overdose of anesthetic in the patient. The unknown degree of tissue uptake of anesthetic makes it difficult for the anesthesiologist to estimate the concentration of anesthetic the patient is inhaling. (140–141; **86–88**)

CHECKING THE ANESTHESIA MACHINE AND CIRCLE SYSTEM FUNCTION

66. The anesthesia machine should be checked out completely each day before the administration of an anesthetic. In 1993 the Food and Drug Administration published their Anesthesia Apparatus Checkout Recommendations, which are still widely followed today. The recommendations include checks for emergency ventilation equipment, checks of the high pressure system and low pressure system, and checks of the breathing system, scavenging system, and the manual and automatic ventilation systems. Among the most important checks of the anesthesia machine are the oxygen analyzer calibration, the low-pressure leak test, and the circle system test. (141, Table 11–4; **201–204, Figs. 7–29, 7–30**)

67. Anesthesia machine checks that should be made before the delivery of each anesthetic during the course of the day include a test of circle system integrity. The test of the circle system includes a leak test and a flow test. The leak test can be performed by closing the adjustable pressure limiting valve, occluding the Y-piece, and pressuring the circuit to 30 cm H_2O by depressing the oxygen flush valve. The pressure measured by the airway pressure gauge should not decline over 10 seconds. Proper functioning of the inspiratory and expiratory valves by a flow test should also be confirmed because a stuck valve may provide for a leak test whose outcome is falsely considered acceptable. (141, Table 11–4; **201–204, Figs. 7–29, 7–30**)

ELIMINATION OF CARBON DIOXIDE

68. Carbon dioxide can be eliminated in an open anesthetic breathing system by allowing the gas to vent to the atmosphere. (141; **193–194**)

69. Carbon dioxide cannot be eliminated to the atmosphere in a semi-closed or closed anesthetic breathing system because, by definition, the rebreathing of gases occurs in both these systems. Carbon dioxide must therefore be neutralized chemically to eliminate it from these systems and allow the rebreathing of gases. (141, Table 11–5; **193–194**)

70. Soda lime and baralyme are used to neutralize carbon dioxide. The products formed by their reactions with carbon dioxide are carbonates, water, and heat, making them exothermic reactions. (141, Table 11–5; **193–194**)

71. Soda lime consists of approximately 94% calcium hydroxide, 5% sodium hydroxide, and 1% potassium hydroxide. The sodium hydroxide and potassium hydroxide act as activators. (143; **193–194**)

72. Silica is added to soda lime to make the soda lime granules harder, minimizing the formation of alkaline dust. Alkaline dust can be irritating to the airways if inhaled. (143; **193–194**)

73. The water that is formed from the reaction of soda lime with carbon dioxide is very alkaline, such that its contact with skin can result in burns. (143; **193–194**)

74. Baralyme consists of 80% calcium hydroxide and 20% barium hydroxide. (144; **193–194**)

75. The size of the carbon dioxide absorbent granules can confer a resistance to air flow if too small, or there can be inadequate surface area for absorptive availability if too large. The present size of the carbon dioxide absorbent granules represents a compromise of these two that was established by trial and error to maximize the efficiency of carbon dioxide neutralization. (144; **193–194**)

76. The optimal absorbent granule size is 4 to 8 mesh. (144; **193–194**)

77. Optimal carbon dioxide neutralization requires that a patient's entire tidal volume be accommodated within the canister containing the carbon dioxide absorbent. (144; **193–194**)

78. Carbon dioxide absorbent granules change color from colorless to violet with use as a result of the pH indicator dye ethyl violet that is added to the granules. The indicator dye changes from colorless to violet in response to the carbonic acids that are formed by the neutralization reaction of the absorbent granules. This provides the anesthesiologist with an indication of how many of the granules have been exhausted by neutralization reactions with carbon dioxide. (144; **193–194**)

79. A maximum volume of 26 L of carbon dioxide can be absorbed per 100 g of absorbent granules. (144; **193–194**)

80. The passage of exhaled gases through pathways of low resistance in the carbon dioxide canister that results in granules being bypassed is termed *channeling*. This can result in absorbent granules never coming into contact with exhaled gases and in a decrease in the efficiency of carbon dioxide neutralization. (144; **193–194**)

81. The most frequent cause of channeling is loose packing of the carbon dioxide absorbent granules. Channeling can be minimized by shaking the canister gently before use. (144; **193–194**)

82. A potentially toxic interaction between the carbon dioxide absorbent and sevoflurane is the production of compound A. This can occur with either soda lime or baralyme, but the risk appears to be higher with baralyme. Other factors that may increase the risk of compound A production include the low inflow of fresh gases, high concentrations of sevoflurane, higher absorbent temperatures, and fresh absorbent. The concern with compound A is that it has been shown to be nephrotoxic in animals. Even so, no clinical cases of nephrotoxicity have occurred in humans, even with low gas inflows. (7, 144; **194–195**)

83. A potentially toxic interaction between the carbon dioxide absorbent and desflurane is the clinically significant production of carbon monoxide. Carboxyhemoglobin concentrations can reach as high as 30%. This can occur with either soda lime or baralyme, but the production of carbon monoxide appears to be greater with baralyme. Other factors that appear to increase the production of carbon monoxide include higher anesthetic concentrations, an increased

temperature, and greater dryness of the absorbent. The majority of cases of carbon monoxide toxicity occurred after 2 days of disuse of the absorbent, particularly with continued air flow through the circle system. The diagnosis is often difficult because the toxicity may be masked by the anesthesia itself and the pulse oximetry readings are likely to be unchanged. (6–7; **194–195**)

HUMIDIFICATION

84. Inhaled gases delivered to the patient can be humidified by the addition of water vapor to the gases. (144; **2405–2406**)

85. Inhaled gases are normally humidified in an awake patient breathing through his or her native airway by their passage through the nares, mouth, and trachea. The air becomes saturated with water vapor and is warmed to body temperature by the time it reaches the carina in these patients. (144; **2405–2406**)

86. The humidification of gases delivered to a patient from an anesthesia machine can be accomplished by the placement of specially designed humidifiers in the anesthetic breathing circuit. Humidification of inspired gases can also be achieved by the rebreathing of exhaled gases that have passed through the canister used for the neutralization of carbon dioxide. The water formed by the neutralization of carbon dioxide serves to humidify the gases passing through the canister. (144; **192–193**)

87. Benefits of the humidification of inspired gases include the preservation of respiratory epithelium from damage, the prevention of the drying of secretions, and the prevention of water and heat loss from the patient. This is especially important in pediatric patients in whom heat loss can occur rapidly under general anesthesia. (144, Fig. 11–11; **2405–2406**)

BACTERIAL CONTAMINATION OF ANESTHESIA EQUIPMENT

88. Anesthesia equipment is rarely implicated as a cause for respiratory infection because the environment in the anesthesia machine and anesthetic breathing system is an unsuitable host for organisms. Characteristics that make it unsuitable include the shifts in humidity and temperature, the presence of metallic ion metals, and the presence of oxygen. In addition, most of the anesthetic breathing systems are disposable. Nevertheless, the anesthesia machine and anesthetic breathing systems may still be sources of bacterial contamination to patients. (146)

89. During anesthesia it is infrequent that airborne bacteria from patients with known respiratory infections become transmitted to the anesthesia machine. This is because during anesthesia there is typically quiet breathing. In addition, oxygen even at low concentrations is often lethal to airborne bacteria. (146)

90. Maintenance of the anesthesia machine when used for a patient with suspected or known tuberculosis should include the use of filters during the use of the anesthesia machine, the disposing of the anesthesia breathing circuit after anesthesia, and disinfection of the nondisposable equipment before its use for another patient. (146–147; **2707–2709**)

POLLUTION OF THE ATMOSPHERE WITH ANESTHETIC GASES

91. The National Institute of Occupational Safety and Health recommends that the maximum atmospheric concentrations of nitrous oxide be lower than 22 parts per million (ppm), and volatile anesthetic atmospheric concentrations should be lower than 5 ppm. (146; **2701–2702**)

92. A concentration greater than 200 parts per million of nitrous oxide should alert personnel to examine the anesthesia machine for leaks. (146; **2701–2702**)

93. A high pressure leak of nitrous oxide may occur from the escape of the gas from nitrous oxide cylinders or from faulty tubing or connections used to connect the nitrous oxide from the central supply source to the pipeline inlets on the anesthesia machine. (143)

94. A low pressure leak of nitrous oxide may occur from the leakage of nitrous oxide from sites anywhere between and including the flowmeters and the patient. (143)

95. Potential spillage of anesthetic gases can be controlled by the periodic maintenance of anesthesia equipment, the scavenging of excess anesthetic gases, adequate ventilation in the operating rooms, and attention to anesthetic technique. A substantial source of anesthetic gas pollution in the operating room is when spillage occurs with filling of the anesthetic vaporizer. (143)

96. Gases are scavenged from the anesthesia breathing system at the adjustable pressure limiting valve. Gases that normally exit the anesthetic breathing system through this valve are captured by a slight suction device and usually delivered to a central vacuum system in the hospital for disposal. (143; **198–201, Fig. 7–25**)

Chapter 11

Tracheal Intubation

PREOPERATIVE EVALUATION

1. What are some things that should be considered in the preoperative evaluation of a patient's airway?

EXAMINATION FOR PREDICTING THE TECHNICAL EASE OF TRACHEAL INTUBATION

2. What examinations of the airway should be included in the preoperative evaluation to predict the technical ease of tracheal intubation?

3. How is the size of the tongue versus the size of the oropharyngeal cavity assessed? What are the Mallampati classifications of airways that may be assigned to the patient based on this examination? Which classes are correlated with a poor laryngoscopic (grade III or grade IV) view?

4. How is the degree of atlanto-occipital joint extension assessed? What degree of atlanto-occipital joint extension is correlated with a poor laryngoscopic (grade III or grade IV) view?

5. How is the anterior mandibular space assessed? What are some patient physical characteristics that would result in a short thyromental distance? What thyromental distance is correlated with a poor laryngoscopic (grade III or grade IV) view?

6. Why is a preoperative dental examination important to include during assessment of the airway? What should be included in the preoperative dental examination? What finding on the preoperative dental examination may indicate that direct laryngoscopy may be difficult?

INDICATIONS FOR OROTRACHEAL INTUBATION

7. Name some absolute indications for orotracheal intubation during surgery.

TECHNIQUE FOR OROTRACHEAL INTUBATION

8. What are some equipment and drugs the anesthesiologist should have available for orotracheal intubation of the trachea via the direct laryngoscopy approach?

9. How should the patient's head be positioned to facilitate orotracheal intubation of the trachea via direct laryngoscopy? What is the advantage of placing the patient's head in this position?

10. How does extension of the head without raising the head off the bed misalign the oral, pharyngeal, and laryngeal axes?

11. What should the height of the operating room table be to facilitate orotracheal intubation of the trachea via direct laryngoscopy?

12. What is cricoid pressure? When should it be applied?

13. How should the laryngoscope be manipulated during direct laryngoscopy? Describe the procedure for direct laryngoscopy.

14. Where should the curved MacIntosh blade be placed during direct laryngoscopy? What size MacIntosh blade is used for most adult patients?

15. What are some advantages of the MacIntosh blade over other laryngoscope blades for direct laryngoscopy?

16. Where should the straight (Jackson-Wisconsin or Miller) blade be placed during direct laryngoscopy? What size straight blade is used for most adult patients?

17. What are some advantages of the straight blade over other laryngoscope blades for direct laryngoscopy?

18. What are some characteristics of an endotracheal tube? What size endotracheal tube is typically used in adult patients?

19. What are some purposes of the cuff at the end of the endotracheal tube? How is the risk of tracheal mucosa ischemia secondary to the cuff pressure minimized?

20. How should placement of the endotracheal tube during direct laryngoscopy be executed?

21. How is inflation of the cuff of the endotracheal tube after placement confirmed?

22. Name at least five ways to confirm tracheal placement of the endotracheal tube. Which sign may be the most reliable confirmation of tube placement?

23. What is the typical depth of insertion of an endotracheal tube for midtracheal position in a man? What is the typical depth of insertion of an endotracheal tube for midtracheal position in a woman?

24. Why is it important to grade the airway with respect to the degree of visualization of the glottic opening that was achieved with direct laryngoscopy?

25. With what approximate frequency does a grade III airway occur? With what approximate frequency does a grade IV airway occur?

26. If intubation of the trachea via direct laryngoscopy is not possible, how should the anesthesiologist proceed?

ALTERNATIVES TO OROTRACHEAL INTUBATION DURING GENERAL ANESTHESIA

27. Name some alternatives to orotracheal intubation via direct laryngoscopy for intubation of the trachea.

28. What are some conditions in which an awake tracheal intubation may be preferred? What are some advantages to an awake tracheal intubation?

29. Describe the procedure for orotracheal intubation in an awake patient.

30. What are some ways in which the awake patient's airway may be anesthetized for awake orotracheal intubation?

31. What are some possible indications for an awake nasotracheal intubation under fiberoptic guidance?

32. What preparations should be made before initiating the procedure for awake nasotracheal intubation under fiberoptic guidance? Describe the procedure for an awake nasotracheal intubation under fiberoptic guidance.

33. How does the ease of fiberoptic guidance of nasotracheal intubation compare with the ease of fiberoptic guidance of orotracheal intubation? Why?

34. What are some advantages of nasotracheal intubation versus orotracheal intubation?

35. What are some complications that are unique to nasotracheal intubation? What are some contraindications to nasotracheal intubation?

36. What is the Bullard intubating laryngoscope? When might it be useful?

37. What is the lightwand or lighted stylet? When might it be useful?

38. What are some methods by which nasotracheal intubation of the awake patient might be achieved?

39. When might an awake blind nasotracheal intubation be considered? Describe the procedure for an awake blind nasotracheal intubation.

40. When might nasotracheal intubation under general anesthesia be considered? Describe the procedure for a nasotracheal intubation under general anesthesia.

41. What is the laryngeal mask airway? Describe the procedure for placement of a laryngeal mask airway.

42. What are some situations in which a laryngeal mask airway might be useful?

43. What are some advantages to the laryngeal mask airway?

44. What are some disadvantages to the laryngeal mask airway?

45. Describe the use of the laryngeal mask airway as a conduit for tracheal intubation.

46. When might a cuffed oropharyngeal airway be useful?

UNANTICIPATED DIFFICULT AIRWAY MANAGEMENT

47. What should be done in the event of inability to perform direct laryngoscopy?

48. What defines difficult mask ventilation?

49. What defines difficult tracheal intubation via direct laryngoscopy?

50. What are some alternatives for the immediate oxygenation of a hypoxic patient in whom attempts at tracheal intubation and mask ventilation have failed?

OROTRACHEAL INTUBATION IN CHILDREN

51. What are anatomic differences between the airways of children and adults?

52. What age of pediatric patient does not require a cuffed endotracheal tube? Why?

53. Why is the correct selection of tracheal tube size especially important in pediatric patients? What is a commonly used formula for the selection of endotracheal tube size in pediatric patients?

54. How is the correct selection of tracheal tube size confirmed after tracheal intubation of pediatric patients?

55. Why is careful depth of insertion of the endotracheal tube especially important in pediatric patients?

56. Anesthesia is not required for orotracheal intubation until what age?

57. What type of laryngoscope blade is most frequently used for direct laryngoscopy in the pediatric population? Why?

EXTUBATION OF THE TRACHEA

58. What equipment and supplies must be available to the anesthesiologist during extubation of the trachea of a patient?

59. Describe the procedure for extubation of the trachea while the patient is still deeply

anesthetized. What patients may be candidates for this method of extubation of the trachea? In which patients is this method of extubation of the trachea contraindicated?

60. Describe the procedure for an awake extubation of the trachea. In which patients is an awake extubation of the trachea indicated?

61. What is the purpose of suctioning of the oropharynx before the extubation of the trachea?

62. What is the purpose of placing positive pressure on the reservoir bag simultaneous to extubation of the trachea?

63. Name some potential hazards of extubation of the trachea.

COMPLICATIONS OF TRACHEAL INTUBATION

64. Name some potential complications of tracheal intubation.

65. What is the most frequent complication of direct laryngoscopy?

66. Should dislodgment of a tooth occur during direct laryngoscopy what measures should be taken by the anesthesiologist?

67. What level of anesthesia places the patient most at risk for laryngospasm after extubation of the trachea? How should laryngospasm be treated?

68. Which patient population is most likely to have symptomatic laryngeal or subglottic edema after extubation of the trachea? Why? What can be done to minimize this risk?

69. How should symptomatic laryngeal or subglottic edema after extubation of the trachea be treated?

70. What is the most common complication of prolonged intubation of the trachea?

ANSWERS*

PREOPERATIVE EVALUATION

1. In addition to the routine airway examination, things that should be considered in the preoperative evaluation of the patient's airway include the route of intubation of the trachea appropriate for the surgery and the method by which intubation of the trachea will take place. Other things that should be considered include a history of difficulties with airway management during previous anesthesias, a history of obstructive sleep apnea, and a dental examination. (148; **1417–1419**)

EXAMINATION FOR PREDICTING THE TECHNICAL EASE OF TRACHEAL INTUBATION

2. Airway examinations that should be performed preoperatively to predict the technical ease of tracheal intubation include the Mallampati examination in which the oropharyngeal cavity is assessed, an evaluation of the degree of

---

*Numbers in parentheses: lightface numbers refer to pages, figures, or tables in Stoelting RK, Miller RD: Basics of Anesthesia, 4th ed. Philadelphia, Churchill Livingstone, 2000; **boldface numbers** refer to pages, figures, and tables in Miller RD: Anesthesia, 5th ed. Philadelphia, Churchill Livingstone, 2000.

atlanto-occipital joint extension, and an evaluation of the anterior mandibular space. (148; **1417–1419, Figs. 39–1, 39–2**)

3. The size of the tongue versus the size of the oropharyngeal cavity is assessed visually. The patient is asked to open the mouth the maximal extent while sitting upright in a chair. The head should remain in the neutral position, the tongue should be maximally protruded, and the patient should not phonate. The initial evaluation should be of the degree of mouth opening. The adult mouth should be able to open by at least 40 mm between the upper and lower incisors. Most adults are able to open their mouths 50 to 60 mm. Next, the determination of the Mallampati classification should be made. The Mallampati classification of the patient's airway is based on the degree of visualization of the physiologic structures of the airway. A class I airway is assigned to patients whose entire uvula is visible. A class II airway is assigned to patients whose soft palate and entire uvula are visible but the tonsillar pillars are hidden by the tongue. A class III airway is assigned to patients whose uvula is only partially visible as well as the soft palate. A class IV airway is assigned to patients in whom only the hard palate is visible. Mallampati class III and IV airways are correlated with a poor laryngoscopic (grade III or grade IV) view. The Mallampati classification of the patient's airway is thus a predictor for patients whose anatomy may make intubation of the trachea by direct laryngoscopy technically difficult. (148–149, Figs. 12–1, 12–2; **1417–1419, Figs. 39–1, 39–2**)

4. The degree of atlanto-occipital joint extension is assessed by having the patient sit upright and extend the head on the atlanto-occipital joint to their maximum capacity. Extension of the atlanto-occipital joint by less than 10 degrees is correlated with a poor laryngoscopic (grade III or grade IV) view. The normal degree of extension of the atlanto-occipital joint is approximately 35 degrees. (149, Fig. 12–3; **1417–1419, Fig. 39–3**)

5. The anterior mandibular space is assessed by having the patient maximally extend the head while in the supine position. The distance from the notch of the thyroid cartilage to the tip of the mentum is measured. This distance is commonly referred to as the thyromental distance. A patient with a receding mandible or short muscular neck may have a short thyromental distance. A thyromental distance less than 6 cm is correlated with a large tongue in relation to pharyngeal size and a poor laryngoscopic (grade III or grade IV) view. (149–150, Fig. 12–5; **1417–1419**)

6. The objectives of a preoperative dental examination are to evaluate for any loose teeth, chipped teeth, missing teeth, or any fixed or removable dental prosthetics. Also an important part of the dental assessment is evaluating for any prominent or protuberant teeth that may make direct laryngoscopy difficult. Documentation of the findings on the preoperative dental examination is important so dental abnormalities discovered postoperatively are not erroneously attributed to damage from direct laryngoscopy. (150–151; **1417**)

INDICATIONS FOR OROTRACHEAL INTUBATION

7. Absolute indications for orotracheal intubation during surgery include the prevention of the aspiration of gastric contents or blood in a patient considered to be at risk for this, the need for frequent suctioning, the facilitation of positive pressure ventilation of the lungs, an operative site near or involving the upper airway, an operative position other than supine, and the maintenance of a patent airway. (151; **1425, Table 39–4**)

TECHNIQUE FOR OROTRACHEAL INTUBATION

8. Some equipment the anesthesiologist should have available for orotracheal intubation via the direct laryngoscopy approach includes an endotracheal tube,

a laryngoscope, suction, and the equipment necessary to administer positive pressure ventilation of the lungs with oxygen. Drugs the anesthesiologist should have available for orotracheal intubation include intravenous anesthetic agents and a neuromuscular blocking drug. (151; **1425**)

9. The patient's head should be positioned in a manner that facilitates orotracheal intubation via direct laryngoscopy, often called the sniff position because it simulates the position of a dog's head while sniffing. The sniff position is one in which the patient's head is elevated off the bed by 8 to 10 cm while the shoulders remain on the bed. The head is then extended at the atlanto-occipital joint. The advantage of placing the patient's head in this position for direct laryngoscopy is that it aligns oral, pharyngeal, and laryngeal axes such that there is nearly a straight line from the incisor teeth to the glottic opening. (151, Fig. 12–3; **1430, Figs. 39–3, 39–17**)

10. Extension of the patient's head without elevating the head off the bed does not properly position the patient's head for endotracheal intubation via direct laryngoscopy. This position instead increases the distance from the lips to the glottic opening, anteriorly rotates the larynx, and may lead to the need to lever on the maxillary teeth to gain a view of the glottic opening. (151; **1431**)

11. The operating room table should be at a height such that orotracheal intubation via direct laryngoscopy is facilitated. The optimal height is one that places the face of the patient at the level of the anesthesiologist's xiphoid process. (151)

12. Cricoid pressure, also called Sellick's maneuver, is the application of approximately 5 kg of pressure on the cricoid cartilage by an assistant to the anesthesiologist. Cricoid pressure occludes the esophagus and may prevent the regurgitation of gastric contents during the time between the induction of anesthesia and intubation of the trachea when the airway is not protected. It is important that the assistant not release cricoid pressure until instructed to do so by the anesthesiologist. This should only occur after successful intubation of the trachea has been confirmed by at least two methods. Cricoid pressure does not guarantee that the aspiration of gastric contents will not occur. Indeed, aspiration has occurred despite the correct application of cricoid pressure. Cricoid pressure may also be used to improve the anesthesiologist's view of the larynx during direct laryngoscopy. (151–152, Fig. 12–6; **1432**)

13. The laryngoscope should be held in the left hand of the anesthesiologist. The blade should be placed on the right side of the open mouth of the patient and moved to midline while sweeping the patient's tongue to the left. The patient's tongue should then lie between the patient's left cheek and the long axis of the blade of the laryngoscope. The laryngoscope blade should then be moved toward the epiglottis until the epiglottis is visualized. Once the epiglottis is visualized the anesthesiologist should properly place the laryngoscope relative to the epiglottis depending on the laryngoscope blade being used, and the laryngoscope and hand together as a unit should lift upward and outward at an approximate 45-degree angle in one single motion. The glottic opening should then be visible, and the anesthesiologist should be able to proceed with endotracheal intubation. An attempt should be made by the anesthesiologist to avoid pressure on the patient's teeth, lips, or gums throughout the procedure. (152, Fig. 12–7; **1430–1432, Fig. 39–16**)

14. During direct laryngoscopy, proper placement of the curved MacIntosh blade is with the tip of the blade in the vallecula. The vallecula is the space between the tongue and epiglottis. Visualization of the glottic opening is achieved by stretching the hypoepiglottic ligament with the tip of the laryngoscope blade. A size 3 MacIntosh blade is used for most adult patients. (152–153, Fig. 12–8; **1430–1432, Fig. 39–18**)

15. Advantages of the MacIntosh blade over other laryngoscope blades for direct laryngoscopy include less trauma to teeth, the creation of more room in the mouth to allow for the passage of the endotracheal tube, and less bruising of the epiglottis. (152–153; **1427–1428**)

16. During direct laryngoscopy proper placement of the straight (Jackson-Wisconsin or Miller) blade is with the tip of the blade beyond the epiglottis between the epiglottis and larynx. When the straight laryngoscope blade is lifted, the epiglottis is one of the structures lifted by the blade. A size 2 or 3 straight blade is used for most adult patients. (153, Fig. 12–8; **1430–1432, Fig. 39–18**)

17. Advantages of the straight blade over other laryngoscope blades for direct laryngoscopy include a straighter line of visualization, better exposure of the glottic opening, easier visualization of an anterior larynx, and easier visualization of the larynx in children. (153; **1427–1428**)

18. Endotracheal tubes are characterized by their internal diameter, shape, and whether there is a cuff built into the distal end. They are available in various sizes in increments of 0.5 mm internal diameter. An endotracheal tube with an internal diameter between 7.0 mm and 8.5 mm is typically used in adult patients. Endotracheal tubes can be shaped differently from the regular slightly curved shape to facilitate their positioning in a manner that will not interfere with the surgeon's work, as in otolaryngologic procedures. Endotracheal tubes are made of polyvinyl chloride that is tested to be free of toxins or irritants. In addition, the polyvinyl chloride molds to the shape of the airway on warming to body temperature. The tubes are made to be transparent for visualization through the tube, and a radiopaque line enables the clinician to visualize the endotracheal tube and its placement on a radiograph. (150, Fig. 12–9, Table 12–1; **1425–1427, Fig. 39–14**)

19. The cuff at the end of the endotracheal tube is designed to create a seal in the trachea. The seal facilitates positive pressure of the lungs as well as decreasing the risk of the aspiration of any oral or gastric contents. The endotracheal tube cuffs are designed to be low pressure/large volume. With insufflation of air in the endotracheal tube cuff the pressure on the tracheal wall is distributed over a larger area, minimizing the risk of excessive pressures on a small portion of the tracheal mucosa. This helps minimize the risk of tracheal mucosa ischemia secondary to prolonged endotracheal tube cuff pressure. Furthermore, the cuff on the endotracheal tube can be inflated until there is just enough air in the cuff to prevent air from leaking around the cuff during positive pressure ventilation of the lungs. The minimum pressure exerted on the tracheal mucosa that still does not allow air to leak during positive pressure ventilation of the lungs has been shown to be less than the perfusion pressure of the tracheal mucosa. Nevertheless, ciliary denudation has been seen to occur within only 2 hours of placement of an endotracheal tube. (153–154; **1425–1427**)

20. The endotracheal tube that is being placed during direct laryngoscopy should be held in the anesthesiologist's right hand, advanced in the right side of the mouth, passed through the vocal cords, and advanced another 1 to 2 cm in the adult person's trachea. The laryngoscope blade should then be removed, the cuff inflated, and the position confirmed. (154; **1430–1432**)

21. Confirmation of endotracheal tube cuff inflation can be achieved by assessing the tension of the small pilot balloon attached to the cuff. (154; **1427**)

22. Signs confirming tracheal placement of the endotracheal tube include symmetric, bilateral chest movement with positive pressure ventilation of the lungs, symmetric, bilateral breath sounds with positive pressure ventilation of the lungs, a characteristic feel of normal pulmonary airway resistance with manual ventilation of the lungs with a reservoir bag, condensation of water vapor in the

endotracheal tube, external palpation of the cuff of the endotracheal tube in the suprasternal notch, an adequately maintained oxygen saturation by pulse oximetry, and the detection of exhaled carbon dioxide with an end-tidal P_{CO_2} exceeding 30 mm Hg for each breath by capnography or mass spectrometry for at least 5 breaths. The exhaled carbon dioxide sign is probably the most reliable confirmatory sign of appropriate placement of the endotracheal tube. (154)

23. The typical depth of insertion of an endotracheal tube for the midtracheal position in a man and woman is 23 cm and 21 cm at the patient's teeth, respectively. (154; **1431–1432, Fig. 39–20, Table 39–5**)

24. It is important to grade the patient's airway based on how much of the glottic opening was able to be visualized during direct laryngoscopy after direct laryngoscopy has been completed. This information should be documented because it is valuable information for anesthesiologists who may need to intubate the trachea of the patient at a later date. Documentation should include not only the grade view of the airway but also which laryngoscope blade or blades were used for direct laryngoscopy. Conventionally, the patient's airway has been divided into grades I to IV. A grade I airway is one in which the entire glottic opening is visualized with ease. A grade II airway is one in which visualization of just the posterior portion of the glottic opening is possible. A grade III airway is one in which only the epiglottis is able to be visualized. A grade IV airway is one in which the soft palate is the only structure able to be visualized. (155–156, Fig. 12–2; **1433, Fig. 39–21**)

25. A grade III airway occurs in 1% to 4% of patients. This grade view historically may require multiple attempts and blades and may or may not lead to successful intubation of the trachea via direct laryngoscopy. A grade IV airway occurs in less than 0.35% of patients and represents a majority of the patients in whom direct laryngoscopy failed to lead to endotracheal intubation. (156; **1433**)

26. If intubation of the trachea via direct laryngoscopy is not possible, the anesthesiologist must consider different approaches to securing the airway. The approach to secure the patient's airway must take into consideration the condition of the patient and the urgency of the procedure. Typically, the patient will be allowed to awaken after failed intubation of his or her trachea and the airway is secured with the patient awake. (156; **1433–1436, Figs. 39–22, 39–23**)

ALTERNATIVES TO OROTRACHEAL INTUBATION DURING GENERAL ANESTHESIA

27. Alternatives to orotracheal intubation for intubation of the trachea include awake and asleep orotracheal intubation with fiberoptic guidance, awake and asleep nasotracheal intubation with fiberoptic guidance, awake blind nasotracheal intubation of the trachea, asleep nasotracheal intubation by direct laryngoscopy, the placement of laryngeal mask airway, and tracheostomy. (157)

28. An awake tracheal intubation may be preferred when attempts at intubation of the trachea by direct laryngoscopy, either past or present, have failed. Advantages to an awake tracheal intubation over asleep intubation are that spontaneous ventilation of the lungs, laryngeal reflexes, and the natural skeletal muscle tone of the airway will all be maintained. The maintained tone allows for better separation of the structures and easier identification of the important landmarks of the airway. Finally, the larynx stays in a more posterior position when the patient is awake, making access to it easier. (157; **1437–1438**)

29. Two preparatory things must be fulfilled before orotracheal intubation in an awake patient. First, the patient must have an understanding of what is to occur

and why it is to occur and must agree to cooperate. Second, the patient's airway must be adequately anesthetized. Anesthetizing the airway may be done in conjunction with intravenous sedation that still allows the patient to be oriented and cooperative. After these, the patient's trachea may be intubated via either direct laryngoscopy or with fiberoptic guidance. Care must be taken to be gentle with the patient, and continual conversation with the patient is preferred. (157; **1437–1438**)

30. Anesthesia for intubation of the awake patient's trachea may involve topical anesthesia, nerve blocks, intravenous drying agents, and intravenous sedation. Topical anesthesia can be achieved with pledgets or an atomizer delivering 4% lidocaine. The patient may inhale or gargle the solution to anesthetize the laryngeal structures. The delivery of the topical anesthetic should advance progressively farther toward the larynx. If the nasal approach to the trachea is chosen, 0.25% to 0.5% phenylephrine should be added to the lidocaine to vasoconstrict the nasal passage and minimize bleeding. Long cotton-tipped applicators soaked with the solution can be used as well as pledgets to introduce the lidocaine/phenylephrine topical anesthetic to the nasopharynx. Alternatively, 4% cocaine may be used to topically anesthetize these areas. Cocaine will provide anesthesia as well as vasoconstriction. The total dose of cocaine administered should not exceed 3 mg/kg.

There are several nerve blocks that can be used to anesthetize the awake patient's airway. A transtracheal block anesthetizes the trachea below the area of the vocal cords. The transtracheal block is done by injecting 2 to 3 mL of lidocaine through the cricothyroid membrane with a 23-gauge needle after confirmation of needle placement in the trachea with the aspiration of air. The transtracheal block is contraindicated in patients with a local pathologic process or a coagulopathy. A superior laryngeal nerve block anesthetizes the nerves that supply the epiglottis, aryepiglottic folds, and the laryngeal structures down to the false cords. In patients with a coagulopathy, local pathologic process, or a full stomach this nerve block is contraindicated. The superior laryngeal nerve block can be achieved by injecting 2 to 3 mL of lidocaine between the greater cornu of the hyoid bone and the thyroid cartilage with a 23-gauge needle. A glossopharyngeal nerve block anesthetizes the posterior tongue and may be done in patients in whom an awake direct laryngoscopy will be performed. A glossopharyngeal nerve block can be achieved by injecting 2 mL of lidocaine in the base of the tongue in the area where the tongue opposes the palatoglossal fold. This block is safe in patients with a full stomach, because laryngeal reflexes are preserved. An intravenous drying agent commonly used in preparation of an awake intubation of the patient's trachea is glycopyrrolate at a dose of 0.2 mg. This helps reduce secretions that may otherwise obscure the anesthesiologist's view. Intravenous sedation must be sufficient for patient comfort while still preserving airway reflexes and an ability to communicate with the anesthesiologist. (157, Fig. 12–12; **1437–1440, 1541–1543, Figs. 39–27, 43–23, 43–24**)

31. Possible indications for an awake nasotracheal intubation under fiberoptic guidance include upper airway obstruction as from tumor, abscess, or prior surgery, a mediastinal mass, subglottic stenosis, congenital airway abnormalities, and an immobile cervical vertebrae. (158; **1442–1443**)

32. An awake nasotracheal intubation under fiberoptic guidance begins with discussion with the patient, preparation of the selected naris, sedating the patient, drying the patient's secretions, and anesthetizing the airway. Secretions and blood may obscure the visual field through the fiberoptic laryngoscope to the extent that the fiberoptic guidance of tracheal intubation becomes impossible. Specific preparations for the fiberoptic laryngoscope include focusing the image, defogging the lens of the scope, and lubricating the laryngoscope along its length to facilitate its passage through the endotracheal tube. The procedure for

fiberoptic nasotracheal intubation begins with placing the endotracheal tube in the selected naris and advancing the tube toward the glottic opening. The fiberoptic laryngoscope is advanced through the tube and, after visualization of the vocal cords, passed through the vocal cords to the trachea. The presence of tracheal rings on the posterior portion of the trachea confirms appropriate placement. The endotracheal tube is then advanced through the cords into the trachea with the guidance of the laryngoscope. (157–158, Fig. 12–13; **1442–1443**)

33. The fiberoptic guidance of nasotracheal intubation is technically easier than the fiberoptic guidance of orotracheal intubation. With nasotracheal intubation the fiberoptic scope in the nasopharynx is in alignment with the vocal cords and often merely needs advancement to visualize the cords. In contrast, the oropharynx is not in direct alignment and fiberoptic scope advancement often requires guidance with an oropharyngeal airway or downward displacement of the tongue. Alternatively, a laryngeal mask airway may be placed and used as a channel through which fiberoptic guidance of orotracheal intubation may take place. (158; **1422, 1442–1443, Fig. 39–12**)

34. Advantages of nasotracheal intubation versus orotracheal intubation include a more direct alignment between the direction in which the endotracheal tube is advanced into the pharynx and its passage into the larynx, more stable tube fixation, less chance for tube kinking, greater comfort in awake patients, and fewer oropharyngeal secretions. Nasotracheal intubation is typically performed in patients with anatomic abnormalities by disease or otherwise, patients who will be having intraoral procedures, or patients who are expected to have prolonged intubation of the trachea. (159; **1430**)

35. Complications that are unique to nasotracheal intubation include epistaxis, dislodgment of the adenoids, eustachian tube obstruction, gastric distention due to air swallowing, bacteremia, and maxillary sinusitis. The incidence of sinusitis appears to be increased after 5 days of nasotracheal intubation, and prophylactic antibiotics are indicated for patients in whom endocarditis is a risk. Contraindications to a nasotracheal intubation include coagulopathy, severe intranasal pathology, basilar skull fracture, and the presence of cerebrospinal fluid leakage. (159; **1430**)

36. The Bullard intubating laryngoscope is a rigid fiberoptic laryngoscope blade that is shaped to facilitate the passage of an endotracheal tube through a visualized glottic opening. The Bullard laryngoscope is useful in patients in whom extension of the atlanto-occipital joint is limited or who have limited mouth opening. (159, Fig. 12–15)

37. The lightwand or lighted stylet is a flexible stylet with a light at the distal end that can be placed in the lumen of the endotracheal tube during direct laryngoscopy. The transillumination of the soft tissues of the neck may be used to assist in guiding the endotracheal tube through the vocal cords. The lightwand may be useful in patients whose anatomy makes it difficult to intubate the trachea during direct laryngoscopy. (160, Fig. 12–16)

38. Methods by which nasotracheal intubation of the awake patient might be achieved include a blind nasal procedure, nasotracheal intubation with direct laryngoscopy and Magill forceps, and under fiberoptic guidance. (159; **1430, 1432–1433**)

39. An awake blind nasotracheal intubation is typically performed in patients in whom it appears visualization of the glottic opening via direct laryngoscopy and ventilation of the lungs would be difficult, making the induction of anesthesia a possible hazard. To perform an awake blind nasotracheal intubation the patient must be cooperative and must have adequate topical anesthesia of the selected

naris. The endotracheal tube is then advanced via the naris toward the glottic opening and, on inspiration or panting, the tube is quickly advanced past the vocal cords into the trachea. Confirmation of appropriate tube placement is with the auscultation of breath sounds through the tube, or, if a reservoir bag is attached, appropriate bag movement with spontaneous ventilation. With the cuff of the endotracheal tube inflated, an awake patient whose trachea is intubated is not usually able to phonate. (160; **1441**)

40. Nasotracheal intubation under general anesthesia may be considered for patients in whom the loss of laryngeal reflexes is not contraindicated and it is expected to be possible to ventilate the lungs manually with a mask. The procedure for a nasotracheal intubation under general anesthesia begins the same as that of orotracheal intubation under general anesthesia, with the additional step of preparing the naris to prevent epistaxis. After the induction of anesthesia, the endotracheal tube is advanced through the selected, prepared naris to just before the glottic opening. With direct laryngoscopy to visualize the glottic opening, and if necessary the use of a Magill forceps to assist in directing the endotracheal tube, the tube may then be advanced past the vocal cords into the trachea. (160; **1432–1433**)

41. The laryngeal mask airway may be used as an alternative to intubation of the trachea. It is a shallow mask that is inserted into the laryngeal inlet and inflated to mold to the patient's airway anatomy and provide a seal. The inflatable mask of the laryngeal mask airway is connected to a tube that may connect directly to the anesthesia breathing system on the anesthesia machine. Positive pressure ventilation of the lungs may be provided with a laryngeal mask airway to airway pressures not to exceed 15 cm H_2O. There are various sizes of laryngeal mask airways, such that they can be used in children. Placement of a laryngeal mask airway is usually done in patients after an intravenous induction dose of anesthesia. The head should be placed in the position appropriate for direct laryngoscopy. The laryngeal mask is then introduced into the oropharynx and advanced along the superior portion of the oropharynx and posterior pharynx until it is seated in the laryngeal inlet. It is then inflated with the appropriate volume of air, which causes the laryngeal mask to move outward slightly. Confirmation of appropriate placement should be done by auscultation and visualization of chest rise with the administration of positive pressure to the lungs. (161–162, Figs. 12–17, 12–18, 12–19, 12–20; **1422–1424, Figs. 39–9, 39–10, 39–11**)

42. A laryngeal mask airway is useful under conditions in which ventilation of the lungs with a mask is acceptable. It may also be useful in patients in whom tracheal intubation via direct laryngoscopy and ventilation by mask have been proven to be difficult. Tracheal intubation with fiberoptic guidance via an appropriately placed laryngeal mask is also a potential use of the laryngeal mask airway. (161; **1422–1423, 1436, Fig. 39–12**)

43. Advantages to the laryngeal mask airway are that it provides an adequate airway for spontaneous ventilation of the lungs of an anesthetized patient without necessitating the use of the anesthesiologist's hands as does a mask and without the trauma and complications associated with intubation of the trachea. Patients may tolerate the laryngeal mask airway at lower levels of anesthesia than those required when the patient's trachea is intubated. (161; **1422–1423**)

44. Disadvantages to the laryngeal mask airway include its lack of protection of the patient's airway from aspiration or laryngospasm, the need for extension of the neck for placement, and the inability to provide positive pressure ventilation of the lungs with peak inspiratory pressures greater than 15 cm H_2O. (161–162; **1422–1423**)

45. The laryngeal mask airway can be used as a conduit for tracheal intubation. The endotracheal tube must fit through the lumen of the laryngeal mask airway

and protrude sufficiently from its distal end. For these reasons, a 6.0 microlaryngeal endotracheal tube is best selected for this purpose. The tube can then be advanced to the trachea under fiberoptic guidance. Once the trachea has been successfully intubated, the laryngeal mask airway may be left in place but deflated until the conclusion of the procedure. Alternatively, a tube changer may be used if removal of the laryngeal mask airway is desired. (162; **1422–1423, 1436, Fig. 39–12**)

46. A cuffed oropharyngeal airway, when properly placed with the cuff inflated, provides for forward displacement of the patient's tongue. The cuffed oropharyngeal airway also has a connector on its end to allow attachment to the anesthetic breathing system. Thus, this airway device might be useful in situations similar to those in which a laryngeal mask airway is useful. (162)

UNANTICIPATED DIFFICULT AIRWAY MANAGEMENT

47. In the event of inability to perform direct laryngoscopy after several attempts with different laryngoscope blades, the anesthesiologist should call for help while devising an alternative plan. Airway trauma from recurrent attempts should be avoided. If mask ventilation of the lungs is not possible, alternative methods to avoid morbidity should be instituted. The American Society of Anesthesiologists has endorsed a difficult airway algorithm to follow in such cases. (163; **1433–1434, Fig. 39–22**)

48. Difficult mask ventilation is defined as the inability to maintain arterial oxygenation greater than 90% or the inability of the anesthesiologist alone to reverse the signs of unsuccessful ventilation. These may include lack of chest movement, gastric dilation, cardiopulmonary alterations, and cyanosis. (163)

49. Difficult tracheal intubation via direct laryngoscopy is defined as the inability of the anesthesiologist to perform tracheal intubation via direct laryngoscopy in three attempts, or when successful tracheal intubation requires more than 10 minutes. (163)

50. Oxygen can be supplied through a catheter or airway placed directly through the cricothyroid membrane. This is usually done under conditions in which attempts at intubation of the trachea and mask ventilation have failed. If the oxygen is supplied by a catheter the subsequent ventilation is termed *transtracheal jet ventilation,* because it requires a jet ventilator to provide for oxygen flow via the catheter. If this technique is instituted, intermittent disconnection of the catheter from the oxygen source may be necessary to facilitate passive exhalation of the lungs and to avoid hypercarbia. Other risks of small transtracheal catheters for ventilation include displacement of the catheter and subcutaneous emphysema, pneumomediastinum, and barotrauma, making this technique serve only as a short-term solution. An alternative to transtracheal jet ventilation that avoids these risks is a cricothyrotomy. A cricothyrotomy is the creation of a translaryngeal airway through which a small endotracheal tube can be inserted. Its placement requires a scalpel, dilating stylet, and a wire. A cricothyrotomy is not a permanent solution but a temporizing measure until a tracheostomy can be performed. (163–164, Figs. 12–21, 12–22; **1436–1437, Figs. 39–25, 39–26**)

OROTRACHEAL INTUBATION IN CHILDREN

51. Anatomic differences between the airways of children and adults include a more highly arched palate, a larger tongue in comparison to the oral cavity, a longer, stiffer, U-shaped epiglottis, a more cephalad larynx, and more acutely angled vocal cords. The narrowest portion of the airway is at the cricoid cartilage. In

addition, neonates have a larger occiput and are obligate nose breathers. (164; **1443–1444**)

52. Pediatric patients generally do not require a cuffed endotracheal tube to seal the airway until after the age of 5. In patients younger than 5 years of age, the narrowest diameter of the airway occurs below the vocal cords and an adequate seal can be achieved with an appropriately sized endotracheal tube. (164; **1443–1444, 2103**)

53. The correct selection of tracheal tube size is especially important in pediatric patients because an endotracheal tube too large for the trachea may cause trauma to the larynx or trachea, whereas an endotracheal tube that is too small may not provide an adequate seal. A commonly used formula for selection of endotracheal tube size in pediatric patients is (16 + age)/4. (164; **1443–1444, Table 39–5**)

54. The correct selection of tracheal tube size for pediatric patients is confirmed after its placement by checking the pressure at which a leak will occur around the endotracheal tube when positive pressure is administered to the lungs. A leak should occur between 15 to 20 cm H_2O. (164; **1427, 1443–1444, 2103, Table 39–5**)

55. The careful depth of insertion of the endotracheal tube is especially important in pediatric patients because of the small margin of error between appropriate placement, endobronchial intubation, and extubation. (164; **1443–1444, 2103**)

56. Anesthesia is not required for orotracheal intubation in neonates younger than 2 weeks of age. (164; **1443–1444**)

57. The laryngoscope blade most frequently used for direct laryngoscopy in the pediatric population is a straight blade. The straight blade typically allows for better visualization of the glottis by directly picking up the epiglottis during direct laryngoscopy. Visualization of the glottic opening is especially easier with a straight laryngoscope blade in patients younger than 3 years of age. (164; **1443–1444**)

EXTUBATION OF THE TRACHEA

58. The equipment and supplies that must be available to the anesthesiologist during extubation of the trachea of a patient are the same as those used during intubation, because the anesthesiologist must always be prepared to re-intubate the trachea should it become necessary. (164; **1446**)

59. Extubation of the trachea while the patient is still deeply anesthetized requires the patient to not be at risk of aspiration and to be able to adequately ventilate the lungs spontaneously. The patient must also have an adequate level of anesthesia to prevent laryngospasm or coughing. With these criteria met, the oropharynx should be suctioned, positive pressure to the lungs applied, the pilot balloon deflated, and the endotracheal tube removed from the trachea. Patients who may be candidates for this method of extubation of the trachea are those in whom coughing or bucking on an endotracheal tube may be detrimental to the surgical procedure. Patients in whom intubation of the trachea or ventilation of the lungs with a mask was difficult, or who may have postoperative edema of the airway, are not appropriate candidates for extubation of the trachea while deeply anesthetized. (164; **1446**)

60. Awake extubation of the trachea necessitates both that the patient be able to adequately ventilate the lungs spontaneously and the removal of all anesthetics so that laryngeal reflexes have returned. Often the return of these reflexes is evidenced by the patient bucking or coughing with the tube in the trachea. When these criteria have been met, the oropharynx should be suctioned, positive

pressure to the lungs applied, the pilot balloon deflated, and the endotracheal tube removed from the trachea. Patients who are candidates for an awake extubation of the trachea include any patients in whom aspiration is a risk or patients in whom intubation of the trachea or ventilation of the lungs with a mask was difficult. These patients may also be extubated after a fiberoptic bronchoscope or airway exchange catheter has been placed in the trachea should tracheal reintubation be necessary. (164–165; **1446–1447**)

61. Suctioning of the oropharynx before extubation of the trachea minimizes the risk of pharyngeal secretions draining into the trachea after extubation. It also minimizes the risk of stimulation of the vocal cords from secretions causing laryngospasm after extubation. (164; **1447**)

62. Placing positive pressure on the reservoir bag simultaneous to extubation of the trachea results in exhalation after extubation, possibly facilitating the expulsion of secretions after extubation. (164; **1446**)

63. Potential hazards of extubation of the trachea include laryngospasm, vomiting, and aspiration. (165; **1446–1447**)

COMPLICATIONS OF TRACHEAL INTUBATION

64. There are numerous potential complications of tracheal intubation. Complications that may occur during direct laryngoscopy and intubation include dental and oral soft tissue damage, hypertension, tachycardia, myocardial ischemia, cardiac dysrhythmias, and aspiration. Complications that may occur while the tracheal tube is in place include tracheal tube obstruction, endobronchial intubation, esophageal intubation, tracheal tube cuff leak, barotrauma, disconnection from the breathing circuit, tracheal mucosa ischemia, and accidental extubation. Complications that may occur after extubation of the trachea include laryngospasm, aspiration, pharyngitis, laryngitis, laryngeal or subglottic edema, laryngeal ulceration, tracheitis, tracheal stenosis, vocal cord paralysis, and arytenoid cartilage dislocation. (165; **1444–1446**)

65. The most frequent complication of direct laryngoscopy is dental trauma. Dental trauma occurs in one in every 4500 anesthesias that involve upper airway management. Patients at the greatest risk of dental trauma are patients with poor dentition. (165; **1444**)

66. Dislodgment of a tooth during direct laryngoscopy requires that the tooth be recovered. If necessary, chest and abdomen radiographs must be obtained to ensure that the tooth was not aspirated or swallowed. (165; **1444**)

67. A light level of anesthesia places the patient most at risk for laryngospasm after extubation of the trachea. Laryngospasm should be treated with the application of positive pressure 100% oxygen via a face mask and a head-tilt/jaw-lift that displaces the mandible forward. If laryngospasm persists, the administration of succinylcholine may be necessary. (165; **1444–1445, 2183**)

68. Pediatric patients are most likely to have symptomatic laryngeal or subglottic edema after extubation of the trachea because a small degree of swelling may obstruct a significant portion of the airway. The subglottic area in these patients is the narrowest part of the pediatric patient's airway as well. To minimize the risk of laryngeal or subglottic edema after extubation of the trachea, an appropriately sized endotracheal tube as evidenced by the leak pressure should be chosen in pediatric patients. (165; **1445**)

69. Symptomatic laryngeal or subglottic edema after extubation of the trachea should be treated with warmed, humidified oxygen, nebulized racemic epinephrine, and intravenous corticosteroids if necessary. For severe, persistent, or

progressive obstruction, re-intubation of the trachea may be necessary. (161–162; **1432**)

70. The most common complication of prolonged intubation of the trachea is tracheal stenosis as an end result of damage to the tracheal mucosa. Tracheal stenosis that results in a tracheal lumen decrease to less than 5 mm causes symptoms for the patient. (162; **2192**)

Chapter *12*

Spinal and Epidural Anesthesia

1. What other terms are used to describe spinal and epidural anesthesia?

2. Where is medicine deposited in spinal anesthesia? In epidural anesthesia? In caudal anesthesia?

3. What are some advantages and disadvantages of spinal and epidural anesthesia?

4. What are some drugs that may be administered intravenously for sedation during regional anesthesia?

5. What are some fears and biases patients and surgeons may have concerning regional anesthesia?

6. How effective are opioids introduced into the epidural or subarachnoid space? What is this technique often used for?

ANATOMY

7. What is the number of each type of vertebrae in the vertebral column?

8. Describe the anatomic parts of a vertebra by answering the following questions: What are the two parts that make up a vertebra? From what parts of the vertebra does the transverse process arise? From what parts of the vertebra does the spinous process arise?

9. How is the spinous process oriented relative to the vertical axis of the upright patient in the lumbar region? In the thoracic region? What clinical implications does this have?

10. How are the laminae of adjacent vertebrae connected?

11. How are the posterior spinous processes of adjacent vertebrae connected?

12. How are the tips of the spinous processes of adjacent vertebrae connected?

13. What passes through the intervertebral foramina?

14. Where do the preganglionic nerves of the sympathetic nervous system originate from the spinal cord? What is their course of travel after leaving the spinal cord?

15. Where does the sympathetic chain extend? What are some nerve plexuses and ganglions the sympathetic chain gives rise to?

16. What are the contents of the spinal canal?

17. What are the cephalad and caudad limits of the spinal cord?

18. What is the cauda equina? Where does it extend?

19. Where is cerebrospinal fluid? What is another term for this space?

20. Where is the epidural space? What is it bound by?

21. What is the plica mediana dorsalis? What is its clinical significance?

22. What is contained in the epidural space?

PREOPERATIVE PREPARATION

23. How does a preoperative evaluation for a regional anesthetic differ from that for a general anesthetic?

24. When a patient does not want a regional anesthetic, how should the patient be convinced?

25. What are special considerations on the preoperative physical examination of a patient who is to undergo a regional anesthetic?

26. How should the coagulation status of a patient be determined before administering regional anesthesia? What is the risk of administering regional anesthesia to a patient who is anticoagulated?

27. When should a regional anesthetic be administered to a patient who is anticoagulated?

28. What is the recommendation with regard to regional anesthesia for patients who are to receive heparin or enoxaparin after surgery?

29. What are the risks of administering regional anesthesia to a patient who is septic?

30. What is the risk of administering regional anesthesia to a patient who is hypovolemic?

31. What are the goals of preoperative medication for a patient who is to undergo a regional anesthetic?

32. Why should an intravenous catheter be placed prior to the administration of a regional anesthetic?

33. How do the equipment, monitors, and drugs that the anesthesiologist has present for administering a general anesthetic differ from those present for administering a regional anesthetic?

SPINAL ANESTHESIA

34. What are some anatomic landmarks the anesthesiologist uses to administer a spinal anesthetic?

35. What vertebral level is crossed by a line drawn across the patient's back at the level of the top of the iliac crests? What interspace is represented directly above this line? What interspace is represented directly below this line?

36. What is the anatomic value of placing a spinal anesthetic at a level below L2?

37. What are the two most common positions the patient is placed in for the administration of a spinal anesthetic? What are the circumstances in which each may be preferred?

38. What equipment and drugs are typically prepackaged in a kit used for spinal anesthesia?

39. What preparations should be made to minimize infection when administering a spinal anesthetic?

40. How is the skin anesthetized before the introduction of the spinal needle?

41. How is the subarachnoid space located by the anesthesiologist?

42. What accounts for the "pop" the anesthesiologist may feel when advancing a spinal needle into the subarachnoid space?

43. How is subarachnoid placement of the spinal needle confirmed?

44. How should the spinal needle be handled by the anesthesiologist to stabilize the needle after proper placement into the subarachnoid space is confirmed?

45. After the syringe containing the local anesthetic solution for administration into the subarachnoid space is attached to the spinal needle, how can continued subarachnoid placement of the spinal needle be confirmed?

46. When blood-tinged cerebrospinal fluid initially flows from the spinal needle, should the anesthesiologist proceed?

47. What are some spinal needle types and sizes? What are their potential advantages and disadvantages?

48. What are some disadvantages to using a smaller-gauge spinal needle?

49. Describe the paramedian approach to a spinal anesthetic. When is this approach advantageous?

50. Describe the lumbosacral approach to a spinal anesthetic. When is this approach advantageous?

51. What are the three things that most influence the distribution of the local anesthetic solution in cerebrospinal fluid after its administration into the subarachnoid space?

52. What are the two things that most influence the duration of a spinal anesthetic?

53. What is the relative motor blockade versus sensory blockade that results from the administration of each local anesthetic for spinal anesthesia?

54. How do spinal anesthetics regress during the recovery from spinal anesthesia?

55. Please complete the following table of some local anesthetics used for spinal anesthesia:

LOCAL ANESTHETIC	CONCENTRATION (%)	T10 (mg)	T4 (mg)	VOLUME (mL)	ONSET (min)	NO EPI (duration min)	EPI (duration min)
Lidocaine							
Tetracaine							
Bupivacaine							
Ropivacaine							

56. How is the baricity of a local anesthetic solution to be administered into the subarachnoid space defined? Why is this clinically important?

57. What is the baricity of the most commonly used spinal anesthetics? What is added to local anesthetics for spinal anesthesia to make the solution hyperbaric?

58. How do hyperbaric solutions diffuse in the subarachnoid space?

59. Where would the resultant hyperbaric spinal anesthetic block be most dense for a patient seated upright and for a patient supine just after its administration?

60. What can be added to a local anesthetic solution to make it hypobaric?

61. How do hypobaric solutions diffuse in the subarachnoid space?

62. What type of procedures might make the administration of a hypobaric spinal anesthetic most convenient?

63. What local anesthetic is most commonly administered for isobaric spinal anesthesia?

64. What two vasoconstrictors can be added to local anesthetic solutions to prolong the duration of action of a spinal anesthetic?

65. What are the two ways in which vasoconstrictors are thought to prolong the duration of action of spinal anesthesia?

66. What is a concern regarding the addition of vasoconstrictors to local anesthetic solutions for spinal anesthesia?

67. Which local anesthetics are thought to show the greatest prolongation of duration of action when vasoconstrictors are added to the spinal local anesthetic solution?

68. What spinal dermatomal levels derive the most benefit from the addition of a vasoconstrictor to the spinal local anesthetic solution to prolong its duration of action?

69. How is a continuous spinal anesthetic performed? What are its potential advantages and disadvantages?

70. What is the temporal order of blockade of the motor, sensory, and sympathetic nerves after the administration of a spinal anesthetic? Given that, what is a useful way to gain an early indication of the level of spinal anesthesia?

71. From highest to lowest, what is the dermatomal order of blockade of the motor, sensory, and sympathetic nerves produced by a spinal anesthetic?

72. Explain in physiologic terms two reasons why sympathetic nerve fibers undergo conduction blockade from spinal anesthesia before sensory and motor fibers.

73. Name a useful test for the evaluation of the level of sympathetic nerve blockade.

74. Name a useful test for the evaluation of the level of sensory nerve blockade.

75. Name a useful test for the evaluation of the level of motor nerve blockade.

76. What are the physiologic effects on the respiratory system of an appropriately instituted spinal anesthetic?

77. What are some physiologic effects on the gastrointestinal tract that can result from a spinal anesthetic?

78. What are the physiologic effects on the genitourinary system of an appropriately instituted spinal anesthetic?

79. What is the adrenocortical response to painful stimulation in a patient when the surgical site has been anesthetized with spinal anesthesia?

80. What are some side effects associated with spinal anesthesia?

81. Explain in physiological terms some reasons why a patient may become hypotensive after the sympathetic nervous system blockade that results from the administration of a spinal anesthetic. Which of these is thought to predominate when the hypotension is modest? Which of these is thought to predominate when the hypotension is severe?

82. What influences the degree of hypotension that can occur with a spinal anesthetic?

83. What are two nonpharmacologic methods that can be used to treat the hypotension that can occur with a spinal anesthetic?

84. What pharmacologic methods can be used to treat the hypotension that can occur with a spinal anesthetic?

85. What are two potential benefits of the decrease in systemic vascular resistance that accompanies spinal anesthesia for the patient in the perioperative period?

86. Describe the hallmark features of a postdural puncture headache. Which feature of a headache must be present to qualify it as a postdural puncture headache?

87. Give a physiologic explanation for a postdural puncture headache.

88. What are the risk factors for a postdural puncture headache?

89. What are some conservative treatment methods for a postdural puncture headache?

90. How effective is an epidural blood patch for a postdural puncture headache? How is it thought to work?

91. Describe the epidural blood patch procedure.

92. How effective is the administration of saline in lieu of blood as an epidural patch in patients with postdural puncture headaches?

93. What is a total spinal? How does it present?

94. What is the physiologic explanation for the apnea that occurs with a total spinal? What level of a total spinal will begin to interfere with breathing?

95. What is the treatment for a total spinal?

96. What is the duration of a total spinal relative to the duration of the local anesthetic administered?

97. What are two possible causes of nausea that presents soon after the administration of a spinal anesthetic?

98. How can the nausea after the administration of a spinal anesthetic be treated?

99. Why might urinary retention occur after the administration of a spinal anesthetic?

100. Why might backache occur after the administration of a spinal anesthetic?

101. What are some possible causes of neurologic sequelae after a spinal anesthetic?

102. Why is it important to consult a neurologist when nerve injury presents after a spinal anesthetic?

103. What is transient radicular irritation? What are its risk factors?

104. What were the circumstances under which spinal anesthesia resulted in cauda equina syndrome? What is the explanation for its occurrence?

105. What is the incidence of paralysis with spinal anesthesia?

106. What is the difference in perioperative mortality in relatively healthy patients who underwent a scheduled elective surgery under spinal anesthesia versus those who had general anesthesia?

EPIDURAL ANESTHESIA

107. What is contained in the sterile, prepackaged kits for epidural anesthesia?

108. Describe the procedure for placing an epidural catheter for epidural anesthesia using the loss of resistance technique.

109. Why should the epidural catheter never be pulled back through the Tuohy needle?

110. What is the test dose for an epidural catheter? What is it testing for? How long must the anesthesiologist wait after administering the test dose to be sure the result is negative?

111. What would be seen as a result of the test dose if the epidural catheter were in an epidural vein?

112. What would be seen as a result of the test dose if the epidural catheter were in the subarachnoid space?

113. How should local anesthetic be administered through the epidural catheter for epidural anesthesia?

114. How is the level of anesthesia determined after the administration of an epidural anesthetic?

115. What is the single-shot technique of an epidural anesthetic? When is it appropriate?

116. What are the major influences over the level and duration of epidural anesthesia?

117. Please complete the following table of local anesthetics used for epidural anesthesia:

	CONCENTRATION (%)	ONSET (min)	DURATION (min)
Chloroprocaine			
Lidocaine			
Ropivacaine			
Bupivacaine			

118. Why are tetracaine and procaine rarely used for epidural anesthesia?

119. What are two reasons for the relatively increased cephalad spread of local anesthetic as compared with caudad spread when injected into a lumbar epidural catheter?

120. Why might a unilateral anesthetic block result from an epidural anesthetic, despite proper technique?

121. What is the major site of action of local anesthetic solutions placed in the epidural space?

122. What is the mechanism by which the addition of epinephrine to local anesthetic solutions prolongs the duration of epidural anesthesia?

123. What is an explanation for the often observed delay in onset of epidural anesthesia in the S1–S2 region?

124. How much does diffusion of local anesthetic into the subarachnoid space contribute to the anesthesia produced by an epidural?

125. How does epidural anesthesia compare with spinal anesthesia with regard to the various levels of blockade of the sympathetic, sensory, and motor nerves?

126. How does the vascular absorption of epinephrine from its addition in a local anesthetic solution administered in the epidural space affect blood pressure?

127. How does epidural anesthesia compare with spinal anesthesia with regard to its effects on the respiratory system and gastrointestinal system?

128. What are some potential side effects of epidural anesthesia?

129. What is the risk of epidural hematoma formation resulting from an epidural anesthetic?

130. What are some indications of accidental dural puncture during the performance of epidural anesthesia? How should it be managed?

131. What results from the unrecognized, accidental subarachnoid injection of local anesthetic when administering an epidural anesthetic?

132. What results from the unrecognized, accidental subdural injection of local anesthetic when administering an epidural anesthetic?

133. What is the potential risk of local anesthetic systemic toxicity when administering an epidural anesthetic?

134. How does the hypotension associated with epidural anesthesia compare with that associated with spinal anesthesia?

135. What can result from the unrecognized, accidental intravascular injection of local anesthetic when administering an epidural anesthetic?

136. What is the technique for administering a combined spinal and epidural anesthetic?

CAUDAL ANESTHESIA

137. What position should the patient be in to facilitate the administration of a caudal anesthetic?

138. Where is the sacral hiatus located?

139. Where and how is the needle placed for a caudal anesthetic?

140. How can it be confirmed that the needle tip is appropriately placed in the caudal canal for a caudal anesthetic?

141. Given the proximity of the rectum to the site of needle insertion for a caudal anesthetic, how frequently is infection noted with this technique?

142. What is a potential risk of caudal anesthesia?

143. What is the failure rate of caudal anesthesia?

144. How does technical ease of the administration of a caudal anesthetic in children compare with the ease of its administration in an adult?

Answers*

1. Other terms used to describe spinal and epidural anesthesia include regional or conduction anesthesia. These types of anesthesia are also referred to as neuraxial blocks. (168)

2. In spinal anesthesia, medicine is deposited in the subarachnoid space, most commonly at the lumbar level. In epidural anesthesia, medicine is deposited in the epidural space, most commonly at the lumbar level. In caudal anesthesia, medicine is also deposited in the epidural space but the needle used to inject the medicine approaches the epidural space via introduction through the sacral hiatus. (168; **1491–1492**)

3. Some advantages of regional anesthesia include the provision of surgical anesthesia without affecting the state of consciousness of the patient, skeletal muscle relaxation, and the lack of the need to manipulate the airway or mechanically ventilate the lungs. Spinal anesthesia when compared with epidural anesthesia takes less time to perform and has a quicker onset, provides for intense sensory and motor anesthesia, and may be of less discomfort to the patient. Epidural anesthesia when compared with spinal anesthesia has a decreased risk of a postdural puncture headache, allows for more control over the level of anesthesia and the duration of the anesthetic if prolonged anesthetic times are desired, may lead to better control of associated hypotension due to its slower onset, and provides for an indwelling catheter that can be used for acute postoperative pain management. (168)

4. Some drugs that may be administered intravenously for sedation during regional anesthesia include benzodiazepines, opioids, and propofol. (168)

5. Fears patients may have about regional anesthesia include the fear of needlesticks in their backs and the fear of paralysis resulting from the administration of the anesthetic. Biases surgeons have against regional anesthesia stem from, among other things, their belief that the administration of regional anesthesia will delay the start of the case or will be inadequate for the procedure. (168; **1491–1492**)

*Numbers in parentheses: lightface numbers refer to pages, figures, or tables in Stoelting RK, Miller RD: Basics of Anesthesia, 4th ed. Philadelphia, Churchill Livingstone, 2000; **boldface numbers** refer to pages, figures, or tables in Miller RD: Anesthesia, 5th ed. Philadelphia, Churchill Livingstone, 2000.

6. Opioids introduced into the epidural or subarachnoid space have proven to be very effective in deepening the level of analgesia as well as for postoperative pain control. (168; **2330–2333**)

ANATOMY

7. The vertebral column consists of 7 cervical vertebrae, 12 thoracic vertebrae, 5 lumbar vertebrae, as well as the 5 fused sacral and 4 fused coccygeal vertebrae. (168, Fig. 13–1; **1495, Fig. 42–6**)

8. A vertebra is made up of the vertebral body and the bony arch. The transverse process arises from the junction of the pedicle and laminae. The spinous process arises from the joining of the laminae. (168; **1492–1493, Fig. 42–1**)

9. The spinous processes in the lumbar region are oriented in a nearly horizontal position in the upright patient, whereas in the thoracic region the spinous processes are oriented in a position approaching vertical. Clinically, this implies what the orientation of the long axis of the needle must be to successfully transverse the interspace at these levels to administer an epidural or spinal anesthetic. (168, Fig. 13–1; **1492–1493, Fig. 42–1**)

10. The laminae of adjacent vertebrae are connected by the ligamentum flavum. (168, Fig. 13–2; **1493, Fig. 42–4**)

11. The posterior spinous processes of adjacent vertebrae are connected by the interspinous ligaments. (168, Fig. 13–2; **1493, Fig. 42–4**)

12. The tips of the spinous processes of adjacent vertebrae are connected by the supraspinous ligaments. (168, Fig. 13–2; **1493, Fig. 42–4**)

13. The spinal nerves pass through the intervertebral foramina and supply a specific dermatome. (168, Fig. 13–3; **1492–1493**)

14. Preganglionic nerves of the sympathetic nervous system originate from the spinal cord at the T1 to L2 levels. From there they travel with the spinal nerves before separating to form the sympathetic chain. (168, Fig. 13–4; **526–529, Fig. 14–6**)

15. The sympathetic chain sits on the anterolateral aspects of the vertebral bodies along the entire length of the spinal column. The sympathetic chain gives rise to the stellate ganglion, the splanchnic nerves, and the celiac plexus. (168; **529, Fig. 14–6**)

16. Contents of the spinal canal include the spinal cord, pia, arachnoid, dura mater, and cerebrospinal fluid. (168; **1492**)

17. The cephalad limit of the spinal cord is the foramen magnum, whereas its caudal limit is at the L1–L2 level. (168; **1492**)

18. The cauda equina is the collection of lumbar and sacral nerves that extend from the end of the spinal cord as a collection of nerves in the spinal canal before exiting via the intervertebral foramina at their respective vertebral column levels. (168–169; **1492**)

19. Cerebrospinal fluid is found in the spinal space between the pia and arachnoid, or subarachnoid. Another term for this space is the subarachnoid space. (169; **1492**)

20. The epidural space is found between the connective tissue covering the vertebrae and the ligamentum flavum posteriorly and the dura mater anteriorly. Laterally it is bound by the pedicles and the intervertebral foramina. The epidural space extends from the foramen magnum, where the dura is fused to the base of the skull, to the sacral hiatus. (169; **1493–1494, Fig. 42–3**)

21. The plica mediana dorsalis is a connective tissue band that may extend from the dura mater to the ligamentum flavum. The plica mediana dorsalis may divide the posterior epidural space into two compartments, a right and left compartment. Clinically, this is significant because it may affect the manner in which medicine deposited into the epidural space is distributed. (169; **1493–1494, Fig. 42–5**)

22. The epidural space, a potential space, contains connective tissue, venous plexuses, and adipose tissue. (169; **1507**)

PREOPERATIVE PREPARATION

23. A preoperative evaluation of a patient scheduled to undergo a surgical procedure with a regional anesthetic is no different than the evaluation of the same patient were he or she to undergo the procedure under general anesthesia. Special consideration should be given to possible systemic infections; infections overlying the skin where the introduction of a needle may be necessary to perform the regional anesthetic; and any history of coagulopathy, bleeding dyscrasias, or medicines that may alter normal clotting. Any abnormalities of these special considerations may preclude proceeding with a regional anesthetic technique. (169; **1492**)

24. Patients who do not want a regional anesthetic should not be convinced to have one. (170; **1492**)

25. For the patient who is to undergo a regional anesthetic, in addition to the routine preoperative physical examination, the preoperative physical examination should also include examination of the back for any deformities or evidence of infection. (170; **1492**)

26. The coagulation status of a patient should be determined by either history or laboratory test before administering a regional anesthetic. The administration of a regional anesthetic in the face of clotting abnormalities puts the patient at an increased risk of an epidural hematoma and subsequent serious neurologic symptoms that may be permanent. (170; **1514**)

27. A regional anesthetic should only be administered to an anticoagulated patient if the risk of the alternative outweighs the risk of the regional anesthetic technique. (170; **1514**)

28. For patients who are to receive heparin or enoxaparin after surgery the administration of a regional anesthetic is a controversial issue. If the decision is made to proceed, and a blood vessel is disrupted during the course of placement of the regional technique, it may be prudent to delay the start of surgery for approximately 24 hours. This may allow for healing of the blood vessel to occur. Another alternative is to proceed with surgery but in the case of enoxaparin to delay its administration until 24 hours postoperatively. (170; **1514**)

29. The administration of regional anesthesia to a septic patient is controversial because of the risk of introduction of infected blood into the epidural or subarachnoid space by the needle during the technique. The infected blood may lead to an epidural abscess or meningitis in these patients. If regional anesthesia is to be performed in these patients, appropriate antibiotic therapy must be instituted before the administration of the regional anesthetic. (170; **1492**)

30. The administration of regional anesthesia to a hypovolemic patient is of concern because of the probable inability of the patient to tolerate the peripheral sympathetic nervous system blockade that accompanies the tech-

nique. This could result in hypotension that is difficult to reverse. (170; **1492, 1496–1497**)

31. Preoperative medication for the patient who is to undergo a regional anesthetic technique should make the patient comfortable and help to decrease his or her level of anxiety as necessary. This may include an opioid or a benzodiazepine as needed. Reassurance by the anesthesiologist that the patient will be kept comfortable is also a useful preoperative anxiolytic. (170–171)

32. An intravenous catheter should be placed before the administration of any regional anesthetic technique. There are at least two reasons for this. First, hydration of the patient before the administration of the regional anesthetic helps to attenuate the hypotension that often results from the peripheral sympathetic nervous system blockade that accompanies regional anesthesia. Second, intravenous access must be obtained in the event that the emergent administration of medicines becomes necessary during the course of, or directly after, the administration of regional anesthesia. (171)

33. The equipment, monitors, and drugs that the anesthesiologist has present for a regional anesthetic are not different from those present during a general anesthetic. These must be present in case of the emergent need to administer a general anesthetic, as in the case of a total spinal anesthetic. (171; **1515**)

SPINAL ANESTHESIA

34. Spinal anesthetics are most commonly administered at the lumbar level. Anatomic landmarks that the anesthesiologist uses to administer a spinal anesthetic include the spinous processes and the iliac crests. (171; **1499–1500**)

35. A line drawn across the patient's back at the level of the top of the iliac crests usually crosses the vertebral column at the L4 vertebral level. The interspace palpated directly above this line is the L3–L4 interspace, and the interspace palpated directly below this line is the L4–L5 interspace. (171, Fig. 13–5; **1500**)

36. The anatomic value of placing a spinal anesthetic at a level below L2 is that the spinal cord ends at L2. Thus, risk of trauma to the spinal cord by the spinal needle decreases by placing the spinal anesthetic below this level. (171; **1492**)

37. The two most common positions that the patient is placed in for the administration of a spinal anesthetic are the seated upright and the lateral decubitus positions. The lateral decubitus position may be preferred in ill or sedated patients. The seated upright position may be preferred in patients in whom the midline is difficult to identify, there is difficulty in accessing the vertebral interspaces, or when a low level of spinal anesthesia is desired. Whichever of these two positions the patient is in, the patient is asked to round out his or her back as much as possible to facilitate access to the subarachnoid space through the vertebral interspaces. (172; **1499–1500, Figs. 42–10, 42–11**)

38. Prepackaged spinal anesthesia kits typically contain a local anesthetic such as bupivacaine or tetracaine, lidocaine and a 25-gauge needle for local infiltration, a spinal needle, epinephrine, two syringes, and drapes. (173, Fig. 13–7)

39. Sterility should be maintained with each spinal anesthetic. The technique should involve preparing the skin overlying the selected area with an antiseptic solution such as povidone-iodine (Betadine); the back should be sterilely draped, and sterile gloves should be worn. (172)

40. The skin should be anesthetized with local anesthetic before the introduction of the spinal needle. The local anesthetic should be administered with a

small-gauge needle (e.g., a 25-gauge needle), and the skin wheal created should directly overlie the interspace in which the anesthesiologist wishes to advance the spinal needle. (172; **1500**)

41. The subarachnoid space is located by advancing the spinal needle through the skin between two spinous processes. The spinal needle continues to be advanced traversing the supraspinous and interspinous ligaments between two vertebrae. The advancement of the spinal needle continues through the ligamentum flavum, where increased resistance is felt. Finally, the dura mater is traversed and the subarachnoid space is accessed. (172; **1500, Fig. 42–12**)

42. The anesthesiologist may feel a characteristic "pop" just before accessing the subarachnoid space as the spinal needle is being advanced. This "pop" is the spinal needle passing through the dura mater. (172; **1500**)

43. Subarachnoid placement of the spinal needle is confirmed by the appearance of cerebrospinal fluid in the hub of the spinal needle. The most common reason for the lack of cerebrospinal fluid, and erroneous placement of the needle, is off-midline placement of the needle. (172; **1500**)

44. The spinal needle should be stabilized by the anesthesiologist after proper placement into the subarachnoid space is confirmed. This can be done by holding the hub of the spinal needle between the anesthesiologist's thumb and forefinger and resting the dorsum of the same hand on the patient's back. When the spinal needle is held in this manner, it should remain stabilized even with patient movement. (172; **1500**)

45. After the syringe containing the local anesthetic solution for administration into the subarachnoid space is attached to the spinal needle, the anesthesiologist typically aspirates back on the syringe to confirm continued subarachnoid placement of the spinal needle tip. Confirmation is made by the characteristic swirl in the syringe as cerebrospinal fluid enters the syringe and mixes with the local anesthetic solution. The local anesthetic solution can then be deposited into the subarachnoid space over a period of 3 to 5 seconds. After completion of the deposition of the local anesthetic solution into the subarachnoid space, the spinal needle and syringe should be removed together as a single unit. (172; **1500**)

46. If blood-tinged cerebrospinal fluid appears in the hub of the spinal needle, the anesthesiologist should wait until the fluid clears. If blood-tinged cerebrospinal fluid continues to flow from the spinal needle, the spinal needle should be removed and reinserted at a different interspace. If blood-tinged cerebrospinal fluid is encountered in the second interspace accessed, the attempt at administration of a spinal anesthetic should be discontinued and the patient further evaluated. On the other hand, when blood-tinged fluid initially appears in the hub of the spinal needle but subsequently clears and is free flowing, the local anesthetic solution can be deposited safely into the subarachnoid space. (172)

47. There are a variety of spinal needle types and sizes that are used for spinal anesthesia. Among the needle sizes used are 22-, 24-, 25-, and 27-gauge needles. The advantage of using a smaller-gauge needle is that it may decrease the risk of a postdural puncture headache. There are two main types of spinal needles, those that cut the dura and the newer type that are designed to spread the dural fibers. The cutting needles include the Quincke-Babcock and Pitkin needles. The newer needles, also called pencil-point needles, include the Greene, Sprotte, and Whitacre needles. These newer needles are thought to decrease the risk of a postdural puncture headache by causing less disruption of the dura. In addition, the newer needles may provide for better tactile sense as they pass through the tissues. A Tuohy needle may be used if a

catheter is to be inserted into the subarachnoid space. (172–173, Fig. 13–6; **1499, 1507, Figs. 42–9, 42–17**)

48. Although spinal needles that are 25-gauge or smaller may decrease the risk of a postdural puncture headache, there are some disadvantages associated with their use. First, they are too flexible for easy advancement through the ligaments to access the subarachnoid space. For this reason a larger-gauge introducer needle well embedded in the interspinous ligament facilitates the advancement of the smaller-gauge spinal needle to the subarachnoid space. They also provide the anesthesiologist with poor tactile feedback as the tissue planes are penetrated. Finally, the successful entry of the subarachnoid space may not be immediately known secondary to the slow return of cerebrospinal fluid to the hub of the spinal needle. Aspiration of the needle with an attached syringe hastens the return of cerebrospinal fluid through the spinal needle and provides confirmation of appropriate placement of the spinal needle. (173; **1499**)

49. The paramedian approach to a spinal anesthetic involves introducing the spinal needle through the skin 1 cm lateral to the midline and directed medial and cephalad. The needle meets resistance at the ligamentum flavum, and the remainder of the technique is similar to that of the median approach. The paramedian approach to a spinal anesthetic is less reliant on the patient flexing his or her back. This approach may be useful in patients who are unable to flex their backs, such as parturients. It may also be useful in patients in whom ligaments may be calcified, such as the elderly. (173, Fig. 13–8; **1500–1502, Fig. 42–13**)

50. The lumbosacral approach to a spinal anesthetic involves introducing the spinal needle 1 cm medial and 1 cm caudad to the posterior iliac spine. The needle is then directed in a medial, caudal direction where the L5–S1 interspace is accessed. The L5–S1 interspace is generally the largest interlaminal interspace in the vertebral column. This approach, like the paramedian approach, is advantageous when the patient is unable to flex the back. (173; **1502, Fig. 42–14**)

51. The three things that most influence the distribution of local anesthetic solution in the cerebrospinal fluid in the subarachnoid space are the baricity of the solution, the contour of the spinal canal, and the position of the patient during and for the first few minutes after its administration. (173; **1505–1506, Tables 42–4, 42–5, 42–6**)

52. The two things that most influence the duration of a spinal anesthetic are the drug selected and whether or not a vasoconstrictor is present in the local anesthetic solution, such as epinephrine or phenylephrine. (173–174, Table 13–1; **1503–1505, Tables 42–2, 42–3**)

53. The administration of local anesthetics in the subarachnoid space may lead to a denser blockade of motor or sensory nerves. For example, bupivacaine produces more sensory than motor blockade and tetracaine produces more motor than sensory blockade. It theoretically follows that bupivacaine may be a more appropriate choice of local anesthetic for spinal anesthesia for lower extremity, vascular, or orthopedic operations. Tetracaine may be a more appropriate choice of local anesthetic for spinal anesthesia for abdominal operations in which skeletal muscle relaxation is necessary to optimize surgical results. Spinal anesthesia that results after the administration of lidocaine is of short duration and does not appear to have any preferential blockade of the motor or sensory nerves. The short duration of lidocaine spinal anesthesia dictates in which surgical cases its use would be appropriate. (174; **507, 1504**)

54. During recovery from spinal anesthesia, regression of the anesthetic is from the highest dermatome to a caudad direction. (174)

55. (174, Table 13–1; **1504, Table 42–2**)

LOCAL ANESTHETIC	CONCENTRATION (%)	T10 (mg)	T4 (mg)	VOLUME (mL)	ONSET (min)	NO EPI (duration min)	EPI (duration min)
Lidocaine	5	30–50	75–100	1–2	2–4	45–60	60–90
Tetracaine	0.5	6–10	12–16	1–3	4–6	60–90	120–180
Bupivacaine	0.5–0.75	6–10	12–16	1–2	4–6	90	140
Ropivacaine	0.5–0.75	6–10	12–16	1–2	4–6	90	140

56. Baricity is a ratio that compares the density of two solutions. The baricity of a local anesthetic solution to be administered in the subarachnoid space is the density of the local anesthetic divided by the density of cerebrospinal fluid at 37°C. Local anesthetics are characterized as hyperbaric, hypobaric, or isobaric relative to cerebrospinal fluid. The clinical importance of knowing the baricity of a local anesthetic solution for administration into the subarachnoid space is that, by understanding the baricity, the medicine can be guided to the desired spinal nerves for a given surgical procedure. (174; **1505**)

57. Most administered spinal anesthetics are hyperbaric. Local anesthetics for spinal anesthesia are made hyperbaric by the addition of dextrose to the solution. Dextrose is added to bupivacaine 0.75% and lidocaine 5% commercially. A hyperbaric solution of tetracaine can be made by adding 10% dextrose to equal volumes of 1% tetracaine. The resulting solution will be 0.5% tetracaine plus 5% dextrose. (174; **507, 1504**)

58. Hyperbaric solutions diffuse in the subarachnoid space by settling to the most dependent portion of the space. The most dependent portion of the subarachnoid space is contingent on the position of the patient at the time of and shortly after the administration of the local anesthetic. (174)

59. A patient given a hyperbaric spinal anesthetic in the seated upright position would have an anesthetic block that would be most dense at the caudad level. This type of spinal anesthesia block is appropriate for genitourinary procedures, such as transurethral resection of the prostate. A patient who was placed in the supine position just after the administration of a hyperbaric spinal anesthetic would have an anesthetic block that would be most dense at the kyphotic thoracic level, approximately T6. This level of spinal anesthesia is appropriate for an intra-abdominal surgical procedure. (175, Fig. 13–1; **1499**)

60. Local anesthetics can be made hypobaric by the addition of sterile water to the solution. Another method to achieve hypobaric-like effects is to warm 0.5% bupivacaine. Lidocaine 2% is also believed to have hypobaric-like effects. (175; **1515**)

61. Hypobaric solutions float in the subarachnoid space, bathing nerves in the nondependent portion of the subarachnoid space. The nondependent portion of the space is contingent on the position of the patient at the time of and shortly after the administration of the local anesthetic. (175; **507, 1505**)

62. The administration of a hypobaric spinal anesthetic is useful in procedures such as a hemorrhoidectomy in the jackknife prone position or hip arthroplasty in the lateral position. In both these cases the hypobaric spinal anesthetic is useful because the patient can be placed in the position necessary

to perform the operative procedure before the administration of the anesthetic. (175; **507, 1505**)

63. The local anesthetic most commonly administered for isobaric spinal anesthesia is 0.5% and 0.75% bupivacaine. Tetracaine can be made isobaric by diluting it with cerebrospinal fluid. (175; **507, 1505**)

64. Two vasoconstrictors that can be added to spinal local anesthetic solutions to prolong their duration of action are epinephrine and phenylephrine. The dose used for this purpose is 0.1 to 0.2 mg epinephrine or 2 to 5 mg phenylephrine. There are conflicting data regarding which vasoconstrictor produces the greatest prolongation of the duration of a spinal anesthetic. (175; **1504–1505**)

65. One way in which vasoconstrictors are thought to prolong the local anesthetic duration of action in the subarachnoid space is by causing localized vasoconstriction. The localized vasoconstriction results in decreases in spinal blood flow and therefore a decrease in the vascular absorption of the local anesthetic. This allows the local anesthetic to remain in the subarachnoid space and in contact with the nerves for a prolonged period of time. The second way in which epinephrine is thought to prolong the duration of action is through antinociceptive action by its direct stimulation of spinal cord alpha-adrenergic receptors. (175; **1504–1505**)

66. A concern regarding the addition of vasoconstrictors to local anesthetic solutions for administration in the subarachnoid space is that the vasoconstriction that results might compromise the vascular supply to the spinal cord. Studies evaluating spinal cord blood flow after the administration of vasoconstrictors to the subarachnoid space in dogs has not shown this to be the case, nor is there known to be any unfavorable outcomes in humans. (174; **1504–1505**)

67. All the local anesthetics are thought to have a prolonged spinal anesthetic duration when vasoconstrictors are added to the administered local anesthetic solution. Because lidocaine and bupivacaine have vasodilatory effects, these two local anesthetics were thought to be unaffected by the addition of vasoconstrictors. This has since been shown to be untrue. More recent studies that evaluated the duration by checking for dermatome regression of anesthesia in the lower thoracic dermatomes and by pain at the operative site have shown that lidocaine does have a duration prolonged by the addition of vasoconstrictors. The addition of phenylephrine to bupivacaine has not been shown to prolong the duration of spinal anesthesia, however. It is well accepted that the duration of spinal anesthesia produced by tetracaine with a vasoconstrictor is greater than the duration of spinal anesthesia when tetracaine is administered alone. (174; **1504–1505, Table 42–3**)

68. The addition of a vasoconstrictor to a local anesthetic solution for spinal anesthesia appears to most prolong spinal anesthesia below the L1 level. (174)

69. A continuous spinal anesthetic is performed in a similar manner to a single-shot spinal anesthetic, with two exceptions. First, the needle used is a thin-walled, larger-gauged needle, such as an 18-gauge Tuohy needle. Second, once cerebrospinal fluid freely flows from the needle, a catheter is inserted 2 to 3 cm into the subarachnoid space and secured. The administration of the local anesthetic is through the catheter. The advantages of a continuous spinal anesthetic are that the level and the duration of spinal anesthesia can be better controlled. A disadvantage of this technique is the increased risk of a postdural puncture headache that can result from the tear of the dura created by the larger needle. In the past, microbore spinal catheters were used in an attempt to decrease the risk of a postdural puncture headache. The microbore catheters were associated with cauda equina syndrome. This risk of cauda equina

syndrome was greatest for patients receiving 5% lidocaine via the catheter. It is believed that the pooling of local anesthetic in the most dependent portion of the subarachnoid space led to high concentrations of local anesthetic at those spinal nerves and subsequent irreversible neurotoxicity. Although small microbore catheters for continuous spinal anesthesia are no longer used, caution must be taken with the administration of a continuous spinal anesthetic. Because cauda equina syndrome is still a potential complication, alternatives to 5% lidocaine should be considered for the spinal local anesthetic. (176; **1491, 1499, 1506**)

70. Sympathetic nerves are blocked before both motor nerves and sensory nerves after the administration of a spinal anesthetic. A useful way to gain an early indication of the level of spinal anesthesia is by testing the patient's ability for temperature discrimination in the relevant dermatomes. For example, in an unblocked area an alcohol sponge will produce a cold sensation, whereas in the blocked areas the same alcohol sponge will feel warm or neutral. (174–175)

71. The dermatomal order of blockade produced by a spinal anesthetic, from highest to lowest, is sympathetic nerves, sensory nerves, then motor nerves. Sympathetic nervous system blockade from spinal anesthesia exceeds the level of sensory nerve blockade by at least two dermatomes and sometimes by as many as six dermatomes. For this reason, hypotension may accompany a spinal anesthetic whose sensory level is low. (176; **1496**)

72. There are two reasons why sympathetic nerve fibers undergo conduction blockade from spinal anesthesia before sensory and motor fibers. First, the nerves of the sympathetic nervous system are small-diameter, unmyelinated fibers, as compared with the larger, myelinated fibers of the sensory and motor nerves. Second, the small-diameter unmyelinated nerve fibers of the sympathetic nerves are closest to the surface of the nerve bundle and hence are the first nerve fibers exposed to the local anesthetic solution. (176)

73. A useful test for the evaluation of the level of sympathetic nerve blockade is the evaluation of the patient's ability to discern between temperature changes at various levels with an alcohol sponge. (175)

74. A useful test for the evaluation of the level of sensory nerve blockade is the evaluation of the patient's ability to discriminate sharpness produced by an object touching the patient's abdomen or chest at various levels. (175)

75. A useful test for the evaluation of the level of motor nerve blockade is the evaluation of the patient's ability to do various motor tasks, such as dorsiflexion of the foot (S1–S2), raising the knees (L2–L3), and tensing the abdominal rectus muscles (T6–T12). (175)

76. Appropriately instituted spinal anesthesia has little effect on alveolar ventilation when evaluated by arterial blood gases. There is no change in tidal volume, but the expiratory reserve volume may decrease slightly owing to the inability of paralyzed abdominal muscles to perform forced exhalation. Levels of spinal anesthesia that produce paralysis of the abdominal and intercostal muscles can also result in a decrease in the patient's ability to cough and expel secretions. From the perspective of the patient, however, high levels of spinal anesthesia often produce a sensation of difficulty breathing, or dyspnea. This results from decreased sensory input from the thoracoabdominal muscles during regular breathing. Exaggerated hypoventilation might result after the administration of sedatives to patients who are undergoing surgery with a spinal anesthetic simply because of the lack of external stimulation. The judicious administration of sedatives to these patients is indicated for these reasons. (176; **1497–1498, 1508**)

77. When spinal anesthesia results in sympathetic nervous system blockade above T5, the sympathetic nerves that innervate the gastrointestinal tract are blocked. This results in unopposed parasympathetic nervous system activity in the gastrointestinal tract, whose effect may lead to contracted intestines and relaxed sphincters. (176; **1498**)

78. The effects of sympathetic nervous system blockade on the genitourinary system include contraction of the ureters and relaxation of the ureterovesical orifice. (176; **1498**)

79. The adrenocortical response to surgical stimulation that can occur is blocked in a patient whose surgical site is anesthetized by spinal anesthesia. This is a result of the blocked afferent impulses from the surgical site. (176)

80. Some side effects associated with spinal anesthesia include hypotension, bradycardia, postdural puncture headache, total spinal, nausea, urinary retention, backache, neurologic sequelae, and hypoventilation. (176; **1506–1507**)

81. As a result of the sympathectomy caused by spinal anesthetics, as many as one third of patients receiving a spinal anesthetic become hypotensive with a systolic blood pressure less than 90 mm Hg and 10% to 15% of patients become bradycardic. There are several reasons why hypotension can occur with spinal anesthesia. First, it may be due to decreases in systemic vascular resistance. Second, it may be due to decreased venous return to the heart and subsequent decreases in cardiac output. Finally, if blockade of the cardioaccelerator fibers occurs, bradycardia results and there are even greater decreases in cardiac output. Blockade of the cardioaccelerator fibers occurs when the dermatomal level of the sympathetic nervous system blockade is at or above the T1 level since the cardioaccelerator fibers originate from T1 to T4. When the hypotension is modest it is probably due to decreases in systemic vascular resistance. When hypotension is severe, it is believed to be due to decreases in cardiac output. (177, Fig. 13–9; **1496–1497**)

82. The degree of hypotension that can accompany a spinal anesthetic is most influenced by the level of spinal anesthesia and the intravascular fluid volume status of the patient. (177; **1496–1497**)

83. There are at least two nonpharmacologic methods that can be used to treat the hypotension that can occur with a spinal anesthetic. One is providing the patient with adequate hydration before administering the spinal anesthetic so as to minimize the effects of the decreased systemic vascular resistance that results from the anesthetic. The second is placing the patient in a modest head-down position to provide for an increased venous return of intravascular fluid that may be pooling in the lower extremities. This may not be appropriate in patients who cannot handle the increased intravascular fluid volume load or the dilutional anemia it may cause, such as patients with ischemic cardiac disease and poor cardiac function. (177; **1496–1497**)

84. Sympathomimetics such as ephedrine or phenylephrine can be administered to treat the hypotension that can occur with a spinal anesthetic. Ephedrine in doses of 5 to 10 mg intravenously is the preferred method of treatment because it has positive inotropic as well as venoconstrictor effects, thus correcting the factors responsible for the decrease in blood pressure. Phenylephrine, on the other hand, increases systemic blood pressure by increasing systemic vascular resistance but does not necessarily increase venous return and may in fact result in a reflex bradycardia. For hypotension that is accompanied with bradycardia, atropine may be administered to increase the heart rate. There are reports of hypotension and bradycardia after a spinal anesthetic leading to asystole that does not respond to atropine. For this

reason, when hypotension is not easily reversed with standard treatment the prompt administration of epinephrine must follow. (177; **1496–1497**)

85. There are at least two potential benefits of the decrease in systemic vascular resistance that accompanies spinal anesthesia. First, there may be decreased bleeding during certain types of surgery, such as hip surgery. This is a result of the decreases in arterial blood pressure in the surgical areas anesthetized by a regional anesthetic. Second, there is a decreased incidence of thrombo-embolic complications after hip surgery when a regional anesthetic technique is used. This is believed to be due to the increased blood flow to the lower extremities that results from regional anesthesia. (176; **2132–2133**)

86. The hallmark features of a postdural puncture headache include its postural component and the fact that the headache gets worse with sitting or standing and better in the supine position. The headache must have a postural component to be a postdural puncture headache. The second hallmark of the postdural puncture headache is the location of the headache in the frontal or occipital region. Diplopia, tinnitus, and decreased hearing acuity may also accompany a postdural puncture headache. (177; **1507, Table 42–7**)

87. A postdural puncture headache is believed to occur as a result of leakage of cerebrospinal fluid from the hole in the dura mater caused by the needle. The loss of cerebrospinal fluid results in decreased cerebrospinal fluid pressures and less "cushion" around the brain in the skull. This in turn leads to tension on the meningeal vessels and nerves, causing the headache. It is believed that the diplopia may result from tension on the abducens nerve. (177; **1506–1507**)

88. Risk factors for a postdural puncture headache include patient characteristics and procedure technique. Patients most at risk for a postdural puncture headache include patients who are young, female, and, in particular, parturients. With regard to technique, the larger the needle gauge, the cutting spinal needles, and multiple dural punctures all increase the risk. To minimize the risk of a postdural puncture headache the anesthesiologist may select a 25-gauge or smaller pencil-point spinal needle. (178, Fig. 13–10; **1499, 1506–1507, Table 42–7**)

89. Some conservative methods of treating a postdural puncture headache include bed rest, analgesics, caffeine, and hydration of 3 L or more a day. Hydration may be via the oral or intravenous route and is intended to exceed the rate at which the cerebrospinal fluid is leaking through the hole in the dura mater. Caffeine intake can be by the oral route or intravenous route. If caffeine consumption orally does not provide any relief, the administration of 500 mg intravenously has been shown to provide some benefit. (178; **1507**)

90. An epidural blood patch is highly effective for the treatment of a postdural puncture headache. Over 90% of patients experience relief from their headaches with the administration of the epidural blood patch. A second blood patch will provide relief to over 90% of patients who did not respond to the epidural blood patch on the first attempt. Resolution of a postdural puncture headache after the administration of an epidural blood patch is almost immediate. An epidural blood patch for treatment of a postdural puncture headache is thought to work by providing a "patch" over the hole in the dura mater, thus preventing the further leakage of cerebrospinal fluid through the hole. The sealed dura mater allows for reestablishment of appropriate pressures in the subarachnoid space to support the brain in its confined space, relieving the traction on the meningeal vessels. (178; **1507**)

91. An epidural blood patch is performed first by having the patient appropriately positioned for an epidural anesthetic. The lumbar epidural space is found using the loss of resistance technique, just as with an epidural anesthetic. Once the lumbar epidural space has been located, 10 to 20 mL of blood is

drawn sterilely from the patient's vein, most commonly from a cubital vein. The blood is then, still sterilely, administered into the lumbar epidural space through the needle. The epidural blood patch is most commonly administered at the interspace or one interspace below the interspace at which the dura mater was punctured. Radiographic studies of radiolabeled red blood cells have shown that 15 mL of blood in the epidural space spreads about 9 segments, with the greatest degree of spread in the cephalad direction. An epidural blood patch should be performed no sooner than 24 to 48 hours after the dural puncture to achieve the best results. (178; **1507**)

92. An epidural patch performed with saline is not as effective as an epidural patch performed with blood. (178)

93. A total spinal anesthetic is a spinal anesthetic whose level of sympathetic, sensory, and motor nerve blockade is higher than intended and results in hypotension and difficulty breathing or apnea. Nausea and agitation may also accompany the difficulty breathing seen in a total spinal. Apnea associated with a total spinal will begin to manifest soon after the deposition of the local anesthetic solution into the subarachnoid space. For those whose level of spinal anesthetic leads to apnea, pupils appear dilated. (178; **1497, 1514**)

94. A total spinal anesthetic that begins to interfere with breathing is usually a high thoracic level of anesthesia, and it approaches the lower cervical levels. Usually the cervical nerves are spared, as are the nerves to the diaphragm. The physiologic explanation for why a total spinal causes apnea without affecting the phrenic nerves is related to the hypotension caused by the total spinal. The profound hypotension caused by the total spinal results in hypoperfusion of the medullary ventilatory centers along with a decrease in cerebral blood flow. (178; **1497, 1514**)

95. The treatment for a total spinal anesthetic is supportive. The patient's ventilation can be supported by face mask and hand ventilation with oxygen. The patient's hemodynamic status can be supported by the intravenous administration of fluids and sympathomimetics as indicated. When a total spinal results from the administration of local anesthetic solution in the subarachnoid space, the patient should not be placed in a head-up position in an attempt to decrease the level of the spinal anesthesia. Placing the patient in a head-up position further decreases venous return and exacerbates the hypotension, jeopardizing cerebral blood flow. This further contributes to hypoperfusion of the medullary ventilatory centers. Instead, patients should be placed in a head-down position to facilitate venous return to the heart and possibly reverse medullary ischemia. Patients with a total spinal should have their tracheas intubated for ventilatory support if necessary. Tracheal intubation is also indicated if they are at an increased risk of aspiration, as is a parturient. (178; **1514**)

96. The duration of a total spinal anesthetic is usually short because the concentration of local anesthetic is low at the higher thoracic or lower cervical levels. (178)

97. Two possible causes of nausea that presents soon after the administration of a spinal anesthetic include hypotension sufficient to produce cerebral ischemia and predominant parasympathetic nervous system activity on the gastrointestinal tract resulting in contracted intestines and relaxed sphincters. (178; **1498**)

98. The anesthesiologist should suspect possible hypotension when nausea occurs just after the administration of a spinal anesthetic. In these cases the administration of a sympathomimetic may reverse the hypotension and the nausea. Nausea occurring in the absence of hypotension can be treated by the administration of 0.4 mg of atropine, a muscarinic antagonist, intravenously.

The atropine would counteract the unopposed parasympathetic nervous system activity on the gastrointestinal tract, relaxing the intestines and increasing sphincter tone. (178; **1498**)

99. Urinary retention might occur after the administration of a spinal anesthetic because of the inhibition of bladder tone that results from the anesthesia. This can lead to bladder distention, requiring drainage by a catheter. Bladder distention can be minimized by minimizing the amount of intravenous fluids administered to the patient while undergoing minor surgery with spinal anesthesia. (178–179; **1498**)

100. Backache presenting after spinal anesthesia is frequently due to the position the patient was required to remain in during the surgery. It has been estimated that 25% of patients complain of backache after surgery regardless of the anesthetic technique. However, patients with the decreased sensory perception characteristic of a spinal anesthetic may remain in positions for long periods of time that may otherwise have been uncomfortable to them, thus resulting in ligament strain that might not have otherwise occurred. (179; **1507**)

101. Some possible causes of postspinal neurologic complications are an erroneously placed spinal needle, injection of the wrong substance into the subarachnoid space, transient radicular irritation, exacerbation of co-existing neurologic disease, surgical retractors, pressure on peripheral nerves caused by the patient's position during the procedure, and birth trauma. The occurrences of postspinal neurologic sequelae are extremely rare. (176; **1504, 1506, 1508**)

102. It is important to consult a neurologist when nerve injury presents after a spinal anesthetic to establish a cause. If this is done early in the postoperative course the neurologist will be able to ascertain if the nerve injury is new or preexisting through the performance of electromyography. (176; **1508**)

103. Transient radicular irritation, also called transient neurologic symptoms, is a finding after the administration of a spinal anesthetic in which the patient complains of pain in the legs or buttocks. It appears to be due to direct neurotoxicity from the local anesthetic. Risk factors for transient radicular irritation include the use of lidocaine for spinal anesthesia, lithotomy position during surgery, and outpatient status. Indeed, when these three risk factors are combined the incidence has been found to be as high as 24%. Age, gender, history of back pain, needle type, and lidocaine concentration do not appear to have any influence over the risk of transient radicular irritation, whereas obesity may have some minor influence. To minimize the risk, alternative local anesthetics may be chosen, particularly for patients who will be positioned in lithotomy and will be discharged home after the procedure. (176; **517, 1506**)

104. Cauda equina syndrome has been reported to occur after the administration of continuous spinal anesthesia through a 28-gauge microbore catheter in the subarachnoid space. It is believed now that the slow continuous injection through the catheter resulted in the highly concentrated exposure of unmyelinated neural tissue to hyperbaric local anesthetic solution, causing irreversible damage to the nerve. The microbore catheters are no longer available for use. (176; **1506, 1515**)

105. The incidence of paralysis with spinal anesthesia is extremely rare. One retrospective review of over 582,000 spinal anesthetics cited an incidence of zero. (176; **1506**)

106. There was no difference in perioperative mortality between young, healthy patients who underwent scheduled elective surgery under spinal anesthesia and similar patients who underwent similar procedures under general anesthesia. (176)

EPIDURAL ANESTHESIA

107. The sterile, prepackaged kits for epidural anesthesia typically contain lidocaine for local infiltration, saline for loss of resistance technique, a test dose of lidocaine with epinephrine, a loss of resistance syringe, a 17- or 18-gauge epidural needle and an epidural catheter, various other syringes and needles, drapes, and labels. Epidural catheters may have multiple orifices on the distal end to facilitate aspiration and contribute to the spread of local anesthetic in the epidural space. (179, Fig. 13–11)

108. Epidural anesthesia is instituted in a similar fashion to spinal anesthesia. The patient is placed in a seated upright or lateral decubitus position with the back flexed as much as possible. The back is prepared and draped sterilely, local infiltration of the skin overlying the chosen interspace is administered, and the anesthesiologist proceeds to locate the epidural space. A 17- or 18-gauge Tuohy needle is used to find the epidural space. The needle tip is curved to help prevent accidental puncture of the dura mater and to facilitate threading of the epidural catheter through the needle into the epidural space.

    The epidural space is locatable by the loss of resistance technique for anatomic reasons. First, the tough ligamentum flavum overlies the space posteriorly, providing resistance to the needle as it passes through it. Second, there is negative pressure in the epidural space implying negative resistance. The change in resistance, or loss of resistance, as the needle passes through the ligamentum flavum into the epidural space accounts for the method by which anesthesiologists locate the epidural space. The anesthesiologist can sense the loss of resistance by connecting a syringe on the hub of the Tuohy needle and applying continuous gentle pressure on the plunger of the syringe as the needle is advanced through the ligaments into the epidural space. Once the epidural space is located with the Tuohy needle by the loss of resistance technique the epidural catheter can be threaded into the space, typically 2 to 5 cm. Epidural catheters that are threaded farther into the space are more likely to enter a vein, puncture the dura, or migrate into the intervertebral foramina. After the epidural catheter has been placed and the Tuohy needle has been pulled back, the epidural catheter is best secured in place by taping it to the patient's back. (179–180, Fig. 13–12; **1509–1511, Fig. 42–18**)

109. The epidural catheter, once threaded past the end of the Tuohy needle, must never be pulled back through the Tuohy needle for fear that this may result in shearing of the catheter in the epidural space. Instead, if the epidural catheter must be removed once it has exited the tip of the Tuohy needle, it is generally recommended that the needle and catheter be withdrawn together as a unit. (179)

110. The test dose commonly used for the epidural catheter is 3 mL of 1.5% lidocaine with 1:200,000 epinephrine. The test dose is performed to exclude the possibility that the epidural catheter has been accidentally placed into an epidural vein or into the subarachnoid space. The anesthesiologist must wait at least 3 minutes after the administration of the test dose to safely exclude these two possibilities. (180; **1511**)

111. If the epidural catheter were in an epidural vein there would be a definitive, rapid, self-limited increase in heart rate in response to the intravenous administration of 3 mL of 1:200,000 epinephrine in the test dose. (180)

112. If the epidural catheter were in the subarachnoid space, there would be a saddle area sensory and motor anesthetic block as a result of the subarachnoid injection of 45 mg of lidocaine in the test dose. (180)

113. The appropriate epidural dose of local anesthetic solution for the planned procedure should be estimated for administration. Typically, volumes of 15

to 25 mL of local anesthetic are required in a lumbar epidural catheter to achieve an adequate level of sensory analgesia for an abdominal procedure. The dose should be administered into the epidural space over 1 to 3 minutes. It is prudent to fractionate the administered dose, performing aspiration before the administration of each fraction, in the event that the catheter migrated or the epidural test dose was mistakenly believed to be negative. (180–181; **1511, 1515**)

114. The level of anesthesia after the administration of an epidural anesthetic is determined in a similar manner to that of a spinal anesthetic. The level of sympathetic nervous system blockade can be determined by the discrimination of temperature at various levels by using an alcohol sponge. The level of sensory nerve blockade can be determined by the discrimination of a sharp object at various levels. (181)

115. The single-shot technique of an epidural anesthetic involves the administration of the local anesthetic solution through the Tuohy needle when the duration of anesthetic required for the procedure is short. (181)

116. There are two major influences over the level and duration of epidural anesthesia. First is the volume and concentration, or dose, of local anesthetic administered. Second is the presence or absence of epinephrine in the local anesthetic solution injected. The position of the patient during the administration of the local anesthetic solution in the epidural space has minimal influence on the subsequent level of anesthesia achieved, although the more dependent side may have a more intense block than the nondependent side. The weight, height, and age of the patient and baricity of the local anesthetic solution do not influence the distribution of local anesthetic in the epidural space. (181; **507, 1508, 1513, Table 42–8**)

117. The following are local anesthetics commonly used for epidural anesthesia, their concentration, time of onset, and duration of action. (181, Table 13–4; **1512, Table 42–8**)

	CONCENTRATION (%)	ONSET (min)	DURATION (min)
Chloroprocaine	2–3	5–15	30–90
Lidocaine	1–2	5–15	60–120
Ropivacaine	0.25–1	10–20	120–140
Bupivacaine	0.25–0.75	10–20	120–240

118. Tetracaine and procaine are rarely used for epidural anesthesia because of their slow onset of action. (181; **507**)

119. The cephalad spread exceeds the caudad spread of local anesthesia when injected into a lumbar epidural catheter for two reasons. The first is because of the transmission of negative intrathoracic pressures in the cephalad portion of the space, drawing the anesthetic in a cephalad direction. Second, the resistance of the epidural space increases at the lumbosacral junction because of narrowing, making cephalad spread the path of least resistance. (181)

120. A unilateral anesthetic block may result from the administration of local anesthetic in the epidural space secondary to the plica mediana dorsalis, a connective tissue band in the epidural space that extends in a vertical direction between the ligamentum flavum and dura mater dividing the epidural space in half. (181; **1493–1494, Fig. 42–5**)

121. The major site of action of local anesthetics administered in the epidural space is at the spinal nerve roots. At the spinal nerve roots the dura mater is relatively thin, allowing for the easiest diffusion of local anesthetic through the dura mater to the nerves. (182; **501**)

122. The addition of epinephrine to a local anesthetic solution to be administered in the epidural space prolongs the duration by causing localized vasoconstriction in the area that the drug is administered. This results in decreased vascular absorption of the drug from that area and a prolonged amount of time in which the local anesthetic is in contact with the nerve roots at the administered concentration. The addition of epinephrine to local anesthetic solutions for administration in the epidural space seems to prolong the duration of lidocaine more than bupivacaine. (181; **507, 1512–1513, Table 42–8**)

123. There is often a delayed onset in anesthesia at the S1–S2 nerve root region during an epidural anesthetic. This may be due to the covering of these nerve roots with connective tissue, slowing the diffusion of local anesthetic to these nerve roots. (182; **2129**)

124. The diffusion of local anesthetic from the epidural space to the subarachnoid space is a minor contributor to the anesthetic effects of local anesthetic solutions in the epidural space. (182)

125. Epidural anesthesia results in sympathetic nerve blockade, sensory nerve blockade, and motor nerve blockade just as in spinal anesthesia. In epidural anesthesia, however, the levels of each are different than they are in spinal anesthesia. First, sympathetic nerve blockade is at a level equal to sensory nerve blockade, rather than the two to six segments higher that is seen in spinal anesthesia. Second, motor nerve blockade may average four segments lower than sensory nerve blockade, rather than the two segments seen in spinal anesthesia. (182)

126. The vascular absorption of epinephrine from the epidural space when administered as part of a local anesthetic solution results in very low systemic plasma levels. These low levels may result in primarily beta-agonist effects, augmenting the vasodilation and decrease in blood pressure seen when local anesthetics are administered alone. (182)

127. Epidural anesthesia produces similar effects as spinal anesthesia on the respiratory and gastrointestinal systems. (182)

128. The potential side effects of spinal anesthesia also apply to epidural anesthesia. Additional side effects of an epidural anesthetic that do not apply to spinal anesthesia include the risks of accidental dural puncture, local anesthetic toxicity, subdural injection, and epidural hematoma formation. (182; **1513–1514**)

129. The risk of epidural hematoma formation resulting from an epidural anesthetic is extremely low. Patients on anticoagulants are considered to be at the greatest risk, although the incidence is extremely low even in patients with bleeding abnormalities. There are multiple reviews in the literature of patients who received anticoagulation intraoperatively and postoperatively without any neurologic sequelae. Nevertheless, the American Society of Regional Anesthesia published their consensus statement titled Neuraxial Anesthesia and Anticoagulation in May 1998 with their recommendations on how epidural catheters should be managed in the perioperative period in the presence of anticoagulation. (182; **1514**)

130. Accidental puncture of the dura mater during attempted localization of the epidural space can be recognized by the anesthesiologist by the appearance

of cerebrospinal fluid in the hub of the epidural needle. The flow of cerebrospinal fluid from the large-bore needle is rapid and continuous. Cerebrospinal fluid is warm, distinguishing it from saline used for the loss of resistance technique for localization of the epidural space. Cerebrospinal fluid will also dipstick test positive for glucose. Once accidental dural puncture during attempted epidural anesthesia has occurred, the anesthesiologist may convert to a spinal anesthetic. Alternatively, the needle may be removed and reattempt an epidural anesthetic at another interspace. The development of a postdural puncture headache after accidental dural puncture with an 18-gauge epidural needle is likely, given the size of the hole in the dura mater produced by the relatively large needle. For this reason the patient should be informed about the possibility of a postdural puncture headache and should be instructed as to whom to contact for evaluation and treatment should a postdural puncture headache occur. (182; **1507**)

131. The accidental subarachnoid injection of the large volumes of local anesthetic intended for epidural anesthesia results in a rapidly evolving total spinal. (182; **1514**)

132. The accidental subdural injection of the large volumes of local anesthetic intended for epidural anesthesia results in a slowly evolving total spinal. A subdural injection of local anesthetic may be difficult to recognize. (183; **1514**)

133. The potential for local anesthetic systemic toxicity with epidural anesthesia is high because of the high doses of local anesthetic that must be given to produce epidural anesthesia, coupled with the numerous venous plexuses found in the epidural space that lend themselves to systemic absorption of the local anesthetic. Even so, blood levels of local anesthetic administered in the epidural space are rarely in the toxic range. The risk of systemic toxicity from the systemic absorption of local anesthetic administered in the epidural space is decreased by the addition of epinephrine to the local anesthetic solution. Epinephrine in the local anesthetic solutions slows the rate of systemic absorption of the local anesthetic in the epidural space. (182; **1513**)

134. Epidural anesthesia results in less abrupt hypotension than spinal anesthesia, owing to the slower onset of sympathetic nervous system blockade in epidural anesthesia. The treatment for hypotension resulting from epidural anesthesia is placing the patient in a modest head-down position, the administration of intravenous fluids, and, if necessary, the administration of sympathomimetics. (182; **1497**)

135. The accidental intravascular injection of the large volumes of local anesthetic intended for epidural anesthesia can result in local anesthetic toxicity. This may manifest as cardiovascular collapse, apnea, seizures, and unconsciousness. In the event this occurs, rapid treatment of the seizures and cardiovascular and ventilatory support are indicated. (182; **1513–1514**)

136. A combined spinal and epidural anesthetic is performed by passing a spinal needle through the large-bore Tuohy needle once localization of the epidural space has taken place. When the needle is confirmed to be in the subarachnoid space, local anesthetic and/or narcotic can be deposited into the subarachnoid space. The spinal needle is then removed, and an epidural catheter may be threaded through the Tuohy needle and secured. This technique allows for the rapid onset of anesthesia, while still allowing for a method to extend the duration of the anesthetic and/or provide for postoperative analgesia via the use of the epidural catheter. There are now Tuohy needles designed specifically for this technique. (181–182, Fig. 13-13)

CAUDAL ANESTHESIA

137. To facilitate the administration of a caudal anesthetic the adult patient should be in the prone position, whereas the pediatric patient may be in the lateral decubitus position. (183; **1508, Fig. 42–19**)

138. The sacral hiatus is located between the sacral cornua approximately 5 cm from the tip of the coccyx. (183; **1511–1512, 1525, Fig. 42–21**)

139. For the administration of a caudal anesthetic the needle is first introduced through the sacrococcygeal ligament perpendicular to the skin. After contact with the sacrum, the needle is withdrawn slightly and redirected at a slightly reduced angle about 2 cm into the caudal canal. The needle is then appropriately placed for the administration of the local anesthetic for caudal epidural anesthesia. (183, Fig. 13–14; **1511–1512**)

140. Confirmation that the needle tip is appropriately placed in the caudal canal for the administration of local anesthetic can be made by injecting about 5 mL of saline or air. If the needle is subcutaneously placed, subcutaneous air or a subcutaneous bulge will appear overlying the tip of the needle. Aspiration on the needle before injection would result in the appearance of cerebrospinal fluid in the syringe if the needle were erroneously placed in the subarachnoid space. (183; **1511–1512**)

141. Although the rectum is in close proximity to the point of needle insertion in a caudal epidural anesthetic, the incidence of infection is rare. (183)

142. A potential risk of caudal anesthesia is subarachnoid injection of the local anesthetic. The dural sac ends at S2. The risk of subarachnoid injection of local anesthetic during a caudal anesthetic is therefore limited if the tip of the needle does not extend beyond S2. In addition, the anesthesiologist should aspirate on the needle before the administration of the local anesthetic solution to confirm the absence of cerebrospinal fluid. (183; **1492**)

143. The failure rate of caudal anesthesia is as high as 10% secondary to anatomic anomalies of the caudal canal. If failure of the technique occurs, the anesthesiologist may proceed to do a lumbar epidural anesthetic. (183)

144. The performance of a caudal anesthetic is technically easier in children than in adults. (183; **1508**)

Chapter *13*

Peripheral Nerve Blocks

1. Name some types of peripheral nerve blocks.

2. Other than as anesthesia for a surgical procedure, what are some uses for peripheral nerve blocks?

3. What are some special considerations that should be made in the preoperative evaluation of a patient who is to undergo a peripheral nerve block?

PREPARATION FOR NERVE BLOCKS

4. What is the benefit of preoperative medication for patients who are to undergo a peripheral nerve block?

5. Where should a peripheral nerve block be performed?

6. What type of needle should be used to perform a peripheral nerve block? What are some advantages to using a control syringe for the performance of a peripheral nerve block?

7. During the performance of a peripheral nerve block, what does a paresthesia indicate? What is another method that may be used to locate the nerve?

8. Why are lower concentrations of local anesthetic used for peripheral nerve blocks than for spinal anesthesia?

CERVICAL PLEXUS BLOCK

9. For what surgical procedures is a cervical plexus block most often performed? What areas become anesthetized by a cervical plexus block?

10. What nerves form the cervical plexus?

11. What landmarks are used to locate the cervical plexus for blockade?

12. How is blockade of the deep cervical plexus achieved? What volume of local anesthetic solution is deposited during the performance of a deep cervical plexus block?

13. How is blockade of the superficial cervical plexus achieved? What volume of local anesthetic solution is deposited during the performance of a superficial cervical plexus block?

14. What are four potential complications of a cervical plexus block?

15. Why should bilateral cervical plexus nerve blocks be avoided?

BRACHIAL PLEXUS BLOCK

16. For what surgical procedures is a brachial plexus block useful? What areas become anesthetized by a brachial plexus block?

17. What nerve roots form the brachial plexus?

18. What landmarks are used to locate the brachial plexus for blockade?

19. What local anesthetic solutions are used for brachial plexus blockade?

20. What are three different approaches to blockade of the brachial plexus?

21. How is a brachial plexus block via the interscalene approach achieved? What volume of local anesthetic is deposited with this approach to brachial plexus blockade?

22. How can prolonged brachial plexus blockade be achieved via the interscalene approach?

23. What are some advantages of brachial plexus blockade via the interscalene approach?

24. What is a disadvantage of brachial plexus blockade via the interscalene approach?

25. What are some potential complications of brachial plexus blockade via the interscalene approach?

26. How is a brachial plexus block via the supraclavicular approach achieved? What volume of local anesthetic is deposited with this approach to brachial plexus blockade?

27. What are some advantages of brachial plexus blockade via the supraclavicular approach?

28. What are some potential complications of brachial plexus blockade via the supraclavicular approach?

29. What are two techniques for blockade of the brachial plexus via the axillary approach? What volume of local anesthetic is deposited with this approach to brachial plexus blockade?

30. What is the orientation of the nerves of the brachial plexus relative to the axillary artery in the axilla?

31. Why are frequent aspirations necessary during brachial plexus blockade via the axillary approach?

32. What nerves may require supplementation with blockade of the brachial plexus via the axillary approach? How is this achieved?

33. What are some advantages of brachial plexus blockade via the axillary approach?

34. What are some disadvantages of brachial plexus blockade via the axillary approach?

35. What are some potential complications of brachial plexus blockade via the axillary approach?

DISTAL NERVE BLOCKS OF THE UPPER EXTREMITY

36. Where is the median nerve located in the elbow? Where is the median nerve located in the wrist? What volume of local anesthetic must be deposited in the wrist to achieve a median nerve block?

37. Where is the ulnar nerve located in the elbow? Where is the ulnar nerve located in the wrist? What volume of local anesthetic must be deposited in the wrist to achieve an ulnar nerve block?

38. Where is the radial nerve located in the wrist? What volume of local anesthetic must be deposited in the wrist to achieve a radial nerve block?

INTERCOSTAL NERVE BLOCKS

39. What is the course of the intercostal nerves?

40. What is the sensory distribution of the intercostal nerves? For what procedure is intercostal nerve blockade frequently used?

41. How should an intercostal nerve block be performed? What volume of local anesthetic should be deposited for intercostal nerve blockade?

42. What is the potential problem with administering local anesthetic too far laterally during an intercostal nerve block?

43. What are some potential complications of intercostal nerve blockade?

BLOCKS OF THE LOWER EXTREMITY

44. What are the four major nerves of the lower extremity? What are the two branches of the sciatic nerve?

45. What nerves form the sciatic nerve?

46. For what procedure is sciatic nerve blockade most often used?

47. How is sciatic nerve blockade achieved? What volume of local anesthetic should be deposited for sciatic nerve blockade?

48. What nerves form the femoral nerve?

49. For what procedure is femoral nerve blockade most often used?

50. How is femoral nerve blockade achieved? What volume of local anesthetic should be deposited for femoral nerve blockade?

51. What nerves form the lateral femoral cutaneous nerve?

52. For what procedure is lateral femoral cutaneous nerve blockade most often used?

53. How is lateral femoral cutaneous nerve blockade achieved? What volume of local anesthetic should be deposited for lateral femoral cutaneous nerve blockade?

54. What nerves form the obturator nerve?

55. For what procedure is obturator nerve blockade most often used?

56. How is obturator nerve blockade achieved? What volume of local anesthetic should be deposited for obturator nerve blockade?

57. How is blockade of the femoral, obturator, and lateral femoral cutaneous nerves with a single injection achieved? What volume of local anesthetic should be deposited for this "three-in-one" block?

58. What are the five nerves that supply the foot? What areas do each of these supply?

59. How is an ankle block achieved? What is the total volume of local anesthetic that is typically deposited in an ankle block?

60. For what procedure is an ankle block most often used?

STELLATE GANGLION BLOCK

61. What areas are supplied by the stellate ganglion? What are the most common indications for the performance of a stellate ganglion block?

62. What is the origin of the stellate ganglion?

63. What landmarks are used for blockade of the stellate ganglion?

64. How is blockade of the stellate ganglion achieved? What volume of local anesthetic solution is deposited during the performance of a stellate ganglion block?

65. What are some signs of sympathetic nervous system blockade after the performance of a stellate ganglion block? Which of these provides conclusive evidence that the block has in fact been achieved?

66. What are some potential complications of a stellate ganglion block?

CELIAC PLEXUS BLOCK

67. What areas are supplied by the celiac plexus? What are the most common indications for the performance of a celiac plexus block?

68. What is the origin of the celiac plexus?

69. What landmarks are used for blockade of the celiac plexus?

70. How is blockade of the celiac plexus achieved? What volume of local anesthetic solution is deposited during the performance of a celiac plexus block?

71. What solutions other than local anesthetics may be deposited for celiac plexus blockade that is more permanent?

72. What are some potential complications of a celiac plexus block?

INTRAVENOUS REGIONAL NEURAL ANESTHESIA

73. For what is intravenous regional neural anesthesia (Bier block) commonly used?

74. How is a Bier block achieved? What volume of local anesthetic is used in a Bier block?

75. What local anesthetics are typically used for a Bier block?

76. What are some advantages of a Bier block?

77. What are some disadvantages of a Bier block?

78. What is a potential complication of a Bier block? How can this risk be minimized?

ANSWERS*

1. Types of peripheral nerve blocks include blocks of the cervical plexus, brachial plexus, median nerve, ulnar nerve, radial nerve, intercostal nerves, sciatic nerve, femoral nerve, lateral femoral cutaneous nerve, obturator nerve, stellate ganglion, and celiac plexus. (185)

2. In addition to surgical anesthesia, peripheral nerve blocks may be used for postoperative analgesia and the diagnosis and management of chronic pain syndromes. (185; **1520**)

3. Considerations that should be made in the preoperative evaluation of a patient who is to undergo a peripheral nerve block include the patient's coagulation status, the presence of any neuropathy in the involved nerves, the presence of any skin infection overlying the area where the needle will be inserted, and the presence of any anatomic abnormalities or difficulties with the usual landmarks for the performance of the nerve block. In addition, the patient should be evaluated in the usual manner with regard to history, physical examination, and laboratory analysis. The anesthesiologist must be prepared to administer another anesthetic in the event that the peripheral nerve block is not sufficient for surgical anesthesia and the surgery must proceed. (185; **1520**)

*Numbers in parentheses: lightface numbers refer to pages, figures, or tables in Stoelting RK, Miller RD: Basics of Anesthesia, 4th ed. Philadelphia, Churchill Livingstone, 2000; **boldface numbers** refer to pages, figures, or tables in Miller RD: Anesthesia, 5th ed. Philadelphia, Churchill Livingstone, 2000.

PREPARATION FOR NERVE BLOCKS

4. Preoperative medication for patients who are to undergo a peripheral nerve block may reduce the level of anxiety. Patients are often more receptive to receiving a peripheral nerve block if they are assured they will be made comfortable during the anesthetic and surgical procedures. (185; **1520**)

5. Peripheral nerve blocks that are not performed in the operating room should be performed in an area with the appropriate monitors, drugs, equipment, and oxygen should their use become urgently necessary. (185)

6. Needles that are used to perform a peripheral nerve block should have a blunted needle tip that will push a nerve away rather than traverse it. Advantages to using a control syringe for the performance of a peripheral nerve block are that it may provide for better control, it facilitates aspiration with one hand, and it allows the anesthesiologist to single-handedly refill the syringe without breaking sterility. (185, Fig. 14–1)

7. A paresthesia during the performance of a peripheral nerve block indicates that the nerve has been localized by the needle tip. If the pain persists or escalates during injection, there is a risk of an intraneural injection of the local anesthetic solution. If this occurs, the administration of the solution should be terminated and the patient evaluated. Another method that may be used to locate the nerve is with the delivery of an electrical current from a nerve stimulator. The electrical stimulus will produce a neural impulse that is conducted down the nerve, stimulating the motor end plate. This causes a motor response that will be visibly evident to the anesthesiologist. Proper location of the needle can be guided by the characteristic of the motor response as well as the degree of motor response from a given current. (185)

8. Lower concentrations of local anesthetic are used for peripheral nerve blocks than for spinal anesthesia secondary to the much greater volume of local anesthetic that is necessary to diffuse sufficiently to block nerves. This limits the total dose of local anesthetic delivered and reduces the risk of local anesthetic toxicity. (185–186)

CERVICAL PLEXUS BLOCK

9. A cervical plexus block is most often performed for carotid endarterectomy, lymph node dissection, and plastic surgical procedures. The skin under the mandible extending to the level of the second rib becomes anesthetized with a cervical plexus block. In addition, there is relaxation of the skeletal muscles of the neck. Cervical plexus blockade is achieved by blockade of both deep and superficial nerves of the plexus. The superficial cervical plexus nerves are primarily responsible for cutaneous innervation. (186; **1540–1541**)

10. The cervical plexus is derived from nerves C1 to C4. (186; **1540**)

11. Landmarks that may be used to locate the cervical plexus for blockade include the mastoid process, Chassaignac's tubercle, and the transverse process of C4. (186, Fig. 14–2; **1540–1541, Figs. 43–21, 43–22**)

12. Blockade of the deep cervical plexus can be achieved with either a single injection at C4 or with multiple injections at C2, C3, and C4. The single injection technique relies on cephalad spread of the local anesthetic. Typically 3 to 5 mL of local anesthetic is injected for the performance of a deep cervical plexus block. (186; **1540–1541**)

13. Blockade of the superficial cervical plexus can be achieved by infiltrating a large volume of local anesthetic along the posterior border of the sternocleidomastoid

muscle. Typically about 15 mL of local anesthetic is injected for the performance of a superficial cervical plexus block. (186; **1540–1541**)

14. Complications of a cervical plexus block include intravascular injection into the vertebral artery; blockade of the phrenic, superior laryngeal, and recurrent laryngeal nerves; Horner's syndrome; and injection into the epidural or subarachnoid space. (186; **1540**)

15. Bilateral blockade of the cervical plexus should be avoided so as not to achieve a bilateral phrenic nerve block. (186; **1540**)

BRACHIAL PLEXUS BLOCK

16. Brachial plexus blocks are useful for surgery on the shoulder or upper extremity. Areas anesthetized by a brachial plexus block include all the muscles and most of the sensation of the upper extremity. (186; **1521**)

17. The brachial plexus is derived from the anterior rami of C5 to T1. (186, Fig. 14–3; **1521, Fig. 43–1**)

18. Landmarks that may be used to locate the brachial plexus for blockade include the anterior and middle scalene muscles, the interscalene groove, the transverse process of C6, the clavicle, the axillary artery, and the subclavian artery pulse. (186; **1521**)

19. Among the local anesthetic solutions that may be used for brachial plexus blockade are bupivacaine, mepivacaine, lidocaine, and ropivacaine. (186–187)

20. The three different approaches to blockade of the brachial plexus are the interscalene, supraclavicular, and axillary approaches. (187; **1521**)

21. Brachial plexus blockade via the interscalene approach begins with localization of the interscalene groove by palpation. The patient is placed in the supine position with his or her head turned to the opposite side. The lateral edge of the sternocleidomastoid muscle is located, and posterior palpation will first encounter the belly of the anterior scalene muscle before locating the interscalene groove, which lies between the anterior scalene and middle scalene muscles. The needle is then placed in the interscalene groove at approximately the C6 level. Further localization can then be achieved with either a nerve stimulator or by eliciting paresthesias. Typically, 30 to 40 mL of local anesthetic is deposited, with intermittent aspirations on the syringe to avoid intravascular injection. The administration of 40 mL of local anesthetic has a greater likelihood of achieving blockade sufficient for shoulder surgery. (187–188, Fig. 14–5; **1522–1523, Fig. 43–3**)

22. Prolonged brachial plexus blockade via the interscalene approach can be achieved with the placement of a catheter for the continuous infusion of local anesthetic solution. (187)

23. Advantages of brachial plexus blockade via the interscalene approach include a relatively low risk of pneumothorax, ease of palpation of necessary landmarks, and the ability to perform the block with the patient's arm at his or her side. (188; **1521**)

24. A disadvantage of brachial plexus blockade via the interscalene approach is the inconsistency with which the ulnar nerve is blocked, making it likely that surgery involving the distribution of the ulnar nerve will necessitate supplemental anesthesia. (188; **1522**)

25. Complications of brachial plexus blockade via the interscalene approach include phrenic and recurrent laryngeal nerve blocks; epidural, intrathecal, and intravascular injections; and nerve damage. (188; **1522**)

26. Brachial plexus blockade via the supraclavicular approach can be achieved by injecting local anesthetic where the nerves of the brachial plexus cross the first rib. This is at about the midpoint of the clavicle and can be verified by palpation of the subclavian artery pulse. Once the first rib is encountered care should be taken not to advance the needle into the dome of the lung. When a paresthesia is obtained, 20 to 30 mL of local anesthetic should be deposited, with intermittent aspirations on the syringe to avoid intravascular injection. (188, Fig. 13–6; **1523–1524, Fig. 43–4**)

27. Advantages of brachial plexus blockade via the supraclavicular approach include its rapid onset and density with relatively less volume of anesthetic and the ability to perform the block with the patient's arm at his or her side. (188; **1523**)

28. Complications of brachial plexus blockade via the supraclavicular approach include its relatively increased risk of a pneumothorax. In fact, the incidence of a pneumothorax with this technique is about 1%, making it a poor choice for patients with respiratory compromise. Other complications include phrenic nerve block, Horner's syndrome, and nerve injury. (188; **1523**)

29. Brachial plexus blockade via the axillary approach can be done either by the transarterial approach or by eliciting paresthesias. The axillary artery and brachial plexus run together in the axillary sheath, and this is the basis for this approach to blockade of the brachial plexus. In either approach the arm must be abducted and externally rotated. The axillary artery is palpated, and the needle is advanced toward the artery until either traversing the artery (transarterial approach) or eliciting paresthesias. In the transarterial approach, local anesthetic solution is deposited both anterior and posterior to the axillary artery. Thirty to 40 mL of local anesthetic is deposited with the axillary approach to brachial plexus blockade, with frequent intermittent aspirations on the syringe to confirm the needle tip is not in the axillary artery or vein. (188–189, Fig. 14–8; **1524–1526**)

30. The nerves of the brachial plexus are reliably in a specific orientation to the axillary artery in the axilla. The musculocutaneous nerve has typically exited the axillary sheath at this level. The ulnar nerve lies inferior to the axillary artery, the radial nerve posterolateral, and the median nerve superior to the axillary artery. (189, Fig. 14–7; **1521, 1525, Fig. 43–7**)

31. Frequent aspiration is necessary during brachial plexus blockade via the axillary approach to avoid the injection of local anesthetic into the axillary artery. (189; **1525**)

32. The intercostobrachial and musculocutaneous nerves may require supplementation with blockade of the brachial plexus via the axillary approach. The intercostobrachial nerve, a branch of the T2 intercostal nerve, is easily supplemented with the infiltration of local anesthetic in the subcutaneous tissue over the proximal medial aspect of the axilla. The musculocutaneous nerve frequently requires supplementation because its takeoff from the axillary sheath may be proximal to the injection site. The musculocutaneous nerve can be supplemented with an injection of local anesthetic either between the biceps and brachialis muscles at approximately the mid humerus or within the body of the coracobrachialis muscle. (189; **1526–1527**)

33. Advantages of brachial plexus blockade via the axillary approach are its technical ease, reliable anesthesia of the hand and forearm, and relative safety. (189; **1525**)

34. Disadvantages of brachial plexus blockade via the axillary approach are its insufficient blockade for surgery of the shoulder or upper arm, the need to supplement it with a musculocutaneous nerve block, and the requirement for the patient to abduct and laterally rotate his or her arm. (189; **1525**)

35. Complications of brachial plexus blockade via the axillary approach include intravascular injection and nerve injury. (189; **1525**)

DISTAL NERVE BLOCKS OF THE UPPER EXTREMITY

36. In the elbow crease the median nerve is located 1 cm medial to the brachial artery. In the wrist the median nerve is located just lateral to the flexor palmaris longus tendon. Three to 5 milliliters of local anesthetic must be deposited in the wrist to achieve a median nerve block. (190, Fig. 14–9; **1528–1529, Figs. 43–8, 43–9**)

37. In the elbow the ulnar nerve is located in the groove between the medial condyle of the humerus and the olecranon of the ulna. Blockade of the ulnar nerve at the elbow is associated with a high incidence of neuritis and is not recommended. In the wrist the ulnar nerve is located medial to the ulnar artery. Three to 5 milliliters of local anesthetic must be deposited in the wrist to achieve an ulnar nerve block. (190, Fig. 14–9; **1529, Fig. 43–9**)

38. In the wrist the radial nerve is located lateral to the radial artery. Two to 3 milliliters of local anesthetic must be deposited in the wrist to achieve a radial nerve block. Branches of the radial nerve that innervate the lateral and dorsal aspects of the wrists also require infiltration. (190, Fig. 14–9; **1529, Fig. 43–10**)

INTERCOSTAL NERVE BLOCKS

39. The intercostal nerves arise from the primary rami of T1 to T11. Technically, T12 is not an intercostal nerve but a subcostal nerve. Each of the 12 nerves lies in the inferior costal groove of its corresponding rib. Running together with the nerve in the inferior costal groove are the intercostal vein and artery. The vein and artery lie superior to the nerve in the costal groove. (190; **1544, Fig. 43–26**)

40. The intercostal nerves provide sensation to the skin and innervation of the skeletal muscles of the abdominal wall. Intercostal nerve blockade is frequently used for postoperative analgesia after upper abdominal or thoracic surgery, for rib fracture analgesia, or for the placement of chest tubes. (190–191; **1543–1544**)

41. Intercostal nerve blocks are performed by first positioning the patient prone with a pillow supporting the patient's abdomen. The ribs corresponding to the designated nerve are then palpated. Starting with the lowest nerve to be blocked, the needle is inserted 6 to 8 cm from the midline until it contacts the rib. After contact with the rib the needle is walked off the inferior portion of the rib until it lies in the intercostal groove. After aspiration on the syringe to exclude intravascular injection, 3 to 5 mL of local anesthetic should be deposited for each intercostal nerve block. (190, Fig. 14–10; **1544–1545, Fig. 43–26**)

42. It is recommended that the injection of local anesthetic for an intercostal nerve block be done 6 to 8 cm from midline. If the injection is done too far laterally the intercostal nerve could potentially be blocked distal to the takeoff of its lateral cutaneous branches. (190; **1544–1545**)

43. Complications of intercostal nerve blockade include intravascular injection and pneumothorax. Multiple nerve blocks with a large total dose of administered local anesthetic may also result in significant plasma levels of local anesthetic. The close proximity of the vessels to the nerve in the inferior costal groove make systemic toxicity of local anesthetics an important consideration when performing intercostal nerve blocks. (191; **1544**)

BLOCKS OF THE LOWER EXTREMITY

44. The four major nerves of the lower extremity are the sciatic, femoral, lateral femoral cutaneous, and obturator nerves. The sciatic nerve branches just above

or at the popliteal fossa into the tibial nerve, passing medially, and the common peroneal nerve, passing laterally. (191; **1530**)

45. The sciatic nerve is derived from the anterior rami of L4 to S3. (191; **1534**)

46. Sciatic nerve blockade is most often used together with other nerve blocks for surgery below the knee that does not require a tourniquet. Alone, sciatic nerve blockade provides incomplete anesthesia of the foot and lower leg. (191; **1534**)

47. Sciatic nerve blockade is classically achieved by having the patient lie in the lateral position with the nondependent knee raised. The needle is inserted about 5 cm caudad to a line connecting the posterior superior iliac spine and the greater trochanter of the femur. Confirmation of needle placement can be made by either eliciting paresthesias or with the use of a nerve stimulator. About 25 mL of local anesthetic should be deposited for a sciatic nerve block. (191, Fig. 14–11; **1535–1536, Figs. 43–14, 43–15**)

48. The femoral nerve is derived from L2, L3, and L4. (191; **1531–1532**)

49. Femoral nerve blockade is most often used together with other nerve blocks for surgery in the leg. Alone, femoral nerve blockade provides anesthesia of the anterior thigh and may be used for muscle biopsies in that area. (191; **1532**)

50. Femoral nerve blockade is achieved with the injection of 10 to 20 mL of local anesthetic just below the midpoint of the inguinal ligament and just lateral to the femoral artery. (191; **1532, Fig. 43–13**)

51. The lateral femoral cutaneous nerve is derived from L2 and L3. (191; **1533**)

52. Lateral femoral cutaneous nerve blockade is most often used for anesthesia for the lower extremity in conjunction with other nerve blocks. Alone, lateral femoral cutaneous nerve blockade provides incomplete anesthesia of the anterolateral thigh. (191; **1533**)

53. Lateral femoral cutaneous nerve blockade is achieved by inserting a needle 2 cm medial and 2 cm below the anterior superior iliac spine and depositing 5 to 10 mL of local anesthetic. (191; **1533–1534, Fig. 43–13**)

54. The obturator nerve is derived from L3 and L4, with occasional minor contributions from L2. (191; **1534**)

55. Obturator nerve blockade is most often used for anesthesia for knee surgery in conjunction with other nerve blocks. Alone, obturator nerve blockade provides primarily motor blockade of the thigh adductor muscles. (191; **1534**)

56. Obturator nerve blockade is achieved with the patient in the supine position. The needle is inserted 1 to 2 cm lateral and caudad to the pubic tubercle. The needle is walked 2 to 3 cm laterally and caudad off the inferior pubic ramus until it passes into the obturator canal. Ten to 15 milliliters of local anesthetic should be deposited for obturator nerve blockade. (191; **1534, Fig. 43–13**)

57. Blockade of the femoral, obturator, and lateral femoral cutaneous nerves can be achieved with a single injection. It is done by depositing a large volume of local anesthetic in the fascial envelope around the femoral nerve, applying distal pressure, and relying on the proximal spread of local anesthetic to bathe the lumbar plexus. It is most often done using a 5 cm needle with the patient in the supine position. The needle is advanced lateral to the femoral artery in the cephalad direction until eliciting paresthesias, at which point the local anesthetic is deposited. Twenty to 40 milliliters of local anesthetic should be deposited for this "three-in-one" block with intermittent aspirations on the syringe to minimize the risk of an intravascular injection. The administration of 40 mL of local anesthetic has a greater likelihood of achieving blockade of the obturator nerve. (191–192; **1531, Fig. 43–11**)

58. The posterior tibial, sural, deep peroneal, superficial peroneal, and saphenous nerves supply the entire innervation to the foot. The posterior tibial nerve innervates the sole of the foot, heel, and plantar portion of the toes. The sural nerve innervates the lateral portion of the foot and ankle. The deep peroneal nerve innervates primarily between the first two digits of the foot. The superficial peroneal nerve innervates the majority of the dorsum of the foot. The saphenous nerve innervates the medial foot and ankle. (192; **1535–1536**)

59. An ankle block can be achieved with three separate injections. The posterior tibial nerve is blocked by depositing medicine behind the posterior tibial artery near the border of the medial malleolus and medial to the Achilles tendon. The sural nerve is blocked by depositing medicine lateral to the Achilles tendon near the lateral malleolus. The deep peroneal nerve is blocked by depositing medicine immediately lateral to the anterior tibial artery on the dorsum of the foot. Without withdrawing the needle, a cuff of local anesthetic is deposited both medially and laterally toward the malleoli to block the superficial peroneal and saphenous nerves. Fifteen to 20 milliliters of local anesthetic is deposited for an ankle block. (192, Fig. 14–12; **1536–1537, Figs. 43–17, 43–18**)

60. An ankle block is most often used for surgical procedures of the foot that do not require a tourniquet. (192; **1536**)

STELLATE GANGLION BLOCK

61. The stellate ganglion supplies the sympathetic innervation to the head and arm. The most common indications for the performance of a stellate ganglion block are for the diagnosis and treatment of complex regional pain syndromes and to increase blood flow in patients with vascular insufficiency in the upper extremity. (192–193; **1543, 2362**)

62. The stellate ganglion is derived from the inferior and first thoracic ganglion of the cervical sympathetic chain. (192; **1543**)

63. Landmarks used to identify the location of the stellate ganglion include Chassaignac's tubercle, or the transverse process at C6, the sternocleidomastoid muscle, and the pulse of the carotid artery. (192; **1543, 2362, Fig. 43–25**)

64. Blockade of the stellate ganglion is achieved through the insertion of the needle between the sternocleidomastoid muscle and the trachea over the transverse process of C6 until it is contacted. The needle is then withdrawn 2 to 3 mm, and 8 to 12 mL of local anesthetic solution is deposited. (192, Fig. 14–13; **1543, 2362**)

65. Signs of sympathetic nervous system blockade after the performance of a successful stellate ganglion block include ptosis, miosis, anhidrosis, nasal congestion, injection of the conjunctiva, vasodilation of the vessels in the extremity, and an increase in skin temperature of the extremity. Of all the signs of successful sympathetic nervous system blockade, only the increase in skin temperature of the extremity provides conclusive evidence that the block has in fact been achieved. The other signs may be achieved with the blockade of fibers that course lower than the stellate ganglion. (192–193; **1543, 2362**)

66. Complications of a stellate ganglion block include a pneumothorax, intravascular injection into the vertebral artery, recurrent laryngeal and phrenic nerve blockade, hematoma formation, and epidural and spinal injections. (193; **1543, 2362**)

CELIAC PLEXUS BLOCK

67. The celiac plexus innervates most of the abdominal viscera. The most common indications for the performance of a celiac plexus block is for intractable pain

associated with cancer of the pancreas or upper abdominal viscera. (193; **1545, 2364–2365**)

68. The celiac plexus is derived from nerves from T5 to T12. (193; **1545**)

69. Landmarks used to identify the location of the celiac plexus include the body of the L1 vertebra and the twelfth rib, usually under radiologic guidance. (193, Fig. 14–14; **1545, 2364–2365, Fig. 43–26**)

70. Blockade of the celiac plexus is usually achieved under the guidance of either computed tomography or fluoroscopy. The patient is placed in the prone position, and the needle is inserted lateral to the vertebral body of L1 and walked off the bone in an anterolateral direction until radiological confirmation of needle placement can be made. After aspiration, a 2 mL test dose of local anesthetic solution is deposited before the remaining 25 to 35 mL of local anesthetic solution. (193; **1545, 2364–2365**)

71. Phenol and alcohol solutions may also be deposited for celiac plexus blockade. When phenol or alcohol solutions are used, the intent is for the neurolysis of nerves that are causing intractable pain, as from cancer. Typically, a celiac plexus nerve block with local anesthetic is administered before a block with a neurolytic to establish that blockade of the celiac plexus will in fact alleviate the patient's pain. (193; **1545, 2364–2365**)

72. Potential complications of a celiac plexus block include hypotension; spinal, epidural, or intravascular injection; pneumothorax; puncture of abdominal viscera; and puncture of the inferior vena cava or aorta leading to a retroperitoneal hematoma. (193; **1545, 2365**)

INTRAVENOUS REGIONAL NEURAL ANESTHESIA

73. Intravenous regional neural anesthesia (Bier block) is commonly used for anesthesia for short surgical procedures on an extremity. (193; **1529**)

74. A Bier block is achieved by first placing an intravenous catheter distal in the extremity to be anesthetized. The extremity is then exsanguinated, a double tourniquet is placed proximal in the extremity, and the more proximal cuff is inflated. A dose of local anesthetic based on the patient's weight is administered slowly. The volume of local anesthetic is 25 to 50 mL in the upper extremity and 100 to 200 mL in the lower extremity. The onset of anesthesia is noted within 5 minutes. If the patient starts to develop tourniquet pain during the procedure, the distal cuff may be inflated and the proximal cuff deflated. (193, Fig. 14–15; **1530**)

75. Local anesthetics that can be used for a Bier block include 0.5% lidocaine and prilocaine. The total dose of prilocaine used for a Bier block should be less than 600 mg to minimize the risk of methemoglobinemia that can result from the metabolism of prilocaine. Chloroprocaine is not used because of the concern for thrombophlebitis, nor is bupivacaine, owing to its potential for cardiotoxicity. (193–194; **1530**)

76. Advantages of a Bier block include its ease of administration, rapid onset, rapidity of recovery, and excellent skeletal muscle relaxation. (193–194; **1529–1530**)

77. Disadvantages of a Bier block include the abrupt onset of potentially severe postoperative pain when the cuff is deflated, the difficulty in maintaining a bloodless field, and the potential for pain in an injured extremity during its exsanguination. (194; **1530**)

78. Complications of a Bier block include the risk of excessive, toxic doses of local anesthetic reaching the systemic circulation with accidental deflation of the tourniquet. This risk can be minimized at the conclusion of the case by deflating the tourniquet in increments over time. This allows the local anesthetic to enter the systemic circulation over a greater period of time. (194; **1530**)

Chapter 14

Positioning and Associated Risks

1. How does the absence of pain affect the positions that are tolerated by patients under general anesthesia? What is the clinical implication of this?

2. Whose responsibility is the intraoperative position of the anesthetized patient?

SPECIAL POSITIONS

3. What are the cardiovascular effects of placing the patient in the supine position for a surgical procedure?

4. How does the supine position affect lung perfusion?

5. How much does the functional residual capacity change when a patient's position is changed from standing to supine?

6. How does the administration of skeletal muscle paralysis affect the functional residual capacity of a patient in the supine position?

7. How should the patient's legs be ideally positioned during surgery in the supine position?

8. Why might focal alopecia result from surgery in the supine position?

9. Why might backache result from surgery in the supine position?

10. What are some potential positions the patient's arms may be placed in while the patient is in the supine position for surgery?

11. Describe how the patient's arms should be positioned when the patient is supine and the arms are abducted.

12. Describe how the patient's arms should be positioned when the patient is supine and the arms are adducted.

13. What are the cardiovascular effects of placing the patient in the head-down position, or Trendelenburg position, for a surgical procedure?

14. What are the pulmonary effects of placing the patient in the Trendelenburg position for a surgical procedure?

15. How does the Trendelenburg position affect the patient's intracranial pressure?

16. What is a potential complication of the use of shoulder braces to prevent the patient from sliding off the table while in the steep Trendelenburg position?

17. How does the prone position affect the patient's ventilatory mechanics? How can this effect of the prone position be offset?

18. What are the cardiovascular effects of placing the patient in the prone position for a surgical procedure? How can this potential problem be minimized?

19. What are the potential problems with placing the prone patient's head in the turned position? How can these potential problems be avoided?

20. What are the potential problems with placing the prone patient's head in a forward-facing position, as in a Mayfield headrest? How can these potential problems be minimized?

21. How should the patient's arms be positioned while in the prone position?

22. How can venous pooling in the lower extremities be offset while the patient is in the prone, flexed position, as during a laminectomy?

23. How does the lateral decubitus position affect the patient's ventilatory mechanics and ventilation-perfusion ratio during mechanical ventilation of the lungs? How might these effects of the lateral decubitus position be manifest clinically?

24. What are the cardiovascular effects of placing the patient in the lateral decubitus position for a surgical procedure?

25. What is the purpose of the axillary roll for patients who are placed in the lateral decubitus position? How can the achievement of this goal be confirmed?

26. How should the patient's head and neck be positioned when in the lateral decubitus position?

27. How should the patient's legs be positioned when in the lateral decubitus position?

28. How should the patient's nondependent arm be positioned when in the lateral decubitus position?

29. For what type of surgical procedure is the sitting position most often used?

30. What are the cardiovascular effects of placing the patient in the sitting position for a surgical procedure?

31. What is the principal potential intraoperative complication of positioning a patient in the sitting position for surgery?

32. Which patients are most likely to manifest cardiopulmonary effects from being placed in the lithotomy position for a surgical procedure?

33. How should a patient with a history of low back pain be positioned in the lithotomy position for surgery?

34. What is the principal potential intraoperative complication of positioning a patient in the lithotomy position for surgery? How can this potential problem be minimized?

35. What is a potential problem that can result from placing a patient in the lithotomy position for more than 4 hours during a surgical procedure?

PERIPHERAL NERVE INJURIES

36. What is the usual cause of a peripheral nerve injury? How can this risk be minimized?

37. What are some co-existing medical conditions that place a patient at an increased risk for a peripheral nerve injury?

38. Why is it important to seek early neurologic consultation when a peripheral nerve injury is manifest in the postoperative period?

39. What is the usual recovery time from a peripheral nerve injury?

40. Which peripheral nerve is most likely to manifest a postoperative neuropathy?

41. What are some ways in which the ulnar nerve may be injured intraoperatively? What position should a patient's arm be placed in to minimize this risk?

42. Are males or females more prone to an ulnar nerve injury? Why is this believed to be true?

43. How does injury to the ulnar nerve manifest clinically?

44. Which peripheral nerve is the second most likely to manifest a postoperative neuropathy?

45. Why is the brachial plexus especially susceptible to nerve injury during surgery?

46. What are some ways in which the brachial plexus may be injured intraoperatively?

47. How does injury to the brachial plexus manifest clinically?

48. What are some ways in which the radial nerve may be injured intraoperatively?

49. How does injury to the radial nerve manifest clinically?

50. What are some ways in which the median nerve may be injured intraoperatively?

51. How does injury to the median nerve manifest clinically?

52. What are some ways in which the sciatic nerve may be injured intraoperatively?

53. How does injury to the sciatic nerve manifest clinically?

54. Which peripheral nerve of the lower extremity is most likely to manifest a postoperative neuropathy?

55. What are some ways in which the common peroneal nerve may be injured intraoperatively?

56. How does injury to the common peroneal nerve manifest clinically?

57. What are some ways in which the anterior tibial nerve may be injured intraoperatively?

58. How does injury to the anterior tibial nerve manifest clinically?

59. What are some ways in which the femoral nerve may be injured intraoperatively?

60. How does injury to the femoral nerve manifest clinically?

61. What co-existing disease places patients at a greater risk of having a postoperative femoral nerve injury?

62. What are some ways in which the saphenous nerve may be injured intraoperatively?

63. What are some ways in which the obturator nerve may be injured intraoperatively?

64. How does injury to the obturator nerve manifest clinically?

65. How can the intraoperative use of a tourniquet result in nerve injury?

NON-NEURAL INJURY

66. What areas of skin are especially prone to ischemic damage during surgery? How can this risk be minimized?

67. What damage can occur to a patient's eyes intraoperatively that may have permanent effects? What are some clinical situations in which this may occur? How can this risk be minimized?

68. How can the patient's digits of the fingers or toes be injured during moving of operating table parts?

69. How can a patient's ears be damaged intraoperatively when in the lateral position?

DAMAGE RELATED TO THE ANESTHETIC FACE MASK

70. What are potential injuries to the patient that can be sustained during mask ventilation of the airway?

ANSWERS*

1. Pain cannot be used as an indicator that injury is occurring to a patient secondary to his or her position while under general anesthesia. An awake patient will typically move in response to pain, numbness, or tingling associated with nerve ischemia. Positions that would not be tolerated by an awake patient can be assumed for hours while under general anesthesia, especially when combined with drug-induced skeletal muscle relaxation. Therefore, the anesthesiologist must assume responsibility for the position the patient is placed in during general anesthesia, for appropriate padding of the pressure points, and must be aware of what some of the potential injuries are for various positions. A description of the positioning and padding should also be documented in the anesthesia record. (196; **1017, 1029**)

2. The position the patient is placed in intraoperatively while under general anesthesia is the responsibility of the anesthesiologist, surgeons, and nurses. The responsibility is shared among these operating room personnel. During the course of surgery the responsibility becomes primarily that of the anesthesiologist, who must be aware of any changes in the patient's position that have occurred intraoperatively. (196)

SPECIAL POSITIONS

3. Placement of a patient in the supine position may modestly increase cardiac output secondary to an increase in venous return. This results in a slight, reflex-mediated decrease in heart rate and little change in blood pressure. (197; **1017**)

4. The supine position produces more evenly distributed blood flow throughout the lung. (197; **1018**)

5. The functional residual capacity decreases by about 800 mL when a patient's position is changed from standing to supine, largely because of compression of the lung and cephalad displacement of the diaphragm by the abdominal contents. (197; **1018**)

6. The administration of skeletal muscle paralysis further decreases the functional residual capacity of a patient in the supine position. (197; **1018**)

7. While undergoing surgery in the supine position, the patient's legs should be positioned with slight flexion at both the hips and knees. Not only does this facilitate venous drainage from the lower extremities, it also decreases the amount of anterior abdominal wall tension during surgical closure of the abdomen. (197)

8. Focal alopecia may result from being placed in the supine position during surgery secondary to continued pressure in one area on the back of the head. This risk may be minimized by moving the patient's head slightly during surgery or placing the head on padding. (197)

9. Backache may result from surgery in the supine position because of the loss of the normal curvature of the lumbar spine that can occur during surgery, particularly with skeletal muscle relaxation. (197)

10. The patient's arms may be placed in the abducted or adducted (tucked) positions while in the supine position for surgery. One arm may also be adducted while the other is abducted. (197; **1030**)

11. When the supine patient's arms are abducted they should be placed on well-

---

*Numbers in parentheses: lightface numbers refer to pages, figures, or tables in Stoelting RK, Miller RD: Basics of Anesthesia, 4th ed. Philadelphia, Churchill Livingstone, 2000; **boldface numbers** refer to pages, figures, or tables in Miller RD: Anesthesia, 5th ed. Philadelphia, Churchill Livingstone, 2000.

padded armboards. The arms must be extended 90 degrees or less at the shoulder. Some debate exists regarding the position of the hand when the arm is abducted. It is believed that supination of the forearm may result in greater protection of the ulnar nerve from compression. Supination of the hand may result in greater stretching of the brachial plexus, however. In addition, supination of the forearm in awake patients is uncomfortable. An alternative is leaving the forearm in the neutral position or pronated. The neutral position is the spontaneous position of an awake, supine patient. (197–198, Fig. 15–1; **1030**)

12. When the supine patient's arms are adducted, or tucked in to the patient's side, care should be taken to avoid placing any portion of the arm or fingers against any metal surfaces or hard edges of the operating table. This can be accomplished by padding the arm circumferentially before securing it. Most often the arms are allowed to remain in the neutral position, with the palms facing the patient's side. (198; **1030**)

13. Placement of a patient in the head-down position, or Trendelenburg position, for a surgical procedure results in an increase in central venous pressure and myocardial work. There may be an effective decrease in stroke volume in these patients. A decreased stroke volume can result from the cephalad displacement of the abdominal contents, such that the diaphragm impinges on the heart. In hypovolemic patients placement of the patient in the Trendelenburg position may exacerbate already present hypotension. (198; **1022**)

14. Placement of a patient in the head-down position for a surgical procedure results in an increase in pulmonary venous pressure and a decrease in pulmonary compliance and functional residual capacity. This occurs secondary to an increase in central venous pressure and from the cephalad displacement of the abdominal contents against the lung bases. This may manifest as increased peak inspiratory pressures with mechanical ventilation. (198; **1022**)

15. Placement of a patient in the head-down position for a surgical procedure results in an increase in the intracranial pressure. (198; **1022**)

16. Brachial plexus injury can occur when shoulder braces are used to prevent the patient from sliding down the table when in the steep Trendelenburg position. The brachial plexus injury is due to the weight of the torso and subsequent stretching of the brachial plexus. (198; **1022**)

17. Placement of a patient in the prone position results in cephalad displacement of the diaphragm because of pressure from the abdominal contents against the operating room table. This can lead to a decrease in the functional residual capacity and impairment of diaphragmatic motion manifesting as increased peak inspiratory pressures with mechanical ventilation. This effect of the prone position may be offset by placing firm rolls or bolsters along the patient's sides from the clavicle to the iliac crest. The bolsters relieve the pressure of the abdomen against the table and restore diaphragmatic excursion. (198; **1903**)

18. Placement of a patient in the prone position results in compression of the aorta and inferior vena cava. This, in turn, causes impaired venous return to the heart and an increase in myocardial work. A decrease in cardiac output becomes likely. This effect of the prone position may be offset by placing firm rolls or bolsters along the patient's sides from the clavicle to the iliac crest. The bolsters relieve the compression on the aorta and inferior vena cava, facilitate venous return, and decrease the work of the myocardium. (198; **1903**)

19. Placing the prone patient's head in the turned position can result in jugular venous outflow obstruction, as well as obstruction to vertebral artery blood flow and, rarely, thrombosis. In addition, this position can result in postoperative neck pain, especially in patients with a history of cervical arthritis. These potential problems can be avoided by placing the patient's head in a forward-

facing position on a padded rest, such as a Mayfield headrest. The padded rest typically supports the patient's head around the periphery of the face, leaving the center of the face without contact with the padding. (198; **1903**)

20. Potential problems with placing the prone patient's head in a forward-facing position, as in a Mayfield headrest, is the risk of compression of the face on the table or padding. This can be especially hazardous with unrecognized slipping of the patient during the procedure. Of particular concern is pressure on the globes of the eye, which can result in retinal ischemia and blindness. These potential problems can be minimized by frequently checking the patient's eyes, nose, and ears during the course of the surgical procedure. (198; **1030, 1903**)

21. While in the prone position the patient's arms should be positioned such that abduction of the arms at the shoulder is limited to less than 90 degrees. The patient's arms may be placed at the patient's sides or above the head. This helps to minimize the risk of injury to the brachial plexus. (198, Fig. 15–2)

22. Venous pooling in the lower extremities while the patient is in the prone, flexed position can be offset with the placement of fitted elastic stockings or sequential compression devices. (198)

23. Placement of a patient in the lateral decubitus position can result in significant mismatching of pulmonary ventilation-to-perfusion during mechanical ventilation of the lungs for a number of reasons. First, while in the lateral position the mechanically ventilated patient has relatively better ventilation of the superior lung, while the dependent lung is being ventilated less. The reasons for the dependent lung being ventilated less are secondary to the loss of lung volume from compression by abdominal contents, mediastinal contents, and the structures used to position the patient. The patient concurrently has better perfusion of the dependent lung, primarily secondary to the effects of gravity. Together, these factors result in greater mismatching of ventilation and perfusion of the lungs during mechanical ventilation in a patient in the lateral decubitus position. Clinically, this may manifest as arterial hypoxemia. (199; **578–582, 1686–1689, Figs. 26–6, 26–7, 48–9, 48–10, 48–11, 48–12, 48–13**)

24. Placement of a patient in the lateral decubitus position can result in compression of the inferior vena cava from the pressure of a kidney rest. This can lead to a decrease in venous return to the heart. (199)

25. An axillary roll properly placed under a patient in the lateral decubitus position supports the patient's chest and minimizes the risk of compression of the nerves and vessels in the axilla. The dependent brachial plexus may also be injured should the axilla be compressed sufficiently to compress the brachial plexus. Proper placement of the axillary roll is under the thorax caudad to the axilla. The radial pulse may be checked periodically intraoperatively as a gross measure of compression of the vessels in the axilla. Alternatively, a pulse oximeter may be placed on a finger of the dependent hand to ensure no compression of arteries has occurred. (199; **1019–1021, Fig. 26–6**)

26. The patient's head and neck while in the lateral decubitus position should be positioned such that the cervical vertebrae of the neck are in line with the thoracic vertebrae. This can be accomplished with placing the patient's head on a pillow of the correct height. Insufficient padding under the head of the patient in the lateral decubitus position can result in injury to the nondependent brachial plexus. (193, 199, Figs. 14–4, 15–3; **1019–1021, Figs. 26–6, 26–7**)

27. The patient's legs while in the lateral decubitus position should be positioned such that the dependent leg is flexed at the knee and there is a pillow between the two legs. This helps to minimize stretch of the nerves of the dependent leg and distributes more evenly the weight of the legs, such that discrete pressure

points are avoided. Indeed, there have been case reports of arterial insufficiency of the dependent leg of patients undergoing hip arthroplasty in the lateral position leading to the need for subsequent below-the-knee amputation. (199; **1019–1021, Figs. 26–6, 26–7**)

28. The patient's nondependent arm while in the lateral decubitus position should be positioned on an elevated armboard or pillow above and in front of the patient's face. Alternatively, the arm may be suspended from a support bar that is well-padded. Both positions should limit the extension of the arm to less than 90 degrees at the shoulder. (199; **1019–1021, Figs. 26–6, 26–7**)

29. The sitting position is most often used for neurosurgical procedures, especially in the posterior fossa. The advantages of the sitting position for posterior fossa craniotomies are improved surgical exposure, less required retraction of the brain, and facilitated jugular venous drainage leading to less bleeding. (199–200; **1024, 1903, Figs. 26–14, 52–7, Table 26–1**)

30. Patients placed in the sitting position for a surgical procedure may become hypotensive, especially if hypovolemic. Additionally, patients may have decreases in cardiac output and cerebral perfusion pressures. Hypotension can be avoided by positioning the patient in gradual steps to allow for accommodation, by ensuring adequate hydration, and through the temporary administration of small doses of vasopressors. (200; **1024, 1904–1905**)

31. The principal potential intraoperative complication of positioning a patient in the sitting position for surgery is a venous air embolism. Placing the head above the level of the heart during the procedure facilitates the entrainment of room air. Patients undergoing craniotomies are especially at risk, given that veins in the bony cranium do not collapse after being transected. (200; **1027–1029, 1906**)

32. Patients with a large abdominal mass, parturients, or obese patients are most likely to manifest cardiovascular effects when placed in the lithotomy position for a surgical procedure. These patients are more likely to have obstruction of the inferior vena cava in this position. In addition, the lithotomy position leads to the cephalad displacement of the diaphragm by the abdominal viscera, potentially impairing spontaneous ventilation. Again, this may be augmented in patients with a large abdominal mass, parturients, or obese patients. (200)

33. Patients with a history of low back pain may suffer from exacerbation of their pain after being placed in the lithotomy position for surgery. These patients may benefit from assuming the position themselves in the awake position and choosing the position that is most comfortable for them. An alternative position for surgery may also be considered. (200–201)

34. The principal potential intraoperative complication of positioning a patient in the lithotomy position for surgery is peripheral nerve injury. Injury can occur to the sciatic, common peroneal, femoral, saphenous, or obturator nerves in this position. This potential problem can be minimized by ensuring that the patient's legs are well padded in areas where they could potentially be compressed against metal braces. While positioning the patient, the legs should be lifted simultaneously, flexed no more than 90 degrees at the hip, and then simultaneously rotated for placement into the stirrups. (200–201, Figs. 15–5, 15–6; **1018–1019, Figs. 26–2, 26–3, 26–4, 26–5**)

35. Compartment syndrome secondary to inadequate circulation can result from placing a patient in the lithotomy position for more than 4 hours during a surgical procedure. The common initiating event is probably direct local muscle pressure. This can occur from inadequate padding, tight leg straps, or the surgeon leaning on the leg for a prolonged period of time. The direct pressure may lead to arterial insufficiency, tissue necrosis and edema, and rhabdomyolysis. (201, Fig. 15–7; **1018**)

PERIPHERAL NERVE INJURIES

36. Peripheral nerve injuries have occurred in patients after regional anesthesia or sedation as well as general anesthesia. There are several causes of a peripheral nerve injury. Injury occurring to a nerve intraoperatively is usually due to compression or stretching of the nerve. The injury usually sustained to the nerve is neurapraxic, which is a loss of function without corresponding anatomic injury. The risk of sustaining an intraoperative nerve injury can be minimized by carefully positioning patients and by using padding when and where appropriate. There is evidence to suggest that patients who experience intraoperative nerve injury may have preexisting conditions that made the injury unavoidable, even with proper positioning and padding. (202; **1029–1030**)

37. Co-existing medical conditions that place a patient at an increased risk for a peripheral nerve injury include occupational trauma, congenital anomalies, cubital entrapment syndrome, hematomas, hypothermia, hypotension, prolonged tourniquet time, cigarette smoking, and diseases such as diabetes mellitus, vitamin deficiency, alcoholism, or cancer. (202; **1030**)

38. Neurologic consultation obtained early after a peripheral nerve injury manifests in the postoperative period may be useful in detecting between acute injury and chronic injury. This can be accomplished through nerve conduction velocity and electromyographic studies. Signs of denervation from acute nerve injury are detected by an electromyogram 18 to 21 days after the injury, emphasizing the importance of obtaining neurologic consultation before this time. It may also be useful to test the same nerve in the limb opposite the symptomatic one to exclude any preexisting nerve injury that is asymptomatic. (202)

39. The usual recovery time from an intraoperative peripheral nerve injury is 3 to 12 months. In rare cases, injury can be permanent, particularly with stretch injury that results in disrupted axons. (202–203; **1029–1030**)

40. The most common peripheral nerve to manifest a postoperative neuropathy is the ulnar nerve. (203, Fig. 15–10; **1030**)

41. The ulnar nerve may be injured intraoperatively secondary to compression of the nerve against the posterior aspect of the medial epicondyle of the humerus or in the cubital tunnel. There appears to be an increased incidence of ulnar nerve injury associated with sternal retraction during cardiac surgery. The ulnar nerve is at a greater risk of injury when the elbow is flexed or the forearm is pronated. Supination of the forearm intraoperatively may provide some protection to the ulnar nerve, although this may increase the risk to the brachial plexus. Flexion of the arm should be avoided, because this may increase the risk of injury to the ulnar nerve. (203–204; **1030, Fig. 26–19**)

42. Males are five times more likely to acquire an ulnar neuropathy than females, lending evidence to the possibility that males are more prone to an ulnar nerve injury. It may be an anatomic predisposition that makes males more likely to get an ulnar nerve injury. (204; **1072**)

43. Ulnar nerve injury manifests clinically as decreased sensation over the ventral and dorsal portions of the medial one and one-half fingers and an inability to abduct or oppose the fifth finger. Over time, ulnar nerve injury results in the appearance of a "claw hand" secondary to atrophy of the intrinsic muscles. (203)

44. The second most common peripheral nerve to manifest a postoperative neuropathy is the brachial plexus. (204; **1030**)

45. The brachial plexus is especially susceptible to nerve injury during surgery

because its course is superficial and fixed between two points. In addition, it lies close to the clavicle and humerus, which are very mobile. (204, Fig. 15–11)

46. The brachial plexus may be injured intraoperatively through both stretching and compression of the plexus. Stretching of the brachial plexus can occur with neck extension, with turning the head to the opposite side, or with the patient in the lateral decubitus position with inadequate padding to support the neck in the midline position. It can also occur in any position when the arm is abducted more than 90 degrees. Compression of the brachial plexus may occur with inappropriately placed shoulder braces or by spreading of the sternum during cardiopulmonary surgery. (204, Fig. 15–12; **1019**)

47. Injury to the brachial plexus manifests as a limply hanging arm at the side, rotated medially, with a pronated forearm. This position of the arm is commonly referred to as "waiter's tip." (204)

48. The radial nerve may be injured intraoperatively if the arm slips off the surgical table or if pressure is applied to the humerus where the radial nerve runs in the spiral groove. A rare cause of radial nerve injury is the mechanical effects of an automated blood pressure cuff. (204, Fig. 15–13)

49. Injury to the radial nerve manifests as decreased sensation over the dorsal surface of the lateral three fingers and an inability to extend the metacarpophalangeal joints or abduct the thumb. It is also characterized by wristdrop. (204)

50. The median nerve may be injured intraoperatively by needle injury in the antecubital fossa or by the extravasation of injected medicines. (206)

51. Injury to the median nerve manifests as decreased sensation on the palmar surface of the lateral three fingers and an inability to oppose the first and fifth digits. (206)

52. The sciatic nerve may be injured intraoperatively by compression of the nerve or during intramuscular injections in the upper, outer quadrant of the buttocks. Injury may also occur by stretching with external rotation of the leg, which most often occurs while in the lithotomy position. The risk of sciatic nerve stretching can be minimized by the avoidance of excessive rotation of the legs at the hip while in the lithotomy position. Injury of the sciatic nerve may be mistaken as injury to the peroneal nerve, because the peroneal nerve is a branch of the sciatic nerve. (206)

53. Injury to the sciatic nerve manifests as decreased sensation over the lateral leg and foot and weakness of all the skeletal muscles below the knee. (206)

54. The most common peripheral nerve in the lower extremity to manifest a postoperative neuropathy is the common peroneal nerve. (206)

55. The common peroneal nerve may be injured intraoperatively by compression between the patient's fibula and the metal support for the lithotomy position. The risk of this nerve injury can be minimized with appropriate padding. (206; **1018**)

56. Injury to the common peroneal nerve manifests as a loss of dorsal extension of the toes, inability to evert the foot, and footdrop. (206)

57. The anterior tibial nerve may be injured intraoperatively with prolonged plantarflexion of the feet. This risk can be avoided by placing a roll under the ankles of patients in the prone position. (206)

58. Injury to the anterior tibial nerve manifests as footdrop. (206)

59. The femoral nerve may be injured intraoperatively by compression by a pelvic retractor against the pelvic brim. It may also occur with excessive flexing and external rotation at the groin while in the lithotomy position. (206)

60. Injury to the femoral nerve manifests as a decreased sensation over the superior aspect of the thigh, as well as on the medial and anteromedial side of the leg. (206)

61. Diabetes mellitus appears to place patients at a greater risk of developing a femoral neuropathy. (206)

62. The saphenous nerve may be injured intraoperatively by compression against the medial tibial condyle and a metal support for the lithotomy position when the brace is placed medial to the patient's leg. The risk of a saphenous nerve injury may be minimized with the appropriate use of padding. (206; **1018**)

63. The obturator nerve may be injured intraoperatively during a difficult forceps-assisted vaginal delivery or by excessive flexion of the thigh to the abdomen, as during vaginal delivery. (207)

64. Injury to the obturator nerve manifests as decreased sensation over the medial thigh and an inability to adduct the leg. (206–207)

65. The intraoperative use of a tourniquet can result in nerve injury, particularly if the inflation time of the tourniquet exceeds 2 hours or with the application of excessive tourniquet pressures. For this reason, after about 2 hours if there is a continued need for the tourniquet it may be prudent to deflate it for 15 minutes and re-inflate it. (207; **2132**)

NON-NEURAL INJURY

66. Skin that is subject to excessive or prolonged pressure is at risk for ischemic damage. Areas of skin that are especially prone to ischemic damage during surgery include the heels, supraorbital ridge, and the skin at the corner of the mouth in contact with the endotracheal tube. The risk of skin ischemia can be minimized with adequate padding at potential pressure points. (207)

67. Pressure on a patient's eyes intraoperatively can result in permanent blindness. Pressure on the eyes may occur during procedures in the prone position. Patients with pressure on the eyes are especially prone to central retinal artery thrombosis and blindness when hypotension occurs intraoperatively. The risk of blindness can be minimized with frequent checking of the eyes and maintenance of an adequate blood pressure. (207; **1030, Fig. 26–20**)

68. A patient's digits of the fingers or toes can be injured intraoperatively during moving of operating table parts. Movement of the table into a space where the fingers or toes lie could lead to crushing of the digit. (207; **1018–1019, Fig. 26–5**)

69. A patient's ear can be damaged intraoperatively when in the lateral position by being folded onto itself and compressed between the patient's head and surgical table. (207)

DAMAGE RELATED TO THE ANESTHETIC FACE MASK

70. Potential injuries to the patient that can be sustained during mask ventilation of the airway include damage to the facial nerve and necrosis to the bridge of the nose. Facial nerve injury can be caused by the face strap on the anesthetic mask compressing the buccal branch of the nerve or by the anesthesiologist's fingers on the ascending ramus of the patient's mandible. Both of these risks are rare, however. (207)

Chapter 15

Monitoring

1. What is the purpose of intraoperative patient monitoring?

2. What are some monitors that have been mandated for use by the American Society of Anesthesiologists? How frequently is it mandated that intraoperative blood pressures be measured?

COMMONLY EMPLOYED NONINVASIVE MONITORS

3. How does an automated oscillometric blood pressure measuring device, such as the Dinamap, work?

4. What is the appropriate-sized cuff for use with an automated oscillometric blood pressure measuring device?

5. When using an automated oscillometric blood pressure measuring device, will the blood pressure be falsely increased or decreased with a cuff that is too small? When using an automated oscillometric blood pressure measuring device, will the blood pressure be falsely increased or decreased with a cuff that is too loose?

6. What is a potential problem that can result from too frequent cycling of an automated oscillometric blood pressure measuring device?

7. What can be monitored through the use of a precordial or esophageal stethoscope?

8. What are some potential intraoperative problems during anesthesia that can be detected early by an anesthesiologist through the routine use of a precordial or esophageal stethoscope?

9. What is an advantage of an esophageal stethoscope over a precordial stethoscope?

10. What are some potential intraoperative problems during anesthesia that can be detected by an anesthesiologist through the use of an electrocardiogram?

11. What is the advantage to the anesthesiologist in having an audible beep indicator for each QRS complex during surgery?

12. Which lead is selected on the electrocardiogram for continuous tracing on the monitor to best detect cardiac dysrhythmias? Why?

13. Which lead is selected on the electrocardiogram for continuous tracing on the monitor to best detect inferior wall myocardial ischemia? Which lead is selected for continuous tracing on the monitor to best detect anterior or lateral wall myocardial ischemia?

14. How can the equivalent of a V5 lead be achieved with a three-electrode electrocardiogram?

15. How will the electrocardiogram appear in a patient with pulseless electrical activity?

16. The use of a continuous pulse oximeter is valuable for the detection of what?

17. What is the SpO_2? What is the SaO_2? Which of these does a pulse oximeter measure?

18. How does a pulse oximeter work?

19. What is the PaO_2 value likely greater than when the pulse oximeter is calculating a maintained SpO_2 greater than 90%?

20. What are at least five factors that influence the accuracy of pulse oximetry?

21. What are some low flow conditions that can result in difficulty obtaining an oxygen saturation by pulse oximetry?

22. Is the SpO_2 read by the pulse oximeter falsely high or falsely low in the presence of carboxyhemoglobin?

23. What is the SpO_2 read by the pulse oximeter in the presence of methemoglobinemia?

24. How does the presence of fetal hemoglobin affect the SpO_2 read by the pulse oximeter?

25. What is the potential hazard with the use of pulse oximetry during magnetic resonance imaging?

26. A transcutaneous PO_2 ($PtcO_2$) monitor is useful for the detection of what? In what patient population is this monitor most frequently used?

27. What does a $PtcO_2$ monitor measure?

28. How does a $PtcO_2$ monitor work?

29. What influences the accuracy of a $PtcO_2$ monitor?

30. What is the most common complication associated with the use of a $PtcO_2$ monitor? How can this risk be minimized?

31. What is a capnograph?

32. What portion of the ventilatory cycle is represented by each letter in the following figure?

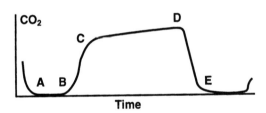

Figure 15–1. From Stoelting RK, Miller RD: Basics of Anesthesia, 4th ed. Philadelphia, Churchill Livingstone, 2000, p 212.

33. What does the absence of carbon dioxide in a person's exhaled gases indicate during endotracheal intubation? What does the absence of carbon dioxide in a person's exhaled gases indicate after proper and confirmed endotracheal intubation?

34. What are some possible causes of a decrease in the concentration of carbon dioxide in a person's exhaled gases?

35. What are some possible causes of an increase in the concentration of carbon dioxide in a person's exhaled gases?

36. What does the presence of carbon dioxide in a person's exhaled gases during cardiopulmonary resuscitation indicate?

37. How does the end-tidal carbon dioxide concentration measured on a capnogram compare with the $PaCO_2$? Why?

38. How does the carbon dioxide concentration measured transcutaneously compare with the $PaCO_2$? Why?

39. What are some methods by which the exhaled concentrations of multiple gases, including respiratory and anesthetic gases, may be measured?

40. What are some advantages and disadvantages of infrared absorption techniques for measuring a patient's exhaled gases?

41. What are some advantages and disadvantages of mass spectrometry techniques for measuring a patient's exhaled gases?

42. What are some advantages and disadvantages of Raman spectrometry techniques for measuring a patient's exhaled gases?

43. Where is the respirometer commonly placed in the anesthetic breathing system? What information does it provide?

44. A low airway pressure alarm is useful for the detection of what?

45. A high airway pressure alarm is useful for the detection of what?

46. What is the maximum airway pressure that can be delivered to a patient who is spontaneously ventilating into the gas reservoir bag? Why?

47. What are some methods by which the anesthesiologist can monitor a patient's spontaneous breathing efforts, pattern, and efficacy during general anesthesia?

48. The intraoperative measurement of urine output is useful for the detection of what?

49. When should the status of the neuromuscular junction be monitored by the anesthesiologist?

50. How does a patient's body temperature usually change under anesthesia?

51. What are some sites for measurement of a patient's body temperature? When is a nasopharyngeal temperature not accurate?

52. What is the purpose of measuring the inspired concentration of oxygen of a patient under general anesthesia?

INVASIVE MONITORING OF THE CARDIOVASCULAR SYSTEM

53. What are some possible indications for intra-arterial blood pressure monitoring?

54. What are some arteries that may be used for intra-arterial blood pressure monitoring? Which of these is most commonly selected?

55. What is the Allen test? When should it be performed? What does it test for?

56. What gauge catheters are typically used for cannulation of the radial artery?

57. How should a radial artery catheter be managed after its placement?

58. What are some indications for the placement of a central venous catheter?

59. What veins are used for central venous access? What are some potential complications of the cannulation of veins for central access?

60. Which is the preferred jugular vein for cannulation? Why?

61. What are some advantages and disadvantages of cannulation of the internal jugular vein over other central veins?

62. What are some advantages and disadvantages of cannulation of the subclavian vein over other central veins?

63. What does the central venous waveform look like? What do each of the peaks and descents represent relative to the cardiac cycle?

64. Why is the central venous pressure able to be used to estimate a patient's intravascular fluid volume status?

65. Under which circumstances does central venous pressure not estimate a patient's intravascular fluid volume status? What invasive monitor can be used instead of a central venous catheter under these conditions?

66. Name six possible indications for the placement of a pulmonary artery catheter. What information can be obtained regarding the patient's status with the use of a pulmonary artery catheter?

67. What distance of advancement of the catheter, in centimeters, typically indicates the right ventricular tracing and the pulmonary capillary wedge pressure tracing?

68. What is the pulmonary capillary wedge pressure a reflection of? What other measurement derived by the pulmonary artery catheter can also be used in lieu of the pulmonary capillary wedge pressure?

69. How is estimation of the cardiac output accomplished through the use of a pulmonary artery catheter?

70. What are some potential complications of pulmonary artery catheterization?

71. Please complete the following table illustrating the usefulness of central venous catheters and pulmonary artery catheters in the evaluation of various hemodynamic disorders. (PAEDP, pulmonary artery end-diastolic pressure; PAo, pulmonary artery occlusion pressure)

	CENTRAL VENOUS PRESSURE ↑ OR ↓	PAo ↑ OR ↓	PAEDP RELATION TO PAo
Hypovolemia			
Left ventricular failure			
Right ventricular failure			
Pulmonary embolism			
Cardiac tamponade			

72. What is some information that can be derived intraoperatively through the use of a transesophageal echocardiogram?

MONITORING OF THE NERVOUS SYSTEM

73. What are some uses of an electroencephalogram intraoperatively? During which surgical procedures is the intraoperative use of an electroencephalogram most common?

74. How does the electroencephalogram appear when the patient is under general anesthesia? What is the potential problem with this?

75. What factors may influence the tracings obtained by an intraoperative electroencephalogram?

76. What is the bispectral index monitor?

77. What are some potential clinical uses of a bispectral index monitor?

78. What is an evoked potential?

79. What are some intraoperative uses of evoked potentials? What is the most common procedure for which evoked potentials are used intraoperatively?

80. How do evoked potentials appear when the patient is under general anesthesia? What is the potential problem with this?

81. What factors may influence the results of evoked potentials, thereby limiting their usefulness in the intraoperative period?

ELECTRICAL HAZARDS

82. How might a patient sustain thermal injury or cardiac dysrhythmias as a result of faulty electrical monitoring equipment?

83. What is a line isolation monitor?

84. Why does the electrosurgical unit used by surgeons not cause thermal injury to the patient? What is one way in which the electrosurgical unit can cause thermal injury to the patient?

ANSWERS*

1. The most direct purpose for intraoperative patient monitoring is to gather data regarding the status of the patient and equipment. There are several ways in which this gathered data may be applied. First, it provides the anesthesiologist with information regarding the patient's physiologic status. Second, it provides the anesthesiologist with more information with which to promptly recognize any adverse reactions. Third, the patient's response to therapeutic interventions can be assessed. Finally, intraoperative monitoring may also give early information regarding the malfunction of anesthetic equipment. (209)

2. The American Society of Anesthesiologists has mandated that qualified anesthesia personnel shall be present in the room to administer anesthesia and monitor the patient throughout the conduct of all general anesthetics, regional anesthetics, and monitored anesthesia care. The standard adopted by the American Society of Anesthesiologists is that during all anesthetics the patient's oxygenation, ventilation, circulation, and temperature shall be continually evaluated. The full description of these standards also provides an explanation of each of these objectives and specific methods by which they can be achieved. In brief, the use of pulse oximetry, capnography, an oxygen analyzer, a disconnect alarm, and a visual display of the electrocardiogram are all addressed. In addition, the blood pressure and heart rate are to be evaluated at least every 5 minutes during the course of anesthesia. (209)

COMMONLY EMPLOYED NONINVASIVE MONITORS

3. Automated oscillometric blood pressure monitoring devices work by inflating a pneumatic cuff that encircles a peripheral artery until blood flow through the artery is occluded. The computer then deflates the cuff a little bit and maintains it at a lower pressure while the computer senses for oscillations. The automated oscillometric blood pressure monitoring device continues to do this until oscillations are sensed and then sensed no longer. It has been determined that the most reliable blood pressure parameter measured by this noninvasive blood pressure monitoring device is the mean arterial blood pressure. (209–210; **1062, 1120–1123, Figs. 28–14, 30–3**)

4. The appropriate cuff size for use with a noninvasive blood pressure measuring device is one whose width is between 30% and 40% the circumference of the patient's limb. (210; **1062, 1122–1123, Fig. 30–2**)

5. When using an automated oscillometric blood pressure measuring device, the blood pressure will be falsely increased when the blood pressure cuff is too small or is wrapped too loosely around the patient's limb. (210; **1062, 1122–1123, Fig. 30–2**)

6. Cycling an automated oscillometric blood pressure measuring device too frequently can result in limited perfusion to the extremity distal to the cuff. Complications such as edema, nerve paresthesias, superficial thrombophlebitis,

---

*Numbers in parentheses: lightface numbers refer to pages, figures, or tables in Stoelting RK, Miller RD: Basics of Anesthesia, 4th ed. Philadelphia, Churchill Livingstone, 2000; **boldface numbers** refer to pages, figures, or tables in Miller RD: Anesthesia, 5th ed. Philadelphia, Churchill Livingstone, 2000.

and compartment syndrome have all been reported as a result of noninvasive blood pressure devices that have been repeatedly cycled. These complications are rare. (210; **1123**)

7. A precordial or esophageal stethoscope can be used to monitor cardiac and ventilatory sounds of the patient. This monitor should be immediately available to the anesthesiologist, although its routine use today is mainly among pediatric anesthesiologists. (215; **1118**)

8. Through the routine intraoperative use of a precordial or esophageal stethoscope the anesthesiologist may detect early changes in heart rate, heart rhythm, airway resistance, or ventilatory pattern. (215; **1118**)

9. Esophageal stethoscopes may also have a temperature sensor as part of the instrument, enabling simultaneous core temperature monitoring. (214; **1118**)

10. Potential intraoperative problems such as cardiac dysrhythmias, myocardial ischemia, and electrolyte abnormalities may all be detected through the use of an electrocardiogram. (210–211; **1231**)

11. An audible beep indicator for each QRS complex allows the anesthesiologist to auscultate the cardiac rate and rhythm while attending to other intraoperative duties. (211)

12. Lead II provides for the best visualization of the P wave on the electrocardiogram, making it the best lead for the detection of cardiac dysrhythmias on a continuous tracing. (211; **1231, 1239–1240**)

13. Lead II on the electrocardiogram provides for the best detection of inferior wall myocardial ischemia on a continuous tracing. The V5 precordial lead on the electrocardiogram provides for the best detection of anterior or lateral wall myocardial ischemia. (211; **1233–1235, 1245–1246, Fig. 35–15, Table 32–5**)

14. In a three-electrode electrocardiogram, the equivalent of the V5 lead can be achieved by placing the left arm electrode in the V5 position, then selecting the aVL lead for continuous tracing on the monitor. (211; **1233–1234, Fig. 32–6**)

15. A patient with pulseless electrical activity by definition still has electrical activity through the heart, although no blood pressure will be palpable. Therefore, there will be some electrical tracing on the electrocardiogram, although it may or may not be a sinus rhythm. (211; **2551–2554**)

16. The continuous use of a pulse oximeter is valuable for the detection of arterial hypoxemia. (211; **1264–1265**)

17. The Spo_2 is the hemoglobin oxygen saturation in the peripheral arteries. The Sao_2 is arterial hemoglobin saturation. The pulse oximeter measures the Spo_2 and is a reliable measure of the Sao_2. (211; **1264–1265**)

18. A pulse oximeter works by emitting a light through a diode and sensing the light, usually on the opposite side of a digit. The wavelength of light that is absorbed by oxyhemoglobin relative to reduced hemoglobin in the pulsatile (and therefore arterial) vessel allows the computer to calculate the saturation of oxygen in the peripheral artery. (211; **1073–1075, 1264–1265, Figs. 28–33, 28–34, 33–8**)

19. The Pao_2 is likely greater than 60 when the pulse oximeter is calculating a maintained Spo_2 greater than 90% based on the usual shape and position of the oxyhemoglobin dissociation curve. (211; **595–597; Fig. 15–25**)

20. Factors that influence the accuracy of pulse oximetry include low flow conditions, motion artifact, nail polish, ambient light interference, dysfunctional hemoglobins, methylene blue, and a shift in the oxyhemoglobin dissociation curve. (211; **1073–1075, 1265–1267, Fig. 36–8, Table 36–1**)

21. Conditions that may result in low blood flow through a peripheral artery may also result in difficulty in obtaining an oxygen saturation by pulse oximetry. Such low flow conditions include hypotension, hypothermia, and vasoconstriction. (211; **1267**)

22. The SpO_2 read by the pulse oximeter in the presence of carboxyhemoglobin is falsely high. This occurs because carboxyhemoglobin has an absorbance of light that is markedly similar to oxyhemoglobin. (211; **1265–1266**)

23. The SpO_2 read by the pulse oximeter in the presence of methemoglobinemia approaches 85% regardless of the true arterial hemoglobin oxygen saturation. (211; **1266**)

24. The SpO_2 read by the pulse oximeter in the presence of fetal hemoglobin is normal. This occurs because fetal hemoglobin has an absorbance of light that is markedly similar to that of hemoglobin A. (211; **1266**)

25. Severe burns are a potential hazard with the use of pulse oximetry during magnetic resonance imaging. (211; **2250–2251, 2691**)

26. A transcutaneous PO_2 ($PtcO_2$) monitor is useful for the detection of arterial hypoxemia. This monitor is most frequently used in the neonatal population. Transcutaneous PO_2 monitors do not operate efficiently through thick adult skin. (211–212; **1263**)

27. The $PtcO_2$ monitor directly measures the PO_2 from capillaries in the skin on which the monitor is placed. (211–212; **1263**)

28. The $PtcO_2$ monitor is a heated Clark electrode that is placed on the skin surface. Oxygen from capillaries diffuses into the electrode, which then directly measures the PO_2. In areas where local oxygen requirements are minimal the PO_2 measured by the $PtcO_2$ monitor closely correlates with the PaO_2. (211–212; **1263**)

29. The accuracy of a $PtcO_2$ monitor is influenced by the perfusion of the skin on which the monitor is placed. It is also influenced by the thickness of the skin itself. (212; **1263**)

30. The most common complication associated with the use of a $PtcO_2$ monitor is that of skin burns. Because the monitor is actually a heated electrode, the monitor site should be changed every 2 hours in neonates to minimize the risk of burns. (212; **1263**)

31. A capnograph is a waveform display that illustrates the patient's inhaled and exhaled concentrations of carbon dioxide. (212, Fig. 16–2; **1272–1277, Figs. 33–15, 33–16**)

32. In the capnogram, the point A designates the exhalation of anatomic deadspace gas just before the exhalation of alveolar gas. Point B designates the beginning of exhalation of alveolar gas that contains carbon dioxide. Phase C–D designates the exhalation of alveolar gas, while point D designates the end-tidal carbon dioxide concentration. Phase D–E designates the beginning of inspiration and the entrainment of gases. (212, Fig. 16–2; **1273–1276, Fig. 33–16**)

Figure 15–1. From Stoelting RK, Miller RD: Basics of Anesthesia, 4th ed. Philadelphia, Churchill Livingstone, 2000, p 212.

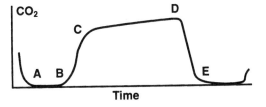

33. The absence of carbon dioxide in a patient's exhaled gases just after attempted endotracheal intubation with properly functioning equipment provides evidence

that the patient's lungs are not being ventilated. That is, the endotracheal tube may not be in the trachea. The absence of carbon dioxide in a patient's exhaled gases after intubation of the trachea has been confirmed may indicate that there is either a malfunction of equipment, a malfunction in the interface between the patient and the equipment (as in disconnection from the anesthesia circuit), movement or dislodgment of the endotracheal tube from its previously proper position, or a physiologic patient problem such as a cardiac arrest. (212; **1276, 1445**)

34. Possible causes of a decrease in the exhaled concentration of carbon dioxide include hyperventilation, hypothermia, low cardiac output, pulmonary embolism, accidental disconnection, tracheal extubation, or cardiac arrest. (212; **1274–1275**)

35. Possible causes of an increase in the exhaled concentration of carbon dioxide include hypoventilation, hyperthermia, sepsis, rebreathing, the administration of bicarbonate, and the insufflation of carbon dioxide during laparoscopy. (212; **1274–1275**)

36. The presence of carbon dioxide in a patient's exhaled gases during cardiopulmonary resuscitation indicates that there is some degree of lung perfusion with external compressions. The corollary is that there may also be some perfusion to the brain and heart. (212; **2536–2537**)

37. The end-tidal carbon dioxide concentration measured on a capnogram is less than the true Pa_{CO_2}, typically by a 2- to 5-mm Hg gradient. This occurs as a result of the alveolar-to-arterial difference for carbon dioxide concentrations secondary to deadspace ventilation. (212; **1275**)

38. The carbon dioxide concentration measured on a Ptc_{O_2} monitor is approximately equal to the Pa_{CO_2}. This is because the value obtained by the Ptc_{O_2} monitor is not influenced by deadspace ventilation. (212; **1073, 1263**)

39. Multiple gas analysis can be achieved by infrared absorption, mass spectrometry, and Raman spectroscopy. (212; **1073, 1269–1271**)

40. An advantage of infrared absorption techniques for measuring a patient's exhaled gases is that it provides a rapid response time, leading to real-time concentrations of gases. A disadvantage of the infrared absorption technique is that it works by infrared wavelength absorption. Because carbon dioxide and nitrous oxide have overlapping infrared wavelengths, these two gases cannot be measured easily when mixed together. In addition, infrared absorption techniques do not work for symmetrical molecules such as oxygen and nitrogen. (212–213; **1271**)

41. Advantages of mass spectrometry techniques for measuring a patient's exhaled gases are that it can measure the gases continuously, it can measure all gases including inhaled anesthetics, oxygen, and nitrogen, and it can measure the inspired gas concentrations as well as the exhaled concentrations. A disadvantage of mass spectrometry technique is that they have traditionally been large and expensive monitors. (213; **1269–1270, Fig. 33–12**)

42. Advantages of Raman spectrometry techniques for measuring a patient's exhaled gases are that it can measure all gases including inhaled anesthetics, oxygen, and nitrogen and it does not alter the gas molecule so that it can be returned to the anesthetic delivery system. A disadvantage of Raman spectrometry technique is that it requires a very high intensity light source to work, such as a laser. (213; **1270–1271**)

43. The respirometer, which is commonly placed on the exhalation limb of the anesthetic breathing system, measures the patient's tidal volume. With this information the patient's minute ventilation can be calculated. (213; **197**)

44. A low airway pressure alarm on the mechanical ventilator is triggered if the patient's maximum peak inspiratory pressure does not reach the predetermined level. This alarm is useful for the detection of a large pressure leak or disconnection of the patient from the anesthetic breathing system. (213; **177–178, 197, Fig. 7–4**)

45. A high airway pressure alarm on the mechanical ventilator is triggered if the patient's maximum peak inspiratory pressure exceeds the predetermined level. This alarm is useful for the detection of changes in the patient's airway resistance or an obstruction in the anesthetic breathing system. (213; **197–198**)

46. The maximum airway pressure that can be delivered to a patient who is spontaneously ventilating into the gas reservoir bag is 50 cm H_2O. Pressures exceeding this will lead to expansion of the bag into a sphere with minimal changes in pressure. (213)

47. The routine use of pulse oximetry, capnography, and a precordial or esophageal stethoscope as well as vigilant observation are all methods by which the anesthesiologist can monitor a patient's spontaneous breathing efforts, pattern, and efficacy. (213)

48. The intraoperative measurement of urine output is useful as an indicator of the adequacy of the intravascular fluid volume status of a patient. The early detection of hemoglobinuria due to a hemolytic transfusion reaction may also be facilitated. (213; **1308–1309**)

49. The status of the neuromuscular junction should be monitored with a peripheral nerve stimulator any time neuromuscular blocking drugs have been administered to a patient. (213; **1351–1352**)

50. Patients will typically have a passive decrease in body temperature by 1°C to 4°C during anesthesia. (214; **1371–1373, Figs. 37–7, 37–8**)

51. Sites for body temperature monitoring include the esophagus, nasopharynx, rectum, bladder, and tympanic membrane. A nasopharyngeal temperature probe is only accurate when a cuffed endotracheal tube is present in the trachea preventing respiratory gases from artificially cooling the temperature probe. (214; **1384–1385**)

52. The purpose of measuring the inspired concentration of oxygen of a patient under general anesthesia is to ensure the patient is not breathing a hypoxic mixture. (214; **201**)

INVASIVE MONITORING OF THE CARDIOVASCULAR SYSTEM

53. Possible indications for intra-arterial blood pressure monitoring include the need for continuous blood pressure monitoring, access for frequent arterial blood gas samplings, need for monitoring intentional pharmacologic cardiovascular manipulation, and failure of indirect blood pressure measurement. (214; **1124–1125**)

54. Arteries that may be used for intra-arterial blood pressure monitoring include the radial, ulnar, brachial, axillary, femoral, dorsalis pedis, and the superficial temporal arteries. Of these, the radial artery is the most frequently used artery for cannulation. (214; **1127–1128**)

55. The Allen test is performed before cannulation of the radial artery to ensure the adequacy of collateral flow to the hand from the ulnar artery. The test is intended to determine in advance which patients may be at risk of ischemia of the hand with cannulation of the radial artery. The test is performed by asking the patient to close the hand as tightly as possible into a fist while the examiner holds simultaneously pressure on the ulnar and radial arteries, thus occluding

them and exsanguinating the hand. Pressure on the ulnar artery alone is then released as the patient opens the hand. The return of blood flow into the hand within 5 to 15 seconds is a negative Allen test. If the Allen test is positive, that is, if blood flow does not return to the hand within 15 seconds, there is a relative contraindication to the cannulation of the radial artery. Despite this, even in the presence of a positive Allen test cannulation of the radial artery rarely leads to complications. (214–215; **1125**)

56. Catheters used for cannulation of the radial artery are typically 20-gauge in adults and 22- to 24-gauge in children. (215; **1125**)

57. After placement of a radial artery catheter and connection to the appropriate tubing, the site of cannulation should be cleaned and securely fastened. The catheter should then be continually or intermittently flushed with heparinized saline to minimize the potential for thrombus formation and to maintain proper arterial waveforms. (215; **1125–1127**)

58. Indications for the placement of a central venous catheter include the measurement of central venous pressures, access through which to provide long-term intravenous feedings, access for the administration of large volumes of fluids, intravascular access when no peripheral access is available, the administration of vasoactive or caustic drugs, to initiate transvenous cardiac pacing, for temporary hemodialysis, and for the aspiration of air emboli. (215; **1144, Table 30–3**)

59. Veins that are cannulated for central venous access include the internal jugular, subclavian, femoral, and antecubital veins. Potential complications of cannulation of the central veins include arterial puncture, hematoma, hemothorax, pneumothorax, nerve injury, emboli, cardiac dysrhythmias, thrombosis, and infection. Accidental arterial puncture while attempting cannulation of the jugular vein can result in the need to surgically explore and repair the artery. A pneumothorax occurs more frequently after placement of a subclavian catheter. This is the basis for the recommendation that a chest radiograph be done after failed subclavian catheterization and before attempting catheterization on the other side. (215; **1148–1153, Table 30–4**)

60. The right jugular vein is preferred over the left jugular vein for cannulation because of its short, straight, valveless route to the superior vena cava. (215; **1146**)

61. Advantages of cannulation of the internal jugular vein include its predictable anatomic location with palpable landmarks, its location at the head of the patient's bed allowing the anesthesiologist easy access to the catheter intraoperatively, and the relatively decreased complications associated with cannulation of this central vein. Disadvantages of cannulation of the internal jugular vein include the potential for puncture of the carotid artery and pleural cavity and trauma to the brachial plexus. (215; **1146**)

62. Advantages of cannulation of the subclavian vein include its landmarks, its capacity to remain patent despite hypovolemia, easier nursing care, and the relative increase in patient comfort associated with cannulation of this central vein. Disadvantages of cannulation of the subclavian vein include the potential for puncture of the subclavian artery and pleural cavity and for thoracic duct damage on the left. (215; **1148–1149**)

63. The central venous pressure waveform has a typical trace in a normally functioning heart. The a wave correlates with atrial contraction, the c wave correlates with closure of the tricuspid valve and its bulging into the right atrium, and the v wave correlates with blood accumulation in the vena cava and right atrium against a closed tricuspid valve. The x descent correlates with atrial relaxation, and the y descent correlates with opening of the tricuspid valve and right ventricular filling. (216, Fig. 16–5; **1153–1156, Fig. 30–27, Table 30–5**)

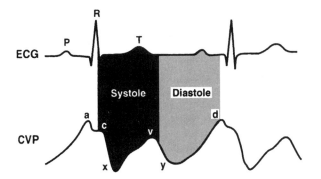

Figure 15–2. Central venous pressure (CVP) waveforms in relationship to electrical events on the electrocardiogram (ECG). (From Stoelting RK, Miller RD: Basics of Anesthesia, 4th ed. Philadelphia, Churchill Livingstone, 2000, p 217.)

64. The central venous pressure parallels right atrial pressure in a patient with normal cardiovascular physiology. In these patients the central venous pressure can be used to estimate the patient's intravascular fluid volume status. (216–217; **1142–1143, 1153**)

65. The central venous pressure does not estimate the patient's intravascular fluid volume status in the face of right-sided heart dysfunction, left ventricular dysfunction, or pulmonary hypertension. Under these conditions a pulmonary artery catheter may be used for cardiovascular monitoring. (216–217; **1156–1157, 1178–1179**)

66. Possible indications for the placement of a pulmonary artery catheter perioperatively include poor left ventricular function, valvular heart disease, recent myocardial infarction, adult respiratory distress syndrome or any pulmonary vascular disease process, massive trauma, and major vascular surgery. In general, the pulmonary artery catheter allows for more accurate assessment of cardiac filling pressures than a central venous monitor in the presence of pulmonary vascular disease, left-sided heart dysfunction, or potential left-sided heart dysfunction due to myocardial ischemia. The pulmonary artery catheter also measures cardiac output and calculates systemic and pulmonary vascular resistance. (217; **1178–1179**)

67. On advancement of a pulmonary artery catheter via a central vein, the right ventricular tracing is typically seen at about 30 cm and the pulmonary capillary wedge pressure is typically seen at 45 to 50 cm. (217; **1158–1159**)

68. The pulmonary capillary wedge pressure is a reflection of left atrial pressure. The pulmonary artery diastolic pressure may be used as an approximation of left atrial pressure in lieu of the pulmonary artery wedge pressure. This allows for continuous monitoring. The pulmonary artery diastolic pressure does not accurately reflect left atrial pressure in conditions in which pulmonary vascular resistance is increased, as with hypoxia, hypercarbia, hypothermia, and various forms of pulmonary disease. (217; **1166–1167**)

69. Cardiac output can be estimated through the use of a pulmonary artery catheter via the thermodilution method. To do this, cold saline is rapidly injected through the proximal central venous port. A thermistor located at the distal end of the pulmonary artery catheter senses the change in temperature. Because blood flow is the source of dilution of temperature, the flow, or cardiac output, can be calculated. It is the right ventricular cardiac output that is actually measured by this technique, whereas left ventricular cardiac output can only be estimated based on the results. (217; **1180–1183**)

70. Potential complications of pulmonary artery catheterization include pulmonary ischemia or infarction from prolonged wedging of the catheter, cardiac dysrhythmias, infection, catheter knotting, and, rarely, pulmonary artery rupture. (217; **1160–1164, Table 30–6**)

71. (218, Table 16–5)

	CENTRAL VENOUS PRESSURE	PAo	PAEDP RELATION TO PAo
Hypovolemia	Decreased	Decreased	PAEDP = PAo
Left ventricular failure	Increased	Increased	PAEDP = PAo
Right ventricular failure	Increased	No change	PAEDP = PAo
Pulmonary embolism	Increased	No change	PAEDP > PAo
Cardiac tamponade	Increased	Increased	PAEDP = PAo

72. Intraoperative cardiac imaging with a transesophageal echocardiogram is now widely accepted as a monitor for cardiac function during surgery, especially cardiac surgery. Information that can be derived from an intraoperative echocardiogram includes regional ventricular and atrial wall motion, ejection fraction, cardiac valve function, the presence of intracardiac air, and the effects of surgery and anesthesia on cardiac function. The use of a transesophageal echocardiogram requires advanced technical training. Complications associated with the use of transesophageal echocardiography include pharyngeal and esophageal injury and bleeding, but these occurrences are rare. (218; **1207**)

MONITORING OF THE NERVOUS SYSTEM

73. Intraoperative uses of an electroencephalogram include monitoring for cerebral ischemia and monitoring the depth of anesthesia. The electroencephalogram is most commonly used during carotid endarterectomy or cardiopulmonary bypass procedures. (218; **1332–1333**)

74. The wave traces obtained by an electroencephalogram decrease in amplitude and frequency when the patient is under general anesthesia. The potential problem with this is that the same occurs during periods of cerebral ischemia, making it more difficult to interpret the data during anesthesia. (218; **1328–1332, Fig. 35–6, Table 35–2**)

75. Among the factors that influence the tracings obtained by an electroencephalogram and limit its usefulness intraoperatively are anesthetics, changes in body temperature, and alterations in the Pa_{CO_2}. (218–219; **1328–1335, Table 35–1**)

76. The bispectral index monitor performs a bispectral analysis of the electroencephalogram and provides the clinician with a processed evaluation of its analysis through its display of a number between 0 to 100. The analysis is done through superficial scalp electrodes typically on the forehead of the patient. The number provided by the bispectral index monitor reflects the state of wakefulness of the central nervous system. (219; **1328**)

77. The bispectral index monitor may be used clinically to predict loss of consciousness and lack of recall during anesthesia. A numerical value of 60 or less corresponds to a low probability of recall or awareness. Thus the use of the bispectral index monitor for the titration of medicines to achieve adequate but not excessive loss of consciousness may result in more rapid awakening at the end of the procedure. The bispectral index has not been shown to be well correlated with the hemodynamic or movement responses to noxious stimuli. (219; **1328–1329**)

78. An evoked potential is a measured low amplitude signal from the central

nervous system that occurs in response to sensory or motor nerve stimulation. (219; **1325**)

79. Evoked potentials can be used intraoperatively to assess the integrity of the neural pathways during anesthesia. Evoked potentials are typically used as a monitoring tool in patients undergoing Harrington rod procedures for the treatment of scoliosis. During these procedures intactness of the sensory nerve pathways from the periphery to the somatosensory cortex via the spinal cord can be confirmed. (219; **1336–1338**)

80. Evoked potentials may undergo changes in the latency period and amplitude while patients are under general anesthesia. These changes are similar to the changes that are seen with neural ischemia, thereby limiting the intraoperative usefulness of evoked potentials. (219; **1340–1343, Figs. 35–12, 35–13, 35–14, 35–15, 35–16, 35–17, Table 35–8**)

81. Factors that may limit the intraoperative usefulness of evoked potentials because of their influence on the results include age and gender of the patient, arterial blood gas tensions, and body temperature. In addition, the cost and complexity of performing evoked potentials intraoperatively contribute to its limitations. (219; **1343**)

ELECTRICAL HAZARDS

82. Faulty electrical monitoring equipment can result in thermal injury or cardiac dysrhythmias through the delivery of leaked current directly to the patient. Monitors are therefore designed to conduct leaked currents to the ground rather than to the patient. Periodic preventive maintenance of electrical monitoring equipment to evaluate for extraneous currents may minimize the risk of extraneous electrical currents. (219–220; **2691, 2698–2699**)

83. A line isolation monitor tests to confirm that power output lines are isolated from the ground. Power output lines that are not isolated from ground may provide for a completed circuit through contact with a patient and ground. The line isolation monitor will alarm when the short circuit has the potential to allow current flow of 2 mA to leak to ground. (220; **2692–2693, Figs. 83–2, 83–3**)

84. The electrosurgical unit used by surgeons does not cause thermal injury to the patient because the energy is focused in a small area and then the current exits the body through a large area formed on a ground plate. Because the current density is distributed widely, thermal injury does not occur. If the ground wire were to become disconnected or broken, alternative exit sites for the current such as metal electrocardiogram electrodes or contact sites with the metal table would result. If the exit sites were a small area, the high-density current flowing through these small areas could result in burns. (220–221; **2697–2698**)

Chapter *16*

Acid-Base Balance and Blood Gas Analysis

1. What is the importance of maintaining a physiologic acid-base status?

2. What is the normal plasma H^+ concentration? What is the normal plasma HCO_3^- concentration?

3. What is the normal arterial pH of blood?

REGULATION OF THE HYDROGEN ION CONCENTRATION

4. How is normal arterial pH maintained?

5. What are some of the buffering systems in the blood? Which buffering system has the greatest contribution to the total buffering capacity of blood?

6. How does the bicarbonate buffering system work? What enzyme facilitates this reaction?

7. How does hemoglobin act as a buffer?

8. How quickly does the buffering system of the blood respond to changes in arterial pH?

9. How quickly does alveolar ventilation respond to changes in arterial pH?

10. How quickly do the kidneys respond to changes in arterial pH?

DIFFERENTIAL DIAGNOSIS OF ACID-BASE DISTURBANCES

11. How is acidemia defined? How is alkalemia defined?

12. What is the difference between a primary disturbance or a compensatory disturbance in acid-base status?

13. What defines primary respiratory acidosis or alkalosis?

14. What defines primary metabolic acidosis or alkalosis?

15. Which affects myocardial contractility more, acidemia or alkalemia?

16. Which affects myocardial function more, respiratory or metabolic acidosis?

17. What is the definition of respiratory acidosis?

18. What are some causes of respiratory acidosis?

19. What are some compensatory responses to arterial acidemia produced by respiratory acidosis?

20. How can acute respiratory acidemia be distinguished from chronic respiratory acidemia?

21. How can acidemia from respiratory acidosis be distinguished from a mixed respiratory and metabolic cause for the acidemia?

22. What are some adverse physiologic effects of respiratory acidosis?

23. What is the treatment for respiratory acidosis?

24. What is the definition of respiratory alkalosis?

25. What are some causes of respiratory alkalosis?

26. What are some compensatory responses to arterial alkalemia associated with respiratory alkalosis? What is the time course for each of these responses?

27. What are some adverse physiologic effects of respiratory alkalosis?

28. What is the treatment for respiratory alkalosis?

29. What is the definition of metabolic acidosis?

30. What are some causes of metabolic acidosis?

31. What are some compensatory responses to arterial acidemia associated with metabolic acidosis?

32. How much does the arterial pH change in response to a 10 mm Hg deviation from 40 mm Hg in the Pa_{CO_2}?

33. How can acidemia from primary metabolic acidosis be distinguished from a mixed respiratory and metabolic cause for the acidemia?

34. What are some adverse physiologic effects of metabolic acidosis?

35. What is the treatment for metabolic acidosis?

36. What is the definition of metabolic alkalosis?

37. What are some causes of metabolic alkalosis?

38. What are some compensatory responses to arterial alkalemia associated with metabolic alkalosis?

39. What are some adverse physiologic effects of metabolic alkalosis?

40. What is the treatment for metabolic alkalosis?

MEASUREMENT OF ARTERIAL BLOOD GASES

41. When obtaining blood for an arterial blood gas sample, what would result from excessive amounts of heparin in the syringe?

42. When obtaining blood for an arterial blood gas sample, why is the syringe placed in ice?

43. When obtaining blood for an arterial blood gas sample, what would result from air bubbles in the syringe?

44. Why do arterial blood gas samples need to be corrected for temperature? What is an estimate for the correction of the P_{O_2} in an arterial blood gas sample from a patient whose temperature was not 37°C?

45. Which electrode measures oxygen, the Clark electrode or the Severinghaus electrode?

46. What are some methods by which the adequacy of ventilation and oxygenation can be assessed?

47. What are some causes of arterial hypoxemia?

48. How does a ventilation-perfusion mismatch result in arterial hypoxemia?

49. How does a right-to-left shunt result in arterial hypoxemia?

50. Will arterial hypoxemia secondary to a right-to-left shunt improve with the administration of 100% oxygen?

51. What is the $A - aDo_2$? How is it calculated?

52. What is the normal $A - aDo_2$? Why?

53. What is a benefit of using the Pao_2/PAo_2 ratio instead of the $A - aDo_2$ for an estimate of the magnitude of the venous admixture?

54. What is the mixed venous Po_2 useful as an indicator of?

55. What mixed venous Po_2 is indicative of tissue hypoxemia? Why might a patient have a high mixed venous Po_2 despite inadequate tissue oxygenation?

56. What is the difference between the arterial and venous content of oxygen useful as an indicator of? What is the normal difference?

57. Draw the oxyhemoglobin dissociation curve. What does the oxyhemoglobin dissociation curve illustrate? What are some points on the curve?

58. What are some events that shift the oxyhemoglobin dissociation curve to the right? What does a rightward shift of the curve reflect physiologically?

59. What are some events that shift the oxyhemoglobin dissociation curve to the left? What does a leftward shift of the curve reflect physiologically?

60. What are some compensatory mechanisms for arterial hypoxemia? Which of these is most efficient?

61. What is the respiratory quotient? What is the respiratory quotient reflective of physiologically?

62. What is the deadspace-to-tidal volume ratio useful as an indicator of? What is a normal deadspace-to-tidal volume ratio?

63. What does an increased deadspace-to-tidal volume ratio indicate?

64. How does a right-to-left shunt affect the deadspace-to-tidal volume ratio?

ANSWERS*

1. A physiologic acid-base status ensures the optimal function of enzymes, the proper distribution of electrolytes, optimal myocardial contractility, and an optimal saturation of hemoglobin with oxygen. The acid-base balance is representative of a balance between the production of hydrogen ions and the excretion of hydrogen ions. There are two types of acids produced by the body. One is carbonic acid, which is produced by the hydration of carbon dioxide and is eliminated by alveolar ventilation. The other acids are metabolic acids, which are primarily eliminated by the kidneys. Deviations from normal levels of each of these ions results in acid-base abnormalities. In general, a deviation of carbonic acids from normal results from respiratory causes and a deviation of metabolic acids from normal results from metabolic causes. (222; **1391**)

2. The normal plasma H^+ concentration is 36 to 44 nmol/L. The normal plasma HCO_3^- concentration is about 24 mEq/L. (222; **1392–1393**)

3. The normal arterial pH of blood is between 7.36 and 7.44. (222; **1392**)

REGULATION OF THE HYDROGEN ION CONCENTRATION

4. Normal arterial pH is maintained through the buffer systems, ventilatory responses, and renal responses. The ventilatory response involves alterations in

alveolar ventilation and therefore the blood and tissue carbon dioxide concentrations. The kidneys allow for near-complete restoration of the arterial pH through the reabsorption of bicarbonate ions and the secretion of hydrogen ions by the renal tubules. (222; **1391, 1393**)

5. When there is a disturbance in the concentration of acid in the blood, buffering systems in the blood help to decrease the degree of disturbance in the pH. A buffer is defined as a solution that maintains its hydrogen ion concentration when a strong acid or base is added to the solution. The buffering systems in the blood include bicarbonate, hemoglobin, phosphate, and plasma proteins. The bicarbonate buffering system is responsible for about 50% of the total buffering capacity of the body. Hemoglobin is responsible for about 35% of the total buffering capacity, and the remainder is by phosphate and the plasma proteins. (222; **1393–1396**)

6. The bicarbonate buffering system works by hydrating carbon dioxide in the plasma and in the erythrocytes. In erythrocytes the enzyme carbonic anhydrase facilitates this reaction. The hydration of carbon dioxide results in H_2CO_3, which spontaneously dissociates to form H^+ and HCO_3^-. The H^+ that is formed is buffered by the hemoglobin, whereas the HCO_3^- that is formed enters the plasma to function as a buffer. With the entry of HCO_3^- in the plasma to act as a buffer, chloride ions enter the erythrocytes to maintain electrical neutrality. This is termed a *chloride shift*. (222, Fig. 17–1; **1393–1394**)

7. Hemoglobin exists as a weak acid and a salt in erythrocytes, allowing it to serve as a buffer. It acts as a buffer through its reduced form binding with the hydrogen ion. Carbon dioxide can also be transported by hemoglobin, forming carbaminohemoglobin and further contributing to its buffering capacity. (222; **1395–1396**)

8. The buffering system of the blood responds to changes in arterial pH almost instantly. (222; **1393**)

9. Compensatory changes in alveolar ventilation in response to changes in arterial pH occur within minutes. (222; **1393, 1403**)

10. Compensatory changes by the kidneys in response to changes in arterial pH require 12 to 48 hours to complete. (222–223; **1400–1401**)

DIFFERENTIAL DIAGNOSIS OF ACID-BASE DISTURBANCES

11. Acidemia is defined as an arterial pH less than 7.35. Alkalemia is defined as an arterial pH greater than 7.45. (223; **1404**)

12. A primary disturbance in acid-base status is the initial deviation in the arterial pH secondary to either respiratory or metabolic causes. A compensatory response occurs in an attempt to reverse the alteration in the arterial pH. Typically the compensatory response is not adequate to completely reverse the deviation in arterial pH but is sufficient to result in near-normal pH levels. (223; **1402–1403**)

13. Primary respiratory acidosis is defined as acidosis secondary to an inadequate minute ventilation. Primary respiratory acidosis is accompanied by a P_{CO_2} above normal, usually greater than 43 mm Hg. Primary respiratory alkalosis is defined as alkalosis secondary to an excessive minute ventilation. Primary respiratory alkalosis is accompanied by a P_{CO_2} below normal, usually lower than 37 mm Hg. (223; **1402–1403**)

14. A primary metabolic disturbance is characterized by a deviation of the HCO_3^- concentration from normal. A primary metabolic acidosis is defined as acidemia in the presence of a HCO_3^- concentration markedly less than 24 mEq/L. A

primary metabolic alkalosis is defined as alkalemia in the presence of a HCO_3^- concentration markedly greater than 24 mEq/L. (223; **1403**)

15. Acidemia has a more pronounced effect on myocardial contractility than alkalemia, particularly when the arterial pH is less than 7.1. Acidemia with a pH greater than 7.1 has attenuated effects of direct myocardial depression. This is due to the myocardial response to the increased levels of circulating catecholamines that is induced by this level of acidemia. Beta-adrenergic receptor blockade interferes with this protective effect of catecholamines. Patients with ischemic heart disease are more sensitive to the effects of acidemia on the heart. (223–224; **1407–1408**)

16. Respiratory acidosis has a greater effect on myocardial function than metabolic acidosis. This increased sensitivity is believed to be due to the ability of carbon dioxide to diffuse across cell membranes and further exacerbate myocardial acidosis. (224; **1404**)

17. Respiratory acidosis is defined as an arterial pH less than 7.35 with a Pa_{CO_2} greater than 45 mm Hg. (224; **1404**)

18. Respiratory acidosis may occur secondary to a decrease in carbon dioxide elimination or an increased metabolic production of carbon dioxide. Causes of a decrease in carbon dioxide elimination include central nervous system depression as from anesthetics, a decrease in skeletal muscle strength, intrinsic pulmonary disease, or the rebreathing of exhaled carbon dioxide gases. Causes of an increased metabolic production of carbon dioxide include hyperthermia and an increased glucose load as from hyperalimentation. (224; **1404**)

19. Respiratory acidosis results in a decrease in pH in the cerebrospinal fluid as well as the blood. The decrease in pH in the cerebrospinal fluid is caused by the diffusion of carbon dioxide across the blood-brain barrier. Physiologic responses to respiratory acidosis occur as a result of these two changes. The decreased pH of the cerebrospinal fluid stimulates the medullary ventilatory centers of the brain, thus stimulating the patient's alveolar ventilation. The arterial acidemia causes stimulation of ventilation via the carotid bodies as well. This effect of the carotid bodies is attenuated in the presence of volatile anesthetics.

    Arterial acidemia results in a secondary increase in HCO_3^- concentration by the hydration of carbon dioxide within seconds of the increase in P_{CO_2}. There is also a compensatory response by the kidneys. The kidneys secrete hydrogen ions into the urine and reabsorb HCO_3^-. This compensation by the kidneys requires 12 to 48 hours to complete. With the increase in the plasma HCO_3^- concentration there is a corresponding active transport of HCO_3^- into the cerebrospinal fluid, thus increasing the pH of the cerebrospinal fluid. The net result is an increase in the plasma HCO_3^- concentration by about 3 mEq/L for every 10 mm Hg increase in the Pa_{CO_2}. Respiratory acidosis is thus reflected as a near-normal arterial pH, an increase in the Pa_{CO_2}, and a mild to moderate increase in the plasma HCO_3^- concentration. (224; **1404**)

20. Acute respiratory acidemia can be distinguished from chronic respiratory acidemia by the degree of elevation of the HCO_3^- concentration. A HCO_3^- concentration that has only slightly increased in response to arterial acidemia reflects the effects of the hydration of carbon dioxide in the acute phase of acidemia. The renal effects of chronic respiratory acidemia require 12 to 48 hours to take effect and are reflected by a more marked increase in the plasma HCO_3^- concentration. (224; **1404**)

21. Acidemia from respiratory acidosis alone can be distinguished from a mixed respiratory and metabolic cause for the acidemia by the plasma HCO_3^- concentration. A plasma HCO_3^- concentration that has not increased by 3 mEq/L in

the presence of chronic respiratory acidosis is reflective of a probable mixed respiratory and metabolic acidosis. (224; **1404**)

22. Adverse physiologic effects of respiratory acidosis include anxiety, confusion, hypertension, pulmonary hypertension, tachycardia and cardiac dysrhythmias, and an increased serum potassium concentration. With very high P_{CO_2} levels, central nervous system depression can progress to stupor or coma. This is termed *CO₂ narcosis*. (224; **1404**)

23. The treatment for respiratory acidosis is treatment of the underlying disorder. The use of mechanical ventilation to decrease an acutely increased Pa_{CO_2} may be indicated. If the respiratory acidosis has been chronic, it is recommended that the Pa_{CO_2} not be lowered too rapidly. This would result in a metabolic alkalosis, because the kidneys have increased their secretion of hydrogen ions into the urine. (224; **1405**)

24. Respiratory alkalosis is defined as an arterial pH greater than 7.45 with a Pa_{CO_2} less than 35 mm Hg. (224; **1405**)

25. Respiratory alkalosis may occur secondary to an increase in carbon dioxide elimination or by a decreased metabolic production of carbon dioxide. Causes of an increase in carbon dioxide elimination include iatrogenic or self-induced hyperventilation due to pain, anxiety, decreased barometric pressure, central nervous system injury, arterial hypoxemia, pulmonary vascular disease, cirrhosis of the liver, sepsis, and hyperthermia. Causes of a decreased metabolic production of carbon dioxide include hypothermia and skeletal muscle paralysis. (224; **1405**)

26. Respiratory alkalosis initially results in arterial alkalemia secondary to the decreased production of hydrogen ions corresponding to the decrease in hydration in carbon dioxide. The decrease in the Pa_{CO_2} and the increase in the arterial pH together decrease the stimulus of the carotid bodies and the medullary ventilatory center for alveolar ventilation. Active transport of bicarbonate ions out of the cerebrospinal fluid leads to a normal pH in the cerebrospinal fluid. This results in the resumption of normal ventilation, or a relative increase in ventilation, despite continued decreased Pa_{CO_2} levels.

There are three physiologic effects of respiratory alkalosis that occur to compensate for the increase in the arterial pH. First, there is an immediate response to the increase in pH by the bicarbonate buffer system, which results in an increase in carbon dioxide. Second, there is stimulation of the activity of the enzyme phosphofructokinase in response to the alkalosis. This results in glycolysis and a rapid increase in lactic acid production. Finally, the renal tubules of the kidney decrease the degree of reabsorption of HCO_3^-, with maximal compensation by the kidneys requiring 12 to 48 hours. With the decrease in the plasma HCO_3^- concentration there is a corresponding active transport of HCO_3^- out of the cerebrospinal fluid, thus decreasing the pH of the cerebrospinal fluid. The net result is a decrease in the plasma HCO_3^- concentration by about 5 mEq/L for every 10 mm Hg decrease in the Pa_{CO_2}. Respiratory alkalosis is thus reflected as a near-normal arterial pH, a decrease in the Pa_{CO_2}, and a mild to moderate decrease in the HCO_3^- concentration. (224–225, Fig. 17–2; **1405**)

27. Adverse physiologic effects of respiratory alkalosis include impaired judgment, confusion, coma, neuromuscular irritability, decreased cerebral blood flow, cardiac dysrhythmias, decreased availability of oxygen to the tissues due to a leftward shift of the oxyhemoglobin dissociation curve, and decreased serum potassium concentrations. (225; **1405**)

28. The treatment for respiratory alkalosis is treatment of the underlying disorder. For a patient under anesthesia the minute ventilation may be decreased to

decrease the elimination of carbon dioxide and decrease the arterial pH. (225; **1405**)

29. Metabolic acidosis is defined as an arterial pH less than 7.35 with a HCO_3^- concentration less than 20 mmol/L. (225; **1407**)

30. Metabolic acidosis may occur secondary to a decrease in the elimination of the hydrogen ions from the renal tubules or an increase in the metabolic production of hydrogen ions. The elimination of hydrogen ions may be decreased secondary to renal failure or a decrease in the conversion of lactate to glucose by a cirrhotic liver. The metabolic production of hydrogen ions may be increased secondary to anaerobic glycolysis from inadequate oxygen delivery to the tissues, diabetic ketoacidosis, the metabolism of amino acids in hyperalimenta- tion solutions, excessive gastrointestinal losses distal to the pylorus, and renal tubular acidosis. A rare cause of metabolic acidosis is hyperchloremic or dilutional acidosis. This may occur when the plasma bicarbonate concentration becomes diluted by the administration of large volumes of 0.9% saline solutions. (225; **1407, Table 38–3**)

31. Compensatory responses to arterial acidemia associated with metabolic acidosis include an increase in the renal tubular secretion of hydrogen ions into the urine and stimulation of the carotid bodies to cause an increase in the minute ventilation. The increase in minute ventilation is abated temporarily by the decrease in $Paco_2$ and increase in cerebrospinal fluid pH that results from the initial increase in minute ventilation. The active transport of bicarbonate ions into the cerebrospinal fluid normalizes the cerebrospinal fluid pH, and the increase in minute ventilation then resumes. In addition, in response to metabolic acidosis there is a neutralization of noncarbonic acids in the circulation by buffers in the bone. This explains why there is a loss of bone mass associated with chronic metabolic acidosis, as in patients with chronic renal failure. Interestingly, patients with metabolic acidosis due to lactic acid production tend to hyperventilate to a greater extent than patients with metabolic acidosis due to other causes. This may occur secondary to the production of lactic acids by the brain and the subsequent direct exposure to decreases in pH by the chemore- ceptors in the cerebrospinal fluid. (226; **1407**)

32. The arterial pH changes by 0.08 for every 10 mm Hg deviation from 40 mm Hg in the $Paco_2$. This provides a useful measure to determine the degree of increase in the arterial pH that is due to a compensatory increase in the minute ventilation. In turn, it also allows for a determination of the degree of acidemia that is due to metabolic acidosis. (226)

33. Acidemia from primary metabolic acidosis can be distinguished from a mixed respiratory and metabolic cause for the acidemia by evaluation of the $Paco_2$. For every 1 mEq/L decrease in the plasma HCO_3^- concentration there is a corresponding decrease in the $Paco_2$ by about 1 mm Hg. When the $Paco_2$ does not decrease by the expected amount, there is likely a mixed respiratory and metabolic cause for the acidemia. (226; **1407**)

34. Adverse physiologic effects of metabolic acidosis include cardiovascular depres- sion, cardiac dysrhythmias, peripheral vasodilation resulting in hypotension, central nervous system depression progressing from fatigue to coma, muscle weakness possibly compromising respiratory function, and an increase in serum potassium levels. Initially, the effects of metabolic acidosis on the heart are offset by increases in systemic catecholamines. As the pH declines to levels less than 7.2, direct myocardial depression progressively worsens. (226; **1407**)

35. The treatment for metabolic acidosis is treatment of the underlying disorder. Mechanical ventilation may need to be instituted to provide for respiratory compensation. For metabolic acidosis that is sufficiently severe to exert effects

on the myocardium, sodium bicarbonate may be considered for intravenous administration. There are nomograms describing the appropriate dose of sodium bicarbonate under these conditions. The dose is based on the degree of alteration in the pH and the patient's body weight. Each milliequivalent of sodium bicarbonate administered is estimated to produce 180 mL of carbon dioxide. When 1 mEq/kg is administered intravenously, sufficient carbon dioxide is produced to necessitate a temporary doubling of alveolar ventilation to prevent hypercarbia. Care should be taken with the administration of sodium bicarbonate, because it is very hypertonic and may result in alkalemia. (226, Table 17–2; **1408**)

36. Metabolic alkalosis is defined as an arterial pH greater than 7.45 with a HCO_3^- concentration greater than 30 mmol/L. (227; **1405**)

37. Metabolic alkalosis may occur secondary to upper gastrointestinal losses secondary to vomiting or nasogastric suction, diuretic-induced chloride and/or potassium losses, the metabolism of lactate in lactated Ringer's solution, the metabolism of citrate administered in blood products, the metabolism of acetate in hyperalimentation solutions, a depletion of the intravascular fluid volume, and hyperaldosteronism leading to an increase in renal tubular hydrogen ion secretion. (227; **1406**)

38. Arterial alkalemia associated with metabolic alkalosis results in an increase in the reabsorption of hydrogen ion by the renal tubules, a decreased secretion of hydrogen ions by the renal tubules, an increase in the excretion of HCO_3^-, and a decrease in alveolar ventilation. Of note, the kidneys are only able to compensate for arterial alkalemia associated with metabolic alkalosis if there is sufficient plasma levels of sodium, potassium, and chloride to excrete excess HCO_3^-. These compensatory mechanisms are typically never enough to compensate for more than 75% of the deviation in the arterial pH. (227; **1406**)

39. Adverse physiologic effects of metabolic alkalosis include hypercapnia due to compensatory responses and the potential effects of hypercapnia, cardiac dysrhythmias, and decreases in the serum potassium and calcium levels that could lead to neuromuscular irritability. (227; **1406**)

40. The treatment for metabolic alkalosis is treatment of the underlying disorder, including the correction of the electrolyte disorders. (227; **1406**)

MEASUREMENT OF ARTERIAL BLOOD GASES

41. Because heparin is acidic, excessive amounts of heparin in the syringe containing blood for arterial blood gas and pH analysis may result in a falsely decreased arterial pH reading. (228)

42. The syringe containing blood for an arterial blood gas sample is placed in ice to decrease the rate of metabolism in the blood. Metabolism in the blood could result in a decrease in the oxygen tension in the blood and an increase in the carbon dioxide tension. (228; **1263**)

43. Air bubbles in the syringe containing blood for an arterial blood gas sample could result in the diffusion of oxygen and carbon dioxide between the air bubble and the blood in the syringe. Typically this results in a decrease in the oxygen and carbon dioxide tensions in the blood sample. (228; **1263**)

44. By convention, most blood gas electrodes are maintained at 37°C. Because the temperature of the patient is rarely exactly 37°C, arterial blood gas analysis can be corrected for temperature. Blood gas analysis from patients whose temperature is above or below 37°C can result in artificial results. For example, if a patient's body temperature is less than 37°C, warming of the sample to 37°C

after its collection will result in artificially elevated P_{O_2} and P_{CO_2} values. The opposite also occurs for samples taken from hyperthermic patients. An estimate for the correction of the P_{O_2} in an arterial blood gas sample from a patient whose temperature was not 37°C is to decrease the P_{O_2} by 6% for every 1°C the patient's body temperature was below 37°C and to increase the P_{O_2} by 6% for every 1°C the patient's body temperature was above 37°C. Temperature correction of blood gases is not universally practiced, however. This is based on the recognition that the pH must be altered with alterations in body temperature to maintain electrochemical neutrality. For instance, as body temperature increases, the pH necessarily decreases to maintain electrochemical neutrality. (228; **1261–1262**)

45. The Clark electrode measures the P_{O_2} in the blood sample, and the Severinghaus electrode measures the P_{CO_2}. (228; **1260**)

46. The adequacy of ventilation and oxygenation can be assessed by the measurement of the partial pressures of oxygen and carbon dioxide in the arterial blood, measurement of the gradient between the arterial and alveolar oxygen concentrations, measurement of the ratio between the arterial and alveolar partial pressures of oxygen, measurement of the mixed venous P_{O_2}, measurement of the arterial and mixed venous content of oxygen, determining the position of the oxyhemoglobin dissociation curve, and measurement of the deadspace-to-tidal volume ratio. (229; **1257–1260**)

47. Causes of arterial hypoxemia include a low inspired concentration of oxygen, hypoventilation, and an increase in the venous contribution to arterial blood. An increase in the venous contribution to arterial blood involves blood that passes from the pulmonary circulation to the systemic circulation without passing by ventilated alveoli. These right-to-left shunts can be intrapulmonary, as with atelectasis, pneumonia, or one-lung ventilation. These shunts can also be intracardiac, as with congenital heart disease. Ventilation-perfusion mismatching for any reason, such as with chronic obstructive pulmonary disease, may also result in arterial hypoxemia. (229)

48. A ventilation-perfusion mismatch results in arterial hypoxemia by the passage of blood via alveoli that is underventilated. This blood enters the systemic circulation and mixes with blood that has been replenished with oxygen by passing through ventilated alveoli. The resultant mixture of blood in the systemic circulation has a Pa_{O_2} that is less than that which would have been expected had all the blood passing through the pulmonary circulation passed through ventilated alveoli. (229; **1259**)

49. In a right-to-left shunt venous, desaturated blood enters the systemic circulation without replenishing its oxygen supply by contacting alveolar gases. This results in blood with decreased oxygen tensions from the venous system mixing with arterial blood and a decrease in the oxygen tension in the systemic circulation. The net effect on the oxygen tension depends on the magnitude of the shunt. (229; **597–598, 1258–1260, Figs. 15–26, 33–4**)

50. Arterial hypoxemia secondary to ventilation-perfusion mismatch that is not caused by a right-to-left shunt improves with the administration of 100% oxygen. The administration of 100% oxygen under these circumstances replaces nitrogen with oxygen in alveoli that are poorly ventilated. This results in an increase in the partial pressure of oxygen that blood passing via these alveoli is exposed to and an improvement in the Pa_{O_2}. The administration of 100% oxygen to patients with arterial hypoxemia secondary to a right-to-left shunt will not lead to an improvement in the Pa_{O_2}. The administration of 100% oxygen to a

patient with arterial hypoxemia may help to delineate between these two causes of arterial hypoxemia. (229; **597–598, 607, 1258–1260, Figs. 15–26, 33–4**)

51. The $A - aDo_2$ is the alveolar-to-arterial difference for oxygen. It is calculated by the difference between the PAo_2 and the Pao_2. The partial pressure of oxygen in the alveoli is influenced by the arterial concentration of carbon dioxide and the inspired concentration of oxygen. (229, Table 17–3; **896, 1259**)

52. The normal $A - aDo_2$ is 5 to 10 mm Hg when breathing room air. The normal $A - aDo_2$ reflects the cardiac output that is normally shunted from the right-to-left side of the circulation without passing via the alveoli. This portion of the cardiac output returns to the heart through the bronchial, pleural, and thebesian veins. (229; **896, 1259**)

53. A benefit of using the Pao_2/PAo_2 ratio instead of the $A - aDo_2$ for an estimate of the magnitude of the venous admixture is that the Pao_2/PAo_2 ratio, or a/A ratio, remains constant even with changes in the inhaled concentration of oxygen. In contrast, the $A - aDo_2$ will vary with changes in the inhaled concentration of oxygen. For example, when the inspired concentration of oxygen increases the $A - aDo_2$ will become higher. This makes interpretation of the $A - aDo_2$ in patients inspiring supplemental oxygen difficult. (229, Table 17–4; **896, 1259**)

54. The mixed venous Po_2 is useful as an indicator of the adequacy of the cardiac output. The mixed venous Po_2 is dependent on both the cardiac output and tissue oxygen consumption, as well as the hemoglobin concentration and the saturation of oxygen. Typically, the hemoglobin concentration and oxygen saturation are constant. Given this, if the consumption of oxygen from the tissues has not greatly changed, a decrease in the mixed venous Po_2 is indicative of a decrease in the cardiac output because of the greater extraction of oxygen that is required during times of decreased blood flow to maintain tissue oxygenation. (229–230; **1267–1268, Fig. 33–4**)

55. A mixed venous Po_2 of lower than 30 mm Hg is indicative of tissue hypoxemia. A patient may have a high mixed venous Po_2 despite inadequate tissue oxygenation secondary to the presence of a high arterial-to-venous admixture, as can be present in disease states such as portal hypertension and sepsis. (230; **1267–1268**)

56. The difference between the arterial and venous content of oxygen is also useful as an indicator of the adequacy of cardiac output for the provision of oxygen to the tissues. The normal difference between the arterial and venous oxygen contents is 4 to 6 mL of oxygen per dL of blood. If the extraction of oxygen from the tissues has not greatly changed, an increase in the difference between the arterial and venous content of oxygen indicates a decrease in the cardiac output because of the greater extraction of oxygen that is required during times of decreased blood flow to maintain tissue oxygenation. (230, Table 17–5; **596–598**)

57. The oxyhemoglobin dissociation curve illustrates the affinity of hemoglobin for oxygen over various partial pressures of oxygen, making it representative of the saturation of hemoglobin with oxygen. Some points on the oxyhemoglobin dissociation curve include the P_{50}, P_{75}, and P_{90}. These are the partial pressures of oxygen that result in the hemoglobin being 50%, 75%, and 90% saturated. The partial pressures of oxygen that correspond to each of these are 26, 40, and 60 mm Hg, respectively. (230–231, Fig. 17–3; **595–597, Fig. 15–25**)

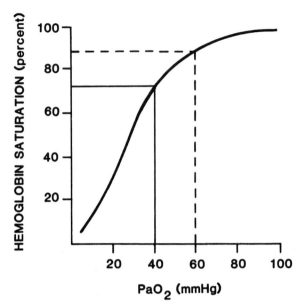

Figure 16–1. The oxyhemoglobin dissociation curve describes the relationship of the hemoglobin saturation with oxygen (%) to the P_{O_2}. The P_{50} is the P_{O_2} that results in 50% saturation of hemoglobin with oxygen. In the presence of a normal pHa (7.4) and body temperature (37°C), hemoglobin is 50% saturated with oxygen at a P_{O_2} of 26 mm Hg (P_{50}). Events that shift the oxyhemoglobin dissociation curve to the left (P_{50} <26 mm Hg) may jeopardize tissue oxygenation since the Pa_{O_2} must decrease further to permit release of oxygen from hemoglobin. Conversely, a shift of the oxyhemoglobin dissociation curve to the right (P_{50} >26 mm Hg) permits unloading of oxygen from hemoglobin at a higher P_{O_2} and thus favors tissue oxygenation. The mixed venous P_{O_2} is near 40 mm Hg, and the associated hemoglobin saturation with oxygen is about 75%. Saturation of hemoglobin with oxygen is about 90% when the Pa_{O_2} is 60 mm Hg. The saturation of hemoglobin with oxygen can be assumed to be 100% when the Pa_{O_2} is >150 mm Hg. (From Stoelting RK, Miller RD: Basics of Anesthesia, 4th ed. Philadelphia, Churchill Livingstone, 2000, p 230.)

58. The oxyhemoglobin dissociation curve shifts to the right in response to acidosis, hypercapnia, hyperthermia, and an increased 2,3-diphosphoglycerate value, as can occur with chronic arterial hypoxemia or anemia, and during exercise. A rightward shift of the curve reflects a decreased affinity of hemoglobin for oxygen at a given partial pressure, such that the unloading of oxygen at the tissues is facilitated. (231, Table 17–6; **596–597**)

59. The oxyhemoglobin dissociation curve shifts to the left in response to alkalosis, hypocapnia, hypothermia, a decreased 2,3-diphosphoglycerate value, as can occur with the transfusion of old bank blood or in diabetic ketoacidosis, and carbon monoxide poisoning. A leftward shift of the curve reflects an increased affinity of hemoglobin for oxygen at a given partial pressure, such that a lower partial pressure of oxygen is required to saturate the hemoglobin. This results in the necessity of a lower oxygen concentration in the tissues for the oxygen to unload from hemoglobin. (231, Table 17–6; **596–597**)

60. Compensatory mechanisms for arterial hypoxemia include an increase in cardiac output and an increase in the minute ventilation. The increase in cardiac output is the most efficient compensatory mechanism for arterial hypoxemia. The increase in cardiac output is achieved through increases in heart rate, stroke volume, and myocardial contractility. (231; **611–612, Table 15–4**)

61. The respiratory quotient is 0.8. This respiratory quotient reflects the ratio between the production of carbon dioxide and the consumption of oxygen, such that only 80% as much the volume of carbon dioxide is produced when compared with the volume of oxygen consumed. Put another way, when the volume of oxygen consumed per minute is 250 mL, the volume of carbon dioxide produced per minute is about 200 mL. (231; **599**)

62. The deadspace-to-tidal volume ratio is useful as an indicator of the proportion of the minute ventilation that ventilates airways that are not perfused. Another term for this is *wasted ventilation*. The normal deadspace-to-tidal volume ratio is less than 30%, reflecting a volume of about 2 mL/kg. (231, Table 17–7; **593–594, 1259–1260, Figs. 15–21, 15–22**)

63. An increased deadspace-to-tidal volume ratio indicates that a greater volume of the minute ventilation is wasted or does not come in contact with blood vessels for oxygen and carbon dioxide exchange. An increased deadspace-to-tidal volume ratio may result in elevations in the Pa_{CO_2}. Patients with a pulmonary embolus or chronic obstructive pulmonary disease are examples of patients who may have an increased deadspace-to-tidal volume ratio. (231; **593–594, 1259–1260**)

64. A right-to-left shunt has very little to no effect on the deadspace-to-tidal volume ratio. A right-to-left shunt is indicative of blood that passes by unventilated alveoli or directly to the systemic circulation without passing by alveoli at all. This has no effect on the deadspace-to-tidal volume ratio, which reflects airways, possibly alveoli, that are ventilated but not involved in gas exchange. A right-to-left shunt may affect oxygenation but has little or no effect on the Pa_{CO_2}. (231; **1259–1260**)

Chapter 17

Fluid and Blood Therapy

1. What are some factors that influence the intraoperative management of fluid administration?

BODY FLUID COMPARTMENTS

2. What body fluid compartments can total body water be divided into?

3. What is the plasma volume? What percent of body weight is made up by the plasma volume?

4. What is the interstitial fluid? What percent of body weight is made up by the interstitial fluid volume?

5. How does total body water weight differ between men and women? How does total body water weight differ between obese and nonobese patients? How does total body water weight differ between infants and adults?

6. How can a patient's intravascular fluid volume status be assessed preoperatively?

7. Why is it important to assess a patient's intravascular fluid volume status before the delivery of anesthesia?

8. What is the tilt test? What constitutes a positive tilt test?

9. What is orthostatic hypotension?

10. How can orthostatic hypotension be distinguished from autonomic nervous system dysfunction?

11. What are some reasons why a patient may have intravascular fluid volume overload? What are some clinical consequences that can result?

12. How do serum sodium concentrations and serum osmolarity change with alterations in the extracellular fluid volume?

13. What are some reasons for hypovolemic, normovolemic, and hypervolemic hyponatremia?

14. What are some manifestations of hyponatremia? At what serum sodium level do central nervous system signs of hyponatremia become manifest?

15. How can hyponatremia be treated?

16. What is the most common cause of hypernatremia? What are some other causes of hypernatremia?

17. What are some manifestations of hypernatremia? How can hypernatremia be treated?

18. What are some causes of hyperkalemia when due to an increased total body potassium content?

19. What are some causes of hyperkalemia when due to an altered distribution of potassium between extracellular and intracellular sites?

20. Are the adverse effects of hyperkalemia more likely to occur with acute or chronic increases in serum potassium concentrations?

21. What are some adverse effects of hyperkalemia?

22. How can hyperkalemia be treated?

23. What serum potassium level is often considered to be the upper limit acceptable for patients who are scheduled to undergo elective operative procedures?

24. What are some potential causes of hypokalemia? What is acute stress-induced hypokalemia?

25. What are some adverse effects of hypokalemia? How might hypokalemia manifest on the electrocardiogram?

26. How can hypokalemia be treated? How effective is oral potassium replacement?

27. What is the concern regarding patients with hypokalemia who are scheduled to undergo elective surgery?

28. What are some causes of hypermagnesemia?

29. What are some manifestations of hypermagnesemia? How can hypermagnesemia be treated?

30. What are some causes of hypomagnesemia?

31. What are some manifestations of hypomagnesemia? How can hypomagnesemia be treated?

32. What are some causes of hypercalcemia?

33. What are some manifestations of hypercalcemia? How can hypercalcemia be treated?

34. What are some causes of hypocalcemia?

35. What are some manifestations of hypocalcemia? How can hypocalcemia be treated?

INTRAOPERATIVE FLUID REPLACEMENT

36. What are some sources of insensible fluid losses that can occur in patients during surgery? What volume of fluid should be administered intraoperatively to replace insensible water losses in patients?

37. What volume of fluid should be administered intraoperatively to replace third space losses of fluids?

38. What day postoperatively do third space fluid losses become mobilized?

39. What are crystalloids?

40. What volume of crystalloid fluid should be administered to patients to correct intraoperative blood loss?

41. What are colloids? How should they be administered to correct blood loss?

42. What are some potential adverse effects of using hetastarch and dextran for volume replacement?

43. What is the primary indication for the transfusion of 5% albumin? What is the primary indication for the transfusion of 25% albumin?

44. What is Plasmanate? When should it be administered?

45. When might glucose-containing solutions be administered?

46. What are some clinical signs of blood loss? What urine output intraoperatively lends evidence that the patient's intravascular fluid volume is adequate?

47. How well can vasoconstriction compensate for intraoperative blood loss?

48. What are the indications for the transfusion of blood?

49. How should the acute loss of large volumes of blood be managed?

50. How can the adequacy of blood replacement be assessed?

BLOOD THERAPY

51. What is the recipient's blood tested for during the routine typing of blood? What is the risk of transfusing blood to patients without typing the recipient's blood?

52. How is the crossmatching of blood accomplished?

53. How does the transfusion of O-negative packed red blood cells in an emergency situation affect the patient's subsequent transfusions?

54. What does type-specific blood refer to? What is the chance of a significant hemolytic reaction with the transfusion of type-specific blood to a patient?

55. What does a type and screen refer to? When is a type and screen typically ordered? What is the chance of a significant hemolytic reaction with the transfusion of typed and screened blood to a patient?

56. What is contained in preservative solutions for the storage of blood? What is the benefit of adding adenine to the preservative solution?

57. How long can blood be stored?

58. What is the temperature at which blood is stored? Why?

59. What is the volume of blood, the volume of citrate-containing preservative, and the hematocrit in a given unit of whole blood?

COMPONENT THERAPY

60. Name the components that can be derived from whole blood. What is the advantage of using components for blood therapy instead of whole blood?

61. What is the hematocrit and total volume in a unit of packed red blood cells?

62. What is the indication for the administration of packed red blood cells?

63. How much will adult hemoglobin concentrations increase with the administration of a single unit of packed red blood cells?

64. What solutions may be used to reconstitute packed red blood cells for administration?

65. What potential complication associated with the administration of whole blood is less likely to occur with the administration of packed red blood cells?

66. Why is the risk of allergic reactions increased with the administration of whole blood than it is with the administration of packed red blood cells?

67. When is the administration of platelets indicated during surgery?

68. How much will the platelet count increase after the administration of 1 unit of platelets?

69. What are some of the risks associated with the administration of platelets?

70. What is fresh frozen plasma? What is contained in fresh frozen plasma?

71. When is the administration of fresh frozen plasma indicated during surgery?

72. What are some of the risks associated with the administration of fresh frozen plasma?

73. What is cryoprecipitate? What is contained in cryoprecipitate?

74. What is cryoprecipitate useful for treating?

COMPLICATIONS OF BLOOD THERAPY

75. Name some potential complications of blood therapy.

76. What is the risk of the transmission of viral diseases with the transfusion of blood?

77. What are the various types of transfusion reactions that may occur with blood therapy?

78. Why are febrile transfusion reactions thought to occur? How do febrile transfusion reactions manifest?

79. How are febrile transfusion reactions treated?

80. Why are allergic transfusion reactions thought to occur? How do allergic transfusion reactions manifest?

81. How are allergic transfusion reactions treated? How are allergic transfusion reactions distinguished from hemolytic transfusion reactions?

82. Why are hemolytic transfusion reactions thought to occur?

83. What are the clinical signs that a hemolytic transfusion reaction has occurred? Which of these are masked by anesthesia?

84. What diagnostic tool provides evidence that a hemolytic transfusion reaction has occurred?

85. What are some consequences that can follow a hemolytic transfusion reaction?

86. What is the treatment for a hemolytic transfusion reaction?

87. What is transfusion-related acute lung injury?

88. Describe the immunosuppression that may accompany blood transfusions.

89. What are some metabolic abnormalities that may accompany blood transfusions?

90. How does the transfusion of blood affect the patient's arterial pH?

91. How much does the serum potassium level increase in patients after the transfusion of blood?

92. How do concentrations of 2,3-diphosphoglycerate change with the prolonged storage of blood? How does this affect oxygen delivery to the tissues?

93. How does the administration of citrate in blood products affect the recipient's serum calcium concentration?

94. How does the administration of citrate in blood products affect the recipient's arterial pH?

95. What do microaggregates in whole blood consist of? What is the risk of the administration of these microaggregates?

96. What is the potential risk of hypothermia with the administration of blood products?

97. What are some ways in which massive blood transfusions can result in coagulation disorders?

98. What is dilutional thrombocytopenia? What is the treatment of dilutional thrombocyopenia?

99. Which clotting factors may decrease in concentration in the patient's blood with massive transfusions? What percent of each of these clotting factors is necessary to maintain hemostasis during surgery? How can this clotting factor deficiency be treated?

100. What is disseminated intravascular coagulation? What is the treatment of disseminated intravascular coagulation?

AUTOLOGOUS BLOOD

101. What is the advantage of the administration of autologous blood over homologous blood for necessary blood transfusions?

102. What is an acceptable schedule for the collection of pre-deposited blood for autologous blood transfusion? How can anemia secondary to the donation of autologous blood be minimized?

103. What are some complications that can occur with autologous blood transfusions of pre-deposited blood?

104. How is the intraoperative salvage of blood for autologous blood transfusions accomplished? What are some relative contraindications to the intraoperative salvage of blood?

105. What are some complications that may accompany the intraoperative salvage of blood for autologous blood transfusions?

106. What is the hemodilution technique for autologous blood transfusions? What are some advantages of this technique?

ANSWERS*

1. Factors that influence the intraoperative management of fluid administration include the patient's intraoperative fluid status, any co-existing disease, knowledge of fluid shifts, quantitation of blood loss, and the selection of the appropriate fluids for the replacement of losses. (233; **1601**)

BODY FLUID COMPARTMENTS

2. Total body water can be divided into the extracellular and intracellular fluid compartments. Included in the extracellular fluid compartments are the interstitial fluid and the plasma volume. (233, Fig. 18–1; **1587–1588**)

3. The plasma volume is the fluid contained within the vasculature excluding the erythrocytes. About 5% of body weight is made up of the plasma volume. (233; **1588**)

4. The interstitial fluid is the fluid that is external to the blood vessels and cells. About 15% of body weight is made up of the interstitial fluid volume. The interstitial fluid volume serves as a reservoir from which water and/or electrolytes can be taken into the plasma volume at times of need. (233; **1588**)

5. Total body water is about 55% of a man's weight and 45% of a woman's weight. Obese patients have less total body water per weight than nonobese patients. Infants have more total body water than adults, with total body water being about 80% of an infant's weight. (233; **1587**)

6. A patient's intravascular fluid volume status can be assessed preoperatively by evaluating the patient's mental status, history of recent intake and output, supine and upright arterial blood pressures and heart rates, skin turgor, mucous membranes, urine output, arterial gas pH and base deficit, hematocrit, electrolytes, and central venous pressure. Certain disease states or medicines may also provide an indication of possible intravascular fluid depletion.

*Numbers in parentheses: lightface numbers refer to pages, figures, or tables in Stoelting RK, Miller RD: Basics of Anesthesia, 4th ed. Philadelphia, Churchill Livingstone, 2000; **boldface numbers** refer to pages, figures, or tables in Miller RD: Anesthesia, 5th ed. Philadelphia, Churchill Livingstone, 2000.

Examples include prolonged losses from the gastrointestinal tract, chronic hypertension, trauma, sepsis, and diuretic therapy. (233)

7. Assessment of a patient's intravascular fluid volume status may help to predict and avoid potentially adverse effects of anesthesia on a hypovolemic patient. Anesthetics can cause hypotension secondary to systemic vasodilation and/or myocardial depression, and this effect may be more pronounced in the hypovolemic patient. This is particularly important given that preoperatively patients frequently fast, have blood drawn, or have their bowels cleared in preparation for surgery. Patients who appear to have an intravascular fluid volume deficit preoperatively should have their volume augmented with the administration of intravascular fluids before the induction of anesthesia. (233; **1601–1602**)

8. The tilt test measures heart rate and systolic blood pressure when the patient stands upright. A positive tilt test is defined by an increase in heart rate by more than 20 beats per minute and a decrease in the systolic blood pressure by more than 20 mm Hg. (233)

9. Orthostatic hypotension is a physical examination finding that indicates a patient may be hypovolemic. The test for orthostatic hypotension involves taking a patient's blood pressure and heart rate first while the patient is supine and then repeating blood pressure and heart rate measurements after the patient stands. Orthostatic hypotension is defined as a decrease in blood pressure by greater than 20 mm Hg. This may correspond to a fluid volume deficit of 6% to 8% of body weight, but there is a great degree of variability among patients. This limits the usefulness of this test, particularly among the young and healthy or the elderly. (233; **567–568**)

10. Orthostatic hypotension should be distinguished from autonomic nervous system dysfunction because they have two different implications. In the case of orthostatic hypotension, an intravascular fluid volume deficit should result in a decrease in blood pressure as well as a corresponding increase in heart rate. If the decrease in blood pressure is not accompanied by an increase in heart rate the patient may have dysfunction of the autonomic nervous system. There are several causes of autonomic dysfunction, including medications, diabetes, advanced age, and spinal cord injury. (234; **566–567**)

11. Intravascular fluid volume overload may be due to co-existing disease or iatrogenic causes. These patients are likely to have hypertension. Patients with intravascular fluid volume overload and co-existing cardiopulmonary disease are at an increased risk of congestive heart failure and/or pulmonary edema. (234)

12. Serum sodium concentrations and serum osmolarity change with alterations in the plasma volume if the volume lost or gained is electrolyte free. A decrease in the electrolyte-free plasma volume results in an increase in serum sodium concentrations and serum osmolarity. The opposite is also true. That is, an increase in the electrolyte-free plasma volume results in a decrease in serum sodium concentrations and serum osmolarity. (234; **978–979, 1587–1588**)

13. Hypovolemic hyponatremia can result from vomiting, diarrhea, third space sequestration of fluids, osmotic diuresis, renal failure, diuretics, or adrenal insufficiency. Normovolemic hyponatremia can result from the syndrome of inappropriate secretion of antidiuretic hormone, renal failure, and water intoxication. Hypervolemic hyponatremia can result from congestive heart failure, liver failure, or nephrotic syndrome. (234; **978–979, 1588–1589, Tables 25–43, 45–4**)

14. Manifestations of hyponatremia are generally nonspecific. These include

nausea, malaise, and lethargy. Central nervous system signs secondary to cerebral edema caused by hyponatremia become manifest at a serum sodium level less than 110 mEq/L. Mental status changes may occur with serum sodium levels higher than 110 mEq/L when the onset of hyponatremia is acute. (234; **978–979, 1588–1589**)

15. The treatment of hyponatremia ranges from fluid restriction to the administration of hypertonic saline with osmotic and loop diuretics, depending on the severity of the symptoms. Of great importance is the time course for correction of the serum sodium levels during treatment. Correction of the serum sodium levels too rapidly can result in neurologic damage and central pontine myelinolysis. Cerebral edema typically resolves when the serum sodium level is 130 mEq/L or greater. (234; **978–979, 1588–1589**)

16. The most common cause of hypernatremia is water deficiency secondary to excessive loss or inadequate intake, which may be iatrogenic in origin. Excess total body sodium leading to hypernatremia can result from exogenous loads, primary hyperaldosteronism, diabetes insipidus, and renal dysfunction. Hypernatremia may occur in conjunction with cirrhosis of the liver or congestive heart failure. (234; **978–979, 1589–1590, Table 45–5**)

17. Manifestations of hypernatremia include tremulousness, irritability, ataxia, and mental confusion. Severe hypernatremia can result in coma due to cerebral water loss. Hypernatremia can be treated with renal tubular diuretics or hemodialysis. Central diabetes insipidus may be treated with vasopressin. Patients who are depleted intravascularly may benefit from the administration of hypotonic saline. Correction of the serum sodium level too rapidly can result in neurologic damage secondary to cerebral edema. (234; **978–979, 1589–1590**)

18. Hyperkalemia due to an increased total body potassium content is commonly caused by renal failure. It can also be caused by potassium-sparing diuretics, from the excessive administration of intravenous potassium supplements, or from the excessive ingestion of salt substitutes. (234; **979–981, 1590–1591, Table 45–7**)

19. Hyperkalemia due to an altered distribution of potassium between extracellular and intracellular sites can be caused by metabolic or respiratory acidosis, digitalis intoxication, insulin deficiency, hemolysis, and tissue and muscle damage after burns or may occur after the administration of succinylcholine to patients with muscle denervation injuries. (234; **979–981, 1590–1591**)

20. Adverse effects of hyperkalemia are more likely to occur with acute increases in serum potassium concentrations. Chronic hyperkalemia is better tolerated by patients. Chronic hyperkalemia allows for the equilibration of extracellular and intracellular potassium, thus maintaining the resting membrane potential. (234; **979–981, 1590–1591**)

21. Adverse effects of hyperkalemia include areflexia, weakness, paralysis, paresthesias, and cardiac conduction abnormalities. The potential effects of hyperkalemia on the heart are of the most concern for the anesthesiologist. Sequential changes that may be seen on the electrocardiogram as the serum potassium level rises are narrowing and peaking of the T waves, first-degree atrioventricular block, QRS widening, and ST segment depression progressing to merging of the QRS and T waves to a sine wave. Tachycardia and ventricular fibrillation may also occur. Low serum levels of sodium and calcium will augment the adverse effects of hyperkalemia. (234–235; **979–981, 1590–1591**)

22. The primary goal of the treatment of acute hyperkalemia is the avoidance of the adverse cardiac effects of hyperkalemia. The treatment of acute hyperka-

lemia with insulin and glucose causes a shift of potassium from the serum into cells and increases the membrane threshold. Hyperkalemia may also be treated with the intravenous administration of calcium to antagonize the adverse effects of hyperkalemia on the heart. Systemic alkalosis, as is produced by hyperventilation of the lungs or the administration of intravenous sodium bicarbonate, may also be used to treat acute hyperkalemia. (235; **979–981, 1590–1591**)

23. Because of the potential morbidity and mortality that can result from intraoperative hyperkalemia, a serum potassium level of 5.5 mEq/L is often considered to be the upper limit acceptable for patients who are scheduled to undergo elective operative procedures. (234; **979–981, 1590–1591**)

24. Causes of hypokalemia include losses from the gastrointestinal tract, as from diarrhea or nasogastric suction, systemic alkalosis, diabetic ketoacidosis, diuretic therapy, sympathetic nervous system stimulation, and the administration of beta-adrenergic receptor agonists. Acute stress-induced hypokalemia is probably secondary to the shift of potassium from the extracellular spaces into cells secondary to sympathetic nervous system stimulation. Acute stress-induced hypokalemia may be seen in the immediate preoperative period. (235, Fig. 18–2; **979–981, 1590, Table 45–6**)

25. Adverse effects of hypokalemia include an autonomic neuropathy, decreased myocardial contractility, skeletal muscle weakness, and electrical conduction abnormalities that can result in arrhythmias, tachycardia, and ventricular fibrillation. In addition, patients with hypokalemia are more sensitive to the potential cardiovascular effects of digoxin. Hypokalemia manifests on the electrocardiogram as a prolonged PR interval, a prolonged T interval, widening of the QRS complex, and flattening of the T wave. (235; **979–981, 1590**)

26. The treatment of hypokalemia is by the slow intravenous administration of potassium supplements, especially when there is evidence of changes on the electrocardiogram consistent with hypokalemia. Oral potassium replacement may be ineffective in patients in whom the underlying cause of hypokalemia has not been corrected. (235–236; **979–981, 1590**)

27. The concern regarding hypokalemia in patients scheduled to undergo elective surgery is their increased risk of intraoperative myocardial irritability. The incidence of cardiac dysrhythmias has not been shown to be increased with serum potassium levels greater than 2.6 mEq/L, however. Nevertheless, patients with mild hypokalemia undergoing surgical procedures should be managed without hyperventilation of the lungs and without the addition of glucose to intravenous fluids because these can lead to further decreases in serum potassium levels. Potassium supplementation may be added to the intravenous solution, but care must be taken that the inadvertent rapid administration of the intravenous solution does not occur. (236; **979–981, 1590**)

28. Hypermagnesemia is defined as a serum magnesium level greater than 2.5 mEq/L. Causes of hypermagnesemia include iatrogenic administration, as for the treatment of preeclampsia, and intake from antacids or laxatives. Because magnesium is cleared by the kidneys patients with renal failure may be at an increased risk of hypermagnesemia. (236; **1593–1594**)

29. Manifestations of hypermagnesemia include central nervous system depression from sedation to stupor and coma, skeletal muscle weakness up to respiratory failure, decreased peripheral vascular tone, decreases in myocardial contractility, and tocolysis. Hypermagnesemia manifests on the electrocardiogram as a prolonged PQ interval and widened QRS complexes. The treatment of hypermagnesemia includes supportive treatment, fluid loading, and diuresis. In the acute situation intravenous calcium may be administered

to more rapidly counter the effects of elevated magnesium levels. (236; **1593–1594**)

30. Hypomagnesemia is defined as a serum magnesium level less than 1.5 mEq/L. Causes of hypomagnesemia include inadequate intake; total parenteral nutrition; gastrointestinal losses, as with prolonged nasogastric suction or diarrhea; pancreatitis; parathyroid hormone disorders; hyperaldosteronism; ketoacidosis; syndrome of inappropriate antidiuretic hormone secretion; chronic alcoholism; increased renal excretion; and therapy with amphotericin B, diuretics, theophylline, and aminoglycosides. (236; **1593, Table 45–10**)

31. Manifestations of hypomagnesemia include central nervous system irritability, such as seizures and hyperreflexia, and skeletal muscle spasm. The treatment of hypomagnesemia is with the intravenous administration of magnesium sulfate. (236; **1593**)

32. Causes of hypercalcemia include calcium mobilization from bone due to immobility, tumors, or hyperparathyroidism. (236; **1592, Table 45–8**)

33. Manifestations of hypercalcemia include anorexia, nausea, constipation, and cognitive depression. Manifestations on the electrocardiogram include a prolonged PR interval, a shortened QT interval, and premature ventricular contractions. The treatment of hypercalcemia is by treatment of the underlying cause and volume expansion. Sodium inhibits the renal tubular absorption of calcium, making its administration useful in hypercalcemia. Intraoperative hypercalcemia should be managed with the administration of adequate fluids and maintenance of the urine output. (236; **1592**)

34. Causes of hypocalcemia include decreased serum albumin concentrations, the chelation of calcium by citrate, rhabdomyolysis, hypoparathyroidism, pancreatitis, and renal failure. (236; **1592–1593, Table 45–9**)

35. Manifestations of hypocalcemia include neuromuscular irritability, weakness, vasodilation, myocardial dysfunction, bradycardia, and heart block. Neuromuscular irritability may manifest as tetany, laryngospasm, and hyperactive deep tendon reflexes. The treatment of hypocalcemia is by calcium replacement. Intraoperatively, hypocalcemia may also be treated with the institution of hyperventilation and respiratory alkalosis. (236; **1592–1593**)

INTRAOPERATIVE FLUID REPLACEMENT

36. Sources of insensible fluid losses that can occur in patients during surgery include water loss through the urine, feces, sweat, and the respiratory tract. Typically, the correction of insensible water losses intraoperatively requires the administration of about 2 mL/kg per hour of crystalloid solution. (236; **1601, 1605–1606**)

37. Third space losses of body fluids refers to the transfer of fluids from the extracellular space to the interstitial space or other non-intravascular spaces. The volume of fluid that is transferred corresponds to the degree of manipulation of tissues intraoperatively. The replacement of third space losses of fluids intraoperatively is therefore dependent on the type of surgical procedure the patient is undergoing. For procedures that cause minimal trauma, 3 to 4 mL/kg per hour is recommended. For procedures that cause moderate trauma, 5 to 6 mL/kg per hour is recommended. Finally, for procedures that cause severe trauma, 7 to 8 mL/kg per hour is recommended. (236–237; **1606**)

38. Third space fluid losses become mobilized on about the third day postoperatively. Clinically, this may manifest as an increase in the intravascular fluid volume on this day. Patients with limited cardiac reserve or with renal

dysfunction may have hypervolemia or pulmonary edema if the mobilization of fluids is sufficiently large. (237)

39. Crystalloids are a class of fluids that can be administered intraoperatively to maintain normal body fluid composition and replace losses. Crystalloids contain water and electrolytes. Crystalloids cross plasma membranes easily and may dilute plasma proteins, resulting in a reduction of the plasma oncotic pressure. Although crystalloids are effective at increasing the intravascular fluid volume, the administration of crystalloids may be associated with an increased risk of pulmonary edema than that of colloids if administered in sufficient volumes. (237, Table 18–3; **1602–1603**)

40. It is recommended that the volume of crystalloid fluid administered to replace intraoperative blood loss be three times the volume of the estimated blood loss. This is because volume replacement is not just to replenish the volume lost from the intravascular space but also to replenish volume that is transferred from the extravascular spaces to the intravascular spaces to maintain the plasma volume during times of acute blood loss. (237)

41. Colloids include albumin, Plasmanate, hetastarch, and dextran. These all contain large molecules that do not readily cross plasma membranes. For this reason they can be administered in a 1:1 ratio to replace blood loss. Colloids may be advantageous in that they may maintain the plasma oncotic pressure and remain in the intravascular space for longer than crystalloids. About 20 mL of water is held in the circulation for every gram of colloid administered. There is no evidence that colloids are superior than crystalloids for replacing the intravascular fluid volume. The main advantage of colloids for transfusion is their lack of risk of the transmission of disease. The risk of transmission of hepatitis is eliminated by the pretreatment with heat to 60°C for 10 hours. Disadvantages of colloids include their lack of oxygen-carrying capacity and coagulation factors and their increased cost. (237, 241; **1602–1603**)

42. The administration of hetastarch and dextran in large volumes can result in a dilutional coagulopathy. Hetastarch can cause a decrease in factor VIII when administered in a volume greater than 1000 mL in a 70-kg patient. Dextran appears to decrease platelet adhesiveness and has the potential to cause an anaphylactoid or anaphylactic reaction. Dextran has the added disadvantage of interfering with the ability to subsequently crossmatch a patient's blood secondary to the agglutination of red blood cells. (239; **1604**)

43. The primary indication for the transfusion of 5% albumin is for rapid intravascular fluid volume expansion, and the primary indication for the transfusion of 25% albumin is hypoalbuminemia. (241; **1639**)

44. Plasmanate, or plasma protein fractions, are 5% solutions of albumin and alpha and beta globulins in isotonic saline. Plasmanate should be reserved for situations in which there is documented hypoproteinemia, such as with burns or peritonitis. The administration of plasma protein fractions can result in hypotension due to a decrease in systemic vascular resistance. (241; **1603–1604, 1639**)

45. Glucose-containing solutions are typically not administered intraoperatively, owing to the hyperglycemic response associated with surgery. An exception to this would be for the prevention of hypoglycemia in diabetic patients who have been administered insulin. (237; **1603**)

46. Clinical signs of blood loss include tachycardia, hypotension, a decrease in central venous pressure, and oliguria. Intraoperatively, these may be used as an indication of the patient's intravascular fluid volume status and as a guide to the administration of fluids. A urine output of 0.5 to 1 mL/kg per hour is typically indicative of an adequate intravascular fluid volume, although the

administration of medicines such as diuretics may interfere with the utility of monitoring the urine output. The systolic blood pressure variation with the respiratory cycle in mechanically ventilated patients may also be used to assess intravascular fluid volume. The normal variation in systolic blood pressure is 8 to 10 mm Hg, owing to the decrease in venous return that occurs with inspiration. Variations greater than 10 mm Hg may be an indication of hypovolemia. These clinical signs may be altered in the presence of anesthesia. Also of note, young healthy patients may lose up to 20% of their blood volume without any clinical signs of hypovolemia. (238; **1306–1309**)

47. Vasoconstriction of the splanchnic and venous capacitance vessels occurs in response to blood loss. A loss in blood volume of approximately 10% or greater can be masked by this compensatory change. This compensatory mechanism may be interfered with by the administration of anesthetics. (238)

48. The primary indication for the transfusion of blood is to increase the oxygen-carrying capacity of the blood. Because there are no direct measures of the oxygen-carrying capacity, other measures must be used. Typically, the hemoglobin concentration is the basis on which the decision to transfuse is made. Blood transfusion is almost always justified when the hemoglobin value is less than 6 g/dL and is rarely justified when the hemoglobin value is greater than 10 g/dL. Oxygen transport is maximized when the hemoglobin level is 10 g/dL, such that the transfusion of blood at hemoglobin levels above 10 g/dL may provide no further benefit to the patient. The threshold for the transfusion of blood between hemoglobin values of 6 g/dL and 10 g/dL is further modified by several factors. These include the patient's age and medical status, the surgical procedure and the potential for ongoing losses, and the extent to which the patient's current anemia is chronic or is due to blood loss that is acute. For example, patients with coronary artery disease and who are at risk for myocardial ischemia may benefit from keeping the hemoglobin level no less than 10 g/dL, whereas a young healthy patient may not be transfused with a hemoglobin level of 7 g/dL. The decision to transfuse must therefore be made on an individual basis. (238; **1613–1614**)

49. The acute loss of large volumes of blood should be managed with the administration of blood because the administration of crystalloids to these patients in volumes necessary to replace the intravascular volume will result in an inadequate oxygen-carrying capacity of the blood. Typically, this corresponds to a blood loss of greater than one third of the entire blood volume and/or blood loss leading to hypovolemic shock. Whole blood is preferable to packed red blood cells in these situations because the blood loss is sufficiently large to warrant the expansion of blood volume as well as the administration of red blood cells. (238; **1634–1635, Table 46–13**)

50. The adequacy of blood replacement may be assessed through the evaluation of the systemic blood pressure, heart rate, central venous pressure, urine output, arterial oxygenation, arterial pH, base deficit, and serial hematocrit levels. (239)

BLOOD THERAPY

51. Routine typing of the recipient's blood tests for the presence of A or B or both A and B antigens on the recipient's red blood cells and for the presence of anti-A or anti-B antibodies in their serum. It also tests for the presence or absence of Rh(D) antigen on the red blood cell. The purpose of typing the recipient's blood is to avoid the transfusion of incompatible blood to the recipient. This may occur if the patient has antibodies to A or B or to A and B in their serum and they are transfused red blood cells that have the corresponding antigen on the red blood cells. Likewise, if a recipient lacks

the Rh(D) antigen, the transfusion of the Rh(D)+ blood would be incompatible. The risk of transfusing patients who have not had this typing done, or who have had it done incorrectly and the blood is incompatible, is a transfusion reaction. In this case, the transfusion would result in disastrous, rapid intravascular hemolysis. (239; **1615, Table 46–2**)

52. Crossmatching of blood is done to test for a serious transfusion reaction before the administration of the blood to the recipient. A crossmatch test is accomplished by incubating the recipient's plasma with the donor's red blood cells. There are three steps to the process, which in its entirety takes about 45 minutes to perform. The first phase is the immediate phase, in which the blood is tested for ABO compatibility at room temperature. It also tests for incompatibilities in the M, N, P, and Lewis groups. The second phase is the incubation phase, which tests for the presence of antibodies at 37°C. Albumin or a low ionic strength saline solution is added to the products of the first phase to cause the agglutination of weak or incomplete antibodies that are present. The last phase is the antiglobulin phase, in which antiglobulin is added to the products of the second phase. Incomplete antibodies in the Rh, Kell, Duffy, and Kidd systems will be detected by this step. In each phase, incompatible blood will result in agglutination during the crossmatch test. (239; **1616, Fig. 46–1**)

53. In emergency situations in which acute large volume blood loss requires the immediate replacement with blood products, there may be inadequate time to perform a type-and-cross or even to wait for type-specific blood. In these situations, O-negative packed red blood cells are administered because they lack the A, B, and Rh(D) antigens. This type of blood cannot be hemolyzed by anti-A or anti-B antibodies that may be present in the patient's blood and is therefore termed the *universal donor*. After the administration of 2 units of O-negative packed red blood cells subsequent blood transfusions may have to be continued with O-negative blood. It is center specific and dependent on how well the red blood cells are washed free of plasma and how they are preserved in the units of O-negative blood. The concern is that the transfusion of blood that is the patient's type may result in major intravascular hemolysis of donor red blood cells by increasing titers of transfused anti-A and anti-B antibodies. The risk of continued use of O-negative packed red blood cells under these conditions is minor hemolysis of donor red blood cells and hyperbilirubinemia. In most centers, however, subsequent transfusions with the patient's own blood type is possible and preferred. (239; **1618**)

54. Type-specific blood refers to blood that has only been typed for the A, B, and Rh antigens. Type-specific blood testing is merely the first phase, or the immediate phase, of the crossmatch. It requires only about 5 minutes to perform. The chance of a significant hemolytic reaction with the transfusion of type-specific blood to a patient is about 1 in 1000. Type-specific blood is most frequently transfused in emergent situations during which time does not allow for a formal crossmatch. (239; **1617–1618**)

55. A type and screen refers to a recipient's blood that, in addition to being typed for the A, B, and Rh antigens, has been screened for the most common antibodies. A type and screen is performed by incubating the recipient's plasma with commercially prepared type O red blood cells that contain all the antigens able to cause a hemolytic reaction. Agglutination would designate a positive antibody screen, and the recipient's serum is further tested for identification of the antibodies responsible for the agglutination. If, however, no agglutination results, the patient is said to be antibody screen negative. In a type and screen the patient's blood is not matched to a specific unit of donor blood. This allows for 1 unit of blood to be available for more than one patient. A type and screen is typically ordered for surgical procedures in

which the risk of transfusion is remote. If the patient subsequently requires transfusion, the immediate phase of a crossmatch blood test is performed to exclude blood type incompatibilities before its administration to the patient. The chance of a significant hemolytic reaction with the transfusion of typed and screened blood to a patient is 1 in 10,000. (239–240; **1617**)

56. Solutions used to preserve blood include phosphate, dextrose, and adenine. The addition of adenine to the preservative solution of blood allows red blood cells to resynthesize adenosine triphosphate. This allows red blood cells to continue to fuel their metabolic requirements and increases their survival time in storage. Phosphate acts as a buffer, and dextrose provides energy to the red blood cells. (240; **1618–1619**)

57. Blood can be stored for 21 to 35 days. The duration of the storage of blood is determined by the requirement that at least 70% of the red blood cells be viable for more than 24 hours after transfusion. (240; **1618–1619**)

58. Blood is stored at a temperature of 1°C to 6°C. This slows down the rate of glycolysis in red blood cells and increases their survival time in storage. (240; **1618–1619**)

59. In a given unit of whole blood the volume of blood is 450 mL, the volume of citrate-containing preservative is 65 mL, and the hematocrit is about 40%. The total volume of a unit of whole blood is about 515 mL. (240; **1618–1619**)

COMPONENT THERAPY

60. Components that can be derived from whole blood include packed red blood cells, platelet concentrates, fresh frozen plasma, cryoprecipitate, albumin, plasma protein fraction, leukocyte-poor blood, factor VIII, and antibody concentrates. The advantage of using components for blood therapy instead of whole blood is that a patient's specific deficiency can be directly corrected. It also allows for prolonged storage, the retention of unnecessary components for other patients who may need them, and the avoidance of transfusing unnecessary components that could potentially contain antigens or antibodies. (240; **1634, Fig. 46–11**)

61. In a given unit of packed red blood cells the total volume is about 300 mL and the hematocrit is about 70%. (240; **1634–1636, Table 50–8**)

62. The administration of packed red blood cells is indicated for the treatment of anemia that is not associated with acute hemorrhage or shock. The purpose of transfusing packed red blood cells is to augment the oxygen-carrying capacity of the blood. (240; **1634–1636**)

63. Hemoglobin concentrations will increase by approximately 1 g/dL with the administration of a single unit of packed red blood cells to a 70-kg adult. (240; **1634–1636**)

64. Packed red blood cells can be administered either alone or reconstituted in crystalloid or colloid. Reconstitution with 50 to 100 mL of saline facilitates the administration of packed red blood cells. Crystalloid solutions that are hypotonic should not be used to reconstitute packed red blood cells. Hypotonic solutions can result in red blood cell swelling and lysis. Examples of hypotonic solutions include glucose-containing solutions and Plasmanate. The reconstitution of packed red blood cells in solutions containing calcium may result in clotting. (240; **1634–1636**)

65. The potential for citrate toxicity that can result from the administration of whole blood is less likely to occur with the administration of packed red blood cells simply because there is less volume of citrate infused with each unit of packed red blood cells. (240; **1626–1627**)

66. The risk of allergic reactions is increased with the administration of whole blood than it is with the administration of packed red blood cells secondary to the greater volume of plasma that is infused with whole blood. (240; **1624–1625**)

67. The administration of platelets during surgery is usually indicated for platelet counts less than 50,000 cells/mm³. Both laboratory analysis and the clinical situation must be taken into consideration. For instance, in cases of surgical trauma or in cases of bleeding in the brain, eye, or airway the transfusion of platelets at a higher number may be warranted. (240; **1636–1637, Table 46–5**)

68. The platelet count will increase by 5,000 to 10,000 cells/mm³ after the administration of 1 unit of platelets to a 70-kg adult. (240; **1636–1637**)

69. Risks associated with the administration of platelets include the transmission of viral diseases and sensitization to the human leukocyte antigens present on the platelet cell membranes. Platelets may also cause bacterial infection in 1 in 12,000 transfusion. Although the risk is small, platelet-related sepsis should be considered in a patient who develops a fever after receiving platelet therapy. (240–241, Table 18–6; **1636–1637**)

70. Fresh frozen plasma is the plasma portion of 1 unit of donated blood. The plasma is frozen within 6 hours of collection. All plasma proteins are contained in fresh frozen plasma. Included are all the coagulation factors except platelets. This includes factors V and VIII, which decrease in concentration during the storage of packed red blood cells. (241; **1637**)

71. The administration of fresh frozen plasma is indicated during surgery when the prothrombin time and/or partial thromboplastin times are greater than one and one-half times normal and there is a clinical indication of the need to transfuse. Other indications include the need to reverse warfarin therapy or for the correction of known factor deficiencies. (241; **1637**)

72. Risks associated with the administration of fresh frozen plasma include sensitization to foreign proteins, the transmission of viral diseases, and allergic reactions. (241; **1637**)

73. Cryoprecipitate is the plasma fraction that precipitates when fresh frozen plasma is thawed. Cryoprecipitate contains high concentrations of factor VIII, von Willebrand factor, factor XIII, fibrinogen, and fibronectin. (241; **1637–1638**)

74. Cryoprecipitate is useful for the treatment of factor VIII deficiency as in hemophilia A, von Willebrand factor deficiency, and fibrinogen deficiency. (241; **1637–1638**)

COMPLICATIONS OF BLOOD THERAPY

75. Complications of blood therapy include transfusion reactions, metabolic abnormalities, citrate intoxication, the transmission of viral diseases, microaggregates, hypothermia, coagulation disorders, acute lung injury, and immunosuppression. (242, Table 18–6; **1619–1634**)

76. Viral diseases that may be transmitted with the administration of blood include infection with the human immunodeficiency virus (HIV), hepatitis virus, cytomegalovirus, and *Yersinia enterocolitica.* The implementation of routine screening for the hepatitis virus and HIV, as well as the use of volunteer instead of paid donors, has significantly decreased the risk of transmission of these viruses. For example, the risk of infectivity with hepatitis in 1980 was 1 in 10 transfusions, whereas now it is about 1 in 60,000 transfusions. The risk of the transfusion of the HIV may be 1 in 1

million with the implementation of new tests. Although the risk of transmission of these viruses is small, the potential for transmission still exists and must be discussed with the patient as part of informed consent for transfusion. It must also be a consideration of the anesthesiologist before the administration of blood products. (242, Table 18–6; **1636–1637, 1640–1641, Tables 46–9, 46–10**)

77. The types of transfusion reactions that may occur with blood therapy include febrile, allergic, and hemolytic transfusion reactions. (242; **1628–1631**)

78. Febrile transfusion reactions are thought to occur as a result of antibodies in the recipient's serum interacting with antigens from the donor's cells. Febrile transfusion reactions are the most frequently occurring transfusion reaction. A febrile transfusion reaction may manifest as fever, chills, headache, myalgias, nausea, and a nonproductive cough occurring after the initiation of the transfusion of blood. When a fever occurs after a transfusion has been started, a febrile transfusion reaction can be distinguished from a hemolytic transfusion reaction by evaluating the serum and the urine for hemolysis. (242; **1630–1631**)

79. Febrile transfusion reactions are treated by decreasing the rate of the infusion of blood and administering antipyretics. (242; **1630–1631**)

80. Allergic transfusion reactions are thought to occur as a result of the presence of incompatible plasma proteins in the donor blood. Allergic transfusion reactions manifest as urticaria, pruritus, and occasional facial swelling. (242; **1630–1631**)

81. The treatment of an allergic transfusion reaction is through the intravenous administration of antihistamines. There are more severe cases of allergic transfusion reactions that are anaphylactic without red blood cell destruction. Those cases are believed to be due to the transfusion of IgA to patients who are IgA deficient. In such situations the blood transfusion should be discontinued. The differentiation between allergic reactions and hemolytic reactions can be made by checking the urine and plasma for free hemoglobin. (242; **1630–1631**)

82. Hemolytic transfusion reactions are thought to occur as a result of the administration of an erroneous unit of blood to a patient. Transfused donor cells are attacked by the recipient's antibody and complement, resulting in intravascular hemolysis. As little as 10 mL of donor blood can result in a hemolytic transfusion reaction, which can be fatal. The severity of a transfusion reaction is proportional to the volume of transfused blood. (242; **1629–1630, Fig. 46–10**)

83. Clinical signs of a hemolytic transfusion reaction include fever, chills, chest pain, hypotension, nausea, flushing, dyspnea, and hemoglobinuria. All of these are masked by anesthesia except for hemoglobinuria and hypotension. (242; **1629–1630, Table 46–7**)

84. The diagnosis of a hemolytic transfusion reaction can be made by a direct antiglobulin test. Other laboratory analysis should be performed, including plasma and urine hemoglobin and bilirubin analysis. The plasma bilirubin concentration will peak at 3 to 6 hours after starting the blood transfusion. Hemoglobinuria or hemolysis in the presence of a transfusion and suspected hemolytic transfusion reaction should be treated as one until proven otherwise. (242; **1629–1630**)

85. Hemolytic transfusion reactions can result in renal failure and disseminated intravascular coagulation. (242; **1629–1630**)

86. The first step in the treatment of a hemolytic transfusion reaction is to

stop the transfusion. Subsequent treatment interventions are geared toward preventing renal failure by maintaining urine output. It is believed that renal failure occurs as a result of precipitates in the renal tubules. The urine output is recommended to be maintained at about 100 mL/hr through the administration of lactated Ringer's solution and mannitol and/or furosemide as necessary. The urine may also be alkalinized with bicarbonate. Laboratory analysis should be performed, including diagnostic tests of urine and plasma hemoglobin concentrations as well as baseline coagulation studies. Finally, unused blood should be sent to the blood bank along with a sample from the patient for a repeat type and crossmatch analysis. (242; **1629–1630, Table 46–8**)

87. Transfusion-related acute lung injury is acute, noncardiogenic pulmonary edema associated with dyspnea and arterial hypoxemia that occurs within 4 hours of a transfusion. Treatment for the patient is supportive. Most episodes of transfusion-related acute lung injury spontaneously recover. (242; **1633**)

88. A nonspecific immunosuppressive effect of homologous blood transfusions has been established. It appears that this effect is related to the volume of plasma transfused, because whole blood appears to have a greater immunosuppressive effect than packed red blood cells. This immunosuppressive effect may be beneficial to patients who are transplant recipients, but concern for patients with malignancy has been an issue of debate. It was believed that the transfusion of homologous blood resulted in an increased risk of the recurrence of tumor or decreased survival in cancer patients. Studies comparing cancer patients and their risk of tumor recurrence with the administration of homologous blood versus autologous blood, which has no immunosuppressive effects, have yielded no difference between these two groups. It may be that the underlying reason for the blood transfusion itself is the cause of the increased risk of tumor recurrence or the decreased survival in cancer patients receiving blood transfusions. Nevertheless, it may be prudent to administer packed red blood cells rather than whole blood to these patients. (242–243; **1633–1634, Tables 46–11, 46–12**)

89. Metabolic abnormalities that may accompany blood transfusions include increased levels of serum hydrogen and potassium, decreased 2,3-diphosphoglycerate levels, metabolic alkalosis, and hypocalcemia. (243; **1631–1632**)

90. The pH of a unit of blood is about 7.1 after collection and is 6.9 after being stored for 21 days. This is partly due to a high PCO_2 of the blood being stored, but it is also due to the addition of acidic preservatives. Although it would seem that the recipient's arterial pH might decrease with the administration of blood products, it actually increases. This probably occurs for two reasons. First, the elevated PCO_2 of blood can be quickly corrected on transfusion through the ventilation of the lungs of the recipient. More significantly, blood products contain the preservative citrate that metabolizes to bicarbonate on transfusion. The increased bicarbonate levels actually increase the arterial pH of the recipient, frequently resulting in a metabolic alkalosis with the transfusion of large volumes of blood. Therefore, any treatments of the recipient's arterial pH should be based on laboratory analysis and not be done empirically. (243; **1628, Fig. 46–9**)

91. Potassium concentrations in blood stored for 21 days may be as high as 20 to 30 mEq/L. Even after the transfusion of large volumes of blood, serum potassium levels rarely increase with the transfusion of blood. This is in part because the high concentration of potassium exists in a small volume and the total potassium content is small. Nevertheless, hyperkalemia resulting from blood transfusions is occasionally reported. In most cases it was associated with large volumes of blood rapidly infused, typically at rates greater than 120 mL/min. (243; **1627**)

92. Concentrations of 2,3-diphosphoglycerate in erythrocytes decrease with the prolonged storage of blood. Decreased concentrations of 2,3-diphosphoglycerate are associated with a shift of the oxyhemoglobin dissociation curve to the left and an increase in the affinity of hemoglobin for oxygen. This could result in a decrease in the delivery of oxygen to the tissues. This effect of a decrease in 2,3-diphosphoglycerate could be further compounded by the presence of acidosis and hypothermia. Although of concern for the effect on oxygen delivery to the tissues, there appears to be little clinical consequence of the decreased level of 2,3-diphosphoglycerate. (243; **1620–1621, Fig. 46–2**)

93. The infusion of citrate preservative during the transfusion of blood can result in a metabolic alkalosis and hypocalcemia. The metabolic alkalosis results from the metabolism of citrate in the liver to bicarbonate. Hypocalcemia can result from the binding of citrate to calcium in the intravascular space but is usually attenuated by the mobilization of calcium stores in bone. Hypocalcemia can be augmented by hypothermia, liver disease, or hyperventilation because these will all decrease the rate of metabolism of citrate to bicarbonate. Under these circumstances, the infusion of large volumes of citrate combined with the decreased metabolism of citrate can result in hypocalcemia. Indeed, serum ionized calcium has been found to begin to decrease with a rate of infusion of 1 unit of blood every 10 minutes. Hypocalcemia can result in hypotension, a narrow pulse pressure, and elevated central venous pressures. Findings on the electrocardiogram may include a shortened PR interval and a prolonged QT interval. Hypocalcemia should be treated based on laboratory analysis in combination with the clinical status of the patient. Hypocalcemia after blood transfusion rarely occurs to the extent that it needs to be treated. Patients who may need to be treated with calcium include patients in whom the rate of blood transfusion is greater than 50 mL/min, patients with hypothermia or liver disease, or neonates with immature liver function. (243, Fig. 18–3; **1626–1627, Fig. 46–8**)

94. The infusion of citrate preservative during the transfusion of blood can result in a metabolic alkalosis. The metabolic alkalosis results from the metabolism of citrate in the liver to bicarbonate. This metabolic alkalosis is offset somewhat by the acidic pH of the transfused unit of blood. Metabolic alkalosis can accompany the transfusion of large volumes of blood, however. (243; **1626–1628**).

95. Microaggregates in whole blood consist of platelets and leukocytes. These spontaneously form during the storage of whole blood. The concern is that microaggregates will enter the recipient's blood, accumulate in the lungs, cause vascular obstruction, and contribute to adult respiratory distress syndrome. Whole blood is usually transfused through standard 170-μm diameter filters, but these filters may not filter out microaggregates of smaller size. For this reason 10- to 40-μm micropore filters have been designed. The use of these filters also filters out leukocytes and may decrease the incidence of febrile complications associated with blood transfusions. There is as yet no evidence for the need to use micropore filters for the prevention of the accumulation of microaggregates in the lung. (243–244; **1628**)

96. Intraoperative hypothermia can lead to intraoperative cardiac irritability, especially in the presence of arterial pH abnormalities. Postoperative hypothermia can lead to shivering and increased myocardial oxygen demand. Because blood being stored for transfusion is stored at a temperature below 6°C, the administration of stored blood to a patient can result in decreases in the patient's body temperature. This risk can be minimized by administering the blood through warmers. It is prudent to confirm that the blood is being warmed to an appropriate temperature of 37°C to 38°C because red blood cells will hemolyze if overheated. (244; **1627–1628**)

97. Massive blood transfusions can result in two different coagulation disorders: a dilutional thrombocytopenia and a dilution of some of the coagulation factors necessary to clot blood. In either case, it may manifest clinically as continued frank bleeding without clotting in the surgical site. It may also manifest as hematuria, gingival bleeding, and spontaneous oozing from various puncture areas in both surgical and nonsurgical sites, such as sites of intravenous access. If this clinical situation is noted, the anesthesiologist must also consider disseminated intravascular coagulation and a hemolytic transfusion reaction as a potential source for the bleeding abnormalities. (244; **1621–1625**)

98. Dilutional thrombocytopenia refers to the dilution of platelets from its baseline concentration to a decreased concentration by virtue of the loss of platelets during bleeding without subsequent replacement, as with the administration of crystalloid, colloid, or non–platelet-containing blood products. This occurs even with the transfusion of blood because platelet activity has decreased to about 5% of normal after just 2 days of blood storage. The risk of a dilutional thrombocytopenia is the loss of the ability of blood to clot. When platelet counts decrease to less than 75,000/mm^3, a bleeding disorder is likely to occur. This level of platelets has been seen to occur after the transfusion of 10 to 15 units of non–platelet-containing blood products to previously healthy patients with previously normal platelet counts. Of note is that patients with chronically decreased platelet counts appear to tolerate thrombocytopenia better than patients with an acute decrease in platelets. The treatment of a dilutional thrombocytopenia by transfusing platelets should be instituted when a combination of clinical status and laboratory analysis confirms suspicions of a bleeding disorder secondary to insufficient platelets. (244; **1621–1622, Fig. 46–3, Table 46–5**)

99. Factors V and VIII are necessary for normal blood clotting. For normal blood clotting to occur there must be 5% to 20% of the normal amount of factor V and 30% of the normal amount of factor VIII. When these factors decrease to below these levels, abnormal blood clotting may result. This is manifest on laboratory analysis as a prolongation of the prothrombin time and/or partial thromboplastin time. The importance of factors V and VIII during the transfusion of blood arises from the decrease in concentration of these factors in stored blood. After 21 days of blood storage the concentration of factors V and VIII is 15% and 50% of their normal values, respectively. During times of massive transfusions a decrease in these factors may contribute to bleeding disorders. This is particularly true if the blood being transfused has little plasma volume or has been stored for long periods of time. The treatment of bleeding disorders secondary to a dilution of factors V and VIII is the administration of fresh frozen plasma, which contains all clotting factors. The decision to administer fresh frozen plasma is determined by laboratory analysis and the clinical status of the patient. The administration of fresh frozen plasma is also indicated when laboratory analysis reveals a prolongation of the prothrombin time and/or partial thromboplastin time greater than one and one-half times normal, when normal platelet counts exclude thrombocytopenia as a cause of the bleeding disorder, and when there is uncontrolled bleeding in the surgical field. (244; **1622**)

100. Disseminated intravascular coagulation (DIC) is a condition in which the patient's coagulation and fibrinolytic systems become uncontrollably activated. It causes the uncontrolled consumption of platelets and clotting factors and results in unclottable blood and increased levels of fibrin degradation products in the serum. DIC appears to be triggered by significant patient tissue damage and the corresponding release of toxins to the circulation. Laboratory analysis consistent with DIC includes a prolonged prothrombin

time, a prolonged partial thromboplastin time, a decrease in the serum concentration of fibrinogen, and an increase in the level of fibrin split products. The treatment of DIC is by treating the underlying cause. In addition, the administration of platelets and fresh frozen plasma may be instituted in an attempt to correct the bleeding disorder. (244; **1622–1623, Fig. 46–4**)

AUTOLOGOUS BLOOD

101. Autologous blood donation should be considered for procedures in which significant blood loss is likely to occur. An obvious advantage of the administration of autologous blood rather than homologous blood to patients requiring blood transfusions is the decreased risk of complications associated with homologous blood transfusions, including transfusion reactions and the transmission of blood-borne diseases. In addition, autologous blood donation reserves blood bank stores for other patients, thus decreasing the strain on blood bank resources. (244; **1645**)

102. The collection of pre-deposited blood for autologous blood transfusion must be done in a manner that will not decrease the patient's hemoglobin level to unacceptable levels preoperatively. Because of the risk of preoperative anemia, patients selected for autologous blood donation probably should not have significant cardiac or neurologic disease. A collection schedule that can be employed is the donation of 1 unit of blood every 4 days. This can be done for up to 3 units. The final unit of blood must be donated 72 hours or more before the surgical procedure to ensure that the patient's plasma volume has been restored. Anemia secondary to the donation of autologous blood remains a concern. Patients scheduled to pre-deposit autologous blood for blood transfusions are typically prescribed ferrous sulfate. Studies have shown that the administration of erythropoietin to these patients may be beneficial as well but requires parenteral or subcutaneous administration and is expensive. (244; **1647**)

103. A significant complication that can occur with autologous blood transfusions is the risk of clerical error leading to the erroneous blood being transfused to the patient. Blood should be checked just as meticulously whether autologous or homologous blood is being transfused. Other complications include sepsis from bacterial contamination or hypersensitivity to stabilizers. (244; **1648–1649**)

104. The intraoperative salvage of blood should be considered for surgical procedures that result in blood loss from a clean wound and will likely lead to the need to transfuse blood to the patient. Intraoperative blood salvaging is accomplished by semi-automated systems that collect, wash, and store red blood cells in a reservoir for their future administration. The hematocrit of blood prepared in this manner is 50% to 60%, and the pH is alkaline. Relative contraindications to the intraoperative salvage of blood include malignancy and the presence of blood-borne disease. Blood that has been contaminated with bowel contents should probably not be transfused. (244; **1653–1655, Fig. 47–3**)

105. Complications of intraoperative blood salvaging include a dilutional coagulopathy, the re-infusion of blood treated with anticoagulants, hemolysis, air embolism, fat embolism, sepsis, and disseminated intravascular coagulation. (244–245; **1654–1655**)

106. Hemodilution for autologous blood transfusion should be considered for patients who are expected to lose more than 2 units of blood intraoperatively and who have an adequate preoperative hematocrit. It is probably not appropriate for patients with anemia or severe cardiac or neurologic disease. The hemodilution technique involves the removal of venous or arterial blood from

the patient just before or after the induction of anesthesia and restoration of the plasma volume with crystalloid or colloid. The volume of blood that can be removed from the patient is dependent on the patient's preoperative hematocrit, estimated blood volume, and the lowest hematocrit acceptable for that patient. The blood is stored in the operating room at room temperature in a sterile container that contains anticoagulants, and it can be transfused to the patient when it is indicated or after major blood loss has ceased. The blood does not undergo any other biochemical transformations. There are several advantages to the hemodilution method of autologous blood transfusions. This method is less expensive than autologous blood donations and does not require the patient's cooperation or time that is required for the pre-depositing of autologous blood. In addition, the decreased viscosity and hematocrit of the blood result in a decrease in the concentration and number of red blood cells lost during the procedure. Finally, the blood that is transfused to the patient has platelet and coagulation factor activity that would have been lost in autologous blood that had been stored. (245; **1649–1653**)

Chapter 18

Cardiovascular Disease

CORONARY ARTERY DISEASE

1. What percent of adult patients undergoing surgery are estimated to have, or be at risk for, coronary artery disease?

2. What are some components of a routine preoperative cardiac evaluation? What are some more specialized methods of cardiac evaluation? What is the ultimate purpose of a preoperative cardiac evaluation?

3. What are some important aspects of the preoperative history taken from patients with coronary artery disease with respect to their cardiac status?

4. What are some co-existing noncardiac diseases that are frequently present in patients with coronary artery disease?

5. By what percent can a major coronary artery be stenosed in an asymptomatic patient?

6. What is the best indicator for a patient's cardiac reserve?

7. When is angina pectoris considered "stable"?

8. When is angina pectoris considered "unstable"? What is the clinical implication of unstable angina?

9. When dyspnea follows the onset of angina pectoris, what is it likely an indication of?

10. How does angina pectoris due to spasm of the coronary arteries differ from classic angina pectoris?

11. What is silent myocardial ischemia?

12. Approximately what percent of myocardial ischemic episodes are not associated with angina pectoris? Approximately what percent of myocardial infarctions are not associated with angina pectoris?

13. Is hypertension or tachycardia more likely to result in myocardial ischemia in the patient with coronary artery disease? What is the physiologic explanation for this?

14. What is the basis for the common recommendation that elective surgery be delayed until 6 months or more after a prior myocardial infarction?

15. What is the approximate incidence of perioperative myocardial infarction 6 months after a myocardial infarction? What is the approximate incidence of perioperative myocardial infarction in patients who have not had a prior myocardial infarction?

16. What time period after surgery do most perioperative myocardial infarctions occur?

17. What are some cardiac medications that patients with coronary artery disease are likely to be taking? What is the recommendation regarding the patient's preoperative medicine regimen with regard to their regular cardiac medicines?

18. What information can be gained from a preoperative electrocardiogram?

19. How might myocardial ischemia appear on the electrocardiogram?

20. Complete the following table:

ELECTROCARDIOGRAM LEAD	CORONARY ARTERY RESPONSIBLE FOR MYOCARDIAL ISCHEMIA	AREA OF MYOCARDIUM THAT MAY BE INVOLVED
II, III, aVF		
V_3–V_5		
I, aVL		

21. Name some determinants of myocardial oxygen requirements and delivery.

22. What are some intraoperative goals for the anesthesiologist in an attempt to decrease the risk of myocardial ischemia in patients at risk?

23. What are two potential benefits of administering premedication preoperatively to patients with coronary artery disease?

24. How should anesthesia be induced in patients at risk for myocardial ischemia?

25. Why is there an increased risk of myocardial ischemia during direct laryngoscopy? What are some things the anesthesiologist may do during this time to minimize this risk?

26. What are some methods of maintenance of anesthesia that may be employed by the anesthesiologist for the patient with coronary artery disease?

27. What is coronary artery steal syndrome? What is its clinical significance?

28. What is a concern regarding the administration of a regional anesthetic to patients with coronary artery disease?

29. What are some considerations an anesthesiologist should take when selecting a neuromuscular blocking drug for patients with coronary artery disease? What is unique about pancuronium in this situation?

30. How should neuromuscular blockade be reversed in patients with coronary artery disease?

31. What are some factors that influence the intensity of intraoperative monitoring by the anesthesiologist?

32. When might an intraoperative pulmonary artery catheter be useful? What information does it provide?

33. What is some information that may be provided by an intraoperative transesophageal echocardiogram?

34. What are some treatment options when myocardial ischemia is detected intraoperatively?

35. What is the problem with decreases in body temperature that may occur intraoperatively in patients with coronary artery disease?

36. Why is it important to control postoperative pain in the patient with coronary artery disease?

VALVULAR HEART DISEASE

37. What information can be gained from Doppler echocardiography in patients with valvular heart disease?

38. How should anesthetic drugs and neuromuscular blocking drugs be selected for the patient with valvular heart disease?

39. Why is it important to administer antibiotics to patients with known valvular heart disease?

40. What is mitral stenosis? How does it affect left atrial and pulmonary venous pressures? At what chronic left atrial pressure is an increase in pulmonary vascular resistance likely to be seen?

41. What is the most common cause of mitral stenosis? How does it present?

42. Why are patients with mitral stenosis at an increased risk of atrial fibrillation?

43. Why are patients with mitral stenosis at an increased risk of thrombus formation in the left atrium?

44. What are some anesthetic considerations for patients with mitral stenosis?

45. How can the maintenance of anesthesia be achieved in patients with mitral stenosis?

46. How might the adequacy of intravascular fluid replacement be monitored in patients with mitral stenosis? Why is this important?

47. Why might the mechanical support of ventilation be required postoperatively in patients with mitral stenosis?

48. What is mitral regurgitation? How is mitral regurgitation reflected on the recording of pulmonary artery occlusion pressure tracings?

49. What is the most common cause of mitral regurgitation? What other pathologic process is often present under these circumstances? What are some other causes of mitral regurgitation?

50. What are some anesthetic considerations for patients with mitral regurgitation?

51. How can the maintenance of anesthesia be achieved in patients with mitral regurgitation?

52. What is aortic stenosis? How is the severity of aortic stenosis estimated? What is considered to be hemodynamically significant aortic stenosis?

53. Name at least two causes of aortic stenosis. What is the natural course of aortic stenosis?

54. Why might patients with aortic stenosis have angina pectoris despite the absence of coronary artery disease?

55. How is aortic stenosis diagnosed on cardiac auscultation? Why is it important for the anesthesiologist to rule out aortic stenosis by auscultation preoperatively?

56. What are some anesthetic considerations for the patient with aortic stenosis?

57. What would result from tachycardia, bradycardia, or decreases in systemic vascular resistance in the patient with aortic stenosis?

58. How can the maintenance of anesthesia be achieved in patients with aortic stenosis?

59. How should the intravascular fluid status be managed intraoperatively in patients with aortic stenosis?

60. In patients with chronic aortic stenosis, why might the pulmonary artery occlusion pressure not be reflective of the left ventricular end-diastolic pressure?

61. How effective are external cardiac compressions in patients with aortic stenosis during cardiopulmonary arrest?

62. What is aortic regurgitation? What is the effect of chronic aortic regurgitation on the left ventricle?

63. What is acute aortic regurgitation most likely due to? What is chronic aortic regurgitation most likely due to?

64. Why might a patient with aortic regurgitation have angina pectoris despite the absence of coronary artery disease?

65. What are the goals for the anesthetic management of aortic regurgitation? The anesthetic management of aortic regurgitation resembles the anesthetic management for which other valvular disease?

66. What is mitral valve prolapse? What percent of the adult population is estimated to have mitral valve prolapse?

67. What are some other conditions associated with mitral valve prolapse?

68. What symptoms do most patients with mitral valve prolapse have?

69. What are some potential complications of mitral valve prolapse?

70. What is the goal of the maintenance of anesthesia in patients with mitral valve prolapse? How should the intravascular fluid volume status be managed in patients with mitral valve prolapse?

71. What is the potential problem with regional anesthesia in patients with mitral valve prolapse?

CONGENITAL HEART DISEASE

72. What approximate percent of live births are associated with some form of congenital heart disease? What is the most common congenital heart defect?

73. Why do patients with congenital heart disease often receive antibiotics perioperatively?

74. What are some congenital heart defects that result in a left-to-right shunt? What is the net physiologic result of these shunts?

75. How is an atrial septal defect diagnosed? When is surgical closure of an atrial septal defect indicated?

76. How is a ventricular septal defect diagnosed by cardiac auscultation?

77. What symptoms may accompany a small ventricular septal defect?

78. What is the physiologic result of failure of the ductus arteriosus to close after birth? What symptoms do most of these patients have?

79. What is heard on cardiac auscultation in a patient with patent ductus arteriosus?

80. What are the goals of the management of anesthesia in patients with a left-to-right shunt?

81. What is the risk of inadvertently introducing an air bubble into the patient's vascular system via the intravenous tubing used for intravascular fluids when the patient has a left-to-right shunt?

82. What are the physiologic hallmarks of a right-to-left shunt?

83. What is the most common congenital heart defect associated with a right-to-left shunt?

84. Describe the physiologic anomalies in a child with tetralogy of Fallot.

85. What is the usual Pa_{O_2} of a child with tetralogy of Fallot?

86. What happens when children with tetralogy of Fallot squat?

87. What is a "tet spell"? What triggers a "tet spell"? Why does it occur physiologically? How should a "tet spell" be treated?

88. What are some of the goals of the anesthetic management of patients with tetralogy of Fallot?

89. How does positive pressure ventilation of the lungs affect the child with tetralogy of Fallot?

90. How is the induction of anesthesia in a child with tetralogy of Fallot usually achieved?

91. How might anesthesia be maintained in a child with tetralogy of Fallot? Why might the concentration of inhaled nitrous oxide be limited to 50%? What is the potential problem with using a volatile anesthetic for the maintenance of anesthesia in these children?

92. Why might pancuronium be useful as a neuromuscular blocking drug in children with tetralogy of Fallot?

93. How should perioperative fluids be managed in the child with tetralogy of Fallot?

94. What can result from the infusion of an air bubble into the vein of a child with tetralogy of Fallot?

DISTURBANCES OF CARDIAC CONDUCTION AND RHYTHM

95. What are some tools available to the clinician for the diagnosis of disturbances in cardiac conduction and rhythm?

96. What are some types of conduction defects? Are conduction defects above or below the atrioventricular node usually permanent?

97. Is the placement of a prophylactic artificial cardiac pacemaker before surgery indicated in a patient with a bifascicular block? Why or why not? What is the theoretical concern?

98. How is third-degree atrioventricular heart block treated? What are the various methods by which this can be accomplished? How can third-degree heart block be treated pharmacologically?

99. What is sick sinus syndrome? How does it present? How is it treated?

100. What are ventricular premature beats? What are the hallmark features of a ventricular premature beat on an electrocardiogram?

101. When do premature ventricular beats warrant treatment? How are they treated under these circumstances?

102. What may be some causes of ventricular premature beats?

103. When is ventricular tachycardia diagnosed? How can it be treated?

104. What are preexcitation syndromes?

105. What is Wolff-Parkinson-White syndrome? What is the incidence of Wolff-Parkinson-White syndrome in the general population? How is it characterized on the electrocardiogram?

106. What is the most common cardiac dysrhythmia associated with Wolff-Parkinson-White syndrome? How can it be treated?

107. What is the goal of the anesthetic management of a patient with Wolff-Parkinson-White syndrome?

108. What are the various methods by which paroxysmal atrial tachycardia or fibrillation may be treated in the perioperative period in patients with Wolff-Parkinson-White syndrome?

109. What is prolonged QT interval syndrome? What adverse events are associated with a prolonged QT interval? How can they be treated pharmacologically?

110. What is a congenital cause of prolonged QT interval syndrome? How is a stellate ganglion block thought to work for this?

111. What is the goal of the anesthetic management of a patient with a chronically prolonged QT interval?

ARTIFICIAL CARDIAC PACEMAKERS

112. What should be included in the preoperative evaluation of the patient with an artificial cardiac pacemaker?

113. How should the pacemaker be evaluated by the anesthesiologist preoperatively?

114. What intraoperative monitoring is important in a patient with an artificial cardiac pacemaker?

115. What can occur if the ground plate for electrocautery is placed too near the pulse generator of the artificial cardiac pacemaker?

116. How is the selection of drugs or anesthetic techniques altered by the presence of an artificial cardiac pacemaker in a patient?

117. Why should an electric magnet be kept in the operating room intraoperatively for a patient with an artificial cardiac pacemaker undergoing anesthesia?

118. What are some causes of temporary pacemaker malfunction? When is placement of a pulmonary artery catheter in a patient with an artificial cardiac pacemaker a risk?

ESSENTIAL HYPERTENSION

119. What is the definition of essential hypertension? What is the benefit of the long-term treatment of patients with essential hypertension?

120. What should be included in the preoperative evaluation of a patient with essential hypertension?

121. How should blood pressure medications be managed in the perioperative period in the patient with essential hypertension?

122. What other medical problems are frequently seen in patients with essential hypertension? Approximately what percent of patients with peripheral vascular disease can be assumed to have 50% or greater stenosis of one or more coronary arteries even in the absence of symptoms?

123. How is the curve for the autoregulation of cerebral blood flow altered in patients with essential hypertension?

124. What is the value of treating essential hypertension in patients before an elective procedure?

125. How do patients with essential hypertension frequently respond physiologically to the induction of anesthesia with intravenous medications? Why is this thought to occur?

126. How do patients with essential hypertension frequently respond physiologically to direct laryngoscopy? What are these patients at risk of during this time? How can this response be attenuated?

127. What is the goal for the anesthetic management of patients with essential hypertension?

128. How can the maintenance of anesthesia in patients with essential hypertension be achieved?

129. How might intraoperative hypotension be managed by the anesthesiologist in patients with essential hypertension?

130. What is the potential problem with regional anesthesia in patients with essential hypertension?

131. How frequently does hypertension occur in the early postoperative period in patients with essential hypertension? How can it be managed?

CONGESTIVE HEART FAILURE

132. What is the correlation between congestive heart failure and postoperative morbidity? What does this suggest for the patient scheduled for elective surgery in the presence of congestive heart failure?

133. What is the goal of the anesthetic management of patients with congestive heart failure who are undergoing urgent or emergent surgery? What medicines may be useful to achieve this?

134. Why might ketamine be useful in patients with congestive heart failure?

135. How does positive pressure ventilation of the lungs affect patients in congestive heart failure?

136. For major surgery in patients with congestive heart failure, what monitoring may be necessary?

137. For peripheral surgery in patients with congestive heart failure, can regional anesthesia be selected as an anesthetic option?

HYPERTROPHIC CARDIOMYOPATHY

138. What is another name for hypertrophic cardiomyopathy? What pathophysiology defines hypertrophic cardiomyopathy? What is the stroke volume in patients with hypertrophic cardiomyopathy?

139. What are some symptoms associated with hypertrophic cardiomyopathy?

140. What is the goal of the anesthetic management of patients with hypertrophic cardiomyopathy?

141. How can intraoperative hypotension be treated in patients with hypertrophic cardiomyopathy?

142. How can intraoperative hypertension be treated in patients with hypertrophic cardiomyopathy?

143. What is the problem with using beta agonists for the treatment of hypotension or using nitrates for the treatment of hypertension in patients with hypertrophic cardiomyopathy?

COR PULMONALE

144. What is cor pulmonale?

145. What are some signs and symptoms associated with cor pulmonale?

146. What are some treatment methods for cor pulmonale?

147. What is the recommendation for the patient with cor pulmonale who is scheduled for an elective surgical procedure?

148. What is the goal of the anesthetic management of patients with cor pulmonale? How can this be achieved?

149. What is the advantage of monitoring right atrial pressure during surgery in patients with cor pulmonale?

CARDIAC TAMPONADE

150. What is cardiac tamponade?

151. Name some manifestations of cardiac tamponade.

152. What is the treatment for cardiac tamponade? What are some temporizing measures for patients with cardiac tamponade awaiting definitive treatment?

153. What is the goal of the anesthetic management of cardiac tamponade?

154. What effect can the induction of anesthesia and positive pressure ventilation of the lungs have on patients with cardiac tamponade?

155. What is the recommendation for anesthesia in patients with cardiac tamponade?

156. What pharmacologic agents may be useful in patients with cardiac tamponade?

ANEURYSMS OF THE AORTA

157. What is the most frequent cause of aortic aneurysms? Do most aortic aneurysms involve the thoracic or abdominal aorta?

158. What is a dissecting aneurysm?

159. When is elective resection of an abdominal aortic aneurysm recommended?

160. What are some medical problems frequently associated with aortic aneurysms?

161. What is the goal of the anesthetic management of patients undergoing resection of an abdominal aortic aneurysm? What monitoring is warranted in these procedures?

162. When are patients with coronary artery disease especially at risk of myocardial ischemia during surgery for resection of an aortic aneurysm? How is this manifest on a pulmonary artery catheter? How can it be treated?

163. How should intraoperative fluids be managed during surgery for resection of an aortic aneurysm?

164. Why does hypotension frequently accompany unclamping of the abdominal aorta during surgery for the resection of an aortic aneurysm? What are some methods for minimizing the hypotension?

165. What are some concerns regarding renal function in patients undergoing aortic aneurysm repair?

166. What are some concerns regarding spinal cord function in patients undergoing aortic aneurysm repair?

CARDIOPULMONARY BYPASS

167. How is blood drained from the venae cavae during cardiopulmonary bypass?

168. What are two different types of pumps that are used to return blood to the arterial system during cardiopulmonary bypass? Which produces nonpulsatile flow? Which results in less trauma to blood?

169. How is blood kept from entering the heart from the superior and inferior venae cavae during cardiopulmonary bypass?

170. Under what conditions does the aorta need to be cross-clamped distal to the aortic valve and proximal to the inflow cannula during cardiopulmonary bypass?

171. How can venous drainage from the inferior and superior venae cavae during cardiopulmonary bypass be facilitated?

172. What is the required cardiac index delivered by the roller pump on the cardiopulmonary bypass machine dependent on? What approximate cardiac index is usually sufficient?

173. What is the advantage of low flows when a roller pump is used to deliver blood to the aorta during cardiopulmonary bypass?

174. What PaO_2 is generally maintained in blood that is returning to the arterial system during cardiopulmonary bypass?

175. What are two different types of oxygenators that are used to oxygenate blood that is returning to the arterial system during cardiopulmonary bypass?

176. What is the advantage of a bubble oxygenator? What is the disadvantage of a bubble oxygenator?

177. What is the advantage of a membrane oxygenator? What is the disadvantage of a membrane oxygenator?

178. How can the patient's body be heated or cooled by the cardiopulmonary bypass machine?

179. How is blood loss from the field recirculated to the patient during cardiopulmonary bypass?

180. What is a problem with the cardiotomy suction used during cardiopulmonary bypass?

181. Why might the left ventricle need a vent during cardiopulmonary bypass? How might this be achieved?

182. How are systemic emboli from cellular debris prevented from occurring during cardiopulmonary bypass?

183. What does priming of the cardiopulmonary bypass system refer to? What is the cardiopulmonary bypass system primed with?

184. What is the patient's hematocrit maintained at during cardiopulmonary bypass? Why is it important to hemodilute patient's blood during cardiopulmonary bypass?

185. Why is it important to remove all air from the cardiopulmonary bypass system during cardiopulmonary bypass?

186. Why is heparin-induced anticoagulation of the patient's blood necessary during cardiopulmonary bypass? What dose of heparin is usually administered? How is the adequacy of anticoagulation confirmed?

187. What are some explanations for the low mean arterial pressure often seen after the institution of cardiopulmonary bypass? What blood pressure is typically considered acceptable?

188. Why does blood pressure slowly rise spontaneously after some time on cardiopulmonary bypass?

189. What are the dangers of hypertension while on cardiopulmonary bypass? How can hypertension under these circumstances be treated?

190. What are some methods by which the adequacy of tissue perfusion during cardiopulmonary bypass can be evaluated?

191. Why is diuresis induced during cardiopulmonary bypass?

192. What may be the cause of an increasing central venous pressure with or without facial edema while on cardiopulmonary bypass? How can this be confirmed?

193. What may be the cause of increasing abdominal distention while on cardiopulmonary bypass?

194. What are some complications that require immediate discontinuation of cardiopulmonary bypass and the resumption of the patient's own cardiac output?

195. How should ventilation of the lungs be managed during cardiopulmonary bypass?

196. What is the goal of myocardial preservation during cardiopulmonary bypass? What are some methods by which this can be achieved?

197. What is the oxygen consumption of a normally contracting heart at 30°C? What is the oxygen consumption of a fibrillating heart at 22°C? What is the oxygen consumption of an electromechanically quiet heart at 22°C?

198. How is the effectiveness of cold cardioplegia of the heart measured?

199. What are two potential negative effects of intramyocardial hyperkalemia due to cold cardioplegia after cardiopulmonary bypass? How can it be treated?

200. What are two potential sources for systemic hyperkalemia during cardiopulmonary bypass? How can the hyperkalemia be treated if it were to persist at the conclusion of cardiopulmonary bypass?

201. Why might supplemental intravenous anesthetics be administered during cardiopulmonary bypass?

202. Why might supplemental neuromuscular blocking drugs be administered during cardiopulmonary bypass?

203. Is supplemental anesthesia routinely required during rewarming after the conclusion of cardiopulmonary bypass?

204. What conditions in the patient must be present for cardiopulmonary bypass to be discontinued?

205. When are the aortic and vena cava cannulae removed after cardiopulmonary bypass?

206. What are some potential problems associated with persistent hypothermia after cardiopulmonary bypass?

207. What special precautions must be taken before discontinuing cardiopulmonary bypass in patients who have had the left side of the heart opened, as during valve replacement surgery? What is the potential risk?

208. For each of the following situations, please complete the diagnosis and appropriate therapy:

BLOOD PRESSURE	ATRIAL PRESSURE	CARDIAC OUTPUT	DIAGNOSIS	THERAPY
Decreased	Increased	Decreased	?	?
Decreased	Decreased	Decreased	?	?
Decreased	Decreased	Increased	?	?
Increased	Increased	Decreased	?	?
Increased	Decreased	Increased	?	?

209. Why might a patient have posterior papillary muscle dysfunction after cardiopulmonary bypass? How would this be manifest on the pulmonary artery occlusion pressure tracing?

210. What is a mechanical alternative to the pharmacologic support of cardiac output in

patients with a poor cardiac output after cardiopulmonary bypass? How does it work? What physiologic alterations may interfere with its efficacy?

211. When is protamine administered after cardiopulmonary bypass? Why?

212. What are some possible side effects of protamine administration?

213. What does the perfusionist do with blood and fluid that remains in the cardiopulmonary bypass circuit after cardiopulmonary bypass?

214. Why might there be a gradient between central aortic and radial artery blood pressures in the early period after cardiopulmonary bypass? How long can this effect persist?

Answers*

CORONARY ARTERY DISEASE

1. It is estimated that 40% of adult patients undergoing surgery have, or are at risk for, coronary artery disease. (248; **941**)

2. Components of a routine preoperative cardiac evaluation include the history and physical examination, evaluation of the patient's electrocardiogram, and reviewing or ordering more specialized procedures. Specialized methods of cardiac evaluation include a Holter monitor, exercise electrocardiogram, echocardiogram, radioisotope imaging, cardiac catheterization, and angiography. The ultimate purpose of a preoperative cardiac evaluation is to assess the patient's risk of an adverse cardiac event perioperatively and to determine whether the patient is in optimal medical condition for surgery. (248; **843–846, 941–942, 1753, Figs. 23–6, 25–13, Tables 25–27, 25–28, 25–29, 49–2, 49–3, 49–4**)

3. Important aspects of the preoperative history taken from patients with coronary artery disease with respect to their cardiac status include their exercise tolerance, characteristics of their angina, and the presence of a previous myocardial infarction. It is also important to learn what cardiac medicines the patient may be taking and what the potential interactions of these are with anesthetics that may be administered for surgery. (248; **829–830, 1756–1757, Tables 49–3, 49–4, 49–5**)

4. Noncardiac diseases that are frequently present in patients with coronary artery disease include peripheral vascular disease, chronic obstructive pulmonary disease, renal dysfunction, chronic hypertension, and diabetes mellitus. (248; **941–942, 1756, Table 49–6**)

5. A major coronary artery can be stenosed by as much as 50% to 70% in an asymptomatic patient. (248)

6. The best indicator for a patient's cardiac reserve is by evaluation of their exercise tolerance. A limited exercise tolerance in the absence of significant pulmonary disease gives evidence of a decrease in a patient's cardiac reserve. Alternatively, the cardiac reserve of a patient who is able to climb up two to three flights of stairs without stopping is probably adequate. (248; **941–942, Table 25–30**)

7. Angina pectoris is considered "stable" when there has been no change in the patient's anginal symptoms for at least 60 days. Factors related to the angina

---

*Numbers in parentheses: lightface numbers refer to pages, figures, or tables in Stoelting RK, Miller RD: Basics of Anesthesia, 4th ed. Philadelphia, Churchill Livingstone, 2000; **boldface numbers** refer to pages, figures, or tables in Miller RD: Anesthesia, 5th ed. Philadelphia, Churchill Livingstone, 2000.

that should be evaluated include the precipitating factors, frequency, and duration. (248; **1759–1760**)

8. Angina pectoris is considered "unstable" when there has been a change in the patient's anginal symptoms. Changes that should be evaluated include the degree of activity a patient can do before the onset of angina and the duration of each anginal episode. Another symptom of unstable angina is chest pain occurring at rest. The clinical implication of unstable angina is that the patient may be at risk of an impending myocardial infarction. (248; **1759–1760**)

9. Dyspnea after the onset of angina pectoris is likely an indication of acute left ventricular dysfunction due to myocardial ischemia and acute, transient cardiac failure. (248; **1759–1760**)

10. Angina pectoris due to spasm of the coronary arteries differs from classic angina pectoris in that the pain may occur at rest but may not occur during periods of exertion. Angina of this type is associated with ST segment changes on the electrocardiogram. This type of angina is referred to as Prinzmetal's or variant angina. (248; **1759–1760**)

11. Silent myocardial ischemia is myocardial ischemia that occurs in the absence of angina. This type of angina is more common in patients with diabetes mellitus and carries the same prognosis as myocardial ischemia associated with angina. (248–249; **1759–1760**)

12. Approximately 70% of myocardial ischemic episodes are not associated with angina pectoris, and myocardial infarctions are not associated with angina pectoris approximately 15% of the time. (249; **941, 1759–1760**)

13. Tachycardia is more likely than hypertension to result in myocardial ischemia in the patient with coronary artery disease secondary to the greater strain on the heart associated with tachycardia. Tachycardia results in an increased myocardial oxygen requirement in the presence of decreased myocardial perfusion time. Myocardial perfusion on the left side of the heart, and thus myocardial oxygen supply, occurs mostly during diastole. Hypertension, on the other hand, may lead to an increased myocardial oxygen requirement, but it may also lead to increased myocardial perfusion. (249; **1762, Table 49–12**)

14. The basis for the common recommendation that elective surgery be delayed until 6 months after a prior myocardial infarction is based on numerous epidemiologic studies. These studies have shown that there is a 5% to 86% reinfarction rate in the perioperative period if previous myocardial infarction preceded the surgical procedure by less than 6 months. This rate of myocardial infarction is 1.5 to 10 times higher than if more than 6 months separated the previous myocardial infarction and the surgical procedure. (249; **942–946, Table 25–22**)

15. The approximate incidence of perioperative myocardial infarction 6 months or more after a myocardial infarction is 5% to 6%, whereas the approximate incidence of perioperative myocardial infarction in patients who have not had a prior myocardial infarction is 0.13%. (249, Table 19–1; **942–946, Table 25–22**)

16. Most perioperative myocardial infarctions occur in the first 48 to 72 hours postoperatively. (249; **945, Table 25–23**)

17. Cardiac medications that patients with coronary artery disease are likely to be taking include beta antagonists, nitrates, calcium channel blockers, antihypertensives, and diuretics. The recommendation is that patients continue taking their regular cardiac medicines throughout the perioperative period. (249; **941, 1756–1757, Table 49–7**)

18. Preoperative electrocardiograms may provide evidence of myocardial ischemia, prior myocardial infarction, cardiac hypertrophy, abnormal cardiac rhythm or conduction disturbances, and electrolyte abnormalities. (249; **843–846, 946, Tables 23–11, 23–12**)

19. Myocardial ischemia may appear as ST segment changes or T wave changes on an electrocardiogram. (249; **843–846, 946, 1763, 1858–1859**)

20. (250, Table 19–2; **620, 1761–1763, Fig. 49–1**)

ELECTROCARDIOGRAM LEAD	CORONARY ARTERY RESPONSIBLE FOR MYOCARDIAL ISCHEMIA	AREA OF MYOCARDIUM THAT MAY BE INVOLVED
II, III, aVF	Right coronary artery	Right atrium, atrioventricular node, right ventricle
V_3–V_5	Left anterior descending coronary artery	Anterolateral portion of left ventricle
I, aVL	Circumflex coronary artery	Lateral aspects of the left ventricle

21. Determinants of myocardial oxygen requirements and delivery are related to factors that affect myocardial oxygen supply or myocardial oxygen demand. Myocardial oxygen supply is decreased by tachycardia, hypotension, increased preload, hypocapnia, coronary artery spasm, anemia, and hypoxemia. Myocardial oxygen demand is increased by tachycardia, increased wall tension, and increased myocardial contractility. A goal of the anesthetic management of patients with coronary artery disease is maintenance of the balance between myocardial oxygen supply and demand to minimize the risk of myocardial ischemia. (250; **1762, 1857–1858, Fig. 51–3, Table 49–12**)

22. In an attempt to decrease the risk of a perioperative myocardial infarction in patients at risk the anesthesiologist should attempt to maintain stable patient hemodynamics. In general, the desired hemodynamics to minimize the risk of intraoperative ischemia include slower heart rates, lower filling pressures, and normal systolic blood pressures. A common recommendation for patients at risk of myocardial ischemia is that heart rate and blood pressure be maintained within 20% of awake values intraoperatively. Even so, approximately 50% of all new perioperative myocardial ischemic episodes are not preceded by or associated with changes in heart rate or blood pressure. Nevertheless, the anesthesiologist may choose to closely monitor the patient's more limited hemodynamic status using invasive monitors to achieve these goals. He or she should also be prepared to intervene quickly with pharmacologic interventions should they become necessary. (250; **1762–1765, 1858–1860**)

23. Two benefits of administering premedication preoperatively to patients with coronary artery disease are the decrease in the secretion of potentially harmful catecholamines and the potential to prevent the increase in myocardial oxygen requirements that may occur with tachycardia and hypertension related to anxiety. (250; **1762–1763**)

24. The induction of anesthesia in patients at risk for myocardial ischemia is typically achieved with the administration of etomidate or the judicious administration of thiopental or propofol to minimize hemodynamic alterations associated with these drugs. Ketamine is not an appropriate choice for the

induction of anesthesia in patients with coronary artery disease because of its potential to cause tachycardia and hypertension, which lead to increases in myocardial oxygen requirements. (251; **242–243, 1764**)

25. Direct laryngoscopy is associated with an increased risk of myocardial ischemia because it often produces intense sympathetic nervous system stimulation leading to tachycardia and hypertension. To minimize this risk there must be adequate levels of anesthesia to suppress sympathetic nervous system stimulation. Volatile anesthetics, intravenous anesthetics other than ketamine, opioids, and lidocaine may all be used to blunt the response to direct laryngoscopy. Alternatively, beta antagonists may be administered just before direct laryngoscopy to attenuate the increase in heart rate and blood pressure that can occur. (251; **1444–1445**)

26. The maintenance of anesthesia for the patient with coronary artery disease may be achieved through the administration of volatile anesthetics and opioids in conjunction with nitrous oxide. (251; **1780–1784**)

27. Coronary artery steal syndrome is a theoretical risk in which administration of a coronary artery vasodilator to a patient with coronary artery disease could result in diversion of blood flow from the ischemic areas, in which stenotic coronary arteries are maximally dilated, to areas in which the coronary arteries are patent and able to vasodilate. Isoflurane, of all the volatile anesthetics, is the most potent coronary vasodilator. It is therefore believed that isoflurane is the volatile anesthetic that is most likely to result in this syndrome. Clinically, however, the administration of isoflurane to patients with coronary artery disease has not been shown to increase the risk of myocardial ischemia through the coronary artery steal syndrome. (251; **107–108, 642–643, 1764, 1782**)

28. The administration of a regional anesthetic to patients with coronary artery disease can result in hypotension, which may in turn lead to decreased blood flow through pressure-dependent stenosed coronary arteries. For this reason it is important for the anesthesiologist to be prepared to treat decreases in blood pressure in excess of 20% of the patient's resting blood pressure. An advantage of regional anesthesia for patients with coronary artery disease is that the anesthesiologist may continue to monitor the patient for symptoms of angina and treat them accordingly. (252; **1785**)

29. Considerations in the selection of a neuromuscular blocking drug for patients with coronary artery disease should take into account the effects of the neuromuscular blocking drug on the cardiovascular system. For example, a neuromuscular blocking drug that may lower blood pressure through the release of histamine should be administered slowly to minimize those effects. Pancuronium causes mild increases in heart rate and blood pressure that may or may not be beneficial, depending on the status of the patient. (252; **441–443, 1784–1785**)

30. Neuromuscular blockade may be reversed in patients with coronary artery disease in the usual manner with an anticholinesterase-anticholinergic drug combination. Glycopyrrolate has less of a chronotropic effect on the heart, but either glycopyrrolate or atropine is acceptable for the reversal of neuromuscular blockade. (252; **469**)

31. The intensity of intraoperative monitoring the anesthesiologist chooses to implement for a surgical procedure in a patient with coronary artery disease is influenced by the type of procedure the patient is undergoing, the severity of the patient's disease, and a cost-benefit analysis of each type of potential monitoring. (252; **1777–1778**)

32. A pulmonary artery catheter may be useful in patients with poor left ventricu-

lar function, valvular heart disease, a recent myocardial infarction, or pulmonary vascular disease, in situations of massive trauma, or in major vascular surgery. Information provided by a pulmonary artery catheter includes more accurate assessment of cardiac filling pressures than a central venous monitor in the presence of pulmonary vascular disease, left-sided heart dysfunction, or potential left-sided heart dysfunction due to myocardial ischemia. The pulmonary artery catheter also measures cardiac output and calculates systemic vascular resistance. (252–253; **1156–1158**)

33. Information provided by a transesophageal echocardiogram includes early detection of myocardial ischemia through the presence of new onset regional wall motion abnormalities, an assessment of the intravascular fluid volume status of the patient, an estimation of the cardiac output, an estimation of left ventricular afterload, and an evaluation of the cardiac valves. (252–253; **1216–1219**)

34. The detection of intraoperative myocardial ischemia should promptly lead to the treatment of any hemodynamic alterations in an attempt to increase myocardial oxygen supply while decreasing myocardial oxygen demand. Tachycardia may be treated with a beta-adrenergic antagonist. These drugs decrease the demand of the myocardium for oxygen through its effects of decreases in heart rate and myocardial contractility. Its administration should be judicious in patients with left ventricular dysfunction. Hypertension may be treated with a nitrate. Nitroglycerin may also be used in a situation in which there are ischemic changes on the electrocardiogram but blood pressure remains normal to high. Intravenous nitroglycerin administration may lead to reflex tachycardia. Hypotension may be treated with a sympathomimetic and intravascular fluids. (252–253; **1763**)

35. Decreases in body temperature that may occur intraoperatively in patients with coronary artery disease can result in shivering on awakening. Shivering can significantly increase myocardial and systemic oxygen requirements and can be especially detrimental to patients with coronary artery disease because it is often accompanied by tachycardia. (253; **1376–1378**)

36. It is important to control postoperative pain in the patient with coronary artery disease because pain can increase myocardial oxygen requirements. Pain is often accompanied by tachycardia and hypertension as a result of sympathetic nervous system discharge. These can be detrimental to the patient with coronary artery disease. (253; **1798–1799**)

VALVULAR HEART DISEASE

37. Information that can be gained from Doppler echocardiography in patients with valvular heart disease includes the significance of cardiac murmurs, hemodynamic abnormalities, transvalvular pressure gradients, the orifice area of the cardiac valve, and the evaluation of prosthetic valve function. (253; **1208–1210, 1221–1224**)

38. Anesthetic drugs and neuromuscular blocking drugs should be selected for the patient with valvular heart disease based on the effects they may have on cardiac rhythm, heart rate, blood pressure, systemic vascular resistance, and pulmonary vascular resistance. The objective is to choose anesthetic drugs and neuromuscular blocking drugs that will not compromise cardiac output with their administration. (253; **955–956, 1766**)

39. Antibiotics are administered to patients with known valvular heart disease prophylactically to protect the patient from infective endocarditis. Prophylaxis is recommended to minimize the risk of infection from a bacteremic event, such as surgical or dental procedures. Bacteremia does not seem to occur

with orotracheal intubation, but it may occur with nasotracheal intubation independent of any surgical event. There are recommended prophylaxis regimens that vary depending on the site of surgery, mechanism of administration, and any history of allergies to antibiotics the patient may have. (253; **957–958, Tables 25–34, 25–35**)

40. Mitral stenosis is a mechanical obstruction to left ventricular diastolic filling secondary to a decrease in the orifice of the mitral valve. Measurement of the mitral valve area provides for the best indication of the severity of the disease. Mitral stenosis is classified as severe when the mitral valve area is less than 1 cm². Left atrial and pulmonary venous pressures are increased in patients with mitral stenosis. An increase in pulmonary vascular resistance is likely to be seen when the left atrial pressure is higher than 25 mm Hg on a chronic basis. (253; **1767–1768, Fig. 49–3**)

41. The most common etiology for mitral stenosis is rheumatic heart disease. The mitral valve leaflets often fuse, scar, and fibrose during the healing process of acute rheumatic carditis. Mitral stenosis presents after a prolonged course of development, usually after about 20 years after the initial episode of rheumatic fever. Often the disease presents with atrial fibrillation or when there is an increased demand for cardiac output, as may occur during pregnancy or exercise. Patients with mitral stenosis may have recurrent episodes of pulmonary edema, dyspnea, paroxysmal nocturnal dyspnea, chest pains, palpitations, and fatigue. (253; **1767**)

42. Patients with mitral stenosis are at an increased risk of atrial fibrillation secondary to the distention of the left atrium. (253; **1767**)

43. Patients with mitral stenosis are at an increased risk of thrombus formation in the left atrium because of the stasis of blood in that heart chamber. Thrombi in the left atrium may be ejected from the heart as systemic emboli. (253)

44. Considerations for the anesthetic management of patients with mitral stenosis include maintenance of a normal sinus rhythm and heart rate, maintenance of a normal intravascular fluid volume, and the avoidance of increases in pulmonary vascular resistance. Patients with mitral stenosis have a greater reliance on atrial contraction for left ventricular filling. Alterations from sinus rhythm should be promptly treated chemically or with cardioversion. Tachycardia and bradycardia may both result in decreases in left ventricular filling. The intravascular fluid volume should be maintained at near-normal or maximally tolerated levels, while avoiding pulmonary edema. Increases in pulmonary vascular resistance and pulmonary hypertension may place the patient at an increased risk for pulmonary artery rupture with placement of a pulmonary artery catheter and repeated wedge pressure measurements. Care should be taken to avoid overtransfusion or the head-down position in these patients. Arterial hypoxemia or hypercarbia may exacerbate pulmonary hypertension and precipitate right ventricular failure and should be avoided. Central venous pressure monitoring may be useful to detect changes in the right ventricular pressure. (254; **1767–1768**)

45. The maintenance of anesthesia can be achieved in patients with mitral stenosis through the administration of volatile anesthetics, nitrous oxide, and opioids. Of greater importance is the management of the cardiovascular effects of these drugs to achieve the goal of the anesthetic management of patients with mitral stenosis and treatment of the unfavorable effects of these drugs accordingly. For example, pancuronium may not be an appropriate choice for neuromuscular blockade in patients with mitral stenosis secondary to the increased speed of transmission of cardiac impulses through the atrioventricular node that result from this drug. This increased speed of transmission

may be detrimental to patients prone to atrial fibrillation. Likewise, the administration of ketamine to these patients should be avoided. The increase in pulmonary vascular resistance that is associated with nitrous oxide is not usually sufficient enough to detract from its utility in patients with mitral stenosis. Drugs that are being administered for heart rate control should be continued throughout the perioperative period. (254; **1767–1768**)

46. Intraoperative monitoring of the right atrial pressure may be useful in assessing the adequacy of intravascular fluid replacement in patients with mitral stenosis. The monitoring of intraoperative fluid therapy in these patients is important because they are prone to intravascular fluid overload, leading to right heart failure and pulmonary edema. (254; **1767–1768**)

47. The mechanical support of ventilation may be required postoperatively in patients with mitral stenosis because they are susceptible to developing pulmonary edema and right-sided heart failure. This may be especially true in patients with mitral stenosis after major thoracic or abdominal surgery. (254; **1767–1768**)

48. Mitral regurgitation occurs as a result of an incompetent mitral valve. Physiologically, there is left atrial overload and a decreased left ventricular stroke volume in these patients. When mitral regurgitation develops over time, left ventricular dilation and left ventricular hypertrophy develop to maintain the left ventricular stroke volume. With progression of the disease, however, congestive heart failure can occur. Patients with chronic mitral regurgitation are frequently in atrial fibrillation. Acute mitral regurgitation results in acute increases in left atrial pressure and pulmonary artery pressures and can present as pulmonary congestion, pulmonary hypertension, and right-sided heart failure. Measurement of the regurgitant fraction provides for an estimate of the severity of the disease. For instance, a regurgitant fraction of 0.6 or greater is typically associated with congestive heart failure. A recording of pulmonary artery occlusion pressure tracings in a patient with mitral regurgitation would show prominent v waves that are characteristic of mitral regurgitation. (254, Fig. 19–2; **1768, Fig. 49–4**)

49. The most common etiology of mitral regurgitation is rheumatic heart disease. When mitral regurgitation is secondary to rheumatic heart disease it is often chronic, is accompanied by mitral stenosis, and progresses over years. The most common cause of isolated mitral regurgitation is papillary muscle dysfunction, which is usually acute in onset with a corresponding acute onset of symptoms. Papillary muscle dysfunction usually occurs after a myocardial infarction or after rupture of the chordae tendineae secondary to infective endocarditis. (254; **1768**)

50. Considerations for the anesthetic management of patients with mitral regurgitation include the avoidance of sudden decreases in heart rate, the avoidance of sudden increases in systemic vascular resistance, and minimizing drug-induced myocardial depression, because each of these will increase regurgitant flow. The size of the v wave on the pulmonary artery catheter tracing may be monitored as a reflection of mitral regurgitant flow. (254; **1768**)

51. The maintenance of anesthesia in patients with mitral regurgitation can be achieved through the administration of a volatile anesthetic, nitrous oxide, and an opioid. Of greater importance is the management of the cardiovascular effects of these drugs to achieve the goal of the anesthetic management of patients with mitral regurgitation and treatment of the unfavorable effects of these drugs accordingly. The goals include maintenance of normal to increased heart rate, normal to reduced systemic vascular resistance, and myocardial contractility. Nondepolarizing neuromuscular blocking drugs, including pancuronium, may be safely used in patients with mitral regurgitation.

The increase in heart rate that can result from the administration of pancuronium can be beneficial to patients with mitral regurgitation. (254–255; **1768**)

52. Aortic stenosis is the mechanical obstruction to the ejection of blood from the left ventricle secondary to a decrease in the orifice of the aortic valve. Increased left ventricular systolic pressure necessarily results from the chronic attempt of this chamber to maintain an adequate stroke volume through a narrowed aortic valve in aortic stenosis. The increased thickness of the left ventricular wall that is often seen in patients with aortic stenosis occurs in response to chronically increased intraventricular pressures. The severity of aortic stenosis is estimated by the degree of stenosis of the valve. A pressure gradient across the aortic valve that is in excess of 50 mm Hg is considered hemodynamically significant aortic stenosis. (255; **1770–1771, Fig. 49–6**)

53. Two causes of aortic stenosis are rheumatic heart disease and the progressive calcification and stenosis of a congenitally abnormal valve. The congenital valve abnormality most often associated with aortic stenosis is a bicuspid valve. The natural course of aortic stenosis is one of an insidious, long progression of asymptomatic disease before the onset of symptoms. Symptoms may include angina, syncope, dyspnea on exertion, and congestive heart failure. (255; **1770–1771**)

54. Patients with aortic stenosis may have angina pectoris, which typically occurs with exertion despite the absence of coronary artery disease. This occurs because of an increased demand and decreased supply of myocardial oxygen. The increase in myocardial oxygen demand is due to left ventricular hypertrophy. The decrease in myocardial oxygen delivery results from compression of subendocardial coronary blood vessels by increased left ventricular systolic pressures. (255; **1770–1771**)

55. A systolic murmur heard best in the second right intercostal space characterizes the murmur of aortic stenosis heard on cardiac auscultation. It is important for the anesthesiologist to rule out aortic stenosis by auscultation preoperatively to best manage the patient. For instance, a precipitous drop in systemic vascular resistance, as may occur with a regional anesthetic, could be lethal to the patient with aortic stenosis. (256)

56. Considerations for the anesthetic management of a patient with aortic stenosis are the maintenance of a normal sinus rhythm and normal heart rates, the maintenance of myocardial contractility, the avoidance of sudden decreases in systemic vascular resistance, and the optimizing of the intravascular fluid status. (256; **1770–1771**)

57. Tachycardia in the patient with aortic stenosis decreases the amount of time for left ventricular filling leading to a decrease in the stroke volume. Bradycardia can lead to an acute overdistention of the left ventricle in these patients. Sinus rhythm is desired because the contribution of the atrial contraction to left ventricular filling is greater in these patients. Decreases in systemic vascular resistance in patients with aortic stenosis can lead to decreases in coronary blood flow and an increase in the pressure gradient across the aortic valve. (256; **1770–1771**)

58. The maintenance of anesthesia in patients with aortic stenosis can be achieved through the administration of a narcotic-based anesthetic in conjunction with nitrous oxide. Volatile anesthetics in minimal concentrations may be administered as long as excessive decreases in systemic vascular resistance and tachycardia are minimized. Of greater importance is the management of the cardiovascular effects of administered drugs to achieve the goal of the anesthetic management of patients with aortic stenosis. (256; **1770–1771**)

59. Management of the intravascular fluid status of patients with aortic stenosis

should be geared toward the maintenance of an adequate intravascular volume through the prompt, liberal correction of blood and fluid losses. (256; **1770–1771**)

60. The pulmonary artery occlusion pressure may not be reflective of the left ventricular end-diastolic pressure in patients with chronic aortic stenosis secondary to the decrease in left ventricular compliance seen in these patients. (256; **1770–1771**)

61. External cardiac compressions administered during cardiopulmonary arrest are not effective in patients with aortic stenosis because of the greater pressures that are necessary to create forward flow through the stenosed aortic valve. (256; **1770–1771**)

62. Aortic regurgitation results from an incompetent aortic valve. Patients with aortic regurgitation have a decreased left ventricular stroke volume due to regurgitation of part of the ejected stroke volume from the aorta back into the left ventricle. This places an increased volume load on the left ventricle. Chronic aortic regurgitation results in eccentric hypertrophy of the left ventricle in an attempt to compensate for the regurgitation by increasing the stroke volume. Symptoms may include dyspnea, fatigue, and palpitations. (256; **1769–1770, Fig. 49–5**)

63. Acute aortic regurgitation is most likely due to infective endocarditis, trauma, connective tissue disease, or a dissecting thoracic aortic aneurysm. Chronic aortic regurgitation is most likely due to prior rheumatic fever, but it may also be due to hypertension, syphilis, and other causes. (256; **1769–1770**)

64. Angina pectoris despite the absence of coronary artery disease in a patient with aortic regurgitation may occur as a result of increased myocardial oxygen requirements in the presence of a decreased supply. The increase in myocardial oxygen requirements is due to left ventricular hypertrophy. The decrease in myocardial oxygen supply is due to a decrease in aortic diastolic pressure that decreases coronary blood flow. Angina resulting from aortic regurgitation is typically a late and dismal sign. (256)

65. The anesthetic management of aortic regurgitation resembles the anesthetic management for mitral regurgitation. Considerations for the anesthetic management of patients with aortic regurgitation include the avoidance of sudden decreases in heart rate, the avoidance of sudden increases in systemic vascular resistance, and minimizing drug-induced myocardial depression. (256; **1769–1770**)

66. Mitral valve prolapse is a valvular disease in which the valve prolapses into the left atrium during contraction of the left ventricle. This is caused by an abnormality of the valve support structure. Mitral valve prolapse on cardiac auscultation is characterized by a systolic murmur with a clicking sound. It has been estimated that 5% to 15% of the adult population has mitral valve prolapse, also called click-murmur syndrome. Currently, this estimate is believed to be higher than the true prevalence. The diagnosis of mitral valve prolapse can be confirmed through echocardiography. (256; **956–957**)

67. Mitral valve prolapse is associated with atrial secundum defects, von Willebrand's syndrome, and polycystic kidney disease, as well as with musculoskeletal abnormalities such as Marfan's syndrome, pectus excavatum, and kyphoscoliosis. Females are more likely than males to have mitral valve prolapse. (256; **956–957**)

68. Patients with mitral valve prolapse typically are asymptomatic. Symptoms that can be associated with mitral valve prolapse include palpitations, dyspnea, atypical chest pain, dizziness, and syncope. (256; **956–957**)

69. Potential complications of mitral valve prolapse include mitral regurgitation, infective endocarditis, transient cerebral ischemic events, cardiac dysrhythmias, and sudden death. Sudden death is extremely rare, however. Cardiac dysrhythmias associated with atrioventricular bypass tracts and the preexcitation syndrome are fairly common in these patients. Transient cerebral ischemic events may lead to the prescription of aspirin or anticoagulants to patients with mitral valve prolapse. (256; **956–957**)

70. The maintenance of anesthesia in patients with mitral valve prolapse should be geared toward the avoidance of cardiac emptying. Cardiac emptying results in increased prolapse of the mitral valve into the left atrium. Intraoperative avoidance of sympathetic nervous system stimulation, decreases in systemic vascular resistance, and the performance of surgery with patients in the head-up or sitting position will all minimize cardiac emptying. The intravascular fluid volume of the patient should be maintained at normal or high normal for the same reason. Hypotension in patients with mitral valve prolapse can be treated with phenylephrine. Cardiac dysrhythmias that occur intraoperatively should be promptly treated. Ketamine is not recommended in patients with mitral valve prolapse because of its propensity to increase myocardial contractility and heart rate. (257; **956–957**)

71. The potential problem with regional anesthesia in patients with mitral valve prolapse is the decrease in systemic vascular resistance that can be detrimental to these patients. (257; **956–957**)

CONGENITAL HEART DISEASE

72. Approximately 0.8% of live births are associated with some form of congenital heart disease. The most common congenital heart defect is a ventricular septal defect, comprising about 28% of all congenital heart disease. (257, Table 19–4)

73. Patients with congenital heart disease often receive antibiotics perioperatively to protect against potential endocarditis. (257)

74. Congenital heart defects that result in a left-to-right shunt include atrial septal defects, ventricular septal defects, and a patent ductus arteriosus. The net physiologic result of all these shunts is increased pulmonary blood flow with pulmonary hypertension, right ventricular hypertrophy, and eventual congestive heart failure. (257; **1809–1810, Table 50–2**)

75. Atrial septal defects are diagnosed by cardiac auscultation of a systolic murmur over the area of the pulmonary valve during a routine physical examination or by a history of frequent pulmonary infections. Surgical closure of an atrial septal defect is indicated when the pulmonary blood flow is two or more times greater than systemic blood flow. Atrial septal defects may also be corrected under nonoperative conditions through interventional cardiac techniques. Uncorrected shunting results in pulmonary vascular vasoconstriction, which is reversible, followed by eventual, irreversible pulmonary vascular smooth muscle hypertrophy. (257–258; **1772, 1809, 1841**)

76. A ventricular septal defect murmur is pansystolic, auscultated at its greatest intensity along the left sternal border. (258; **1772**)

77. Patients with a small ventricular septal defect are usually asymptomatic. Ventricular septal defects that are large enough to produce symptoms typically produce symptoms of congestive heart failure that are characteristic of symptomatic left-to-right shunts. (258; **1772, 1809**)

78. Failure of the closure of the ductus arteriosus after birth results in oxygenated

blood flowing from the aorta into the pulmonary artery. Most patients with a patent ductus arteriosus are asymptomatic. (258; **1809**)

79. On cardiac auscultation a patent ductus arteriosus is a continuous systolic and diastolic murmur. (258)

80. The goals of the management of anesthesia in patients with a left-to-right shunt are aimed toward the avoidance of hemodynamic changes, such as an increase in systemic vascular resistance, that will increase the magnitude of the shunt. Decreases in the magnitude of the shunt can be achieved through decreases in the arterial pressure and increases in the pulmonary vascular resistance, as with positive pressure ventilation. (257–258; **1819–1820**)

81. Inadvertent introduction of an air bubble into the patient's vascular system via the intravenous tubing used for intravascular fluids can result in an air embolus into the systemic circulation in a patient with a left-to-right shunt. Ultimately, this could lead to emboli in the coronary or cerebral arteries. Although the risk is greater in patients with right-to-left shunts, patients with left-to-right shunts may have reversal of their shunt during certain phases of the cardiac cycle, during cardiopulmonary interventions as during manual manipulation of the heart during cardiac surgery, or with coughing in the awake patient. (258; **1815**)

82. Right-to-left shunting occurs when the resistance to outflow from the right ventricle is greater than systemic vascular resistance. The result is a decrease in pulmonary blood flow. The systemic circulation thus receives blood that has been oxygenated mixed with deoxygenated blood that passes through the shunt. The physiologic hallmark of a right-to-left shunt is arterial hypoxemia leading to cyanosis. (258; **1809–1810**)

83. The most common congenital heart defect associated with a right-to-left shunt is tetralogy of Fallot. (258; **1809, Table 50–2**)

84. Physiologic anomalies that are present in a child with tetralogy of Fallot include a ventricular septal defect, an aorta that overrides the pulmonary artery outflow tract, obstruction to blood flow through the pulmonary artery outflow tract, and right ventricular hypertrophy. Because of the obstruction of blood flow through the pulmonary outflow tract, blood is shunted through the ventricular septal defect to the left ventricle. This leads to deoxygenated blood mixing with oxygenated blood in the left ventricle and its delivery to the systemic circulation. The degree of arterial hypoxemia and peripheral cyanosis depends on the amount of blood shunted relative to the pulmonary blood flow. (258; **1809–1810**)

85. The Pao_2 of a child with tetralogy of Fallot is usually less than 50 mm Hg, even while breathing oxygen. (258)

86. Squatting in children with tetralogy of Fallot increases systemic blood pressure and systemic vascular resistance by compressing the large arteries in the inguinal area. The increase in systemic vascular resistance results in a decrease in the magnitude of the right-to-left shunt and an increase in pulmonary blood flow. The net result of squatting is an increase in arterial oxygenation. (258)

87. A "tet spell" is a hypercyanotic attack that occurs in about 35% of patients with tetralogy of Fallot. It usually occurs in response to crying or exercise but can occur spontaneously. A "tet spell" may also occur in the crying child presenting for surgery or with placement of an intravenous catheter. Physiologically these spells are probably triggered by a decrease in systemic vascular resistance or a spasm of cardiac muscle in the region of the pulmonary artery outflow tract resulting in an increase in the magnitude of the

right-to-left shunt. The appropriate treatment of a "tet spell" depends on the cause of the spell. If the spell is due to a decrease in systemic vascular resistance, it can be treated with phenylephrine or intravenous fluids. Sympathomimetics are not recommended in these patients because the sympathetic nervous system stimulation that results could increase cardiac muscle spasm. If the hypercyanotic attack is due to cardiac muscle spasm, propranolol or esmolol may be used to treat the spell. (258)

88. The goals of the management of anesthesia in patients with tetralogy of Fallot are aimed toward the avoidance of worsening arterial hypoxemia by increasing the magnitude of the shunt. Decreases in systemic vascular resistance and increases in pulmonary vascular resistance should be avoided. (258)

89. Positive pressure ventilation of the lungs of a child with tetralogy of Fallot can result in an increase in pulmonary vascular resistance and an increase in the magnitude of the right-to-left shunt. Nevertheless, the benefits of intraoperative controlled ventilation of the lungs of these children outweigh the potential harm, and positive pressure ventilation of the lungs is typically instituted during the surgical procedure. It is important, however, that the PaO_2 be closely monitored throughout the procedure. (258–259)

90. The induction of anesthesia in a child with tetralogy of Fallot can be achieved with the intravenous administration of ketamine or by an inhalation induction. Ketamine is advantageous in that it increases systemic vascular resistance. When an inhalation induction is chosen, phenylephrine should be readily available to treat decreases in the systemic vascular resistance. (258–259; **1819–1820**)

91. The maintenance of anesthesia in a child with tetralogy of Fallot can be achieved by the administration of low concentrations of a volatile anesthetic in combination with nitrous oxide. The concentration of inhaled nitrous oxide should be limited to 50% to maximize arterial oxygenation and to minimize the increase in pulmonary vascular resistance that can result from its administration. Volatile anesthetics should be used with the awareness that the decrease in systemic vascular resistance that they cause may worsen the magnitude of the shunt. Clinically, however, at lower concentrations the administration of volatile anesthetics often improves arterial oxygenation. This may be due to relaxation of cardiac muscle spasm in the region of the pulmonary outflow tract and improved pulmonary blood flow or a decrease in total body oxygen consumption. Of greater importance than the specific agents used is the management of the hemodynamic effects of administered drugs to achieve the goal of the anesthetic management of patients with tetralogy of Fallot. (259; **1819–1820**)

92. Pancuronium might be useful as a neuromuscular blocking drug in children with tetralogy of Fallot because the increase in heart rate that is an effect of this drug may be helpful in maintaining cardiac output. (259; **443–444**)

93. It is important to avoid hypovolemia in children with tetralogy of Fallot because of the potential of hypovolemia to worsen the shunt. Preoperatively the patient should be well hydrated, and their intravascular fluid status should be maintained intraoperatively. Should hypotension occur it can be treated with fluids and the administration of phenylephrine. (259)

94. The infusion of an air bubble into the vein of a child with tetralogy of Fallot can result in a direct air embolus to the coronary or cerebral arteries by crossing to the left-sided circulation directly via the shunt. (259; **1815**)

DISTURBANCES OF CARDIAC CONDUCTION AND RHYTHM

95. Tools available to the clinician for the diagnosis of disturbances in cardiac conduction and rhythm include an electrocardiogram and a Holter monitor. A

Holter monitor is an ambulatory electrocardiogram that can be worn for days to document the occurrence of cardiac dysrhythmias and to assess the efficacy of treatment interventions. (259; **1239–1240, 1248**)

96. The conduction system of the heart includes the sinoatrial node, atrioventricular node, the bundle of His, and Purkinje fibers of the right and left bundle branches. Types of conduction defects include sinus node block, atrioventricular conduction defects, and intraventricular conduction defects. Atrioventricular conduction defects are classified as first-, second-, or third-degree heart blocks. Intraventricular conduction defects include right bundle branch block, left bundle branch block, and left fascicular hemiblock. Heart block below the atrioventricular node is usually progressive and permanent, whereas heart block above the atrioventricular node is usually transient and benign. (259; **1246–1248, Table 32–6**)

97. The placement of a prophylactic artificial cardiac pacemaker before surgery is not indicated in a patient with a bifascicular block. The theoretical concern in preoperative patients with a bifascicular block is that the single remaining intact fascicle will become compromised by perioperative events, such as changes in hemodynamics, oxygenation, or electrolytes. This would lead to acute third-degree atrioventricular heart block. Third-degree atrioventricular block is also referred to as complete heart block because all the electrical activity from the atria fails to be conducted to the ventricles. Ventricular contractions in patients with third-degree atrioventricular block occur at a rate of about 40 beats per minute, typically too slow to maintain an adequate cardiac output. Fortunately, there is no evidence that bifascicular blocks proceed to third-degree atrioventricular block with enough consistency to warrant the prophylactic placement of a pacemaker. (259; **959, 1247**)

98. Third-degree atrioventricular heart block is treated by the placement of an artificial cardiac pacemaker. There are various methods by which this can be accomplished. An endocardial pacemaker lead may be inserted intravenously, an epicardial or myocardial lead may be placed by the subcostal approach, or noninvasive transcutaneous cardiac pacing can be started. The pharmacologic treatment of third-degree heart block involves a continuous infusion of isoproterenol, which can act as a medical pacemaker until artificial electrical cardiac pacing is implemented. (259; **1247**)

99. Sick sinus syndrome occurs as a result of degenerative changes in the sinoatrial node and is associated with an inappropriate sinus bradycardia. In sick sinus syndrome rapid heart rates inhibit the normal pacemaker activity of the sinoatrial node and lead to periods of asystole. Sick sinus syndrome therefore usually presents as bradycardia with episodes of supraventricular tachycardia. Treatment is by administering medicines to control tachycardia. When these medicines result in bradycardia, medical management is said to have failed and artificial cardiac pacemakers become the next line of treatment. Patients with sick sinus syndrome may be at a high risk for pulmonary embolism and may therefore be started on anticoagulants. (260; **627, 1240, 1773, Fig. 32–13**)

100. Ventricular premature beats occur as a result of ectopic pacemaker activity at a level below the atrioventricular node. The premature ventricular contraction then spreads through the ventricular conducting system. The premature ventricular contraction often blocks the sinoatrial node's subsequent depolarization, leading to a characteristic pause until the next normal sinus beat is generated. The hallmark features of a ventricular premature beat on an electrocardiogram are representative of the aberrant conduction associated with the ventricular contraction. They include a premature occurrence, the absence of a P wave preceding the QRS complex, a wide and bizarre

appearing QRS complex, an inverted T wave, and a compensatory pause after the premature beat. (260; **959, 1244**)

101. Premature ventricular beats warrant treatment when they occur more frequently than six times a minute, are multifocal, occur in a train of three or more, or take place during the ascending limb of the T wave, that is, during the refractory period of the ventricle. Treatment is typically with lidocaine at a dose of 1 to 2 mg/kg. Recurrent premature ventricular beats can be treated with a lidocaine infusion. Additional therapy, if necessary, may include beta-antagonists, bretylium, procainamide, quinidine, verapamil, or overdrive pacing. A search for the underlying cause of the premature beat should also be sought. (260; **959, 1244**)

102. Causes of ventricular premature beats include myocardial ischemia, arterial hypoxemia, hypercarbia, hypertension, hypokalemia, and mechanical irritation of the ventricles. (260; **1244**)

103. Ventricular tachycardia may be diagnosed with the appearance of three or more consecutive, wide QRS complexes on the electrocardiogram occurring at an effective heart rate higher than 120 beats per minute. The QRS complexes must be greater than 0.12 second. The P waves have no fixed relationship to the QRS complex because the beat originates in the ventricle. The acute onset of ventricular tachycardia can be life threatening. Ventricular tachycardia can be treated with intravenous lidocaine as a bolus and an infusion in the absence of any hemodynamic changes. Hemodynamic changes such as hypotension may require immediate cardioversion. (260; **1244–1245**)

104. Preexcitation syndromes are defined as an activation of a portion of the ventricles by cardiac impulses that have originated in the atria but were conducted to the ventricles by an accessory conduction pathway. Activation of the ventricles during this syndrome occur sooner than it otherwise would have because of the accessory pathway, making the QRS complex appear sooner than it would have if sinus rhythm were maintained. (260; **960**)

105. Wolff-Parkinson-White syndrome is the most commonly occurring preexcitation syndrome. The incidence of this syndrome is 0.3% in the general population. These patients may have sporadic supraventricular tachycardia or atrial fibrillation. In extreme cases the rapid heart rate may be associated with syncope or congestive heart failure. On the electrocardiogram Wolff-Parkinson-White syndrome is characterized by a short PR interval and a wide QRS complex. There is also a characteristic delta wave that appears on the electrocardiogram. The delta wave together with the QRS complex represent the composite of cardiac impulses conducted by both the normal and accessory pathways. (260)

106. The most common cardiac dysrhythmia associated with Wolff-Parkinson-White syndrome is paroxysmal atrial tachycardia. Wolff-Parkinson-White syndrome is most frequently treated by catheter ablation of the accessory pathway. Identification of the accessory pathway is accomplished by electrophysiologic mapping. (260; **960, 1773**)

107. The goal of the anesthetic management of a patient with Wolff-Parkinson-White syndrome is the avoidance of any events, such as anxiety or drugs, that can result in sympathetic nervous system stimulation. Any cardiac antidysrhythmic drugs should be continued throughout the perioperative period. An adequate depth of anesthesia should be achieved before direct laryngoscopy to ensure that the patient does not respond to the noxious stimulus with sympathetic nervous system activity, placing the patient at an increased risk of tachyarrhythmias. This can be achieved with adequate doses of an intravenous induction agent other than ketamine, with opioids, or with a bolus of lidocaine

just before direct laryngoscopy. The duration of laryngoscopy should also be as short as possible. (260; **960–961, 1773–1774**)

108. Methods for the treatment of paroxysmal atrial tachycardia or fibrillation that can occur in the perioperative period in patients with Wolff-Parkinson-White syndrome include the administration of adenosine or procainamide. Adenosine acts by prolonging the refractory period of the atrioventricular node, whereas procainamide acts by increasing the refractory period of the accessory pathways. When the tachydysrhythmias become life threatening, emergent electrical cardioversion is indicated. Of note, drugs such as verapamil and digitalis may actually result in an increase in ventricular response during the dysrhythmia by accelerating the conduction in the accessory atrioventricular pathway. (260–261)

109. Prolonged QT interval syndrome can be congenital or acquired. Acquired prolonged QT interval syndrome can be due to quinidine, tricyclic antidepressants, subarachnoid hemorrhage, hypokalemia, hypocalcemia, or hypomagnesemia. It may also present in the postoperative period after right radical neck dissection. The diagnosis of prolonged QT interval syndrome is made when the QT interval is chronically greater than 0.44 second. Adverse events that are associated with a prolonged QT interval include ventricular dysrhythmias, syncope, and sudden death. The pharmacologic treatment of a chronically prolonged QT interval can include beta antagonists or a left stellate ganglion block. These treatments are empirical. (261; **2543–2544**)

110. A congenital cause of prolonged QT interval is thought to be due to an imbalance of autonomic innervation to the heart caused by decreases in right cardiac sympathetic nerve activity. A left stellate ganglion block is thought to work by decreasing left cardiac sympathetic nerve activity, thereby balancing the autonomic innervation to the heart. (261; **638, 1589**)

111. The goal of the anesthetic management of a patient with a chronically prolonged QT interval includes the avoidance of any events or drugs that are likely to cause sympathetic nervous system stimulation. General anesthesia has triggered life-threatening ventricular dysrhythmia and cardiac arrest in patients with this syndrome. Beta-adrenergic blockade may be instituted preoperatively to minimize this risk. Although thiopental prolongs the QT interval in normal patients, it has been used for the induction of anesthesia in patients with the syndrome without any problems. Direct laryngoscopy should be performed with the patient deeply anesthetized. Should acute ventricular dysrhythmias occur, they can be treated with a beta antagonist. Procainamide and quinidine are both known to prolong the QT interval in normal patients and should probably be avoided. Lidocaine, which also prolongs the QT interval in normal patients, has been used to successfully treat ventricular dysrhythmias in these patients. Electrical cardioversion may be necessary in the event of dysrhythmias that become life threatening. (261; **2543–2544**)

ARTIFICIAL CARDIAC PACEMAKERS

112. The preoperative evaluation of a patient with an artificial cardiac pacemaker should include an understanding of the underlying cardiac condition that required placement of the pacemaker and an assessment of the current function of the pacemaker. (261; **961–962**)

113. A pacemaker should be evaluated by the anesthesiologist preoperatively so that the anesthesiologist has a good understanding of the pacemaker and its programming. For instance, the anesthesiologist should be aware of what the default rhythm is should the pacemaker not capture, the type of pacemaker (i.e., demand or fixed or radiofrequency), the chamber paced, the chamber

sensed, how to detect deterioration in battery function, how to change the mode or to fire a radiofrequency type of pacemaker, and the current rate and sensitivity settings of the pacemaker. (261; **961–962**)

114. Intraoperative monitoring that is important in a patient with an artificial cardiac pacemaker include the electrocardiogram, pulse palpation, and auscultation of cardiac sounds through an esophageal stethoscope. Each of these will give the anesthesiologist information regarding the cardiac rhythm or lack thereof. Alternatively, an intra-arterial catheter or a pulse oximeter not affected by electrocautery may be placed because interference of the electrocardiogram by electrocautery may lead to a time of an unmonitored cardiac rhythm during which asystole could develop. The intra-arterial catheter or pulse oximeter would provide a measure of blood flow during that period. (261; **961–962**)

115. If the ground plate for electrocautery is placed too near the pulse generator of the artificial cardiac pacemaker there could be electromagnetic interference that is interpreted as spontaneous cardiac activity by the pacemaker. This may result in asystole due to an inhibition of pulse generator activity by the pacemaker. The ground plate should be placed as far away as possible from the pulse generator but at least 15 cm away. Other potential sources of mechanical interference include electroconvulsive shock therapy, succinylcholine-induced fasciculations, and myoclonic movements. (261; **961–962**)

116. The selection of drugs or anesthetic techniques for a patient should not be altered by the presence of an artificial cardiac pacemaker. (261; **961–962**)

117. An electric magnet should be kept in the operating room intraoperatively for patients with artificial cardiac pacemakers to convert the pacemaker to an asynchronous mode, or fixed rate, should it become necessary. For instance, if the patient's pacemaker stops functioning intraoperatively, placement of an external converter magnet over the pulse generator should convert the pacemaker to an asynchronous mode. This should be demonstrated to the anesthesiologist and confirmed before surgery. Newer designs of pacemakers and their pulse generators have resulted in pacemakers that will convert to an asynchronous mode in the presence of continuous use of electrocautery. This may decrease the need to use an electric magnet intraoperatively, although the anesthesiologist should still be aware of how to convert the pacemaker to an asynchronous mode if necessary. (261; **961–962**)

118. The most common cause of temporary pacemaker malfunction is the disruption of contact between the pacemaker electrode wires and the endocardium. Some causes of this disruption include muscular exertion, blunt trauma, cardioversion, and positive pressure ventilation. When this occurs, pacemaker spikes will continue to be seen on the electrocardiogram, although there is no myocardial activity or pulse. Placement of a pulmonary artery catheter in a patient with an artificial cardiac pacemaker may disrupt the placement of transvenous endocardial electrodes if they have been placed in the 2 weeks preceding the procedure. (261; **961–962**)

ESSENTIAL HYPERTENSION

119. Essential hypertension has been defined as a sustained elevated blood pressure on more than one reading without any known cause. Systolic blood pressures greater than 160 mm Hg or diastolic blood pressures greater than 90 mm Hg have been arbitrarily defined as the limits at which hypertension begins. The benefits of the long-term treatment of patients with essential hypertension include decreases in the incidence of cerebrovascular accidents, congestive heart failure, and renal disease. (261; **935–936, Fig. 25–8, Tables 25–14, 25–15**)

120. The preoperative evaluation of a patient with essential hypertension should include a determination of the adequacy of blood pressure control, a review of the pharmacology of the antihypertensive drugs, and an evaluation of effects of the hypertension on other organs. (262; **935–941**)

121. Antihypertensives include angiotensin-converting enzyme inhibitors, calcium channel blockers, beta-adrenergic antagonists, diuretics, and vasodilators. It is generally recommended that blood pressure medications be administered on their routine schedule in the perioperative period in the patient with essential hypertension. This includes medicines on the morning of the surgical procedure. A possible exception to this may be angiotensin-converting enzyme inhibitors. It is the preference of some anesthesiologists that this antihypertensive not be taken on the morning of surgery, owing to its potential to result in exaggerated hypotension that may be difficult to control after the induction of anesthesia. (262; **935–941, 1852**)

122. Medical problems that are frequently seen in patients with essential hypertension include congestive heart failure, coronary artery disease, cerebral ischemia, renal dysfunction, and peripheral vascular disease. Approximately 50% of patients with peripheral vascular disease can be assumed to have 50% or greater stenosis of one or more coronary arteries, even in the absence of symptoms. (262; **935–941, 1852**)

123. The curve for the autoregulation of cerebral blood flow in patients with essential hypertension is shifted to the right, such that autoregulation occurs at higher pressures than it would for a normotensive patient. This implies that the same degree of absolute hypotension in patients with a history of hypertension may be more harmful than the same blood pressure would be for a normotensive patient. Thus, maintenance of blood pressure in the perioperative period should be relative to what the preoperative resting blood pressure is specific to that patient. (262; **721–722, 1852**)

124. Treating essential hypertension in patients before an elective procedure has been shown to be beneficial in decreasing the risk of intraoperative hypotension and myocardial ischemia. There have been multiple studies conducted regarding this topic. Studies have also shown that there is not an increased incidence of cardiac complications in hypertensive patients in the perioperative period as long as the diastolic blood pressure was not higher than 110 mm Hg preoperatively. (262; **935–941, 1852, Fig. 27–8, Tables 25–14, 25–15, 25–16, 25–17**)

125. Patients with essential hypertension frequently respond to the induction of anesthesia with an exaggerated decrease in blood pressure. This hypotension is thought to occur as a result of an unmasking of a decreased intravascular fluid volume status. (262; **935–941, 1852**)

126. Patients with essential hypertension are especially likely to respond to direct laryngoscopy with exaggerated increases in blood pressure, placing them at risk of myocardial ischemia. This response can be attenuated with adequate levels of anesthesia. It must be done with caution in hypertensive patients, because an excessive depth of anesthesia may produce hypotension in these patients as well. Other methods may be used to attenuate the sympathetic nervous system response to direct laryngoscopy and the associated exaggerated hypertension. For instance, esmolol or lidocaine may be administered just before direct laryngoscopy. In addition, the duration of direct laryngoscopy should be minimized. (262; **935–941, 1852**)

127. The goal for the anesthetic management of patients with essential hypertension is to minimize the fluctuations in blood pressure characteristic of these patients with anesthetics and antihypertensive medications as appropriate.

The patient should also be continually monitored for evidence of myocardial ischemia via a continuous electrocardiogram. (262; **935–941, 1852**)

128. The maintenance of anesthesia in patients with essential hypertension can be achieved through the administration of a volatile anesthetic in conjunction with nitrous oxide and an opioid. A dose sufficient to attenuate hypertensive responses to surgical stimulation should be administered. The maintenance of normotension intraoperatively may also require the administration of other medicines, such as beta antagonists or nitrates. (262)

129. Intraoperative hypotension in patients with essential hypertension can be managed by the administration of intravenous fluids, by decreasing the concentration of volatile anesthetics, and by the administration of vasopressors as necessary. (262–263)

130. The administration of regional anesthesia in patients with essential hypertension has the potential problem of causing excessive decreases in systemic blood pressure. This can occur owing to the corresponding vasodilation associated with the sympathetic nervous system blockade in combination with the decreased intravascular fluid volume status often seen in patients with chronic hypertension. The anesthesiologist must be prepared to support the blood pressure as necessary when a regional anesthetic is administered to these patients. (263)

131. Hypertension occurs frequently in the early postoperative period in patients with a diagnosis of essential hypertension. Hypertension secondary to inadequate pain control should be considered. If hypertension persists despite adequate analgesia, the administration of antihypertensives may be necessary. (263; **2315–2316, Fig. 68–13**)

CONGESTIVE HEART FAILURE

132. Congestive heart failure is highly correlated with postoperative morbidity. In fact, preoperative congestive heart failure is the single greatest preoperative risk factor for predicting postoperative morbidity. This suggests that the preoperative patient with congestive heart failure scheduled for elective surgery should have his or her surgery delayed until treatment of the congestive heart failure can be instituted and the patient's medical status optimized. (263; **803, 829, 949**)

133. The goal of the anesthetic management of patients with congestive heart failure who are undergoing urgent or emergent surgery is the optimization of cardiac output. Optimal cardiac output in patients with congestive heart failure undergoing anesthesia may be best achieved with the administration of an opioid-based anesthetic. Volatile anesthetics may produce a dose-dependent depression of cardiac muscle function that is greater in patients with congestive heart failure than in patients without congestive heart failure. In addition, the maintenance of myocardial contractility may necessitate the continuous administration of dopamine or dobutamine in the perioperative period. (263)

134. Ketamine may be useful in patients with congestive heart failure because of its effect of increased myocardial contractility and increased cardiac output. (263)

135. Positive pressure ventilation of the lungs of patients in congestive heart failure may be beneficial because of its effect of decreasing pulmonary vascular congestion and improvement in arterial oxygenation. (263)

136. Monitors in the patient with congestive heart failure undergoing major surgery might include an intra-arterial catheter as well as a pulmonary artery catheter

to monitor central filling pressures and cardiac output. Monitors chosen should be influenced by the patient's status and the surgical procedure. (263)

137. Regional anesthesia for peripheral surgery in patients with congestive heart failure can be administered safely but is not proven to have reliably better outcomes than general anesthesia for these patients. Mild decreases in the systemic vascular resistance produced by an epidural or spinal anesthetic may provide for an improved cardiac output in the patient with congestive heart failure. Greater decreases in the systemic vascular resistance can lead to hypotension that is unpredictable and difficult to control. (263)

HYPERTROPHIC CARDIOMYOPATHY

138. Hypertrophic cardiomyopathy is a genetically transmitted disease also known as idiopathic hypertrophic subaortic stenosis. The pathology that defines hypertrophic cardiomyopathy is the obstruction to left ventricular outflow produced by asymmetric hypertrophy of the intraventricular septal muscle. As a result of the obstruction to ventricular outflow, left ventricular hypertrophy develops to the degree that the volume of the left chamber is decreased. As the disease advances, the increased muscle mass in the subaortic region can lead to complete obstruction of left ventricular outflow. The stroke volume in patients with hypertrophic cardiomyopathy remains normal despite the physiologic changes. The normal stroke volume is reflective of the hypercontractile state of the myocardium. (263–264; **1771**)

139. Symptoms associated with hypertrophic cardiomyopathy include angina pectoris, syncope, tachydysrhythmias, and congestive heart failure. Patients with hypertrophic cardiomyopathy experiencing angina may have relief of their symptoms by assuming the supine position. This is believed to be due to the increase in left ventricular size that ccompanies lying supine. Patients known to have hypertrophic cardiomyopathy are generally advised not to play competitive sports, owing to the risk of sudden death. (264; **1771**)

140. The goal of the anesthetic management of patients with hypertrophic cardiomyopathy is geared toward decreasing the pressure gradient across the obstructed left ventricular outflow tract. There are several methods of decreasing the left ventricular outflow obstruction in patients with hypertrophic cardiomyopathy. These include decreasing myocardial contractility, as with the administration of beta antagonists, increasing preload with increased intravascular fluid volume or medical bradycardia, and increasing afterload with alpha-adrenergic stimulation as is produced by phenylephrine. (264; **1771**)

141. Intraoperative hypotension in patients with hypertrophic cardiomyopathy can be treated with the administration of intravascular fluids as well as phenylephrine. (264; **1771**)

142. Intraoperative hypertension in patients with hypertrophic cardiomyopathy can be treated with the administration of increased concentrations of volatile anesthetics. (264; **1771**)

143. The administration of beta agonists for the treatment of hypotension in patients with hypertrophic cardiomyopathy can result in an increase in myocardial contractility and a corresponding increase in left ventricular outflow obstruction. Likewise, the administration of nitrates such as nitroprusside or nitroglycerin to these patients can increase left ventricular outflow obstruction by decreasing systemic vascular resistance, making them an unlikely choice for the treatment of hypertension. (264; **1771**)

COR PULMONALE

144. Cor pulmonale is right ventricular hypertrophy and cardiac dysfunction that occurs as a result of pulmonary hypertension. The most likely cause of cor pulmonale is chronic obstructive pulmonary disease with associated chronic arterial hypoxemia leading to chronic pulmonary vascular vasoconstriction. Vascular smooth muscle hypertrophy and permanently increased pulmonary vascular resistance results from sustained pulmonary vascular vasoconstriction. When systemic acidosis is also present there is a synergistic effect between arterial hypoxemia and acidosis on the pulmonary vasculature. In general, when the cause of the increased pulmonary vasculature resistance is due to arterial hypoxemia from chronic obstructive pulmonary disease, the prognosis is somewhat favorable if the arterial hypoxemia can be reversed with the administration of oxygen. Other causes of increased pulmonary vascular resistance leading to cor pulmonale, such as primary pulmonary hypertension or pulmonary fibrosis, have less favorable outcomes. (264; **963–965, 1669–1670**)

145. Symptoms of cor pulmonale are often masked by the symptoms associated with the existence of co-existing chronic obstructive pulmonary disease. As the right ventricle becomes increasingly impaired, patients may experience syncope with exertion. Patients may also have chronic dependent edema, an enlarged liver, ascites, and dilated neck veins. On the lateral chest radiograph right ventricular hypertrophy may present as a decrease in the retrosternal space. There may also be a decrease in pulmonary vascular markings. Right ventricular hypertrophy on the electrocardiogram would show peaked P waves in leads II, III, and aVF. Often there will also be right-axis deviation. On right-sided heart catheterization the mean pulmonary artery pressure will be elevated, whereas the pulmonary artery occlusion pressure is normal. Pulmonary hypertension is considered mild with mean pulmonary artery pressures between 20 and 35 mm Hg and moderate when pressures are greater than 35 mm Hg. (264; **1669–1670, Table 48–4**)

146. The treatment of cor pulmonale is directed toward decreasing right ventricular work by decreasing the pulmonary vascular resistance. This may be achieved through the correction of the patient's pH and through the administration of oxygen to reverse arterial hypoxemia if possible. Diuretics may also be administered for patients with congestive heart failure. Nitroglycerin administration may result in lowering of the pulmonary artery pressure and a decrease in pulmonary vascular resistance. (264; **963–965, 1669–1670**)

147. Just as in any other patient, the patient with cor pulmonale who is scheduled for an elective surgical procedure should be medically optimized before the procedure. Any pulmonary infections should be treated. Patients should have any bronchospasm reversed, be well hydrated, and have their electrolytes evaluated and corrected if necessary. (264; **963–965, 1669–1670**)

148. The goal of the anesthetic management of patients with cor pulmonale is the avoidance of events or drugs that could result in an increase in pulmonary vascular resistance, thereby worsening right ventricular failure. Events that may result in an increase in pulmonary vascular resistance include arterial hypoxemia, hypercapnia, acidosis, and decreases in body temperature. An abrupt or significant decrease in the systemic vascular resistance should be avoided. Nitrous oxide may be avoided because of its potential for increasing pulmonary vascular resistance. Although positive pressure ventilation may increase pulmonary vascular resistance, its potential benefit for improving arterial oxygenation likely outweighs its risk. Finally, high doses of opioids might be avoided because they decrease the patient's responsiveness to carbon dioxide postoperatively and may lead to decreases in ventilation as well as

hypercapnia and increased pulmonary vascular resistance postoperatively. An intra-arterial catheter allows for arterial blood gas analysis to assess the effects of any interventions on the patient's arterial oxygenation and pH. (264; **963–965, 1994–1995**)

149. The advantage of monitoring right atrial pressure during surgery in patients with cor pulmonale is the ability of the anesthesiologist to assess any adverse effects of the surgical procedure or administered drugs on right atrial pressure. It also provides the anesthesiologist with an ability to assess the effects of any therapeutic interventions. (264; **965**)

CARDIAC TAMPONADE

150. Cardiac tamponade occurs as a result of increased intrapericardial pressure from the accumulation of fluid in the pericardial space. The pathophysiology resulting from this and characterizing cardiac tamponade is decreased diastolic filling of the ventricles, decreased stroke volume, and hypotension. The decrease in stroke volume results in sympathetic nervous system activation in an attempt to maintain cardiac output. Cardiac output and systemic blood pressure in these patients become dependent on heart rate and on a central venous pressure that exceeds the right ventricular end-diastolic pressure. (264; **1772–1773**)

151. Manifestations of cardiac tamponade include hypotension, tachycardia, vasoconstriction, equalization of diastolic filling pressures, increased central venous pressure, and a fixed stroke volume. These patients also have pulsus paradoxus. Pulsus paradoxus is a decrease in the arterial blood pressure by greater than 10 mm Hg during inspiration. This is the opposite of what would be expected in normal patients and reflects the decrease in ventricular stroke volume that occurs with inspiration. On the chest radiograph there may be a change in the cardiac silhouette when 250 mL or greater of fluid has accumulated in the pericardial space. Decreased voltages through all leads is seen in patients with cardiac tamponade. There may also be evidence of myocardial ischemia on the electrocardiogram. Cardiac tamponade is best diagnosed through echocardiography. (264; **1772–1773**)

152. The definitive treatment of cardiac tamponade is the drainage of the pericardial fluid. This can be achieved either percutaneously or by a pericardiotomy in the operating room under general or local anesthesia. Temporizing measures until definitive treatment include the expansion of the intravascular fluid volume, the administration of agents that will increase myocardial contractility such as dopamine, and the correction of metabolic acidosis that may depress myocardial contractility. (264; **1772–1773**)

153. The goal of the anesthetic management of patients with cardiac tamponade is the avoidance of events or drugs that could result in a decrease in cardiac output. Myocardial contractility, arterial blood pressure, increased heart rate, and venous return must all be maintained. (264–265; **1772–1773**)

154. The induction of anesthesia and positive pressure ventilation of the lungs of patients with cardiac tamponade can result in profound, irreversible hypotension. Hypotension that occurs in response to positive pressure ventilation of the lungs of these patients results from anesthetic-induced peripheral vasodilation, direct myocardial depression, and decreases in venous return. The recommendation for patients with cardiac tamponade is that, if at all possible, percutaneous pericardiocentesis be performed under local anesthesia to relieve some of the tamponade before the induction of anesthesia. This should be done in the operating room with the patient spontaneously breathing and continually monitored. Monitors may include an intra-arterial catheter for

continuous arterial blood pressure monitoring and a central venous catheter to monitor central venous pressures. (265; **1772–1773**)

155. The recommendation for anesthesia in patients with cardiac tamponade is that percutaneous pericardiocentesis be performed under local anesthesia before the induction of anesthesia. If that is not possible an awake orotracheal intubation should be performed. The patient should have the urgency of the need to perform the procedure explained, and the airway should be anesthetized topically. After confirmed orotracheal intubation the patient can then be gently sedated while still spontaneously ventilating the lungs. Small doses of ketamine may be administered to the patient to provide analgesia and sedation during pericardiocentesis. The induction of anesthesia and positive pressure ventilation if required for further surgical exploration should not be instituted until drainage of the pericardial space has been achieved. The induction of anesthesia may be accomplished with ketamine. (264–265; **1772–1773**)

156. Sympathetic nervous system stimulants such as isoproterenol, dopamine, and dobutamine as continuous infusions may be useful in patients with cardiac tamponade. (265; **1772–1773**)

ANEURYSMS OF THE AORTA

157. Most aortic aneurysms involve the abdominal aorta. About 95% of abdominal aortic aneurysms are due to atherosclerosis, in contrast to about 50% of thoracic aortic aneurysms. Other causes of aortic aneurysms include trauma, mycotic infection, connective tissue disorders such as Marfan's syndrome, and syphilis. Only about 0.5% of abdominal aortic aneurysms extend into the renal arteries. (265; **1869**)

158. A dissecting aneurysm occurs when a tear in the intima of the aorta separates the layers of the wall of the aorta. Blood is then allowed to enter and penetrate between the intima on one side and the media and adventitia layers on the other, creating a false lumen. The dissection can then reenter the true lumen through another tear in the intima, or it may rupture through the adventitia. Acute dissection may present as excruciating chest pain and patients may appear to be in shock. Peripheral pulses may be difficult to palpate. The treatment for aortic dissection is surgical excision, usually followed by placement of a graft. Short-term management until definitive treatment can take place may include decreasing blood pressure to the lowest acceptable level and the relief of pain. (265; **1860–1861**)

159. The risk of rupture of an abdominal aortic aneurysm is best predicted by the diameter of the aneurysm as well as its rate of expansion. Elective resection of an abdominal aortic aneurysm is recommended when the diameter of the aneurysm is estimated to be 5 cm or greater. This recommendation is made based on the dramatic increase in the likelihood of spontaneous rupture of the aneurysm when the size of the aneurysm exceeds 5 cm. Abdominal aortic aneurysms with a diameter less than 5 cm are typically followed with serial measurements to evaluate its rate of expansion. If the aneurysm expands by more than 0.5 cm in a 6-month period, or if the patient becomes symptomatic, surgical repair is recommended. (265; **1860–1861**)

160. Medical problems frequently associated with aortic aneurysms include hypertension, diabetes mellitus, ischemic heart disease, and atherosclerosis. (265; **1860–1861**)

161. The goal of the anesthetic management of patients undergoing resection of an abdominal aortic aneurysm is aimed toward the maintenance of cardiovascular and hemodynamic parameters at or near normal. Aggressive intraoperative monitoring is necessary to achieve this goal. Patients should have their

intra-arterial and central venous pressures closely monitored throughout the case. Patients with a history of co-existing coronary artery disease, left ventricular dysfunction, or pulmonary hypertension may benefit from the placement of a pulmonary artery catheter as well. (265; **1870–1871**)

162. Patients with coronary artery disease are especially at risk of myocardial ischemia during surgery for resection of an aortic aneurysm during cross-clamping of the aorta. Cross-clamping of the aorta at the suprarenal or supraceliac levels creates the greatest increase in systemic vascular resistance, central venous pressures, and decrease in cardiac output. On the pulmonary artery catheter cross-clamping of the aorta would result in an increase in the pulmonary artery occlusion pressure. In contrast, cross-clamping the aorta below the level of the renal arteries creates minimal hemodynamic changes. The hemodynamic response to aortic cross-clamping is influenced by the patient's cardiac status, intravascular fluid volume, and anesthetic drugs and technique. Management of the patient during aortic cross-clamping should be aimed toward decreasing the systolic blood pressure and cardiac filling pressures. Pharmacologic agents that could be administered might include nitroprusside or nitroglycerin. (265; **1870–1871**)

163. Intraoperative fluid management during surgery for resection of an aortic aneurysm is best guided by the data obtained from the pulmonary artery catheter. For instance, preoperative hydration and adequate blood loss replacement can be confirmed or instituted. (265; **1874**)

164. Hypotension frequently accompanies unclamping of the abdominal aorta during the resection of an aortic aneurysm. The hypotension is believed to occur as a result of the sudden increase in venous capacitance that accompanies unclamping. Even when the aortic cross-clamp is infrarenal, unclamping can result in a decrease in the systolic blood pressure by about 40 mm Hg. Methods for minimizing the hypotension include the maintenance of pulmonary artery occlusion pressures between 10 and 20 mm Hg before unclamping and the gradual removal of the aortic cross-clamp to allow time for the pooled venous blood to circulate. It is prudent to use only short-acting vasodilators such as nitroprusside or nitroglycerin to treat increases in the systemic vascular resistance during aortic cross-clamping so that its effects can be reversed with discontinuation of the infusion before unclamping of the aorta. The systemic vascular resistance may be increased after unclamping with the administration of phenylephrine if necessary. (265; **1870–1872**)

165. Renal function may become impaired postoperatively to the extent that hemodialysis is required after aortic aneurysm repair, particularly if the aortic cross-clamp was suprarenal. Co-existing renal disease appears to place the patient at the greatest risk of postoperative renal dysfunction, but other risk factors include the duration of aortic cross-clamp time, thrombotic or embolic interruption of renal blood flow, hypovolemia, and hypotension. Hypothermia may protect the kidneys during periods of ischemia. In an effort to decrease the risk of postoperative renal dysfunction the intravascular fluid volume should be maintained and the urine output should be closely monitored during aortic aneurysm repair. Mannitol is frequently given just before aortic cross-clamping during these procedures to facilitate diuresis and maintain glomerular function. A loop diuretic may be also be administered in selected cases if the urine output is unsatisfactory. Alternatively, a continuous dopamine infusion at low doses may be started to dilate renal blood vessels to maintain renal blood flow and urine output. (265; **1874**)

166. Spinal cord ischemia and paraplegia can occur after supraceliac aortic cross-clamping for thoracic aortic aneurysm repair. The mechanism for the ischemia is most likely due to an interruption of a portion of the blood supply to the

spinal cord. The spinal cord blood supply is from two posterior arteries and one anterior spinal artery. The greatest contributor to the blood supply of the anterior spinal artery is the artery of Adamkiewicz, whose origin is between T9 and T12 in 75% of patients. The anterior spinal artery supplies the motor tracts in the spinal cord. Mechanisms employed to reduce the risk of spinal cord ischemia include cerebrospinal fluid drainage, intrathecal papaverine injection, naloxone administration, barbiturate administration, hypothermia, and partial bypass. Hypothermia is believed to be the most effective method of neuroprotection through its effects of decreasing oxygen requirements. Cerebrospinal fluid drainage is thought to improve spinal cord perfusion because the spinal cord perfusion pressure is distal mean aortic pressure minus the cerebrospinal fluid pressure. Cerebrospinal fluid drainage to improve spinal cord perfusion during aortic aneurysm repair remains controversial. (265; **1872–1874**)

CARDIOPULMONARY BYPASS

167. Blood is drained from the venae cavae during cardiopulmonary bypass by gravity. The blood then passes through an oxygenator before it is returned to the arterial system. (265, Fig. 19–3; **1786, Fig. 49–7**)

168. The two different types of pumps that are used to return blood to the arterial system during cardiopulmonary bypass are the roller pump and the centrifugal pump. The roller pump produces nonpulsatile flow and trauma to blood. It works by compressing the tubing that contains the fluid between a roller and curved metal back plate, producing sine wave flow. In contrast, the centrifugal pump produces pulsatile flow and less trauma to blood. The flow rate generated by the centrifugal pump is affected by the resistance of the tubing and the patient's systemic vascular resistance. (265–266; **1786**)

169. Blood is kept from entering the heart from the superior and inferior venae cavae during cardiopulmonary bypass by ligatures placed by the surgeons that occlude these structures and separate them from the heart. All returning blood from the patient's venous system therefore enters the cardiopulmonary bypass machine via the large cannulae that are placed in the venae cavae. (265; **1786–1787**)

170. The aorta may need to be cross-clamped distal to the aortic valve and proximal to the inflow cannula during cardiopulmonary bypass if the aortic valve is not competent. An incompetent aortic valve without this cross-clamping would allow blood to flow retrograde from the aorta into the heart. (265; **1786–1787**)

171. Venous drainage from the inferior and superior venae cavae during cardiopulmonary bypass, which is achieved by gravity, can be facilitated by raising the operating table to a higher level, creating a larger vertical distance between the operating room table and the cardiopulmonary bypass machine. (265)

172. The required cardiac index that is delivered to the patient by the roller pump on the cardiopulmonary bypass machine depends on the patient's body temperature and oxygen consumption. A cardiac index of 2 to 2.4 L/min per meter squared is usually sufficient in the normothermic or slightly hypothermic patient. Flows of about half these levels have also been used without adverse effects. (266; **1788**)

173. The advantage of low flows when a roller pump is used to deliver blood to the aorta during cardiopulmonary bypass is that less trauma is sustained to the blood. Less noncoronary collateral blood flow returns to the heart as well, which may lead to better myocardial protection because less warm blood

is entering the heart and counteracting the cold myocardial preservation solutions. (266)

174. A PaO_2 of 100 to 150 mm Hg is generally maintained in blood that is returning to the arterial system during cardiopulmonary bypass. (266; **1788**)

175. Two different types of oxygenators that are used to oxygenate blood that is returning to the arterial system during cardiopulmonary bypass are a bubble oxygenator and a membrane oxygenator. (266; **1786**)

176. Advantages of a bubble oxygenator over a membrane oxygenator include its relative simplicity, less cost, a lower priming volume, and greater oxygenation efficiency. Disadvantages of a bubble oxygenator include an increase in the amount of turbulence and foaming it produces, resulting in trauma to blood that increases with the duration of the bypass time. In fact, when cardiopulmonary bypass time is expected to be greater than 2 hours, the membrane oxygenator is preferred. (266; **1786**)

177. An advantage of a membrane oxygenator includes the relatively less trauma produced to the blood than that produced by a bubble oxygenator. Disadvantages of a membrane oxygenator include its increased complexity and cost. (266; **1786**)

178. In addition to the usual methods of heating a patient's body intraoperatively, the body can also be heated or cooled during cardiopulmonary bypass through the use of heat exchangers that are incorporated into the oxygenators. These heat exchangers are able to heat or cool blood as it circulates through the pump via a countercurrent flow system. (266)

179. Blood loss from the field can be recirculated to the patient during cardiopulmonary bypass by having the blood that is suctioned return to a cardiotomy reservoir. In the cardiotomy reservoir the blood is filtered, defoamed, and returned to the oxygenator. The blood is then recirculated to the patient after oxygenation. (266; **1797**)

180. A problem with the cardiotomy suction used during cardiopulmonary bypass is that it is a significant contributor to the hemolysis that occurs during cardiopulmonary bypass. (266)

181. Venting of the left ventricle may be necessary to prevent harmful left ventricular distention during cardiac surgery in which the heart is not opened. Persistent left ventricular distention may lead to damage to the myocardial contractile elements. There are at least three reasons why the left ventricle might need a vent during cardiopulmonary bypass. First, incompetence of the aortic valve can lead to the retrograde flow of blood from the aorta to the heart. Second, there may be a large degree of blood flow from the coronary sinus and bronchial circulation back to the heart. Third, surgical positioning may result in backward flow from the aorta into the heart, or from the heart into the pulmonary veins. Finally, venting of the ventricle or pulmonary artery can help reduce risks of elevated pulmonary artery pressures during cardiopulmonary bypass. Venting of the left ventricle is achieved through the placement of a catheter into the left ventricle, usually through a pulmonary vein and via the left atrium. (267; **1787**)

182. Systemic emboli from cellular debris are prevented from occurring during cardiopulmonary bypass through the use of filters that are incorporated into the oxygen delivery line prior to the roller pumps and in the arterial delivery system. (267; **1786**)

183. Priming of the cardiopulmonary bypass system refers to the filling of the tubing of the cardiopulmonary bypass system with fluid and sometimes blood. The fluid consists of an osmotically active substance, an osmotic diuretic, an

antibiotic, and electrolyte supplements. Blood is added if the patient's hematocrit necessitates it. (267; **1787**)

184. Hemodilution of the patient's blood to a hematocrit of 20 to 25 during cardiopulmonary bypass lessens the viscosity of the blood. This is important to facilitate circulation through the small vessels during hypothermia. (267; **1788, 1823–1824**)

185. It is essential to remove all air from the cardiopulmonary bypass system during cardiopulmonary bypass to prevent the pumping of air into the arterial system of the patient. (267; **1786, 1790–1794**)

186. Heparin-induced anticoagulation of the patient is mandatory before the institution of cardiopulmonary bypass to prevent patient death through clotting of the blood both in the patient and in the cardiopulmonary bypass machine. The dose of heparin that is usually administered is 300 to 400 units/kg. The adequacy of anticoagulation must be confirmed before the placement of the venous and aortic cannulae used for cardiopulmonary bypass. The adequacy of anticoagulation is usually confirmed by evaluating the activated clotting time, which should remain longer than 400 seconds throughout the course of cardiopulmonary bypass. The activated clotting time should be evaluated periodically during the course of cardiopulmonary bypass and additional heparin administered as necessary. After the cannulae are removed from the patient and cardiopulmonary bypass terminated, the effects of heparin may be reversed with the administration of protamine. The activated clotting time should return to baseline, typically between 90 to 120 seconds, after the administration of protamine. (267; **1787, 1795**)

187. The low mean arterial pressure often seen after the institution of cardiopulmonary bypass is believed to be due to the peripheral vasodilation caused by the decreased viscosity, decreased temperature, and low oxygen content of infused priming solution. What pressures during cardiopulmonary bypass are sufficient to allow for coronary and cerebral perfusion is a subject of great debate. Most institutions prefer mean arterial pressures to be about 50 mm Hg and to administer phenylephrine if blood pressure support is needed. Other institutions allow the mean arterial blood pressure to decrease to 30 mm Hg without any adverse effect. (267; **1788–1790**)

188. Blood pressure slowly rises spontaneously after some time on cardiopulmonary bypass as a result of vasoconstriction. The vasoconstriction may be in response to stimulation of the sympathetic nervous system or the renin-angiotensin system. It may also be an indication of inadequate perfusion to some tissues. (267; **1788**)

189. The potential dangers of hypertension while on cardiopulmonary bypass include intracerebral hemorrhage and an increase in coronary and bronchial artery circulation, leading to increased return of warm blood to the heart during a time of cold cardioplegia. Hypertension under these circumstances can be treated by decreasing the systemic vascular resistance with a nitrate or a volatile anesthetic. Vaporizers have been incorporated into the cardiopulmonary bypass circuit for the administration of a volatile anesthetic to patients while on cardiopulmonary bypass. (268; **1788**)

190. The patient can be monitored for adequate tissue perfusion during cardiopulmonary bypass several ways. First, urine output can be monitored as a guide to renal perfusion. A renal output of 1 mL/kg each hour is considered sufficient. Second, the patient's acid-base status can be monitored for any evidence of a progressive metabolic acidosis. Third, the patient's mixed venous oxygen tension can be monitored for evidence of excessive oxygen extraction. A mixed venous Po_2 lower than 30 mm Hg is generally regarded

as evidence of inadequate tissue perfusion. Finally, the nasopharyngeal temperature can be compared with a core temperature such as the bladder, rectum, skeletal muscle, or skin temperature. Whereas bladder temperature represents core temperature, the nasopharyngeal temperature is an indicator of perfusion to the brain. The greater the discrepancy between these two, the greater the indication of poor cerebral perfusion. (267–268; **1788, 1795–1796**)

191. Diuresis is induced during cardiopulmonary bypass due to the inclusion of mannitol in the priming solution, hypothermia which interferes with renal tubular absorption, and well-perfused renal glomeruli with blood low in oncotic pressure due to hemodilution. For this reason during cardiopulmonary bypass the minimally acceptable urine output is 1 mL/kg per hour. Adequate urine output is important for the excretion of potassium administered in the cardioplegia solution. When the urine output is less than desired, a mechanical obstruction to urine flow in the catheter should be considered before instituting methods to increase the urine output. (267; **1785, 1796**)

192. Causes of an increasing central venous pressure with or without facial edema while on cardiopulmonary bypass include aortic cannula flow into the carotid artery, obstruction of the superior vena cava cannula, and obstruction of jugular venous drainage by either a cannula, head position, or neck compression. Inadequate venous return from the patient to the cardiopulmonary bypass machine is an indication that one of these may have occurred. (267; **1787, Table 49–19**)

193. Causes of increasing abdominal distention while on cardiopulmonary bypass include obstruction of the inferior vena cava cannula, intra-abdominal hemorrhage or ascites, or gastrointestinal distention by gas or fluid. (267; **1788, Table 49–19**)

194. The most serious complications that require immediate discontinuation of cardiopulmonary bypass and the resumption of the patient's own cardiac output include aortic dissection, carotid artery superperfusion, and air in the aortic inflow tubing. (267; **1787**)

195. Ventilation of the lungs of a patient is not necessary during cardiopulmonary bypass. The lungs can be ventilated with oxygen during partial cardiopulmonary bypass, or when there is partial pulmonary blood flow. Evidence of pulmonary blood flow is seen as pulsatile pulmonary artery flow on the pulmonary artery catheter tracing. (267; **1795**)

196. The goal of myocardial preservation during cardiopulmonary bypass is the minimization of the effects of ischemia on the heart. This is achieved a variety of ways, all of which are aimed toward reducing the myocardial oxygen requirement of the heart during that period. Myocardial cooling can be achieved by hypothermic cardiopulmonary bypass, by the direct placement of ice on the epicardium, through pericardial irrigation with iced fluid, and by the intracoronary infusion of a cold cardioplegia solution. Myocardial arrest is achieved by the continuous infusion of cardioplegia solution containing potassium both through a cannula at the aortic root and by retrograde flow through the coronary sinuses. The potassium causes cessation of electrical and mechanical cardiac activity by blocking the initial phase of myocardial depolarization. The prevention of myocardial rewarming during cardiopulmonary bypass can be achieved by placing a vent in the left ventricle or by placing a cross-clamp in the aorta distal to the aortic valve when aortic valve incompetence allows the retrograde flow of blood into the heart. (268; **1790**)

197. The oxygen consumption of a normally contracting heart at 30°C is 8 to 10 mL/100 g of heart muscle in a minute. The oxygen consumption of a fibrillating heart at 22°C is 2 mL/100 g per minute, and the oxygen consump-

tion of an electromechanically quiet heart at 22°C is approximately 0.3 mL/ 100 g per minute. (268)

198. The effectiveness of cold cardioplegia of the heart can be measured by placing a temperature probe in the left ventricle and directly measuring the temperature of the heart. The absence of any electrical activity on the heart is also a good indication that the heart muscle is effectively quiescent. (268; **1790**)

199. Two potential negative effects of the intramyocardial hyperkalemia of the cold cardioplegia solutions after cardiopulmonary bypass are decreased myocardial contractility and an increased incidence of atrioventricular heart block while coming off cardiopulmonary bypass. These can both be treated with the administration of calcium and, if necessary, insulin with or without glucose. In addition, the atrioventricular block can be treated through the use of an artificial cardiac pacemaker. The pacemaker is usually only needed temporarily because the atrioventricular block typically only lasts for 1 to 2 hours after discontinuing cardiopulmonary bypass. (268; **1790**)

200. Two potential sources for systemic hyperkalemia during cardiopulmonary bypass are the recirculation of cardioplegia solution that has drained into the blood and decreased renal function. Hyperkalemia that persists at the conclusion of cardiopulmonary bypass can be treated with the administration of insulin and glucose in addition to calcium. (268; **1790**)

201. Although there is a decreased MAC under hypothermic conditions, the decrease in MAC is not sufficient to offset the sudden dilution of anesthetics that occurs when the patient is placed on cardiopulmonary bypass. For this reason, supplemental intravenous anesthetics should be administered during cardiopulmonary bypass to ensure an adequate depth of anesthesia. (268)

202. There is a sudden dilution of the neuromuscular blocking drug level that occurs when the patient is placed on cardiopulmonary bypass. Supplemental neuromuscular blocking drug might be administered during cardiopulmonary bypass to ensure there is a neuromuscular blocking drug level sufficient to prevent patient movement during this important portion of the procedure. (268)

203. Although supplemental anesthesia is not routinely required during rewarming after the conclusion of cardiopulmonary bypass, it is important that the anesthesiologist be aware that the rewarming patient may be returning to consciousness in a paralyzed state. If supplemental anesthetics are given at this time, those that lack cardiac depressant effects, such as an opioid or benzodiazepine, are ideally chosen. (268; **1790**)

204. Conditions in the patient that must be present for the discontinuation of cardiopulmonary bypass include hemodynamic stability; normothermia; the venting of all arterial air; an adequate cardiac rate, rhythm, and output; normal acid-base status and electrolyte levels; ventilation of the lungs; and an adequate intravascular status and hematocrit. (268; **1790–1795, Table 49–21**)

205. The aortic and vena cava cannulae are removed after an adequate blood pressure and cardiac output have been maintained by the heart for several minutes. The ability to reestablish cardiopulmonary bypass should be maintained for some time after the discontinuation of cardiopulmonary bypass. (268; **1790**)

206. Potential problems associated with persistent hypothermia after cardiopulmonary bypass include coagulopathy, hypertension, tachycardia and sympathetic nervous system stimulation, shivering, metabolic acidosis, and difficulty in defibrillating the heart and maintaining a normal cardiac rhythm. The effects

of persistent hypothermia on the heart are particularly evident at temperatures less than 34°C. Rewarming a patient's body can be achieved more rapidly through the administration of a vasodilator such as nitroprusside or a volatile anesthetic. (268; **1796**)

207. Special precautions that must be taken before discontinuing cardiopulmonary bypass in patients who have had the heart opened, as during valve replacement surgery, is the venting of all air from the heart. This can be accomplished by surgical massage of the left atrium and ventricle. In addition, rotating the table from side-to-side simultaneous with the maintenance of positive pressure ventilation of the lungs and placement of the patient's head at a lower level than the heart may assist in venting any air from the heart. Positive pressure of the lungs should be maintained during the removal of the left ventricle vent cannula. The avoidance of nitrous oxide administration after cardiopulmonary bypass might minimize the potential increase in the size of microemboli that may have occurred. The potential risk of air remaining in the heart at the conclusion of cardiopulmonary bypass is the embolization of air to the arterial circulation, especially the coronary and cerebral circulations. Air is most likely to embolize from the heart after cardiopulmonary bypass during manipulation of the heart and alterations in the anatomy, closure of the sternum, and movement of the patient. (268; **1790–1795**)

208. (269, Table 19–5)

BLOOD PRESSURE	ATRIAL PRESSURE	CARDIAC OUTPUT	DIAGNOSIS	THERAPY
Decreased	Increased	Decreased	Left ventricular dysfunction	Inotrope Vasodilator Mechanical assistance
Decreased	Decreased	Decreased	Hypovolemia	Intravascular fluid administration
Decreased	Decreased	Increased	Vasodilation, low blood viscosity	Erythrocyte administration
Increased	Increased	Decreased	Vasoconstriction, left ventricular dysfunction	Vasodilator Inotrope
Increased	Decreased	Increased	Hyperdynamic	Volatile anesthetic Beta antagonist

209. Posterior papillary muscle dysfunction after cardiopulmonary bypass can occur as a result of inadequate cooling of the posterior myocardium during cardiopulmonary bypass. The posterior myocardium is the portion of the heart muscle that is most vulnerable to inadvertent warming of the heart from the return of blood from the coronary and bronchial circulations, as well as any potential blood that flows retrograde via an incompetent aortic valve. Posterior papillary muscle function impairment would manifest as mitral regurgitation. In addition, prominent v waves would be evident on the pulmonary artery occlusion pressure tracing. (269)

210. In some situations the cardiac output of the patient on discontinuation of cardiopulmonary bypass is inadequate, because of either poor myocardial function or refractory myocardial ischemia. Under these circumstances the intra-aortic balloon pump is a mechanical alternative to the pharmacologic support of cardiac output. An intra-aortic balloon pump is a balloon that is 25 cm long and mounted on a long plastic catheter. The pump is advanced from the left femoral artery to the aorta. The pump inflates and deflates timed to the electrocardiogram. Inflation of the balloon, which occurs during diastole, increases the diastolic blood pressure and increases the coronary

perfusion pressure gradient. Deflation of the balloon occurs just before systole. This allows for a reduction of afterload and the pressure against which the heart has to pump. Overall the intra-aortic balloon pump decreases the work of the myocardium and thus the myocardial oxygen requirement. The efficacy of the balloon pump is altered by rapid heart rates and cardiac dysrhythmias. (269; **1764**)

211. Protamine administration after cardiopulmonary bypass should take place after the removal of the aortic and vena cava cannulae. Protamine is administered to reverse the anticoagulant effects produced by heparin. (269; **1795**)

212. Side effects associated with the administration of protamine include hypotension due to myocardial depression, pulmonary hypertension, histamine release, systemic vasodilation, and, rarely, anaphylactic or anaphylactoid reactions. Anaphylactic and anaphylactoid reactions can be associated with bronchospasm and pulmonary edema. These potential effects of protamine call for the careful, slow titration of protamine over the course of 3 to 5 minutes. (269; **1795**)

213. Blood and fluid that remain in the cardiopulmonary bypass circuit after cardiopulmonary bypass are washed, collected, and placed in plastic bags by the perfusionist. The blood and fluid can then be administered to the patient. (269)

214. A gradient between central aortic and radial artery blood pressures can exist in the early period after cardiopulmonary bypass. Although the exact mechanism for this is not known, it is believed to be due to vasodilation in the extremity. The discrepancy can be determined by the surgical placement of a needle in the aorta and transduction of the pressure. Although the duration of this effect is typically only about 60 minutes, a femoral artery catheter can be placed for the transduction of arterial pressure if the discrepancy is large. (269–270; **1790**)

Chapter 19

Chronic Pulmonary Disease

OBSTRUCTIVE AIRWAY DISEASE

1. What are some examples of obstructive airway disease?

2. What is obstructive airway disease?

3. Why does arterial hypoxemia occur in patients with obstructive airway disease?

4. Why does carbon dioxide retention occur in patients with obstructive airway disease?

5. What physical examination findings, radiographic findings, and pulmonary function results are commonly found in patients with obstructive airway disease?

6. Approximately what percent of the population of the United States is estimated to have bronchial asthma? Are males or females more likely to have bronchial asthma? At what age are patients most likely to develop symptoms of bronchial asthma?

7. What characterizes bronchial asthma?

8. What are some potential stimulants for airway hyperreactivity in patients with bronchial asthma?

9. How is the diagnosis of bronchial asthma made?

10. What are some of the physical examination findings noted in patients with bronchial asthma during periods of normal pulmonary function? What are some of the physical examination findings noted in patients with bronchial asthma during periods of exacerbation of their asthma?

11. What are some findings found in the pulmonary function studies and flow-volume loops of patients with bronchial asthma during an exacerbation?

12. Please complete the following table:

DEGREE OF EXPIRATORY AIR FLOW OBSTRUCTION	FEV_1 (% predicted)	Pao_2 (mm Hg)	$Paco_2$ (mm Hg)
Mild–moderate			
Severe			

13. What agents are commonly used to treat bronchial asthma?

14. How effective is aminophylline for the treatment of bronchial asthma? What are some of the potential side effects of aminophylline?

15. How can an acute asthmatic attack be treated?

16. How should the patient with bronchial asthma be assessed preoperatively?

17. How should a patient with bronchial asthma have his or her pulmonary status assessed before undergoing a thoracic or abdominal procedure?

18. When might corticosteroid supplementation be necessary in patients intraoperatively?

19. Why might regional anesthesia be the preferred anesthetic choice in patients with bronchial asthma who are scheduled to undergo surgery on the extremities?

20. What is the goal of the anesthesia management of patients with bronchial asthma?

21. What agents may be used for the induction of general anesthesia in patients with bronchial asthma? What is an advantage and a disadvantage of ketamine for these patients?

22. Why is it prudent to have a sufficient depth of anesthesia before intubation of the trachea of a person with bronchial asthma? What are some methods by which this can be accomplished?

23. Which neuromuscular blocking drugs are associated with histamine release? What is the concern regarding the use of these neuromuscular blocking drugs in patients with bronchial asthma?

24. What is the benefit of using a slow respiratory rate when mechanically ventilating the lungs of a patient with bronchial asthma?

25. What is the potential drawback of using positive end-expiratory pressure in patients with bronchial asthma during mechanical ventilation of the lungs?

26. What is a benefit of maintaining adequate hydration intraoperatively in patients with bronchial asthma?

27. When surgery has concluded, what are the options for extubation of the trachea that will minimize the degree of airway hyperreactivity in response to manipulation of the endotracheal tube?

28. How does the reversal of nondepolarizing neuromuscular blocking drugs with anticholinesterase drugs affect the airway resistance of patients with bronchial asthma?

29. Name at least five potential causes of intraoperative bronchospasm.

30. How should intraoperative bronchospasm be treated?

31. What characterizes pulmonary emphysema physiologically?

32. Why is the work of breathing increased in patients with pulmonary emphysema? Why are patients with pulmonary emphysema commonly classified as "pink puffers"?

33. For patients with pulmonary emphysema who are scheduled to undergo a surgical procedure, what should the preoperative evaluation include? When might preoperative pulmonary function tests be necessary?

34. What are some pulmonary function test and arterial blood gas measurement results that indicate that the patient is at an increased risk of postoperative respiratory failure? What are some treatment interventions that may be warranted by the preoperative evaluation of the patient's pulmonary function?

35. What is the goal for the anesthetic management of patients with pulmonary emphysema? How can this be achieved?

36. What are some potential disadvantages of using nitrous oxide as part of a general anesthetic in patients with pulmonary emphysema?

37. What are two methods by which anesthesiologists may minimize the drying of secretions in the airways of patients with pulmonary emphysema in the intraoperative period?

38. What ventilatory settings are appropriate for intraoperative mechanical ventilation of the lungs of patients with pulmonary emphysema?

39. What are some indications for surgical bullectomy? How can anesthetic management of patients undergoing surgical bullectomy be achieved?

40. What characterizes chronic bronchitis physiologically? What is the major predisposing factor to the development of chronic bronchitis?

41. Why are patients with chronic bronchitis commonly classified as "blue bloaters"?

42. Please complete the following table comparing pulmonary emphysema to chronic bronchitis:

		PULMONARY EMPHYSEMA	CHRONIC BRONCHITIS
FEV_1	(increased or decreased)		
Total lung capacity	(increased or decreased)		
Arterial hypoxemia	(early or late)		
Hypercarbia	(early or late)		
Cor pulmonale	(early or late)		
Hematocrit	(normal or increased)		
Dyspnea	(moderate or severe)		

43. How does the preoperative evaluation and intraoperative management of anesthesia for patients with chronic bronchitis compare with that for patients with pulmonary emphysema?

RESTRICTIVE PULMONARY DISEASE

44. What characterizes restrictive lung disease?

45. What is the physiologic cause of acute restrictive lung disease? What are some common causes of acute restrictive lung disease?

46. What is the physiologic cause of chronic restrictive lung disease? What are some common causes of chronic restrictive lung disease?

47. Why are patients with restrictive lung disease commonly dyspneic? What is the breathing pattern commonly seen in these patients?

48. What $PaCO_2$ is commonly seen in patients with restrictive lung disease?

49. Please complete the following table comparing normal lungs to the lungs of a patient with restrictive lung disease:

	NORMAL LUNGS	RESTRICTIVE LUNG DISEASE
Total lung capacity	Normal	
Vital capacity	Normal	
Functional residual capacity	Normal	
Tidal volume	Normal	
Inspiratory reserve volume	Normal	
Expiratory reserve volume	Normal	
Residual volume	Normal	
Forced exhaled volume in 1 second	Normal	

50. Why might a regional anesthetic that achieves a sensory level above T10 make ventilation difficult for patients with restrictive lung disease?

51. How does restrictive lung disease influence the choice of drugs to be used for general anesthesia?

52. What are some preoperative indications that patients with restrictive lung disease may require postoperative mechanical ventilation of the lungs?

53. Why are patients with restrictive lung disease at risk of having difficulty clearing their airways of secretions in the postoperative period?

ANESTHESIA FOR THORACIC SURGERY

54. What are some preoperative considerations for the patient scheduled to undergo thoracic surgery?

55. What are some specific preoperative history and physical examination findings that are indicative of an increased risk of postoperative pulmonary complications after thoracic surgery?

56. What are some preoperative prophylactic measures that may be taken in an attempt to minimize postoperative pulmonary complications?

57. How does cigarette smoking affect the lungs physiologically?

58. What is the benefit of the preoperative cessation of cigarette smoking? After what duration of time after the cessation of smoking are these benefits noted to occur?

59. What is the utility of preoperative pulmonary function tests before thoracic surgery? For which patients are preoperative pulmonary function tests indicated?

60. What values derived from pulmonary function tests are indicative of an increased risk of postoperative pulmonary morbidity after pneumonectomy?

61. What value for maximal breathing capacity is indicative of an increased risk of postoperative pulmonary morbidity after pneumonectomy?

62. What ratio of FEV_1 to forced vital capacity is usually noted before an increase in the baseline Pa_{CO_2}?

63. What is the reasoning behind the preoperative institution of digitalis prophylaxis for patients undergoing pulmonary tissue resection? When is it instituted?

64. What is a potential disadvantage of the prophylactic institution of digitalis for patients undergoing pulmonary tissue resection?

65. What are some benefits of the administration of volatile anesthetics for patients undergoing thoracic surgery?

66. What is a disadvantage of the administration of nitrous oxide for patients undergoing thoracic surgery?

67. What is a benefit of the administration of nondepolarizing neuromuscular blocking drugs for patients undergoing thoracic surgery?

68. What intraoperative monitors may be useful during thoracic surgery?

69. How does the lateral decubitus position during mechanical ventilation of the lungs affect the ventilation-to-perfusion ratio in the lungs?

70. What are some absolute indications for single-lung ventilation during surgery and anesthesia? What are some relative indications for single-lung ventilation during surgery and anesthesia?

71. What is the most frequently used double-lumen endotracheal tube used for the isolation of the right or left lung or for single-lung ventilation during thoracic surgery?

72. What is the potential problem with an endobronchial tube placed in the right bronchus for isolation of the right lung? How can this problem be avoided?

73. What depth in centimeters typically places the endobronchial tube in approximately the correct position in most adult patients of average height?

74. How is the proper placement of a double-lumen endotracheal tube best confirmed?

75. What is the single-lumen Univent tube? What is its potential advantage for one-lung ventilation?

76. How does one-lung ventilation compare with two-lung ventilation in a patient in the lateral decubitus position with respect to the pulmonary ventilation-to-perfusion ratio?

77. What are four factors that influence the amount of perfusion that goes to the nondependent, unventilated lung during one-lung ventilation of a patient in the lateral decubitus position with a double-lumen endotracheal tube?

78. How should the patient be monitored for arterial hypoxemia during one-lung ventilation for thoracic surgery?

79. What is the most beneficial intervention that can be made when arterial hypoxemia is noted in a patient during one-lung ventilation for thoracic surgery?

80. How frequently do patients have arterial hypercapnia during one-lung ventilation for thoracic surgery?

81. Why is the placement of chest tubes after thoracic surgery necessary postoperatively?

82. When should extubation of the trachea after thoracic surgery occur?

83. What is the most common postoperative pulmonary complication after thoracic surgery? What are some other serious postoperative complications after thoracic surgery?

84. What is the importance of adequate analgesia after thoracic surgery?

MEDIASTINOSCOPY

85. What is the most frequent reason for the performance of a mediastinoscopy?

86. Why is positive pressure of the lungs recommended during a mediastinoscopy?

87. What vital arterial vessels may be compressed during a mediastinoscopy?

88. What is the explanation for the bradycardia that may be seen during a mediastinoscopy? How should it be treated?

89. What are the most common complications that can occur after the performance of a mediastinoscopy?

THORACOSCOPY

90. What are some indications for the performance of thoracoscopy?

91. How can anesthesia for thoracoscopy be achieved?

BRONCHOPLEURAL FISTULA

92. What is the appropriate anesthetic management of a patient with a bronchopleural fistula?

ANSWERS*

OBSTRUCTIVE AIRWAY DISEASE

1. Examples of obstructive airway diseases include bronchial asthma, emphysema, chronic bronchitis, and cystic fibrosis. Emphysema and chronic bronchitis are

---

*Numbers in parentheses: lightface numbers refer to pages, figures, or tables in Stoelting RK, Miller RD: Basics of Anesthesia, 4th ed. Philadelphia, Churchill Livingstone, 2000; **boldface numbers** refer to pages, figures, or tables in Miller RD: Anesthesia, 5th ed. Philadelphia, Churchill Livingstone, 2000.

examples of chronic obstructive pulmonary disease. These diseases are characterized by the progressive, persistent obstruction to air flow. Bronchial asthma is distinguished from chronic obstructive pulmonary diseases owing to the nature of its airway hyperreactivity and its acute, reversible increases in airway obstruction. Patients with long-standing bronchial asthma may develop irreversible air flow obstruction, resulting in chronic obstructive pulmonary disease. (271; **2436–2437**)

2. Obstructive airway disease is characterized by a decrease in the maximal rate of exhalation due to the obstruction of air flow. These patients may have hyperinflated lungs, an increased work of breathing, and impaired pulmonary gas exchange. Obstructive airway disease is chronic when airway obstruction persists despite aggressive therapy. Obstructive airway disease is the most frequent cause of chronic pulmonary dysfunction. (271; **2436–2437**)

3. Arterial hypoxemia occurs in patients with obstructive airway disease as a result of areas of ventilation-to-perfusion mismatching. Areas of ventilation-to-perfusion mismatching occur from regional differences in airway resistance. (271; **2436–2437**)

4. Carbon dioxide retention occurs in patients with obstructive airway disease as a result of regional hypoventilation. (271; **2436–2437**)

5. Patients with obstructive airway disease often appear dyspneic and use their accessory muscles to breathe. They may have a cough and produce sputum. On chest auscultation these patients may have decreased breath sounds. Patients with obstructive airway disease often wheeze on exhalation. Wheezing is the sound produced by turbulent gas flow through narrowed airways. On the chest radiograph the diaphragm often appears flat and low. The lung fields may appear hyperlucent and the lungs hyperinflated. Pulmonary function studies in patients with obstructive airway disease likely reveal a decrease in the FEV_1, or the volume of gas that can be exhaled in 1 second. The vital capacity is typically decreased as well, but not to as great an extent as the FEV_1. This results in a decrease in the FEV_1/FVC ratio. An FEV_1/FVC value less than 70% reflects mild obstructive airway disease, an FEV_1/FVC value less than 60% reflects moderate obstructive airway disease, and an FEV_1/FVC value less than 50% reflects severe obstructive airway disease. (271; **886, 899–900**)

6. In the United States, 3% to 6% of the population is estimated to have bronchial asthma. Two thirds of patients with asthma are male, and two thirds of the patients with asthma developed symptoms before 5 years of age. (271; **2436**)

7. Bronchial asthma is characterized by the presence of an obstruction to air flow on exhalation that is reversible, increased airway hyperreactivity resulting from bronchial smooth muscle contraction in response to stimuli, chronic inflammatory changes in the submucosa of the airways, and occasional edema of the mucosa and the production of secretions. (271; **2436**)

8. Potential stimulants of airway hyperreactivity may include allergens, exercise, cold weather, viral infections, medicines, or mechanical airway stimulation. Airway hyperreactivity may occur even in patients with a history of bronchial asthma who are currently asymptomatic. (271; **2436**)

9. The diagnosis of bronchial asthma is made primarily clinically. The sputum taken from patients with bronchial asthma often contains eosinophils, in contrast to the neutrophils most commonly found in the sputum of patients with bronchitis. Patients with obstruction to air flow on expiration on spirometry that improves by 15% after bronchodilator therapy is further evidence of bronchial asthma that is suggested by clinical history. (271, Fig. 20–1; **961**)

10. Patients with bronchial asthma during periods of normal pulmonary function are typically devoid of any signs of pulmonary disease on physical examination. During periods of exacerbation, patients with bronchial asthma often have expiratory wheezing, a cough, breathlessness, and a sensation of chest tightness. Patients may also produce tenacious sputum. As the severity of the obstruction to expiratory flow increases, patients become increasingly dyspneic. Whereas initially arterial oxygenation may be normal and slight hypocapnia may be present, worsening obstruction and tiring patients may exemplify arterial hypoxemia and hypercapnia. (271–272; **963–964**)

11. Pulmonary function studies of patients with bronchial asthma during an exacerbation reveal a decrease in the FEV_1 and forced expiratory flow in relation to the vital capacity. The FEV_1 may be used as a measure of the degree of obstruction and the effectiveness of interventions. The flow-volume loop of patients with bronchial asthma during an exacerbation reveals a downward scooping of the expiratory limb of the loop that is characteristic of bronchial asthma. (272, Figs. 20–1, 20–2, Table 20–2; **893–894, 899–900, Figs. 24–12, 24–13, 24–14, 24–15**)

12. (272, Table 20–1; **893–894**)

DEGREE OF EXPIRATORY AIR FLOW OBSTRUCTION	FEV_1 (% predicted)	Pao_2 (mm Hg)	$Paco_2$ (mm Hg)
Mild–moderate	50–80	>60	<45
Severe	<35	<60	>50

13. Agents commonly used to treat bronchial asthma on a chronic basis include anti-inflammatory agents and bronchodilators. Inhaled corticosteroids are considered the first line of therapy to control the consistently present airway inflammation. When inhaled corticosteroids are insufficient to control symptoms, bronchodilators are added to the regimen. Selective beta-2 agonists such as albuterol dilate the bronchial smooth muscle most effectively. Beta-2 agonists are administered chronically using a metered-dose inhaler. Other bronchodilating agents include theophylline and anticholinergics. Anticholinergics act by blocking muscarinic receptors in the smooth muscle of the airways and inhibiting vagal tone. Anticholinergics also increase the viscosity of secretions and can make the elimination of secretions from the airways difficult. Ipratropium is an anticholinergic delivered by metered-dose inhaler. (272; **962–965, 2436**)

14. Theophylline is administered to patients with bronchial asthma for its effects of bronchodilation and improved contractility of the diaphragm. Theophylline is typically used for the treatment of bronchial asthma as a third line of treatment. Aminophylline is a preparation of theophylline used intravenously. Potential side effects of aminophylline include cardiac dysrhythmias and seizures when the plasma concentration is greater than about 20 mg/L. (272; **2436–2437**)

15. An acute asthmatic attack should be treated with the administration of oxygen, the continuous administration of beta-2 agonists, and intravenously administered glucocorticoids. The administration of beta-2 agonists may be either nebulized, subcutaneous, or intravenous. In patients with status asthmaticus in whom this therapy is not sufficient, as evidenced by progressive respiratory distress, mental status changes, or a progressively increasing $Paco_2$, intubation of the trachea and mechanical ventilation of the lungs may become necessary. These patients may also benefit from the administration of a volatile anesthetic such as isoflurane that effectively bronchodilates the airways. (272; **2436–2437, 2465–2466**)

16. The preoperative assessment of patients with bronchial asthma should include a history of any recent exacerbations of bronchial asthma or current symptoms, a physical examination in which dyspnea or wheezing is excluded, and the current medicine regimen. Patients without wheezing or dyspnea are not experiencing an exacerbation of their asthma. These patients should continue their medicine regimen throughout the perioperative period. Chest physiotherapy, antibiotics if necessary, and adequate hydration all may provide some benefit to the patient in the preoperative period. Patients who are symptomatic or display symptoms, or who have had a recent exacerbation, may benefit from postponement of elective surgery until their medical status can be optimized. (273; **899–902, 963–964, 966, 1672–1673, Table 48–5**)

17. The pulmonary status of a patient with bronchial asthma who is scheduled to undergo a thoracic or abdominal procedure may be assessed preoperatively with pulmonary function studies. An evaluation of pulmonary function before and after bronchodilating drugs may indicate what benefit is derived from bronchodilator treatment. In the event of concern regarding the patient's ventilatory status or arterial oxygenation, arterial blood gases may be measured. (273; **899–902, 962–965**)

18. Patients on chronic corticosteroid therapy may need to have supplementation with exogenous corticosteroids intraoperatively during major surgery if chronic adrenal cortex suppression is a possibility. (273; **962–966, 1673, Table 48–6**)

19. Regional anesthesia may be preferred over general anesthesia in patients with bronchial asthma who are scheduled to undergo surgery on the extremities to avoid any instrumentation of the airway that may lead to bronchospasm. (273)

20. The goal of the anesthesia management of patients with bronchial asthma is the avoidance of precipitating bronchoconstriction of the patient's hyperreactive airways. (273; **2436**)

21. All intravenous induction agents may be used for the induction of general anesthesia in patients with bronchial asthma. Propofol and ketamine both appear to have bronchodilating effects. The advantage of ketamine under these circumstances is its sympathomimetic effects of relaxation of bronchial smooth muscle. A potential drawback of ketamine administration in these patients is the increased secretions that are associated with its administration. (273; **2436**)

22. A sufficient depth of anesthesia before intubation of the trachea of a person with bronchial asthma minimizes the risk of hyperreactive airway reflexes leading to bronchospasm. Methods by which the patient can be adequately anesthetized include sufficient intravenous induction doses, the administration of lidocaine as a bolus, and the administration of a volatile anesthetic by hand ventilation. Volatile anesthetics appear to bronchodilate through the release of nitric oxide and prostanoids from normal bronchial epithelium. Because these patients are frequently on beta agonists and aminophylline, the administration of halothane that sensitizes the myocardium to the cardiac dysrhythmic effects of circulating catecholamines may not be as good a choice of inhaled anesthetic as isoflurane or sevoflurane. (273; **898, 2436–2437**)

23. Neuromuscular blocking drugs associated with histamine release include succinylcholine, atracurium, mivacurium, and *d*-tubocurarine. The concern regarding the use of these neuromuscular blocking drugs in patients with bronchial asthma is that the release of histamine may increase airway resistance, although this has not been shown to be significant clinically. (273–274; **442–443, 2436**)

24. A slow respiratory rate during mechanical ventilation of the lungs of a patient with bronchial asthma allows time for the passive exhalation of gases from

potentially obstructed airways. This is especially true in patients whose lungs are obstructed and in whom air trapping in the lungs is a risk. (274; **2436–2437**)

25. A potential drawback of using positive end-expiratory pressure during mechanical ventilation of the lungs of patients with bronchial asthma is that the passive exhalation of the gases from potentially obstructed distal airways may be even further impaired. This can result in air trapping, or the accumulation of air in the distal airways that becomes so voluminous that it can impair venous return to the extent that hypotension results. (274; **2436–2437**)

26. Adequate intraoperative hydration of patients with bronchial asthma may facilitate the removal of secretions from the airways by making the secretions less viscous. (274; **607–608, 966**)

27. Extubation of the trachea at the conclusion of surgery in patients with bronchial asthma can be achieved with the patient still deeply anesthetized. This allows for a sufficient level of anesthesia while manipulating the airway during extubation of the trachea and no instrumentation of the airway with the lightening of anesthesia. If extubation of the trachea while deeply anesthetized is contraindicated, the patient must be allowed to awaken with the endotracheal tube still in place in the trachea. This could potentially lead to bronchospasm. To minimize the risk of bronchospasm under these conditions, intravenous lidocaine as a bolus may be administered to the patient on awakening and before extubation. (274; **1446**)

28. The reversal of nondepolarizing neuromuscular blocking drugs with anticholinesterase drugs does not appear to affect the airway resistance of patients with bronchial asthma, although in theory it could secondary to its effects of stimulation of cholinergic receptors in the airway. The co-administration of an anticholinergic with the anticholinesterase for the reversal of neuromuscular blockade may explain why increases in airway resistance do not occur. (274)

29. Potential causes of intraoperative bronchospasm include mechanical obstruction, an inadequate depth of anesthesia, pulmonary aspiration, endobronchial intubation, pneumothorax, pulmonary embolus, and acute bronchial asthma. (274)

30. Intraoperative bronchospasm requires a search for a possible cause other than acute bronchial asthma, even in asthmatic patients. Indeed, patients with bronchial asthma rarely have acute bronchial asthma exacerbations intraoperatively, particularly if they were asymptomatic preoperatively. Once other causes of bronchospasm have been considered, intraoperative bronchospasm can be treated by increasing the depth of anesthesia with a volatile anesthetic that bronchodilates the airways. For continued bronchospasm, inhaled or subcutaneous beta-2 agonists should be administered. Persistent bronchospasm should be treated with the administration of intravenous corticosteroids. Bronchospasm sufficiently severe to impair ventilation and/or oxygenation may require prompt treatment with intravenous epinephrine. (274; **2436–2437**)

31. Pulmonary emphysema is characterized by the loss of elastic recoil of the lungs due to the destruction of lung parenchyma. The loss of elastic recoil leads to collapse of the airways during exhalation, which in turn leads to an increase in airway resistance. The obstruction of airway outflow can lead to the enlargement of air spaces, or bullae, distal to the terminal bronchioles. (274; **962–965**)

32. A loss of elastic recoil of the lungs leads to an increase in the resistance of the airways, which in turn leads to an increase in the work of breathing in patients with pulmonary emphysema. These patients are commonly classified as "pink puffers" as a result of the high minute ventilation these patients usually need to maintain to overcome the increase in airway resistance. The high minute ventilation maintains arterial blood gases near normal. (274; **966, 2437**)

33. The preoperative evaluation of patients with pulmonary emphysema should include an assessment of the patient's current symptoms of dyspnea, cough, and sputum production. The exercise tolerance of the patient should also be assessed. Based on the clinical history, physical examination findings, and the surgical procedure, preoperative pulmonary function tests and arterial blood gas measurements may be indicated. These studies may help to determine the extent of disease, whether there are any reversible components of the disease such as bronchospasm or infection, and the risk of postoperative respiratory failure. (274; **962–965**)

34. The major concern for patients with pulmonary emphysema who are scheduled to undergo surgical procedures is the risk of postoperative respiratory failure and the need for prolonged intubation of the trachea. Pulmonary function test results that indicate that the patient is at an increased risk for postoperative respiratory failure include a vital capacity less than 50% predicted, an FEV_1 less than 2 L, an FEV_1 less than 50% predicted, or the presence of arterial hypoxemia or hypercarbia. A $PaCO_2$ measurement of 50 mm Hg or higher on arterial blood gas analysis is also an indication that the patient is at an increased risk of postoperative respiratory failure. Arterial hypoxemia and/or the detection of cor pulmonale warrant treatment with supplemental oxygen in an attempt to decrease pulmonary vascular resistance. If antibiotic therapy or bronchodilator therapy has been instituted for any reversible component of disease, preoperative pulmonary function tests may be repeated. (274; **962–965, Table 25–39**)

35. The goal for the anesthetic management of patients with pulmonary emphysema is to minimize the risk of postoperative respiratory failure. Patients whose operative site is an extremity or the lower abdomen may benefit from a peripheral nerve block or regional anesthesia. General anesthesia may be accomplished through the administration of volatile anesthetics, possibly in conjunction with nitrous oxide. Opioids should be administered in minimal doses to avoid decreasing the patient's ventilatory drive postoperatively. (274–275; **1278, 2437**)

36. Disadvantages of using nitrous oxide as part of a general anesthetic in patients with pulmonary emphysema include the potential for nitrous oxide to diffuse into air spaces, or bullae, in the lung and cause expansion of the bullac. Expansion of the bullae could lead to rupture and a tension pneumothorax. Another disadvantage of administering nitrous oxide in thesc patients is that the concentration of oxygen that can be concurrently administered is limited. (275; **84, 1732**)

37. Two methods by which anesthesiologists may minimize the drying of secretions in the airways of patients with pulmonary emphysema in the intraoperative period is through the humidification of inspired gases and the maintenance of adequate hydration intraoperatively. (275; **1674, 2436–2437**)

38. Mechanical ventilation of the lungs intraoperatively in patients with pulmonary emphysema requires large tidal volumes and a slow respiratory rate. The goal is maintenance of normal arterial blood gases with an adequate minute ventilation while still allowing sufficient time for the passive exhalation of gases in the lungs. A slow respiratory rate also allows sufficient time for venous return to the heart. (275; **2436–2437**)

39. Patients with lung cysts and bullae are typically at the end-stage of emphysematous lung disease. Surgical bullectomy is indicated when these patients have incapacitating dyspnea, when expanding bullae compress functional lung tissues, or if there are recurrent tension pneumothoraces. The goal of the anesthetic management of patients undergoing surgical bullectomy is the avoidance of causing rupture of bullae and inducing a tension pneumothorax. This can be

accomplished through the placement of a double-lumen endobronchial tube in the anesthetized, spontaneously ventilating patient. Anesthesia should be maintained with 100% oxygen and volatile anesthetic with minimal opioids. Nitrous oxide should be avoided because of its potential for increasing bullae size and its potential for increasing the size of a pneumothorax should one occur. When positive pressure ventilation is to be instituted, it should be with small tidal volumes and a rapid respiratory rate such that peak positive airway pressures are no greater than 10 cm H_2O. (275; **1731–1732**)

40. Chronic bronchitis is characterized by an increased resistance to air flow caused by excessive secretions of mucus into the bronchi. Acute bronchitis differs from chronic bronchitis in that it is usually induced by an infectious agent and is self-limited. Patients with chronic bronchitis typically have a chronic productive cough in response to the secretions. The major predisposing factor to the development of chronic bronchitis, as with pulmonary emphysema, is a history of cigarette smoking. (275; **963**)

41. The small airways provide only a minimal contribution to the symptoms of chronic bronchitis. Because of this the disease process is often advanced before the onset of symptoms in these patients. Patients with chronic bronchitis are commonly classified as "blue bloaters" because of their tendency to develop arterial hypoxemia. These patients are also likely to have hypercarbia and cor pulmonale earlier than patients with emphysema alone. (275)

42. (273, Table 20–2; **963**)

		PULMONARY EMPHYSEMA	CHRONIC BRONCHITIS
FEV$_1$	(increased or decreased)	Decreased	Decreased
Total lung capacity	(increased or decreased)	Increased	Increased
Arterial hypoxemia	(early or late)	Late	Early
Hypercarbia	(early or late)	Late	Early
Cor pulmonale	(early or late)	Late	Early
Hematocrit	(normal or increased)	Normal	Increased
Dyspnea	(moderate or severe)	Severe	Moderate

43. The preoperative evaluation and intraoperative management of anesthesia for patients with chronic bronchitis is similar to that for patients with pulmonary emphysema. (275; **962–966**)

RESTRICTIVE PULMONARY DISEASE

44. Restrictive lung disease is characterized by a decrease in the total lung capacity due to decreases in lung compliance. The cause of the restrictive component of the lung disease may be due to an intrinsic disease process that alters lung elasticity properties or due to the accumulation of substances in the interstitial tissues of the lung. It is classically defined by a decreased vital capacity in the presence of a normal FEV$_1$. (275; **966**)

45. Restrictive lung disease is caused by inflammation and exudate into the interstitial lung spaces. In the acute process the leakage of intravascular fluid into the interstitial spaces of the lung causing edema is the most common pathophysiology. Common causes of acute restrictive lung disease include adult respiratory distress syndrome, aspiration pneumonitis, neurogenic pulmonary edema, and high-altitude pulmonary edema. (275; **966**)

46. Chronic restrictive lung disease is caused by the presence of chronic changes in the pulmonary interstitium such as fibrosis or the presence of any physical process that interferes with the expansion of the lungs. Common causes of chronic restrictive lung disease include sarcoidosis, idiopathic fibrosis, effusions, kyphoscoliosis, obesity, ascites, and pregnancy. (275; **966**)

47. Patients with restrictive lung disease are commonly dyspneic as a result of the increased work of breathing. These patients must overcome the decrease in lung compliance to ventilate the lungs. With the shallow breathing that results, patients must breathe rapidly to maintain their minute ventilation. (275; **883–884**)

48. Early in the disease the $Paco_2$ commonly seen in patients with restrictive lung disease is normal or decreased as a result of hyperventilation. Only very late in the disease course does the $Paco_2$ in these patients begin to increase. (275)

49. (276, Fig. 20–3)

	NORMAL LUNGS	RESTRICTIVE LUNG DISEASE
Total lung capacity	Normal	Decreased
Vital capacity	Normal	Decreased
Functional residual capacity	Normal	Decreased
Tidal volume	Normal	Decreased
Inspiratory reserve volume	Normal	Decreased
Expiratory reserve volume	Normal	Decreased
Residual volume	Normal	Decreased
Forced exhaled volume in 1 second	Normal	Normal

50. A regional anesthetic that achieves a sensory level above T10 might make ventilation difficult for patients with restrictive lung disease secondary to the reliance of these patients on their respiratory muscles to physically maintain the work of breathing required for an adequate minute ventilation. In addition, with the loss of sensation of these muscles patients with restrictive lung disease may become anxious when they feel that their capacity to breathe is impaired. (276; **1497**)

51. Restrictive lung disease does not greatly influence the choice of drugs to be used for general anesthesia. If the expectation is for the patient to spontaneously ventilate at the conclusion of the anesthetic followed by extubation of the trachea, anesthetics should be administered such that there is minimal depression of ventilation postoperatively. For example, the minimizing of intraoperative opioids may be beneficial for these patients. (276)

52. Patients with restrictive lung disease and a marginal pulmonary status preoperatively may require postoperative mechanical ventilation of the lungs. A preoperative vital capacity lower than 15 mL/kg and a preoperative $Paco_2$ higher than 50 mm Hg are indicators that the patients may require postoperative mechanical ventilation of the lungs. (276; **885–886**)

53. Patients with restrictive lung disease are at risk of having difficulty clearing their airways of secretions in the postoperative period secondary to a decrease in the lung volume these patients can generate to effectively cough. (276)

ANESTHESIA FOR THORACIC SURGERY

54. Preoperative considerations for the patient scheduled to undergo thoracic surgery include the medical management of the pulmonary disease, the evaluation of

co-existing disease and its management, the evaluation of pulmonary function with pulmonary function tests, the selection of intraoperative anesthetics and monitors, the effect of one-lung ventilation and/or the lateral decubitus position that may be required intraoperatively, the plan for postoperative pain control, and the potential need for continued mechanical ventilation of the lungs in the postoperative period. Perhaps the main purpose of the preoperative evaluation of patients scheduled to undergo thoracic surgery is to institute perioperative therapy in an effort to minimize postoperative complications. (276–277; **899– 900, 962–965, 1665–1669, Tables 48–2, 48–3)**

55. Preoperative history and physical examination findings that are indicative of an increased risk of postoperative pulmonary complications after thoracic surgery include dyspnea, cough, sputum production, wheezing, a history of cigarette smoking, obesity, and advanced age. (276; **962–965)**

56. Preoperative prophylactic measures that may be taken in an attempt to minimize postoperative complications include the discontinuation of smoking cigarettes, treatment of any pulmonary infections, treatment of any reversible component of increased airway resistance, mobilization of any secretions, and teaching the patient deep breathing exercises and coughing exercises. These prophylactic measures should be instituted at least 48 to 72 hours before surgery. (276–277, Table 20–3; **899–900, 962–965, 1665–1669, Tables 48–2, 48–3)**

57. Cigarette smoking increases the irritability of the small airways, causes mucus hypersecretion, and decreases mucociliary transport. Carbon monoxide may also have negative inotropic effects. The net effect of this for patients scheduled to undergo thoracic surgery is an increase in the incidence of complications in the postoperative period. (277; **900, 957, 1672)**

58. There are many benefits of the preoperative cessation of cigarette smoking. Twelve to 18 hours after the cessation of cigarette smoking there are significant decreases in the carboxyhemoglobin level, a decrease in nicotine-induced tachycardia, and a normalization of the oxyhemoglobin dissociation curve. The oxyhemoglobin dissociation curve shifts to the right, making more oxygen available at the tissues. One to 2 weeks after the cessation of cigarette smoking there begins to be a decrease in the amount of mucus secretions in the airways. Four to 8 weeks after the cessation of cigarette smoking there is marked improvement in mucociliary transport, small airway reactivity, and secretions in the small airways. This is evidenced by the decrease in postoperative respiratory complications in patients who have quit smoking cigarettes for at least 8 weeks before surgery. (277, Fig. 20–4; **965, 1673)**

59. Preoperative pulmonary function tests enable the anesthesiologist to predict which patients may be at an increased risk for postoperative pulmonary complications after thoracic surgery. Patients with a history of chronic pulmonary disease or with severe, limiting pulmonary symptoms in the presence of abnormal findings on the physical examination or chest radiograph are candidates for preoperative pulmonary function studies. Patients with chest wall or spinal deformities as well as morbidly obese patients may also benefit from preoperative pulmonary function studies. Preoperative pulmonary function tests are also useful in evaluating the effectiveness of interventions administered to improve pulmonary function. The physiologic response to antibiotic and bronchodilator therapies can be assessed preoperatively by evaluating the patient's pulmonary status with pulmonary function studies both before and after the therapeutic interventions. Any improvement seen in the patient's pulmonary status as evidenced by improvement on pulmonary function studies can be attributed to the therapeutic interventions. (277; **899–900)**

60. An FEV_1 lower than 2 L, a vital capacity lower than 15 mL/kg, and an FEV_1/ FVC ratio less than 0.5 on pulmonary function studies are indicative of an increased risk of postoperative pulmonary morbidity after thoracic surgery for pneumonectomy of the right or left lung. If any of these conditions exists, split-lung testing that evaluates the functional contribution of each lung may be indicated. A predicted postoperative FEV_1 of 800 mL is usually required before a pneumonectomy is performed. When the predicted postoperative FEV_1 is less than 800 mL or if more than 70% of pulmonary blood flow goes to the diseased lung on split-function tests, patients are considered to be at an increased risk of postoperative dyspnea and hypercarbia. Finally, if further preoperative evaluation of the patient is desired, the pulmonary artery of the surgical side can be occluded by a balloon while arterial blood gas and pulmonary artery pressure measurements are taken. If preoperative pulmonary function tests indicate that the patient is at an increased risk for postoperative pulmonary morbidity after pneumonectomy, it may be prudent to consider a procedure other than a pneumonectomy, such as a lobectomy. (277; **900–901, 962–965, 1668–1669, Tables 25–39, 48–2, 48–3**)

61. A maximum breathing capacity lower than 50% of the predicted value is indicative of an increased risk of postoperative pulmonary morbidity after pneumonectomy. (277; **1668–1669, Tables 48–2, 48–3**)

62. An FEV_1/FVC ratio less than 0.5 is usually present before an increase in baseline $Paco_2$. (277)

63. The preoperative institution of digitalis prophylaxis for patients undergoing pulmonary tissue resection is aimed toward decreasing the risk of postoperative cardiac dysrhythmias. The patient is believed to be at risk of postoperative cardiac dysrhythmias from the reduction in the pulmonary vascular bed and a corresponding increase in the size of the right atrium and ventricle. This is believed to be especially true in patients with cor pulmonale undergoing a large amount of lung tissue resection. When preoperative digitalis therapy is instituted for this reason, it is typically started on the day before surgery. (277–278; **1675**)

64. A potential disadvantage of the prophylactic institution of digitalis preoperatively for patients undergoing pulmonary tissue resection is that, should postoperative cardiac dysrhythmias occur, it is initially unclear whether it is secondary to right atrial enlargement or digitalis toxicity. (277–278; **1675**)

65. The benefits of the administration of volatile anesthetics for patients undergoing thoracic surgery include the effect of decreasing airway irritability, the apparent lack of influence on regional hypoxic pulmonary vasoconstriction, the high inspired concentration of oxygen that may be delivered concurrently, and the ability to be eliminated postoperatively. (278, Fig. 20–5; **1678–1683**)

66. Disadvantages of the administration of nitrous oxide for patients undergoing thoracic surgery include the limited concentration of oxygen that may be administered as a result, and the apparently small decrease in the hypoxic pulmonary vasoconstriction response of the lung. (278; **132–135, 1678–1683, Figs. 48–6, 48–7**)

67. The benefits of the administration of nondepolarizing neuromuscular blocking drugs for patients undergoing thoracic surgery include improved surgical exposure through rib separation and the facilitation of controlled ventilation of the lungs. (278; **1683–1684**)

68. Intraoperative monitors that may be used for patients undergoing thoracic surgery include an intra-arterial catheter, a central venous pressure catheter, a catheter in the bladder to monitor urine output, and possibly a pulmonary artery catheter or a transesophageal echocardiogram. (278; **1675–1678, Table 48–7**)

69. A patient in the lateral decubitus position undergoing mechanical ventilation of the lungs has an increase in pulmonary ventilation-to-perfusion mismatch. The effects on pulmonary blood flow are primarily due to gravity. The dependent lung receives proportionally more blood flow than the nondependent lung. The dependent lung is also concurrently being ventilated less than the nondependent lung. The dependent lung is ventilated relatively less secondary to the loss of lung volume by compression by the mediastinum, abdominal contents, and positioning support structures. These factors together create an increase in pulmonary ventilation-to-perfusion mismatching. The ventilation-to-perfusion ratio can be improved with the application of positive end-expiratory pressure to the dependent lung. (278–279; **580–581, 1686–1689, Figs. 15–4, 15–5, 15–6, 48–9, 48–10, 48–11, 48–12, 48–13**)

70. Absolute indications for single-lung ventilation during surgery and anesthesia include the need to isolate the lungs from each other to avoid contamination from one lung to the other of infected material or blood, the presence of a bronchopleural fistula, surgical opening of a major airway, a giant unilateral lung cyst or bullae, tracheobronchial tree disruption, life-threatening hypoxemia due to unilateral lung disease, and unilateral lung lavage of pulmonary alveolar proteinosis. Relative indications for single-lung ventilation during surgery and anesthesia include to improve operating conditions during a lobectomy, pneumonectomy, resection of a thoracic aneurysm, or operations on the esophagus. (279; **1690, Table 48–10**)

71. The Robertshaw endobronchial tube is the most frequently used double-lumen endotracheal tube for the isolation of the right or left lung or for single-lung ventilation during thoracic surgery. The left-sided tube has a longer bronchial tube than the right-sided tube. (279, Fig. 20–6; **1691–1693, Figs. 48–14, 48–16**)

72. An endobronchial tube placed in the right bronchus for isolation of the right lung could potentially obstruct the lumen of the right upper lobe bronchus. This easily occurs secondary to the short distance between the carina and the takeoff to the right upper lobe bronchus. This problem can be avoided by using a left endobronchial double-lumen tube. The left endobronchial tube can be placed in the left main stem bronchus, with ventilation only of the right lung and isolation of the lung. If a left pneumonectomy is being performed, a left endobronchial tube may still be used. At the time of clamping of the left main stem bronchus the endobronchial tube can be pulled back from the left main stem bronchus, converting the endobronchial tube to a single-lumen tube equivalent in the trachea. (279; **1693**)

73. Most adult patients of average height will require that an endobronchial tube be placed at approximately 29 cm at the lips for correct positioning of the tube. (279; **1694**)

74. The proper placement of a double-lumen endotracheal tube is best confirmed with fiberoptic visualization through the tracheal portion of the double-lumen tube. The desired position of the tube corresponds to visualization of the superior portion of the bronchial cuff, when inflated, just past the bifurcation of the carina. The bronchial side can be confirmed by its orientation to the tracheal rings, which are complete anteriorly. (**1693–1699, Figs. 48–19, 48–20, 48–21**)

75. The Univent tube is a single-lumen tube with a bronchial blocker that, through the use of a fiberoptic bronchoscope, may be advanced into the right or left main stem bronchus. The advantage of the Univent tube is that it then converts to a single-lumen endotracheal tube with the withdrawal of the bronchial blocker when isolation of the lungs is no longer needed. An example in which this may be advantageous is when postoperative ventilation of the lungs is anticipated and changing a double-lumen tube to a single-lumen tube at the conclusion of

the surgical procedure could be dangerous or difficult. (279, Fig. 20–7; **1701–1703, Fig. 48–26**)

76. A patient in the lateral decubitus position will have a greater mismatch of ventilation-to-perfusion ratio during one-lung ventilation than during two-lung ventilation. This occurs because of a greater shunt fraction during one-lung ventilation as a result of blood flow through the unventilated, nondependent lung. The increase in the right-to-left shunt is reflected as a greater gradient between arterial and alveolar oxygen tensions and a lower PaO_2 during one-lung ventilation than during two-lung ventilation. (279; **1705–1706, Fig. 48–27**)

77. Four factors that influence the amount of perfusion that goes to the nondependent, unventilated lung during one-lung ventilation of a patient in the lateral decubitus position with a double-lumen endotracheal tube include gravity, hypoxic pulmonary vasoconstriction, direct surgical compression of blood flow, and the method of ventilation of the dependent lung. (279; **1706–1709, Figs. 48–27, 48–28, 48–29**)

78. A patient undergoing one-lung ventilation during thoracic surgery should be closely monitored for arterial hypoxemia, particularly because arterial oxygenation can continue to decrease for up to 45 minutes after the initiation of one-lung ventilation. This can be achieved through the continuous use of pulse oximetry and frequent arterial blood gases. In addition, the patient should be administered a high fraction of inspired oxygen to minimize the risk of arterial hypoxemia. (279–280; **1709–1710, Table 48–15**)

79. Arterial hypoxemia noted during one-lung ventilation for thoracic surgery is typically initially treated with the administration of a low level of positive end-expiratory pressure to the ventilated, dependent lung. Although this may improve arterial oxygenation, it may also cause an increase in the pulmonary vascular resistance in the ventilated, dependent lung. The most beneficial intervention that can be made when arterial hypoxemia is noted during one-lung ventilation is the application of continuous positive airway pressure to the nondependent, unventilated lung. This results in oxygenation of the nondependent, unventilated lung as well as increasing the pulmonary vascular resistance in that lung. (280; **1710–1715, Figs. 48–30, 48–31, 48–32, 48–33**)

80. Arterial hypercapnia during one-lung ventilation for thoracic surgery is not typically a significant problem. (280; **1677**)

81. Chest tubes are placed after thoracic surgery to ensure continued expansion of the lung by evacuating air that may leak from alveoli that have been incised. Kinking of a chest tube after thoracic surgery places the patient at risk for a tension pneumothorax. (280)

82. Extubation of the trachea after thoracic surgery should take place when the patient is adequately ventilating spontaneously, has intact protective laryngeal reflexes, and has adequate pain relief. (280; **1719–1721, Tables 48–19, 48–20**)

83. The most common postoperative pulmonary complication after thoracic surgery is atelectasis. Other common postoperative pulmonary complications include pneumonia and arterial hypoxemia. Early serious complications include herniation of the heart when an intrapericardial surgical approach was used, pulmonary torsion, or torsion of the lung parenchyma on the bronchovascular pedicle, hemorrhage, bronchial disruption, right-sided heart failure, and neural injuries. (280; **1717–1719**)

84. Adequate analgesia after thoracic surgery is important not only for patient comfort but also to speed recovery. Patients without adequate analgesia after thoracic surgery tend to contract their expiratory muscles (splint) and are unable

to develop a forceful cough as would be necessary to clear secretions. Adequate analgesia after thoracic surgery minimizes pulmonary complications by allowing the patients to breathe deeply and cough effectively, and allows for earlier ambulation. (280; **1722–1724, Table 48–20**)

MEDIASTINOSCOPY

85. The most frequent reason for the performance of a mediastinoscopy is to determine the diagnosis and/or resectability of lung cancer. (280; **1724, Fig. 48–34**)

86. Positive pressure of the lungs is recommended during a mediastinoscopy because it allows the surgeon better operating conditions, minimizes the risk of a venous air embolus, and facilitates the management of major complications. (280; **1724–1725**)

87. The right subclavian and right carotid arteries may be compressed during a mediastinoscopy. For this reason the systemic blood pressure should be measured in the left arm while arterial pulses can be monitored by palpation to provide early evidence of compression of the innominate or right subclavian arteries. The aorta may also be compressed, but this is less likely to occur. (280; **1725**)

88. Bradycardia may occur during a mediastinoscopy as a result of stretching of the vagus nerve or the trachea or by direct compression of the aorta by the mediastinoscope. This can be treated through repositioning of the mediastinoscope. If bradycardia persists, intravenous atropine should be administered. (280–281; **1725**)

89. The most common complications that can occur after the performance of a mediastinoscopy include hemorrhage and a pneumothorax. Other potential complications include a recurrent laryngeal nerve injury, infection, air embolism, and phrenic nerve injury. (280; **1725–1726**)

THORACOSCOPY

90. Indications for the performance of thoracoscopy include the need to biopsy tissue to aid in the diagnosis of pleural or lung tissue disease, to aid in the staging of neoplasm, or to determine the etiology of recurrent pleural effusions. (281; **1726**)

91. Thoracoscopy can be performed under local or general anesthesia. When local anesthesia is chosen, patients may have intercostal nerve blocks and local anesthetic infiltration of the thoracic wall and pleura. The lung on the side of the procedure partially collapses when the air enters the pleural cavity. A disadvantage of local anesthesia for this procedure is that the patient is often in discomfort. General anesthesia would involve the placement of a double-lumen endotracheal tube to allow for one-lung ventilation with high inspired concentrations of oxygen to facilitate the procedure. These procedures are generally short in duration. (281; **1726**)

BRONCHOPLEURAL FISTULA

92. Causes of a bronchopleural fistula include erosion of a bronchus by disease, the breakdown of a bronchial suture line after pulmonary resection, or the rupture of lung abscess, cyst, bulla, or parenchymal tissue. The appropriate anesthetic management of a patient with a bronchopleural fistula almost always involves placement of a double-lumen endotracheal tube to allow for isolation of the affected lung from the unaffected lung. The risk of a tension pneumothorax can

be minimized by placing the double lumen endotracheal tube in the spontaneously ventilating patient. Alternatively, the patient may already have a chest tube in place, in which case the chest tube should be left unclamped. (281; **1740–1741**)

Chapter 20

Liver and Biliary Tract Disease

PHYSIOLOGIC FUNCTIONS OF THE LIVER

1. What are some physiologic functions of the liver?

2. What are Kupffer's cells? What is their function?

3. How does the liver store glucose?

4. How does the liver maintain glucose homeostasis in times of starvation?

5. Why might patients with cirrhosis be more likely to develop hypoglycemia in the perioperative period?

6. What proteins are synthesized in the rough endoplasmic reticulum of hepatocytes?

7. Approximately how many grams of albumin are synthesized by the liver every day?

8. What is the normal plasma concentration of albumin maintained by a healthy liver? What plasma concentration of albumin may reflect the presence of significant liver disease?

9. What is the half-life of albumin? What implication does this have with regard to acute liver dysfunction?

10. What role does the liver play in drug binding to serum proteins? What is the clinical implication of this for the patient with liver disease?

11. How does liver disease affect the hydrolysis of ester linkages? What is the clinical implication of this for the patient with liver disease?

12. What is the plasma half-life of plasma cholinesterase? How does liver disease affect the hydrolysis of succinylcholine?

13. What role does the liver play in blood coagulation? What is the clinical implication of this for the patient with liver disease?

14. How significant must liver dysfunction be before abnormal blood coagulation is noted? How can this be evaluated preoperatively?

15. What is the half-life of clotting factors synthesized in the liver? What is the clinical implication of this for the patient with acute liver disease?

16. What role does the liver play in drug metabolism? What is the clinical implication of this for the patient with liver disease?

17. What liver enzymes are particularly responsible for drug metabolism? How significant must liver dysfunction be before abnormal drug metabolism is noted?

18. Why may drug metabolism be accelerated?

19. What role does the liver play in the excretion of bilirubin? What is the clinical implication of this for the patient with liver disease?

HEPATIC BLOOD FLOW

20. What is the blood supply to the liver? What percent of the cardiac output goes to the liver?

21. Why might oxygen delivery to the liver be marginal despite its extensive blood supply?

22. What are some determinants of hepatic blood flow?

23. What is hepatic autoregulation? How is hepatic autoregulation affected by surgery and anesthesia?

24. What is the hepatic arterial buffer response? How is this hepatic response affected by anesthesia?

25. What results from sympathetic nervous stimulation of the liver?

26. How does positive pressure ventilation of the lungs affect hepatic blood flow?

27. How does congestive heart failure affect hepatic blood flow?

28. How does hepatic cirrhosis affect hepatic blood flow?

29. How do changes in cardiac output or myocardial contractility affect hepatic blood flow?

30. How do changes in arterial blood pressure affect hepatic blood flow?

31. In the absence of surgical stimulation, how much do regional and inhaled anesthetics decrease hepatic blood flow?

32. In animal studies, which volatile anesthetic decreases hepatic blood flow the most, halothane or isoflurane?

33. What is the extent of the effect of surgical stimulation on hepatic blood flow?

LIVER FUNCTION TESTS

34. What are some commonly ordered liver function tests? What is the utility of liver function tests in the perioperative period?

35. When liver function tests become abnormal postoperatively, what is the most likely mechanism for the postoperative liver dysfunction? In what patients and types of surgeries are liver function tests most likely to become elevated postoperatively?

36. When serum bilirubin increases postoperatively secondary to liver dysfunction, is it the conjugated or unconjugated fraction that increases in prehepatic dysfunction? Intrahepatic dysfunction? Posthepatic dysfunction?

37. Are serum aminotransferase enzymes more likely to become elevated in prehepatic, intrahepatic, or posthepatic causes of postoperative liver dysfunction?

38. Are serum alkaline phosphatase levels more likely to become elevated in prehepatic, intrahepatic, or posthepatic causes of postoperative liver dysfunction?

39. Is the prothrombin time more likely to become prolonged in prehepatic, intrahepatic, or posthepatic causes of postoperative liver dysfunction?

40. Are serum albumin levels more likely to decrease in prehepatic, intrahepatic, or posthepatic causes of postoperative liver dysfunction?

41. What are the most likely causes of prehepatic dysfunction postoperatively? What serum levels of bilirubin result in overt jaundice?

42. For a patient with normal hepatic function, how likely is it that the administration of large amounts of blood will result in an elevation in serum bilirubin levels?

43. What are the most likely causes of intrahepatic liver dysfunction postoperatively?

44. What laboratory values indicate an intrahepatic cause of liver dysfunction?

45. What are the most likely causes of posthepatic liver dysfunction postoperatively?

46. What laboratory values indicate a posthepatic cause of liver dysfunction?

47. What is benign postoperative intrahepatic cholestasis? When is it most likely to occur?

DRUG-INDUCED LIVER DYSFUNCTION

48. How easily can drug-induced hepatitis be distinguished from viral hepatitis histologically?

49. What is halothane hepatitis? Are pediatric patients or adult patients more likely to develop halothane hepatitis?

50. What is the cause of halothane hepatitis? Why is it logical that halothane would be more likely to produce hepatitis than other volatile anesthetics?

51. How is the diagnosis of halothane hepatitis made?

52. Is there cross-reactivity between halothane and other volatile anesthetics with regard to halothane hepatitis?

53. Describe a milder form of hepatotoxicity that can result from the administration of halothane and other volatile anesthetics.

PATHOPHYSIOLOGY OF LIVER DISEASE

54. What are some causes of parenchymal liver disease?

55. What is the pathophysiology of cirrhosis of the liver?

56. What are some signs of hepatic cirrhosis on physical examination?

57. What effect does cirrhosis of the liver have on hepatic blood flow? What does this mean with regard to the delivery of volatile anesthetics to patients with cirrhosis of the liver?

58. Why do gastroesophageal varices develop in patients with hepatic cirrhosis? What associated problem do patients frequently have as a result of gastroesophageal varices?

59. Why is ascites thought to accumulate in patients with hepatic cirrhosis?

60. What is the characteristic hemodynamic status of patients with hepatic cirrhosis?

61. What are some reasons why a patient with hepatic cirrhosis may have arterial hypoxemia?

62. What is the coagulation status of patients with hepatic cirrhosis?

63. Why are patients with alcoholic cirrhosis often anemic?

64. Why are patients with alcoholic cirrhosis particularly prone to infection? What type of infection is more frequently seen in patients with alcoholic cirrhosis?

65. How might renal function be affected in patients with hepatic cirrhosis?

66. How might the central nervous system be affected in patients with hepatic cirrhosis?

67. What are some causes of cholestatic liver disease?

68. What is the pathophysiology of cholestatic liver disease?

MANAGEMENT OF ANESTHESIA FOR PATIENTS WITH PARENCHYMAL LIVER DISEASE

69. What are some preoperative findings in patients with liver disease that are associated with increased postoperative morbidity?

70. What is the purpose of the administration of vitamin K to patients with cirrhosis of the liver?

71. What monitoring may be useful intraoperatively for patients with hepatic cirrhosis undergoing surgical procedures?

72. Why is the intraoperative maintenance of the arterial blood pressure particularly important in patients with hepatic cirrhosis?

73. What impaired physiologic functions of the liver may affect the effective dose and duration of effect of injected drugs?

74. How is the volume of distribution of drugs altered in patients with hepatic cirrhosis?

75. How well is citrate metabolized by the patient with hepatic cirrhosis? What clinical implication does this have?

76. What are the most common postoperative complications for patients with hepatic cirrhosis?

77. What is delirium tremens? How does it usually present? What is the treatment?

78. What is the mortality associated with delirium tremens? What is the usual cause of death in these patients?

79. How does chronic alcohol use affect anesthetic requirements? How does acute alcohol ingestion affect anesthetic requirements?

80. How does acute alcohol ingestion affect the patient's vulnerability to the aspiration of gastric contents?

81. How can acute alcohol ingestion affect platelet activity?

DISEASE OF THE BILIARY TRACT

82. What approximate percent of females and males aged 55 to 65 years are believed to have gallstones?

83. What is the potential problem with the use of opioids intraoperatively during a cholecystectomy or common bile duct exploration?

84. What are some anesthetic considerations for patients undergoing laparoscopic procedures?

ANSWERS*

PHYSIOLOGIC FUNCTIONS OF THE LIVER

1. Physiologic functions of the liver include protein synthesis, drug metabolism, fat metabolism, hormone metabolism, bilirubin formation and excretion, and glucose homeostasis. (282; **984**)

---

*Numbers in parentheses: lightface numbers refer to pages, figures, or tables in Stoelting RK, Miller RD: Basics of Anesthesia, 4th ed. Philadelphia, Churchill Livingstone, 2000; **boldface numbers** refer to pages, figures, or tables in Miller RD: Anesthesia, 5th ed. Philadelphia, Churchill Livingstone, 2000.

2. Kupffer's cells are thin endothelial cells lining the sinuses of the liver. Kupffer's cells phagocytize bacteria that have been absorbed into the portal vein from the gastrointestinal tract. (282; **647, 652**)

3. The liver stores glucose as glycogen in the hepatocytes. (282; **650–652**)

4. Glucose homeostasis is maintained during times of starvation by the breakdown of the glycogen to glucose in the hepatocytes. Glucose is then released into the circulation. Only 75 g of glycogen is stored in the liver, corresponding to 24 to 48 hours of glucose supply during times of starvation. Prolonged starvation that results in depletion of the glycogen stores requires that the liver convert lactate, glycerol, and amino acids to glucose. This is termed *gluconeogenesis*. (282; **651**)

5. Patients with cirrhosis may be more likely to develop hypoglycemia in the perioperative period for two reasons. Preoperative fasting causes depletion of the stores of glycogen, and gluconeogenesis may be impaired. (282; **651**)

6. All proteins are synthesized in the rough endoplasmic reticulum of hepatocytes except for gamma globulins and factor VIII. Proteins synthesized by the liver are responsible for the maintenance of the plasma oncotic pressure. (282; **650–651**)

7. Ten to 15 grams of albumin are synthesized by the liver every day. (282; **650–651**)

8. The normal plasma concentration of albumin maintained by a healthy liver is 3.5 to 5.5 g/dL. Significant liver disease should be suspected when the plasma albumin is less than 3.0 g/dL. (282; **655, 984**)

9. The half-life of albumin is about 20 days. The serum albumin concentration therefore may not be an accurate indicator of acute liver dysfunction. (282; **650–651, 655**)

10. The liver synthesizes albumin, which binds drugs in the plasma. The binding of drugs to albumin decreases the free, or pharmacologically active, portion of the drug. When the liver is diseased the synthesis of albumin becomes impaired, decreasing the albumin available in the plasma for binding. As a result there is an increased concentration of free, unbound drug in the plasma. This can result in a more pronounced effect of a drug in patients with liver disease than in patients with normal liver function after an intravenous injection of a specific drug dose. This effect of a diseased liver usually becomes significant when the plasma albumin level is less than 2.5 g/dL. (282–283, Fig. 21–1; **650–651, 653–654, 1967**)

11. A part of normal liver function is the production of enzymes that hydrolyze ester linkages. Clinically, this implies that liver disease may result in a decrease in enzymatic ester hydrolysis activity. This could result in prolonged effects of drugs that rely on ester hydrolysis for termination of their effects, such as succinylcholine, mivacurium, and ester local anesthetics. (283; **650, 653, 1967**)

12. Plasma cholinesterase is synthesized by the liver. The plasma half-life of plasma cholinesterase is 14 days, making decreased circulating concentrations of this enzyme unlikely in the presence of acute liver failure. Even chronic liver disease must be significant to cause a prolongation in the effects of succinylcholine, however. Prolonged effects of succinylcholine to greater than 30 minutes warrants a search for other causes, even in the presence of chronic liver disease. (283; **419–420, 650, 653, 1967**)

13. A normal liver synthesizes most of the proteins responsible for the coagulation of blood. A diseased liver may therefore manifest as a coagulopathy. (283; **655, 984, 1968**)

14. Bleeding can be prevented with only 20% to 30% of normal levels of clotting factors, so that abnormal blood coagulation manifests only after significant liver disease. The coagulation status of a patient can be evaluated preoperatively by checking the patient's prothrombin time, partial thromboplastin time, and bleeding time. Indeed, the prothrombin time is frequently used as an evaluation of the synthetic function of the liver. (283; **651, 655, 1968**)

15. The half-lives of clotting factors synthesized by the liver are short. This implies that even acute liver dysfunction may be associated with a coagulopathy. (283; **651, 1962**)

16. The liver plays a significant role in drug metabolism, making impairment of the metabolism of drugs a concern for patients with liver disease. (283; **148, 653–654**)

17. The metabolism of drugs by the liver is primarily through the action of microsomal enzymes in the smooth endoplasmic reticulum of hepatocytes. Microsomal enzymes transform lipid soluble drugs to water soluble drugs that can then be excreted renally. With severe, chronic liver disease such as cirrhosis there may be impairment of the metabolism of drugs by the liver for two reasons. The patient may have decreased hepatic blood flow as well as a decrease in the number of microsomal enzyme-containing hepatocytes. (283–284, Fig. 21–2; **148, 653–654**)

18. Accelerated drug metabolism may be noted after the administration of certain drugs such as phenobarbital. It is believed that exposure of the microsomal enzymes to these drugs causes an up-regulation, or induction, of their own synthesis. (284; **148, 152**)

19. The conjugation of bilirubin with glucuronic acid takes place in the liver through the action of glucuronyl transferase. The conjugation of bilirubin allows it to become water soluble for renal excretion. Impairment of this function of the liver, as with liver disease, can lead to increased serum levels of unconjugated bilirubin. The liver is also responsible for the excretion of conjugated bilirubin into bile. This explains the elevated serum levels of conjugated bilirubin in the presence of liver disease. (284; **151–152, 653**)

HEPATIC BLOOD FLOW

20. The liver receives its blood supply via the portal vein and hepatic artery. Approximately 25% of the cardiac output goes to the liver. (284, Fig. 21–4; **148, 647, Fig. 17–1**)

21. Oxygen delivery to the liver is primarily via the hepatic artery, which accounts for about 30% of the blood supply to the liver. The remainder of the blood supply is via the portal vein, which contains desaturated blood after having supplied various other abdominal organs with oxygen. Therefore, oxygen delivery to the liver may be marginal despite its extensive blood supply if hepatic artery blood flow decreases. (284; **647**)

22. Total hepatic blood flow is directly proportional to the perfusion pressure across the liver and is inversely proportional to splanchnic vascular resistance. There are many determinants of hepatic blood flow. Determinants intrinsic to the liver include hepatic autoregulation, metabolic control, and the hepatic arterial buffer response. Determinants extrinsic to the liver include sympathetic nervous system activity and humoral factors. (284–285; **649–650**)

23. Hepatic autoregulation refers to the ability of the hepatic artery to alter its resistance in response to changes in arterial pressure to maintain hepatic artery blood flow. For example, hepatic artery resistance may increase when increases in the arterial perfusion pressure are sensed by hepatic arterial smooth muscle

cells. Hepatic autoregulation is thought to be disrupted when patients are in the fasted state. Because most surgical procedures are performed in the fasted state, hepatic autoregulation is not believed to exist during surgery and anesthesia. Of note, there does not appear to be autoregulation of the portal venous system. Instead portal venous blood flow parallels cardiac output. (284–285; **649**)

24. The hepatic arterial buffer response refers to the capacity of the liver to increase or decrease hepatic artery blood flow in response to decreases or increases in portal venous flow. For example, when portal venous flow decreases, the resistance of the hepatic artery decreases and hepatic artery blood flow increases. This reciprocal relationship allows for the hepatic oxygen supply and total hepatic blood flow to be maintained despite alterations in portal venous flow. This compensatory mechanism does not completely compensate for changes in portal venous flow, however. In addition, the hepatic arterial buffer response can be disrupted by several factors, including neural, humoral, and metabolic changes. This hepatic response is also disrupted by hepatic cirrhosis and volatile anesthetics. (284–285; **649–650**)

25. Innervation of the liver is by both the parasympathetic nervous system and the sympathetic nervous system. Generalized sympathetic nervous system stimulation, as can occur with arterial hypoxia or hypercarbia, results in an increase in the splanchnic vascular resistance. The increase in splanchnic vascular resistance yields a decrease in liver blood flow and blood volume. About 80% of the liver blood volume, or 500 mL, is displaced from the liver into the inferior vena cava with sympathetic nervous system stimulation. The liver thus acts as a reservoir for whole blood. (285; **650**)

26. Positive pressure ventilation of the lungs decreases hepatic blood flow through its increase in hepatic venous pressure. Hepatic blood flow is decreased further by the application of positive end-expiratory pressure through the same mechanism. If hypocarbia is produced, splanchnic vascular resistance increases, augmenting the effect of decreasing hepatic blood flow by positive pressure ventilation. (285; **650, 1964**)

27. Congestive heart failure, particularly right-sided heart failure, decreases hepatic blood flow through its increase in hepatic venous pressure. (285; **649–650**)

28. Hepatic cirrhosis causes a decrease in hepatic blood flow by its associated increase in hepatic resistance. (285; **649–650, 658, 1964**)

29. Decreases in cardiac output or myocardial contractility result in decreases in hepatic blood flow. (285; **649–650**)

30. Decreases in arterial blood pressure result in decreases in hepatic blood flow. (285; **649–650**)

31. In the absence of surgical stimulation, regional and inhaled anesthetics decrease hepatic blood flow by 20% to 30%. Changes in hepatic blood flow in response to regional and inhaled anesthetics are believed to result from decreases in cardiac output, mean arterial pressure, or both. Volatile anesthetics may also decrease hepatic blood flow by impairing intrinsic hepatic mechanisms to maintain hepatic blood flow to varying degrees. (285; **158–159, 649–650, 984, 1964**)

32. In animal studies, halothane decreases hepatic blood flow more than isoflurane. This is believed to result from preservation of the ability of the liver to autoregulate its blood supply by altering hepatic artery resistance when isoflurane is administered. The same appears to be true when desflurane and sevoflurane are administered. In contrast, halothane appears to impair hepatic autoregulation. (285–286, Figs. 21–5, 21–6; **158–159, 649–650, 1964**)

33. Surgical stimulation in and of itself can significantly decrease hepatic blood

flow. In some studies, hepatic blood flow may be decreased by as much as 60% in upper abdominal procedures. In fact, the greatest decrease in hepatic blood flow occurs when the surgical site is near the liver. Decreases in hepatic blood flow can be significant when surgery, anesthesia, positive pressure ventilation, fasting, and alterations in cardiac output and carbon dioxide tensions are all combined. (286; **158–159, 649–650, 984, 1964**)

LIVER FUNCTION TESTS

34. Commonly ordered liver function tests include serum bilirubin, aminotransferase enzymes, alkaline phosphatase, albumin, and the prothrombin time. Liver tests are very nonspecific, and significant liver dysfunction must occur before it is reflected in the majority of tests. Despite this, liver function tests have some utility in the perioperative period. Liver function tests may be useful preoperatively to detect the presence of liver disease. Postoperatively, liver dysfunction may be classified as prehepatic, intrahepatic, or posthepatic through the evaluation of the results of the various liver function tests. (286, Table 21–1; **654–656, 1962, 1969–1970, Table 17–2**)

35. Liver function tests are most likely to become abnormal secondary to an inadequate supply of oxygen to the hepatocytes intraoperatively. This is the most likely mechanism for mild, self-limited postoperative liver dysfunction. Abnormal postoperative liver function tests are most likely to occur in patients with preexisting liver disease whose hepatic oxygenation was marginal preoperatively or after surgery in which the operative site was in close proximity to the liver. (286, Figs. 21–7, 21–8; **1969–1970**)

36. When serum bilirubin levels become elevated postoperatively, prehepatic causes of the liver dysfunction can be distinguished from intrahepatic or posthepatic causes by determining if the elevated serum bilirubin levels are primarily of the conjugated or unconjugated fraction. The unconjugated fraction tends to be elevated in prehepatic dysfunction, whereas the conjugated fraction is most likely to be elevated in intrahepatic or posthepatic dysfunction. (286–287, Table 21–2; **655, 1969**)

37. Serum aminotransferase enzyme levels are more likely to become elevated in intrahepatic causes of postoperative liver dysfunction. (287, Table 21–2; **654–655, 1969–1971**)

38. Serum alkaline phosphatase levels are more likely to become elevated in posthepatic causes of postoperative liver dysfunction. (288, Table 21–2; **655, 1962**)

39. The prothrombin time is most likely to become prolonged in intrahepatic causes of postoperative liver dysfunction. (287, Table 21–2; **655**)

40. Serum albumin levels are more likely to decrease in intrahepatic causes of postoperative liver dysfunction. (287, Table 21–2; **655**)

41. The most likely causes of postoperative prehepatic dysfunction leading to jaundice postoperatively include hemolysis, hematoma reabsorption, and an overload of bilirubin administration secondary to large volumes of transfused whole blood. For every 500 mL of blood that is transfused to the patient, about 250 mg of bilirubin is released to the serum. As the age of the transfused blood increases, the amount of bilirubin released to the serum also increases. A serum bilirubin level greater than 3 mg/dL results in overt jaundice. (286; **655, 1969–1970**)

42. Patients with normal hepatic function are unlikely to have a postoperative elevation in serum bilirubin levels after the administration of large amounts of blood. (286; **1969–1970**)

43. The most likely causes of postoperative intrahepatic liver dysfunction include drugs, arterial hypoxemia, sepsis, congestive heart failure, cirrhosis, and a history of preexisting hepatic viruses. (287–288; **655, 1969–1970**)

44. Elevated aminotransferase enzymes, decreased albumin, and a prolonged prothrombin time are all indicative of an intrahepatic cause of liver dysfunction. These alterations are reflective of direct hepatocellular damage. (287–288; **1969–1970**)

45. The most likely causes of postoperative posthepatic liver dysfunction are sepsis and obstruction due to stones or cancer. (288; **1969–1970**)

46. Elevated conjugated bilirubin and alkaline phosphatase levels are indicative of a posthepatic cause of liver dysfunction. Typically, these are elevated in response to bile duct obstruction. (288; **655**)

47. Benign postoperative intrahepatic cholestasis is a postoperative condition that typically follows a prolonged operative procedure complicated by hypotension, hypoxemia, and blood transfusions. This condition is most likely to occur in the elderly patient. It is characterized by severe jaundice, which can present up to 10 days after surgery but usually presents within 48 hours and can persist for up to 1 month. These patients usually have elevated conjugated bilirubin and alkaline phosphatase levels, without significant elevation of aminotransferase enzymes. When postoperative intrahepatic cholestasis occurs, it must be distinguished from mechanical biliary obstruction. (288; **1970**)

DRUG-INDUCED LIVER DYSFUNCTION

48. It is difficult to distinguish histologically between drug-induced hepatitis and viral hepatitis. (288; **984**)

49. There are two different forms of hepatotoxicity that can result from the administration of halothane. Halothane hepatitis typically refers to the more severe hepatotoxicity that can result in hepatic necrosis and death. Halothane hepatitis is extremely rare, occurring with an incidence of 1 in 22,000 to 35,000 halothane anesthetics. Adult patients are more likely to develop halothane hepatitis than pediatric patients. Patients most likely to be affected are middle-aged, obese women who had repeated administration of halothane anesthesia about 4 weeks after their prior halothane anesthetic. (288–289; **158–159, 984–985**)

50. Although the exact cause of halothane hepatitis is unclear, it is believed to be due to an immunologic response to a toxic metabolite of halothane. Patients typically present with a fever and elevated serum aminotransferase enzyme levels within 7 days of the administration of halothane. Evidence lending support to an immune-mediated mechanism includes the presence of eosinophilia, fever, rash, and arthralgias in patients with halothane hepatitis. In addition, patients who have had halothane hepatitis have frequently had exposure to halothane during previous anesthetics. Oxidative halothane metabolism produces antigens, trifluoroacetylated proteins, that modify liver microsomal proteins on the surfaces of hepatocytes. The altered antigen/liver microsomal proteins are then recognized as antigens by a circulating IgG antibody that is present in patients who have had halothane hepatitis. The assumption is that the antibody interacts with the antigen/liver microsomal proteins produced by the oxidative metabolism of halothane to cause injury to the liver. Other volatile anesthetics such as isoflurane and enflurane undergo oxidative metabolism, producing the same metabolite that is produced by halothane. Halothane undergoes a greater degree of metabolism than the other anesthetics, however. This may explain why patients susceptible to hepatitis as a result of the produced metabolite are

more likely to get the hepatitis after the administration of halothane. (288–289, Fig. 21–9; **158–159, 984**)

51. The diagnosis of halothane hepatitis is made after other causes of hepatitis have been excluded. (288–289; **158–159, 984**)

52. There have been case reports of patients having acute necrosis similar to halothane hepatitis after the administration of enflurane. In all cases the patients had previous exposure to halothane, which presumably sensitized the patient to the low levels of metabolite produced by enflurane. Therefore, it is speculated that there is some cross-reactivity between halothane and other volatile anesthetics with regard to halothane hepatitis. It is believed that anesthetics that metabolize to trifluoroacetylated metabolites pose the greatest risk of halothane hepatitis to the patient and to a degree proportional to their metabolism. In this regard, desflurane would pose very little risk, owing to its minimal metabolism. Sevoflurane does not metabolize to trifluoroacetylated metabolites and would theoretically not be expected to have cross-reactivity with patients previously exposed to halothane. (289; **159**)

53. A milder, self-limited form of hepatotoxicity can result from the administration of halothane as well as the other volatile anesthetics. It is believed to occur secondary to an inadequate supply of oxygen to the liver intraoperatively and is characterized by mild elevations in serum aminotransferase levels. This mild form of hepatitis is thought to be due to a decrease in blood flow associated with the anesthetic or the surgery and is not a direct effect of the anesthetic. (288; **158–159**)

PATHOPHYSIOLOGY OF LIVER DISEASE

54. Causes of parenchymal liver disease include acute and chronic viral hepatitis, autoimmune causes, primary biliary cirrhosis, and alcoholic cirrhosis. (289; **984, 1962–1964**)

55. Cirrhosis of the liver is characterized by the replacement of normal liver tissue with collagen and fatty tissue as the number of hepatocytes decreases. There is impairment of all the physiologic functions of the liver in patients with liver cirrhosis. (289; **1964–1965**)

56. Signs of hepatic cirrhosis that may be noted on physical examination include jaundice, hepatomegaly, ascites, atrophy of skeletal muscles, palmar erythema, and spider angiomas. (289; **1966–1967**)

57. In patients with cirrhosis of the liver there is an increase in the resistance of the portal vein when the normal channels for blood flow become disrupted with fibrous tissue. This results in a corresponding decrease in hepatic blood flow. The administration of volatile anesthetics to patients with cirrhosis of the liver may further decrease the already reduced flow of hepatic blood, leading to an inadequate supply of oxygenated blood to the liver. (289; **1964**)

58. Gastroesophageal varices develop in patients with hepatic cirrhosis as a result of a high portal venous pressure and the development of collateral blood circulation. The collateral blood circulation occurs as blood flow from the portal system is transmitted retrograde to the splanchnic veins to reach the azygous and hemiazygous veins. Submucosal collateral vessels become engorged with blood that would have normally traversed the portal system. The collateral blood flow includes flow through the stomach and esophagus, resulting in gastroesophageal varices. Collateral blood flow also develops via the veins around the rectum, in the retroperitoneal space, and in the abdominal wall. Patients with gastroesophageal varices are at risk of gastrointestinal hemorrhage through the rupture of the engorged, dilated submucosal veins. (289; **1965–1966**)

59. Ascites is thought to accumulate in patients with hepatic cirrhosis secondary to a decrease in plasma oncotic pressure, a corresponding increase in the hydrostatic pressure in the hepatic sinusoids, and an increase in sodium retention by the kidneys due to increased circulating levels of antidiuretic hormone. Ascites is also associated with right-sided pleural effusions. The decrease in plasma oncotic pressure is a direct result of impairment of the liver to synthesize proteins such as albumin that maintain the oncotic pressure. Ascites may mechanically interfere with patients' alveolar ventilation and venous return. Paracentesis, a procedure that removes ascites fluid, may be performed to temporarily reverse impaired ventilation in patients with significant ascites. (289; **1966**)

60. Patients with hepatic cirrhosis and ascites may be intravascularly depleted despite overall body fluid overload. The systemic circulation is altered secondary to humoral vasodilatory substances such as glucagon, the decreased viscosity of blood, and arteriovenous communications. Patients who are able to compensate have a compensatory increase in the cardiac output. The circulatory system of these patients has been described as hyperdynamic, owing to decreased peripheral vascular resistance, increased cardiac output, and normal systemic blood pressure. Eventually these patients may develop congestive heart failure. (289; **1966**)

61. Patients with hepatic cirrhosis may have arterial hypoxemia for several reasons. Often, patients with hepatic cirrhosis have right-to-left pulmonary shunting in response to the portal vein hypertension. Patients with ascites and hepatomegaly may also have impairment of diaphragmatic excursion due to the weight of the abdominal contents, particularly in the supine position. Patients with significant ascites may have pleural effusions impairing lung expansion. Finally, patients with hepatic cirrhosis may have smoked tobacco in the past and may have an element of chronic obstructive pulmonary disease. (289; **1966**)

62. Patients with hepatic cirrhosis often have abnormalities of their coagulation status secondary to the impaired ability of the liver to synthesize proteins necessary for coagulation. Impaired coagulation is reflected as elevated prothrombin times in these patients. Patients with hepatic cirrhosis may also have thrombocytopenia. (289; **1968**)

63. Patients with alcoholic cirrhosis often have a megaloblastic anemia secondary to deficiencies in their diet or through the direct antagonism of folate by alcohol. (289)

64. Patients with alcoholic cirrhosis can be considered to be immunocompromised. It is believed that chronic alcohol ingestion leads to depression of the bone marrow and normal immune mechanisms. Spontaneous bacterial peritonitis is an infection more frequently seen in patients with alcoholic cirrhosis, possibly because the shunting of blood away from the liver interferes with the usual removal of toxins from the blood. The primary source of infection is generally unknown in these patients. Spontaneous bacterial peritonitis is treated with antibiotics, but the mortality remains nearly 50%. (289; **1966**)

65. Patients with hepatic cirrhosis tend to have a decrease in renal blood flow and a decrease in glomerular filtration rate. Patients with hepatic cirrhosis are at risk of developing hepatorenal syndrome, a serious complication that is often fatal. The syndrome is characterized by intravascular fluid depletion, intrarenal vasoconstriction, and worsening hyponatremia, hypotension, and oliguria. (289–290; **1966**)

66. Patients with hepatic cirrhosis are at risk for hepatic encephalopathy, possibly as a result of increased levels of ammonia or other toxins in the systemic circulation. The syndrome is characterized by disturbances in the patient's level

of consciousness and behavior. These patients often manifest a flapping tremor of the hands, or asterixis, and may have cerebral edema. Hepatic encephalopathy may be reversible or may progress despite treatment. Flumazenil, a benzodiazepine antagonist, has been administered to attempt reversal of coma caused by hepatic encephalopathy. Other treatments include oral neomycin, lactulose, and the restriction of exogenous sources of ammonia. (289; **984, 1966**)

67. Cholestatic liver disease results from obstruction of extrahepatic biliary flow, as can occur with gallstones, cancer, or stricture. Cholestatic liver disease can also functionally occur after the administration of some drugs. (290; **1968**)

68. Cholestatic liver disease is characterized by jaundice, pruritus, and elevated serum bilirubin concentrations. As the disease progresses, irreversible hepatic cirrhosis can occur. These patients may be intravascularly fluid depleted and may have cardiovascular responses similar to those with parenchymal liver disease. (290; **1968–1969**)

MANAGEMENT OF ANESTHESIA FOR PATIENTS WITH PARENCHYMAL LIVER DISEASE

69. Preoperative findings in patients with liver disease that are associated with increased postoperative morbidity include marked ascites, poor nutrition, markedly elevated prothrombin time and serum bilirubin level, markedly decreased serum albumin level, the presence of infection, and co-existing chronic obstructive pulmonary disease. (290)

70. Vitamin K is administered to patients with cirrhosis of the liver in an attempt to reverse a prolonged prothrombin time because many of the coagulation factors are dependent on vitamin K for their synthesis. A prolonged prothrombin time may be noted even in acute liver dysfunction given the short half-lives of many of the coagulation factors. A prolonged prothrombin time may be due to the impaired protein synthesis of coagulation factors by the liver, by impaired absorption of fat-soluble vitamin K from the gastrointestinal tract, or both. Patients with severe liver disease and subsequent impairment of the synthetic function of the liver will not have reversal of the prolonged prothrombin time with the administration of vitamin K. (290; **655, 1969**)

71. Intraoperative monitoring for patients with hepatic cirrhosis should be guided by the surgical procedure. In general, monitoring of the arterial blood pressure with an intra-arterial catheter may be useful. This allows for monitoring of the arterial blood gases, pH, coagulation status, and glucose as well as the blood pressure. In addition, the urine output should be closely monitored to decrease the risk of postoperative renal dysfunction that can occur in patients with severe liver disease. The infusion of mannitol or renal doses of dopamine may be needed to augment the urine output of these patients. Finally, central venous pressure or pulmonary artery catheter monitoring might be useful in the fluid management of patients with cardiomyopathy and congestive heart failure. The intravascular fluid balance of patients with liver disease and especially ascites can be difficult. (290–291; **1965–1967**)

72. The intraoperative maintenance of the arterial blood pressure is particularly important in patients with hepatic cirrhosis because these patients are dependent on hepatic arterial blood flow to provide oxygen to the hepatocytes. In the presence of portal hypertension, hepatic arterial blood flow is typically reduced from normal levels. The addition of anesthetics and the surgical procedure can exacerbate this reduction in hepatic blood flow and may contribute to postoperative liver dysfunction. It may be prudent to avoid the administration of halothane to these patients as well. (290–291; **650, 1964, 1970**)

73. Impairment of the liver's ability to metabolize drugs may result in impaired clearance mechanisms for certain drugs and a subsequent prolongation of their duration of effect. Consideration should be given to the administration of reduced doses of drugs to these patients. Drugs that may be susceptible to impaired clearance include opioids and most neuromuscular blocking drugs. Impairment of the liver's synthetic ability could result in a decrease in plasma protein binding sites for injected drugs. This could exaggerate the effect of injected drugs by increasing the pharmacologically active, unbound portion of the drug. The decreased level of plasma proteins does not have marked clinical effects, however. The effect of decreased plasma proteins on the effects of injected drugs may be offset by alterations in the volume of distribution of drugs in patients with liver failure. (291; **148–151, 654, 1967**)

74. The volume of distribution is defined as the dose of drug divided by the plasma concentration of the drug. The volume of distribution is increased in patients with hepatic cirrhosis. With the increase in the volume of distribution, a larger loading dose of a drug may be required to achieve a given effect. The administration of larger doses of drugs in patients with liver failure should be done with caution, because there may be a decrease in plasma proteins and impaired metabolism and clearance of the drugs. (291; **16–17, 1967**)

75. Citrate clearance is decreased in patients with hepatic cirrhosis. Clinically, this implies that the administration of blood products containing citrate may result in the accumulation of citrate and hypocalcemia. (291; **1626–1627, 1967–1968**)

76. The most common postoperative complications for patients with hepatic cirrhosis are bleeding, sepsis, renal failure, and an irreversible progression of hepatic failure. (291–292; **1969–1970**)

77. Delirium tremens is a severe withdrawal syndrome in patients with a history of chronic alcohol abuse. The onset of delirium tremens is typically 48 to 72 hours after cessation of the ingestion of alcohol. Delirium tremens presents clinically as tremulousness, hallucinations, agitation, confusion, disorientation, and increased activity of the sympathetic nervous system. Increased activity of the sympathetic nervous system in these patients is manifest as diaphoresis, fever, tachycardia, and hypertension. In severe cases the syndrome may progress to seizures and death. The treatment of delirium tremens is primarily with the administration of central nervous system depressants, usually a benzodiazepine. If necessary, a beta-adrenergic antagonist may be administered to offset sympathetic nervous system hyperactivity. Cardiac dysrhythmias may be treated with lidocaine. The trachea may be intubated if indicated for airway protection. Other treatment is supportive as necessary, including hydration and the correction of electrolyte disorders. (292; **971**)

78. The mortality associated with delirium tremens can be as high as 10%. The usual cause of death in these patients is cardiac dysrhythmias or seizures. (292; **971**)

79. Although chronic alcohol use may increase anesthetic requirements, acute alcohol ingestion decreases anesthetic requirements. (292; **657–658, 1095–1097, Table 29–1**)

80. Acute alcohol ingestion increases the patient's risk of the aspiration of gastric contents. (292)

81. Acute alcohol ingestion may interfere with the aggregation of platelets. This can manifest as increased bleeding intraoperatively. (292)

DISEASE OF THE BILIARY TRACT

82. Approximately 20% of women and 10% of men aged 55 to 65 years are believed to have gallstones. Elevated serum bilirubin and/or alkaline phosphatase levels

in these patients imply the presence of a stone in the common bile duct causing obstruction to the flow of bile. (292; **658–659**)

83. Opioids such as morphine, meperidine, and fentanyl may produce spasm in the sphincter of Oddi in less than 3% of patients. This increases the pressure in the common bile duct in a dose-dependent manner and may be painful to an awake patient. The administration of these medicines intraoperatively could hinder the passage of contrast medium for exploration of the common bile duct. In clinical practice the administration of opioids to these patients rarely results in difficulty with intraoperative cholangiograms. (292–293, Fig. 21–11; **306–307**)

84. Anesthetic considerations for patients undergoing laparoscopic procedures are multiple. Included are the insufflation of the abdomen with carbon dioxide and the possible impairment of ventilation of the lungs in the presence of increased ventilatory requirements, the probable placement of the patient in the reverse Trendelenburg position, the risk of puncture of bowel or vessels, and the potential for nitrous oxide to expand bowel gas. (293; **2016–2017**)

Chapter 21

Renal Disease

1. What are some essential physiologic functions of the kidneys?

2. What percent of the adult American population is estimated to have co-existing renal disease that may increase the risk of perioperative morbidity?

3. Name some factors that place patients at an increased risk of acute renal failure in the perioperative period.

ANATOMY AND PHYSIOLOGY OF THE KIDNEY

4. What is a nephron? What are the two components of the nephron? How does the number of nephrons change after birth?

5. What does normal physiologic renal function depend on?

6. What percent of the cardiac output normally goes to the kidneys? What fraction of this goes to the renal cortex?

7. Over what range of mean arterial blood pressures do renal blood flow and the glomerular filtration rate (GFR) remain constant? How is this accomplished by the kidneys? Why is it important?

8. Even during normal kidney autoregulatory function, what two factors can alter renal blood flow?

9. What nerve roots supply the sympathetic innervation of the kidneys? How does sympathetic nervous system stimulation affect renal blood flow?

10. What is renin? What is the secretion of renin usually in response to? What effect does renin have on renal blood flow?

11. What is the physiologic effect of the secretion of renin?

12. What triggers the release of prostaglandins that are produced by the renal medulla?

13. What is the effect of prostaglandins released by the renal medulla? How do they act to exert this effect?

14. What is glomerular filtration? What is glomerular filtration dependent on?

15. What is the normal hydrostatic pressure of the glomerular capillaries? What is the normal plasma oncotic pressure in the afferent and efferent arterioles?

16. What is the average normal rate of glomerular filtration?

17. About what percent of the fluid shift from glomerular filtration is reabsorbed from renal tubules and ultimately returned to the circulation?

18. How is the GFR influenced by the renal blood flow?

TESTS USED FOR EVALUATION OF RENAL FUNCTION

19. Name some tests used for the evaluation of renal function. How sensitive are tests of renal function?

20. What degree of renal disease can exist before renal function tests begin to indicate possible decreases in renal function?

21. What is the normal level of blood urea nitrogen?

22. What factors may influence the blood urea nitrogen level?

23. Why does the blood urea nitrogen concentration increase in dehydrated states? What is the serum creatinine level under these circumstances?

24. What do blood urea nitrogen concentrations higher than 50 mg/dL almost always indicate?

25. Where does serum creatinine come from? How is the serum creatinine level related to the glomerular filtration rate (GFR)?

26. How might normal serum creatinine levels be different in muscular males when compared with less muscular females?

27. Why might a normal creatinine level be seen in elderly patients despite a decreased GFR?

28. Why might normal serum creatinine levels not accurately reflect the GFR in patients with chronic renal failure?

29. What time course must pass after the onset of acute renal failure before increases in serum creatinine concentrations are seen?

30. What is the creatinine clearance a measurement of? What is a normal creatinine clearance?

31. Why is the creatinine clearance a more reliable measurement of GFR than serum creatinine levels? What is a disadvantage of creatinine clearance measurements?

32. What creatinine clearance rate is considered an indication of a patient being at risk of developing prolonged effects of drugs that are cleared renally? How should the doses of drugs cleared renally be adjusted in these patients?

33. How are proteins normally filtered by the kidneys? What is the most common cause of massive proteinuria?

34. What can result from severe proteinuria?

35. What are some nonrenal causes of proteinuria?

36. What is the normal urine specific gravity after an overnight fast? What does a normal urine specific gravity under these circumstances indicate with regard to renal function?

37. What are some causes of an inability of the renal tubules to concentrate urine adequately?

38. What is the excessive excretion of sodium reflective of? What are some causes of sodium wasting?

EFFECTS OF ANESTHETICS ON RENAL FUNCTION

39. How do volatile anesthetics affect renal function? How might this be reflected clinically?

40. Which volatile anesthetics are most likely to lead to decreases in renal blood flow?

41. How can the effects of anesthetics on renal function be attenuated?

42. How do regional anesthetics affect renal function?

43. What is the reason for the increased release of plasma antidiuretic hormone that can be seen during surgery and anesthesia? What clinical effect does an increased release of plasma antidiuretic hormone have? How can this response be attenuated?

44. What is the clinical effect of atrial natriuretic factor? How does positive end-expiratory pressure affect the release of atrial natriuretic factor?

45. How is the autoregulation of renal blood flow affected by inhaled anesthetics?

46. How can drug-induced changes in sympathetic nervous system tone affect renal blood flow and GFR?

47. How does ketamine affect renal blood flow and GFR?

48. How do increased plasma concentrations of inorganic fluoride affect the kidneys? Which volatile anesthetics are most likely to be metabolized to inorganic fluoride?

49. What is the concern regarding nephrotoxicity produced by compound A?

CHRONIC RENAL DISEASE

50. What is chronic renal disease? What approximate percent of nephrons are nonfunctioning before patients become symptomatic?

51. What approximate percent of nephrons are nonfunctioning when a patient is said to have chronic renal insufficiency?

52. What approximate percent of nephrons are nonfunctioning before a patient becomes uremic and dialysis dependent?

53. Name some physiologic changes commonly present in the patient with chronic renal disease.

54. Why are patients with chronic renal failure often anemic? How can the anemia be treated?

55. What is the usual nature of the bleeding tendency associated with chronic renal failure? How is this reflected by the prothrombin time, plasma thromboplastin time, platelet count, and bleeding time?

56. How can the bleeding tendency usually associated with chronic renal failure be treated? How well does hemodialysis work for its correction?

57. What is the most serious electrolyte abnormality seen in patients with chronic renal disease? What is the implication of this for patients with chronic renal disease who are scheduled for surgery?

58. What are some methods of treating hyperkalemia in a patient with chronic renal disease before emergent surgery?

59. Why do patients with chronic renal disease often have a metabolic acidosis? How can it be treated?

60. Why do patients with chronic renal disease commonly have hypertension? How can it be treated?

61. For patients with chronic renal disease who are scheduled for elective surgery, how should hemodialysis and antihypertensive therapy be managed in the preoperative period?

62. How can the induction of anesthesia in patients with chronic renal disease be achieved?

63. For patients with chronic renal disease, what is the concern regarding the administration of succinylcholine for neuromuscular blockade?

64. What choice of neuromuscular blocking drug should be made for patients with chronic renal disease undergoing surgery with general anesthesia?

65. How likely are patients with chronic renal disease and hypotension to respond to the induction of anesthesia?

66. Which volatile anesthetic may be used for the maintenance of anesthesia in patients with chronic renal disease? What is the concern regarding the formation of inorganic fluorides in these patients?

67. Which intravenous narcotic agents may be used to supplement the maintenance of anesthesia in patients with chronic renal disease?

68. What should the $Paco_2$ be maintained at in patients with chronic renal disease undergoing controlled ventilation of the lungs during a surgical procedure?

69. How should the intravascular fluid volume status be managed intraoperatively in patients with chronic renal disease?

70. How can patients with chronic renal disease be monitored for hyperkalemia intraoperatively?

71. How should arteriovenous shunts be managed intraoperatively in patients with chronic renal disease?

72. What are some advantages of brachial plexus blockade for anesthesia for the placement of a vascular shunt in patients with chronic renal disease? What considerations should be made preoperatively by the anesthesiologist before administering the anesthetic under these conditions?

73. What are some considerations that should be made by the anesthesiologist when skeletal muscle weakness persists or reappears after the reversal of nondepolarizing neuromuscular blocking drugs in patients with chronic renal disease?

DIFFERENTIAL DIAGNOSIS OF PERIOPERATIVE OLIGURIA

74. What is the definition of oliguria?

75. What are some causes of intraoperative prerenal oliguria?

76. For oliguria that is secondary to prerenal causes, is the urine typically concentrated or dilute? Does the urine typically contain excessive stores of sodium or minimal stores of sodium?

77. What is the treatment for prerenal causes of oliguria?

78. What are some causes of intraoperative renal oliguria?

79. For oliguria that is secondary to renal causes such as acute tubular necrosis, is the urine typically concentrated or dilute? Does the urine typically contain excessive or minimal stores of sodium?

80. What is acute tubular necrosis?

81. Why should serum potassium levels be monitored in patients with acute tubular necrosis?

82. What is the concern regarding the administration of diuretics to maintain urine output?

83. What are some causes of intraoperative postrenal oliguria?

84. What is the treatment of postrenal causes of oliguria?

PHARMACOLOGY OF DIURETICS

85. Please complete the following table summarizing some of the effects of the commonly used diuretics by answering yes or no:

	HYPOKALEMIC, HYPOCHLOREMIC, METABOLIC ALKALOSIS	HYPERKALEMIA	HYPERGLYCEMIA
Thiazide diuretics			
Loop diuretics			
Osmotic diuretics			
Aldosterone antagonists			

86. What are some side effects that are associated with hypokalemia?

87. How do thiazide diuretics exert their effect? What are they typically prescribed for?

88. What are some potential problems with prolonged or excessive administration of thiazide diuretics?

89. How do loop diuretics exert their effect? What are they typically prescribed for?

90. How quickly does the diuretic response occur after the intravenous administration of a loop diuretic?

91. How do osmotic diuretics exert their effect? What are they typically prescribed for? What is the most frequently administered osmotic diuretic?

92. How does the administration of osmotic diuretics acutely affect the intravascular fluid volume?

93. How do aldosterone antagonist diuretics exert their effect? For what are they typically prescribed?

TRANSURETHRAL SURGERY

94. How is the procedure for transurethral resection of the prostate or transurethral resection of a bladder tumor accomplished?

95. What is a benefit of general anesthesia for transurethral surgery? What is a disadvantage of general anesthesia for transurethral surgery?

96. What is a benefit of regional anesthesia for transurethral surgery? What is a disadvantage of regional anesthesia for transurethral surgery?

97. What are some complications of transurethral surgery?

98. How does intravascular absorption of irrigating fluid during transurethral surgery occur? What factors determine the amount of irrigating fluid that is absorbed during the procedure?

99. What fluids may be used as irrigating fluids during transurethral surgery? What are the potential problems with electrolyte-containing fluids or with distilled water?

100. What are the potential complications associated with the use of glycine as an irrigating fluid in patients undergoing transurethral surgery?

101. What is a potential complication associated with the use of Cytal as an irrigating fluid in patients undergoing transurethral surgery?

102. What is transurethral resection of the prostate (TURP) syndrome?

103. Name some manifestations of TURP syndrome.

104. How might a patient be monitored intraoperatively for signs and symptoms of excessive intravascular absorption of irrigating fluid?

105. If excessive intravascular absorption of irrigating fluid is thought to have occurred, how might the patient be treated?

106. How does bladder perforation present in the patient undergoing transurethral surgery?

107. Why might abnormally excessive bleeding follow transurethral resection of the prostate?

108. Why might patients become bacteremic after transurethral resection of the prostate?

ANSWERS*

1. Essential physiologic functions of the kidneys include the excretion of metabolic wastes; the retention of nutrients; the regulation of water, tonicity, and electrolyte and hydrogen ion concentrations in the blood; and the production of hormones that contribute to water regulation and bone metabolism. (294; **663, 1297**)

2. Approximately 5% of the adult American population is estimated to have co-existing renal disease that may increase the risk of perioperative morbidity. (294; **976**)

3. Factors that place patients at an increased risk of acute renal failure in the perioperative period include co-existing renal disease, prolonged renal hypoperfusion, high-risk operative procedures such as abdominal aneurysm resection, cardiopulmonary bypass, advanced age, congestive heart failure, extensive burns, sepsis, jaundice, and certain medicines. (294; **684–686, 1945–1946, Table 53–7**)

ANATOMY AND PHYSIOLOGY OF THE KIDNEY

4. The nephron is the functional unit of the kidney. There are approximately 1.2 million nephrons in each kidney. Each nephron consists of two components, the glomerulus and the renal tubule. Urine is made by a combination of glomerular filtration and renal tubule reabsorption and secretion. The number of nephrons does not change after birth. (294, Fig. 21–1; **663, Fig. 18–1**)

5. Normal physiologic renal function is dependent on adequate renal blood flow, glomerular filtration, and responses to nonrenal and renal humoral substances. Nonrenal humoral substances the kidney responds to include parathyroid hormone and antidiuretic hormone, and renal humoral substances the kidney responds to include renin and prostaglandins. (294; **663**)

6. Although the kidneys typically constitute only 0.5% of body weight, about 20% of the cardiac output normally goes to the kidneys. Of the 20%, more than two thirds goes to the renal cortex and the remaining blood flow supplies the renal medulla. The effect of anesthesia on this relationship is not known. (294; **669, 1308**)

7. Renal blood flow and the glomerular filtration rate (GFR) remain constant when mean arterial blood pressures range between 60 and 150 mm Hg. This autoregulatory function of the kidneys is accomplished by the afferent arteriolar vascular bed. The afferent arterioles are able to adjust their tone in response to changes in blood pressure, such that during times of higher mean

---

*Numbers in parentheses: lightface numbers refer to pages, figures, or tables in Stoelting RK, Miller RD: Basics of Anesthesia, 4th ed. Philadelphia, Churchill Livingstone, 2000; **boldface numbers** refer to pages, figures, or tables in Miller RD: Anesthesia, 5th ed. Philadelphia, Churchill Livingstone, 2000.

arterial blood pressures the afferent arterioles vasoconstrict, whereas the opposite occurs during times of lower mean arterial blood pressures. This is important for two reasons. The ability of the kidneys to maintain constant renal blood flow despite fluctuations in blood pressure ensures continued renal tubular function in the face of changes, especially decreases, in blood pressure. In addition, autoregulatory responses of the afferent arterioles protect the glomerular capillaries from large increases in blood pressure during times of hypertension, as may occur with direct laryngoscopy. When mean arterial blood pressures are less than 60 mm Hg or greater than 150 mm Hg renal blood flow is blood pressure dependent. (294; **665–666, 1936–1937, Fig. 18–3**)

8. Even during normal kidney autoregulatory function, renal blood flow can be altered by sympathetic nervous system activity and by circulating renin. (294–295; **665–666, 678**)

9. Sympathetic innervation of the kidneys is supplied by the T4 to L4 nerve roots. There is no parasympathetic nervous system innervation to the kidney. The sympathetic nervous system is stimulated by a decrease in mean arterial blood pressure that is sensed by baroreceptors at the aortic arch, carotid sinus, and afferent arterioles. This causes stimulation of alpha-adrenergic receptors, which in turn results in renal vascular smooth muscle contraction and vasoconstriction. Renal blood flow is subsequently decreased during times of decreased mean arterial pressures. Of note, sympathetic nervous system stimulation and stimulation of the renin-angiotensin system are closely related. (294–295; **677–678**)

10. Renin is an enzyme secreted by the endothelial cells of the afferent arterioles. There are at least three things that stimulate the release of renin from the endothelial cells of the afferent arteriole. First, a decrease in the renal perfusion pressure is sensed by baroreceptors in the afferent arteriole endothelial cells. The afferent arterioles are part of the juxtaglomerular apparatus of the kidneys. The decrease in renal blood flow can be from actual hypovolemia or effective hypovolemia. Actual hypovolemia can occur from hemorrhage, diuresis, and sodium loss or retention; and effective hypovolemia may be associated with positive pressure ventilation, congestive heart failure, sepsis, and cirrhosis. The secretion of renin therefore occurs in response to decreases in renal blood flow. Second, sympathetic nervous system stimulation results in stimulation of beta receptors in the afferent arterioles. Third, increases in the chloride concentration of the tubular fluid are sensed by the macula densa of the distal tubule. The ultimate effect of renin secretion is vasoconstriction of the afferent arterioles and a subsequent decrease in renal blood flow. (295; **678–679**)

11. Renin is the rate-limiting enzyme in the production of angiotensin II. After its secretion from the juxtaglomerular apparatus of the kidneys, renin acts on angiotensinogen. Angiotensinogen is a large glycoprotein released by the liver to the circulation. After being cleaved by renin, angiotensin I is formed from angiotensinogen. Angiotensin I is in turn cleaved by angiotensin converting enzyme in the lungs to form angiotensin II. Angiotensin II stimulates the release of aldosterone from the adrenal cortex and is a potent vasoconstrictor. It also inhibits renin secretion as part of a negative feedback loop. (295; **678–679**)

12. Prostaglandins are released from the renal medulla in response to angiotensin II and sympathetic nervous system stimulation. (295; **680–681, 1300, Fig. 18–15**)

13. Prostaglandins released by the renal medulla preserve renal function during times of ischemic insult or injury. This protective effect of prostaglandins is

mediated by its effects of renal vascular dilation and the enhancement of sodium and water excretion. Thus, prostaglandins attenuate the actions of the sympathetic nervous system and renin on the kidney. Drugs that inhibit prostaglandins, such as nonsteroidal anti-inflammatory agents and aspirin, may impair this protective effect of prostaglandins. (295–296; **680–681, 1300, Fig. 18–15**)

14. Glomerular filtration is the filtration of water and low molecular weight substances from the blood in the renal afferent arterioles into Bowman's space through the glomerulus. Glomerular filtration is dependent on two things: the permeability of the filtration barrier (the glomerular membrane) and the net difference between the hydrostatic forces pushing fluid into Bowman's space and the osmotic forces keeping fluid in the plasma. (295; **663–664, 1299–1300**)

15. The normal hydrostatic pressure of the glomerular capillaries is about 50 mm Hg. The normal plasma oncotic pressure in the afferent and efferent arterioles is 25 mm Hg and 35 mm Hg, respectively. The increase in oncotic pressure between the afferent and efferent arterioles reflects the effects of filtration. (295; **1299**)

16. The average normal rate of glomerular filtration is 125 mL/min. (295; **672**)

17. About 90% of the fluids that have been filtered by the glomerulus into Bowman's capsule are reabsorbed from renal tubules and ultimately returned to the circulation. (295; **667, 1299, Fig. 18–6**)

18. The GFR is decreased during times of decreased renal blood flow or decreased mean arterial blood pressure. (295; **672, 1299, Fig. 18–3**)

TESTS USED FOR EVALUATION OF RENAL FUNCTION

19. Tests that are commonly used for the preoperative evaluation of glomerular function include a serum creatinine level, a blood urea nitrogen level, creatinine clearance, and urine protein levels. Tests that are commonly used for the preoperative evaluation of renal tubular function include the urine specific gravity, urine osmolarity, and urine sodium excretion. Most tests of renal function are not very sensitive. (296; **670–677, 1305–1306, 1308–1310**)

20. A significant degree of renal disease can exist before it is reflected in renal function tests. It is estimated that more than 50% of nephrons must be nonfunctional, or that the glomerular filtration rate (GFR) must decrease by 75%, before renal function tests become abnormal. (296; **674, 1305–1306, 1309–1310, 1938**)

21. The normal blood urea nitrogen level in serum varies among individuals, typically ranging between 10 and 20 mg/dL. Urea is freely filtered by the glomerulus of the kidney, but its reabsorption from the tubules varies greatly. Although the blood urea nitrogen varies with changes in GFR, it is influenced by multiple other factors that decrease its utility as a measure of the GFR and of renal function. (296; **1302, 1309–1310, 1938**)

22. Factors that may influence the blood urea nitrogen level include dietary protein intake, gastrointestinal bleeding, decreased urinary flow, hepatic function, and increased catabolism as during trauma, sepsis, or febrile illness. (296; **1302, 1305–1306, 1309–1310, 1938, Table 34–4**)

23. The blood urea nitrogen concentration increases in dehydrated states as a result of the corresponding decrease in urinary flow. During low urinary flow rates a greater fraction of the urea is reabsorbed by the kidney. During low urinary flow rates the serum creatinine level remains normal, such that the

ratio of serum blood urea nitrogen to creatinine is increased during times of low urinary flow associated with hypovolemia. (296; **976, 1302, 1305–1306, 1310, 1938**)

24. Blood urea nitrogen concentrations higher than 50 mg/dL are almost always an indication of hypovolemia. (296; **1305–1306**)

25. Serum creatinine is a product of skeletal muscle protein catabolism. Serum creatinine levels are dependent on a patient's total body water, creatinine generation rate, and creatinine excretion rate. The generation of creatinine is relatively constant within an individual, making its release into the circulation relatively constant as well. Serum creatinine levels are believed to be reliable indicators of the GFR, because its rate of clearance from the circulation is directly dependent on the GFR. (296; **672–674, 969, 1309–1310, 1938, Figs. 18–11, 34–7**)

26. Muscular males produce more creatinine by virtue of their greater skeletal muscle mass. Normal serum creatinine levels are therefore higher in muscular males than in less muscular females. (296; **673–674, 1309–1310, 1938**)

27. Elderly patients may have a normal creatinine level despite a decreased GFR secondary to the decrease in muscle mass that commonly accompanies aging. For this reason, even mild increases in the serum creatinine level of elderly patients may be an indication of significant renal dysfunction. (296; **673–674, 1309–1310, 1938**)

28. Normal serum creatinine levels may not accurately reflect the GFR in patients with chronic renal failure for two reasons. First, patients with chronic renal failure may have decreased skeletal muscle mass, resulting in a decrease in creatinine production. Second, the excretion of creatinine occurs via nonrenal means in these patients. (296–297; **673–674, 1309–1310, 1938**)

29. Serum creatinine concentrations begin to increase 8 hours after the onset of acute renal failure. This makes serum creatinine levels unreliable indicators of early acute renal failure. (297; **673–674, 976, 1945–1946**)

30. The creatinine clearance is a measurement of the excretion of creatinine into the urine after being filtered by the glomerulus. A normal creatinine clearance is 110 to 150 mL/min. (297; **672–673, 976, 1311, 1938**)

31. The creatinine clearance is a more reliable measurement of GFR than serum creatinine levels because the clearance of creatinine from the serum is directly dependent on glomerular filtration, whereas creatinine generation varies with muscle mass, protein intake, physical activity, and catabolism. A disadvantage of creatinine clearance measurements is the requirement of accurate, timed urine collections. (297; **672–673, 976, 1311, 1938**)

32. A creatinine clearance rate between 10 and 25 mL/min is considered an indication of a patient being at risk of developing prolonged effects of renally cleared drugs. The doses of drugs cleared renally should be decreased in these patients. (297; **672–673, 1311, 1938, 1940**)

33. Proteins are normally filtered by the kidneys at the glomerulus and are reabsorbed by the renal tubules. Massive proteinuria is usually due to glomerular damage leading to abnormally high filtration. Proteinuria from renal dysfunction may also be due to failure of the renal tubules to reabsorb protein, an abnormally increased concentration of plasma proteins, and the presence of abnormal proteins that are excreted in the urine. (297; **1305, 1938**)

34. Severe proteinuria can result in a decrease in plasma albumin and in an associated decrease in plasma oncotic pressure and plasma binding of drugs. (297; **1938**)

35. Intermittent proteinuria occurs in healthy individuals after standing for long periods of time and after strenuous exercise. Proteinuria may also occur during states of fever and congestive heart failure. (297; **1938**)

36. A normal urine specific gravity after an overnight fast is greater than 1.018. A specific gravity of 1.018 or greater after an overnight fast implies the renal tubules are able to functionally concentrate the urine by conserving sodium and water. (297; **1309, 1937–1938**)

37. Causes of an inability of the renal tubules to concentrate urine adequately are multiple. These include hypokalemia; hypercalcemia; excessive serum concentrations of inorganic fluoride-, glucose-, or dextran-containing solutions; proteins; extremes of age; the administration of radiographic contrast media; chronic pyelonephritis; and the administration of mannitol, diuretics, and some antibiotics. (297; **674–675, 1309, 1937–1938, Table 34–3**)

38. The excessive excretion of sodium reflects an inability of the renal tubules to conserve sodium. Conservation of sodium by the renal tubules typically occurs in response to decreased perfusion. Factors that influence this function of the renal tubules include aldosterone secretion, antidiuretic hormone secretion, adrenal gland function, diuretic therapy, the sodium content of administered intravenous fluids, and sympathetic neural control. An excessively high level of urinary sodium may be an indication of acute tubular necrosis, but this test is nonspecific. (297; **675, 1310–1311**)

EFFECTS OF ANESTHETICS ON RENAL FUNCTION

39. Anesthetics may decrease renal blood flow and renal function secondary to the decrease in mean arterial blood pressure produced by their administration. The decrease in renal blood flow and GFR caused by volatile anesthetics is reflected as a decrease in urine output during anesthesia. (297; **677, 684, 1941–1942**)

40. All volatile anesthetics produce similar, dose-dependent decreases in renal blood flow, GFR, and urine output. (297, Fig. 22–2; **684, 1941, Table 53–4**)

41. The effects of anesthetics on renal function can be attenuated by administering low concentrations of volatile anesthetic and ensuring the patient is adequately hydrated. (297; **684**)

42. Regional anesthetics have minimal effects on renal function as long as the mean arterial blood pressure is maintained. (297; **684**)

43. Antidiuretic hormone secretion results in the tubular conservation of water, an increased urine osmolality, and a decrease in plasma osmolality. It is typically secreted in response to small increases in serum osmolality. It is also secreted in response to stretch receptors in the left atrium and pulmonary veins, and in response to a decreased mean arterial pressure sensed by aortic and carotid body baroreceptors. Anesthetics have little direct effect on the secretion of antidiuretic hormone, but their secretion is directly increased in response to painful surgical stimulation. The secretion of antidiuretic hormone in response to surgery can be attenuated by hydrating the patient before the induction of anesthesia. (297–298, Fig. 22–3; **679–680**)

44. Atrial natriuretic factor is released from atrial myocytes in response to local wall stretch and increased left atrial volume. The secretion of atrial natriuretic factor results in an increase in the GFR and in salt excretion by dilating the afferent arterioles. It also appears to oppose the renin-angiotensin-aldosterone system. Positive end-expiratory pressure alters atrial filling and inhibits the release of atrial natriuretic factor. (297; **681–682, Fig. 18–18**)

45. The autoregulation of renal blood flow does not appear to be affected by inhaled anesthetics. (297; **683**)

46. Drug-induced changes in sympathetic nervous system tone directly affect renal blood flow and the GFR through the sympathetic innervation of the kidney, regardless of the mean arterial pressure or cardiac output. Sympathetic nervous system stimulation causes stimulation of alpha-adrenergic receptors, which in turn results in renal vascular smooth muscle contraction and vasoconstriction. (297; **677–678, 682–684, 1934–1935**)

47. Ketamine decreases renal blood flow and the GFR through its stimulation of the sympathetic nervous system. The decreased renal blood flow and GFR occur secondary to ketamine-induced renal vascular vasoconstriction. (297; **677–678**)

48. Increased plasma concentrations of inorganic fluoride can lead to renal toxicity, manifesting as an inability of the renal tubules to concentrate urine and polyuria. Although concentrations of inorganic fluoride of 50 μm/L or greater were originally considered nephrotoxic, more recent studies have found renal function to be preserved when sevoflurane administration led to inorganic fluoride at these levels. Historically, the volatile anesthetic that was most likely to be metabolized to inorganic fluoride was methoxyflurane. Of the anesthetics currently being used, sevoflurane is the most likely to be metabolized to inorganic fluorides. The plasma inorganic fluoride concentration does not significantly change after the administration of isoflurane, halothane, or desflurane. Inorganic fluorides must be eliminated by glomerular filtration. Patients with decreased GFRs are especially at risk of nephrotoxicity, owing to increased levels of circulating inorganic fluorides, particularly when exposed to high levels of inorganic fluorides for a prolonged duration. In clinical practice, however, the administration of sevoflurane to patients with decreased GFRs has not been shown to increase their risk of postoperative renal dysfunction. (298; **684–685, 1941**)

49. A potentially toxic interaction between the carbon dioxide absorbent and sevoflurane is the production of compound A. This can occur with either soda lime or baralyme, but the risk appears to be higher with baralyme. Other factors that may increase the risk of compound A production include the low inflow of fresh gases, high concentrations of sevoflurane, higher absorbent temperatures, and fresh absorbent. The concern with compound A is that it has been shown to be nephrotoxic in animals. Even so, no clinical cases of nephrotoxicity have occurred in humans, even with low gas inflows. The current recommendation remains to maintain a fresh gas flow of at least 2 L/min when administering sevoflurane to minimize the amount of compound A formation. (7, 144, 298–299, Fig. 22–5; **194–195, 684–685, 1941**)

CHRONIC RENAL DISEASE

50. Chronic renal disease is an irreversible decrease in the GFR as a result of decreasing numbers of functioning nephrons. Approximately 50% or more of nephrons are nonfunctioning before the onset of symptoms associated with chronic renal failure. (299, Table 22–2)

51. Chronic renal insufficiency occurs when 60% to 90% of nephrons are nonfunctioning. Patients with chronic renal insufficiency are typically well compensated with the remaining functioning nephrons until times of renal stress, as with catabolic loads or toxic substances. These stressors can exacerbate renal insufficiency. (299)

52. Uremia and the need for chronic hemodialysis occur when more than 90% of nephrons are nonfunctioning. (299)

53. Physiologic changes commonly present in the patient with chronic renal disease include anemia, increased cardiac output, decreased platelet adhesiveness, hyperkalemia, unpredictable intravascular fluid volume, metabolic acidosis, systemic hypertension, pericardial effusion, and decreased sympathetic nervous system activity. (299; **975–976**)

54. Patients with chronic renal failure are often anemic secondary to the abnormal production of erythropoietin by the diseased kidney. A typical hemoglobin level in these patients is 5 to 8 g/dL. The anemia in these patients is generally well tolerated owing to a compensatory rightward shift of the oxyhemoglobin dissociation curve. Nevertheless, many patients with anemia and chronic renal failure experience fatigue. The anemia associated with chronic renal failure can be treated with the administration of recombinant human erythropoietin. Erythropoietin administration is usually discontinued when a target hematocrit of 30% to 33% is achieved. (299; **975, 1938**)

55. The bleeding tendency associated with chronic renal failure occurs as a result of decreased platelet adhesiveness. This is due in part to a release of dysfunctional von Willebrand factor in these patients. When decreased platelet adhesiveness is the sole cause of the bleeding tendency, there is an increased bleeding time. The prothrombin time, plasma thromboplastin time, and platelet count are all normal. (300; **975**)

56. The bleeding tendency associated with chronic renal failure, or decreased platelet adhesiveness, can be treated with the administration of erythropoietin or red blood cells. Evidence has shown that there is a decrease in the bleeding time of uremic patients when the hematocrit is greater than 26%. Additional methods of decreasing the bleeding time of these patients is with the administration of desmopressin, cryoprecipitate, or estrogen. Desmopressin works acutely, peaking in 1 to 4 hours and lasting up to 8 hours. The effects of estrogen last for up to 14 days. Hemodialysis has not been shown to reliably improve the bleeding time for these patients. (300; **975**)

57. Hyperkalemia is the most serious electrolyte abnormality seen in patients with chronic renal disease. This electrolyte abnormality results from the diseased kidney's inability to eliminate hydrogen ions. Hyperkalemia can result in myocardial dysfunction, both with electrical disturbances and cardiac contractility. Patients with severe hyperkalemia may have a prolonged PR interval, a widened QRS, and peaked T waves on their electrocardiogram. Patients with chronic renal disease who are scheduled for surgery should have their electrolytes evaluated before surgery even after hemodialysis and necessary treatment has been instituted. Elective surgery is often recommended to be delayed when serum potassium levels are in excess of 5.5 mEq/L. (299–300; **979–981**)

58. Hyperkalemia that is present in a patient with chronic renal disease can be treated before emergent surgery with the administration of 10 to 20 units of insulin in combination with 50 g of glucose. Calcium chloride may be administered to facilitate myocardial function in the presence of hyperkalemia. Intraoperatively the patient may be hyperventilated as well. For each 10 mm Hg decrease in the $PaCO_2$, the serum potassium level decreases by about 0.5 mEq/L. (299–300; **979–981**)

59. Patients with chronic renal disease often have a metabolic acidosis as a result of the inability of the kidneys to excrete hydrogen ions. Metabolic acidosis can be treated with hemodialysis. If metabolic acidosis is severe such that the arterial pH is less than 7.15, and the patient is scheduled for emergent surgery, hyperventilation of the lungs should be instituted and the intravenous administration of sodium bicarbonate may be considered. Care should be taken to correct acidemia slowly. The patient should also not be hypocalcemic,

because metabolic acidosis is protective for the effects of hypocalcemia. Correction of the acidemia under these conditions could lead to seizures. (299; **975, 1936**)

60. Patients with chronic renal disease commonly have hypertension. Hypertension associated with chronic renal disease is most likely due to a combination of volume overload and activation of the renin-angiotensin-aldosterone system. Hemodialysis may treat hypertension in these patients through the removal of excess fluid. There exists a subset of patients who may have hypertension that is refractory to hemodialysis, in which case antihypertensives should be administered. Patients with perioperative hypertension may benefit from the administration of vasodilators such as hydralazine, labetalol, or nitroprusside for blood pressure control. Postoperative hypertension is frequently noted in these patients as well. (300; **1949–1950**)

61. Patients with chronic renal disease scheduled for elective surgery should continue their antihypertensive medicine regimen throughout the perioperative period. Hemodialysis should precede surgery in these patients, and serum electrolyte levels should be measured after hemodialysis. (300; **975–976, 1946**)

62. The induction of anesthesia in patients with chronic renal disease can be achieved with the administration of intravenous anesthetics in conjunction with succinylcholine or a nondepolarizing neuromuscular blocking drug. (300–301)

63. Succinylcholine may be used for neuromuscular blockade in patients with chronic renal disease. To avoid dangerous rises in the serum potassium level, succinylcholine should not be administered to patients with hyperkalemia. Potassium release after the administration of succinylcholine is not exaggerated in patients with chronic renal disease. The increase in serum potassium in patients with chronic renal disease in the absence of any neuromuscular impairment after the administration of succinylcholine is 0.5 to 1 mEq/L. (301; **1942**)

64. Nondepolarizing neuromuscular blocking drugs that are not dependent on renal clearance mechanisms are the preferred choice for patients with chronic renal disease. Intermediate- and short-acting neuromuscular blocking drugs may be preferred in patients with renal failure, particularly because long-acting pancuronium relies heavily on renal clearance mechanisms. Vecuronium is slightly prolonged in patients with renal failure. Atracurium metabolizes to laudanosine, which is primarily cleared by renal excretion. Although laudanosine lacks any effects relating to neuromuscular blockade, it may produce central nervous system stimulation and seizures with sufficient plasma levels. The newer nondepolarizing neuromuscular blocking drug cisatracurium does not significantly metabolize to laudanosine. Nondepolarizing neuromuscular blocking drug doses should be titrated to the desired effect with the use of a peripheral nerve stimulator. (301; **457–458, 1942–1944, Table 53–5**)

65. Patients with chronic renal disease and hypotension are likely to respond to the induction of anesthesia regardless of their intravascular fluid volume status. Patients with chronic renal disease may have autonomic nervous system dysfunction as well as impaired baroreceptor-mediated reflex responses. These two changes in conjunction with antihypertensive therapy and positive pressure ventilation of the lungs could lead to exaggerated decreases in blood pressure associated with the induction of anesthesia. An adequate intravascular fluid volume status should be confirmed before the induction of anesthesia. (300–301; **976–977**)

66. All volatile anesthetics may be used for the maintenance of anesthesia in

patients with chronic renal disease. There is concern regarding the metabolism of sevoflurane, like enflurane and methoxyflurane, to an inorganic fluoride that is potentially nephrotoxic. Although there is concern regarding the formation of inorganic fluorides in these patients, the administration of enflurane to patients with chronic renal disease in the past failed to show higher peak concentrations of fluoride or a decreased rate of clearance of fluoride from the plasma when compared with halothane. Nevertheless, it may be prudent to avoid the administration of sevoflurane to patients with chronic renal disease. (298, 301; **684–685, 1941**)

67. Intravenous narcotic agents that are preferred for the maintenance of anesthesia in patients with chronic renal disease are those with minimal renally excreted, pharmacologically active metabolites. Morphine-6-glucuronide, a metabolite of morphine that is pharmacologically active, is excreted renally and may be a poor choice for patients with renal failure. Likewise, the administration of meperidine should be avoided in these patients. Its metabolite normeperidine can cause central nervous system excitation and is excreted renally. (301; **1940–1941**)

68. The Pa_{CO_2} is best maintained near normal in patients with chronic renal disease undergoing controlled ventilation of the lungs during a surgical procedure. An increase in the Pa_{CO_2} can result in respiratory acidosis and a subsequent shift of potassium from the intracellular to extracellular compartments. A decrease in the Pa_{CO_2} can result in respiratory alkalosis, a shift in the oxyhemoglobin curve to the left, and a decrease in oxygen delivery to the tissues. (301)

69. The intravascular fluid volume status of patients with chronic renal disease should be carefully managed intraoperatively. The intravenous fluid solutions administered should not contain potassium. The measurement of central venous pressures may be a useful guide to the replacement of fluids in these patients. Patients who are dialysis dependent have very little reserve between inadequate and excessive volume status, making the controlled administration of fluids to these patients crucial. Hypertension occurring in the postoperative period may be secondary to volume overload and may require hemodialysis for its treatment. (301; **1609–1610**)

70. Patients with chronic renal disease should be closely monitored for hyperkalemia intraoperatively by looking for changes related to hyperkalemia on the electrocardiogram or, if there is concern, by measuring serum electrolytes directly. (301; **979–980**)

71. Arteriovenous shunts in hemodialysis-dependent patients should be protected and monitored frequently intraoperatively to ensure they remain patent. Its patency can be easily evaluated through direct palpation. (301)

72. Brachial plexus blockade for the placement of a vascular shunt in patients with chronic renal disease allows the surgeons excellent working conditions by causing vasodilation and inhibiting vasospasm. Considerations that should be made before administering the anesthetic under these conditions are the adequacy of coagulation, the possibility for a decreased seizure threshold for local anesthetics in the presence of metabolic acidosis, and any evidence of neuropathy in the extremity. (302; **1947**)

73. Persistent skeletal muscle weakness after the reversal of nondepolarizing neuromuscular blocking drugs in patients with chronic renal disease should lead to a search for a cause other than waning effects of the anticholinesterase drug. Anticholinesterase drugs are primarily cleared by the kidneys, such that their effects should not wane any sooner than the effects of the neuromuscular blocking drug themselves. Given that, causes for the persistent skeletal muscle

weakness may include antibiotics, acidosis, electrolyte imbalances, or diuretics. (301; **1943–1944**)

DIFFERENTIAL DIAGNOSIS OF PERIOPERATIVE OLIGURIA

74. Oliguria is defined as a urine output less than 0.5 mL/kg in 1 hour. Prolonged oliguria in the perioperative period requires a search for a cause and treatment because it can lead to acute renal failure. (302, Fig. 22–6; **1303–1304, 1308–1309, 1945**)

75. Prerenal oliguria is indicative of a decrease in renal blood flow, the most common causes of which include a decrease in the intravascular fluid volume and a decrease in the cardiac output. Another cause may be surgical compression of the renal arteries leading to obstructed blood flow to the kidneys, either directly through clamping or inadvertently through retraction or manual traction. Whatever the cause, the duration of oliguria should be minimized to decrease the risk of acute renal failure. (302; **1303–1304, 1945, Table 53–7**)

76. Oliguria that is secondary to prerenal causes in normal kidneys typically results in urine that is concentrated and contains minimal sodium. This is indicative of normal renal function, because the kidneys attempt to conserve water and sodium under these conditions. If a diuretic had been previously administered, urine sodium concentration is increased and attributing the oliguria to prerenal causes becomes difficult. (302, Table 22–3; **1303–1304, 1309, 1945, Table 53–8**)

77. The treatment of prerenal causes of oliguria is dependent on whether the cause is secondary to a decrease in intravascular fluid volume or to a decrease in cardiac output. A crystalloid fluid bolus of 2 to 6 mL/kg would result in a brisk diuresis if in fact the cause was hypovolemia. A lack of response to the fluid bolus would indicate that perhaps the cause of the oliguria is a decrease in cardiac output or is a result of the secretion of antidiuretic hormone in response to surgical stress. A small dose of furosemide, 0.1 mg/kg intravenously, will lead to diuresis if the cause of the oliguria is antidiuretic hormone secretion. If there is no response to the intravenous administration of furosemide, a determination should be made as to whether the patient remains hypovolemic or there is a decrease in cardiac output. If the patient is at risk for a decrease in cardiac output, it may be worthwhile to monitor cardiac filling pressures to guide intravascular fluid replacement. If cardiac filling pressures are high, a cause for the decrease in cardiac output should be sought. To maintain renal blood flow under these conditions renal doses of dopamine may be administered at a rate of 3 to 5 µg/kg per minute. The administration of dopamine is associated with other effects as well, because it stimulates not only dopaminergic receptors but also alpha- and beta-adrenergic receptors. Fenoldopam is a dopamine-1-selective drug recently approved by the U. S. Food and Drug Administration for short-term parenteral administration to patients with severe hypertension. It may be useful for the treatment of oliguria through its mechanism of renal vascular vasodilation through dopamine-1-selective stimulation. The administration of fenoldopam results in increased renal blood flow, glomerular filtration, and diuresis. It does decrease systemic blood pressure and should be reserved for oliguric patients who are hemodynamically stable. (302–303, Fig. 22–7; **682–684, 976, 1297–1299, 1303–1309**)

78. Renal oliguria refers to oliguria in which damaged renal tubules are unable to conserve sodium. Some causes of intraoperative renal oliguria include renal ischemia due to prerenal causes, nephrotoxic drugs, and the deposition

of hemoglobin or myoglobin in the renal tubules. Examples of nephrotoxic drugs include aminoglycoside antibiotics, chemotherapy agents, and radiocontrast dyes. Another term for renal oliguria is *acute tubular necrosis.* (303; **1303–1304, 1945–1946, Table 53–7**)

79. Oliguria secondary to primary renal disease, such as acute tubular necrosis, is characterized by urine that is typically dilute and contains excessive sodium. (303, Table 22–3; **1303–1305, 1309, 1945, Table 53–8**)

80. Acute tubular necrosis is acute renal failure due to primary renal disease. It is characterized as the sudden inability of the kidneys to clear metabolic wastes or maintain electrolyte, acid-base, and volume homeostasis. Acute renal failure secondary to primary renal disease is responsible for nearly 90% of the causes of perioperative renal failure. (303; **1303–1306, 1309–1310, 1945**)

81. Serum potassium concentrations may rise to dangerous levels quickly in patients with acute tubular necrosis. Postoperative serum potassium levels can increase by 0.3 to 2 mEq/L per day under these conditions, making it important to closely monitor the potassium levels in these patients. (303; **979–980, 1945**)

82. The administration of diuretics to maintain urine output remains a controversial issue. Urine output that is augmented with diuretics has not been shown to decrease the risk of acute tubular necrosis. Another drawback to its use is that it may interfere with subsequent diagnosis for treatment of oliguria. Diuretics may impair sodium reabsorption for up to 12 hours, making the measurement of urine sodium appear as if acute tubular necrosis is the cause of oliguria if the urine sodium level were to be measured. Nevertheless, many believe that preventing the stasis of urine flow in the renal tubules may prevent acute tubular necrosis from developing. Diuretics that are often used for this purpose include mannitol and furosemide. It is important to administer intravascular fluids to the patient before the administration of a diuretic to avoid exacerbation of hypovolemia should that be the cause of the oliguria. (303; **682–683, 974–975**)

83. Causes of intraoperative postrenal oliguria include ureteral obstruction, bladder outlet obstruction, and obstruction or kinking of the Foley catheter. (303; **1945, Table 53–7**)

84. Intraoperative postrenal oliguria in which a Foley catheter is already in place requires irrigation of the Foley catheter and confirmation of its proper placement in the bladder. (303; **1945**)

PHARMACOLOGY OF DIURETICS

85. (304, Table 22–3)

	HYPOKALEMIC, HYPOCHLOREMIC, METABOLIC ALKALOSIS	HYPERKALEMIA	HYPERGLYCEMIA
Thiazide diuretics	Yes	No	Yes
Loop diuretics	Yes	No	No
Osmotic diuretics	No	No	No
Aldosterone antagonists	No	Yes	No

86. Side effects associated with hypokalemia include skeletal muscle weakness, autonomic neuropathy, impaired myocardial contractility, cardiac conduction abnormalities including arrhythmia and ventricular fibrillation, an increase in the likelihood to develop digitalis toxicity, and a potentiation of nondepolarizing neuromuscular blocking drugs. On the electrocardiogram, hypokalemia manifests as widening of the QRS complex, ST segment abnormalities, and decreased T wave amplitude. (304; **980–981**)

87. Thiazide diuretics work by inhibiting the reabsorption of sodium and chloride from the renal tubules. Thiazide diuretics are typically prescribed for the treatment of essential hypertension or for states of intravascular volume excess, as might occur with renal, hepatic, or cardiac dysfunction. (303–304; **669**)

88. Potential problems with prolonged or excessive administration of thiazide diuretics include hypochloremia, hypokalemia, and metabolic alkalosis. (304; **980–981**)

89. Loop diuretics work by inhibiting the reabsorption of sodium and chloride from the renal tubule, as well as facilitating the secretion of potassium. Loop diuretics are typically prescribed for the treatment of pulmonary edema, to decrease the intracranial pressure, and to aid in the differential of acute renal failure. (304; **668–669, 1901–1902**)

90. A diuretic response occurs 2 to 10 minutes after the intravenous administration of a loop diuretic. (304; **668–669, 1901–1902**)

91. Osmotic diuretics are filtered by glomeruli but are not reabsorbed from the renal tubules. Osmotic diuretics work by increasing the osmolarity of the fluid in the renal tubules, thus causing an associated decrease in the reabsorption of water from the tubules. Osmotic diuretics are typically prescribed for patients with increased intracranial pressures. The most frequently administered osmotic diuretic is mannitol. (304; **668–669, 1901–1902**)

92. The administration of osmotic diuretics acutely increases the intravascular fluid volume by increasing the osmolarity of the plasma volume. The increased osmolarity of the fluid volume in turn draws fluid from the intracellular spaces and into the intravascular space. This is the basis for the use of mannitol in decreasing intracranial pressures, but it may also acutely exacerbate pulmonary edema secondary to congestive heart failure. (304; **1901–1902**)

93. Aldosterone antagonist diuretics work by blocking the effects of aldosterone on the renal tubules. Aldosterone antagonist diuretics are typically prescribed for fluid overload secondary to cirrhosis of the liver. (304; **679**)

TRANSURETHRAL SURGERY

94. Transurethral resection of the prostate or transurethral resection of a bladder tumor is accomplished by the placement of a cystoscope through the urethra into the bladder. Fluids are continuously infused into the bladder for irrigation, to distend the bladder, and to improve visualization. The tissue is then excised, bleeding vessels are coagulated, the cystoscope is removed, and a Foley catheter is placed. (304; **1947**)

95. General anesthesia for transurethral surgery is advantageous in uncooperative patients or in patients who require hemodynamic or ventilatory support. A disadvantage of general anesthesia for transurethral surgery is the inability to monitor the patient's level of mentation for signs of alteration, as may occur with the excessive absorption of irrigating fluid. (305; **1949**)

96. A T10 level is necessary for regional anesthesia in patients undergoing

transurethral resections of tumor or prostate. A benefit of regional anesthesia for transurethral surgery is the ability to detect earlier any signs of central nervous system alteration or bladder perforation. Bladder perforation in patients under regional anesthesia often manifests as referred pain to the shoulder as a result of subdiaphragmatic irritation by irrigating fluid. A disadvantage of regional anesthesia for transurethral surgery is the requirement for cooperation. (305; **1949**)

97. Complications of transurethral surgery include the intravascular absorption of irrigating fluid, hemorrhage, hypothermia, transient bacteremia, nerve injury, and perforation of the bladder or urethra. (304; **1947–1949**)

98. Intravascular absorption of irrigating fluid during transurethral surgery occurs via open venous sinuses. Factors that determine the amount of irrigating fluid that is absorbed during the procedure include the number of venous sinuses opened, the size of the venous sinuses opened, the duration of the procedure, and the hydrostatic pressure of the fluid, as determined by the height of the fluid relative to the patient. Typically, 10 to 30 mL of fluid is absorbed per minute of resection time. The duration of transurethral procedures using irrigating fluid is recommended to be no greater than 1 hour. (305; **1947–1948**)

99. Fluids that may be used as irrigating fluids during transurethral surgery include glycine and Cytal, a fluid containing sugars, mannitol, and sorbitol. These fluids satisfy the criteria that they not contain electrolytes, be nontoxic, be transparent, and nearly isotonic. Because of its hypotonicity, the absorption of distilled water into the intravascular space can result in hemolysis. Fluids that contain electrolytes can disperse high-frequency electrical currents from the area where the surgeons are working. (305; **1947–1948**)

100. Potential complications associated with the use of glycine as an irrigating fluid in patients undergoing transurethral surgery include prolonged central nervous system depression and transient blindness. The central nervous system depression can occur with excessive concentrations of plasma ammonia, a metabolite of glycine. Transient blindness can occur as a result of the intravascular absorption of glycine, which is an inhibitory neurotransmitter at the retina. (305; **1947–1948**)

101. A potential complication associated with the use of Cytal as an irrigating fluid in patients undergoing transurethral surgery is bacterial contamination. Bacterial contamination secondary to Cytal absorption can occur because the sugars in the Cytal solution make it a rich culture medium for bacteria. (305; **1948**)

102. Transurethral resection of the prostate (TURP) syndrome refers to symptoms and signs that are caused by the absorption of large volumes of isotonic irrigating fluids. TURP syndrome is characterized by hypervolemia, hyponatremia, and hypo-osmolarity. (305; **1949**)

103. Manifestations of TURP syndrome are the manifestations of hypervolemia, hyponatremia, and hypo-osmolarity. These manifestations include hypertension, bradycardia, increased central venous pressure, pulmonary edema, congestive heart failure, cerebral edema, headache, restlessness, confusion, obtundation, and seizures. (305; **1949**)

104. Intraoperative monitoring for signs and symptoms of excessive intravascular absorption of irrigating fluid includes the monitoring of blood pressure, heart rate and the electrocardiogram tracing. Central venous pressures and/or laboratory blood analysis for the sodium concentration and serum osmolarity may be useful. In addition, in the awake patient undergoing the procedure under regional anesthesia the patient's mental status may be monitored as well. (305; **1949**)

105. If excessive intravascular absorption of irrigating fluid is thought to have occurred, the procedure should be discontinued and fluid restriction instituted. The administration of mannitol or furosemide may be indicated. For severe hyponatremia, the administration of hypertonic saline may be considered. (305; **1949**)

106. Bladder perforation in the patient undergoing transurethral surgery can be extraperitoneal, which is more common, or intraperitoneal. Extraperitoneal perforation in the awake patient leads to pain in the umbilical, inguinal, or suprapubic regions. Intraperitoneal perforation leads to pain that is more generalized, including pain in the upper abdomen and referred from the diaphragm to the shoulder. Patients with an intraperitoneal bladder perforation may also have pallor, sweating, abdominal rigidity, nausea and vomiting, and hypotension. (305; **1948**)

107. The prostate is a highly vascular organ and operative bleeding is generally quantified to be 2 to 4 mL/min during resection. Abnormally excessive bleeding may follow transurethral resection of the prostate in approximately 1% of patients undergoing the procedure. The excessive bleeding is thought to be due to a coagulopathy resulting from the excessive release of plasminogen activator from the prostate. The plasminogen activator released converts plasminogen to plasmin, which causes systemic fibrinolysis. A second explanation for the fibrinolysis is disseminated intravascular coagulation in response to systemically absorbed prostate tissue rich in thromboplastin. It may be prudent to evaluate the patient's hemoglobin after the procedure if excessive, ongoing bleeding is noted or after prolonged resection times. (306; **1948**)

108. Bacteremia may follow transurethral resection of the prostate due to the bacteria normally harbored in the prostate being released to the circulation. Generally, the bacteremia is asymptomatic, with fever being the only identifying factor. Patients are typically treated with antibiotics in the perioperative period to reduce the risk of subsequent septicemia. (306; **1948**)

Chapter 22

Endocrine and Nutritional Disease

DIABETES MELLITUS

1. What approximate percent of the population of the United States has diabetes? How is it most commonly manifest and thus diagnosed?

2. What are the two major classifications of diabetes? The majority of diabetics fall into which classification?

3. What are the available treatments for diabetes?

4. Name eight acute or chronic complications that can occur as a result of diabetes.

5. What is ketoacidosis? How is it diagnosed?

6. What are some causes of ketoacidosis? How is it treated?

7. What is autonomic neuropathy?

8. Name some signs and symptoms that indicate that a patient with diabetes has autonomic neuropathy. What is the clinical importance of this for the anesthesiologist managing the patient with autonomic neuropathy in the perioperative period?

9. How common are peripheral neuropathies in diabetic patients? What is the clinical implication of this?

10. What are some goals of the anesthetic management of patients with diabetes?

11. What are some considerations in the preoperative evaluation of the diabetic patient?

12. What co-morbid condition is often seen in diabetic patients that also accounts for the most common cause of perioperative morbidity in these patients?

13. What information does a serum glycohemoglobin level provide before surgery?

14. What time of the day is preferred for surgery to be scheduled for the insulin-dependent diabetic patient?

15. What are some indications for admission of the diabetic patient to the hospital on the night before surgery?

16. How should exogenous insulin be managed perioperatively in patients with diabetes?

17. Which patients may benefit from tightly controlled plasma glucose levels in the perioperative period? What benefit might these patients derive from tightly controlled plasma glucose levels?

18. How should oral hypoglycemic therapy be managed in the perioperative period?

19. What induction and maintenance anesthetic drugs can be used in patients with diabetes?

20. How do volatile anesthetics affect the secretion of insulin?

21. What physical examination findings are important to note before the administration of a regional anesthetic in diabetic patients?

HYPEROSMOLAR HYPERGLYCEMIC NONKETOTIC COMA

22. Name some signs and symptoms of hyperosmolar hyperglycemic nonketotic coma.

23. Which patients are vulnerable to hyperosmolar hyperglycemic nonketotic coma?

24. How should patients with hyperosmolar hyperglycemic nonketotic coma be managed?

HYPERTHYROIDISM

25. What is hyperthyroidism?

26. How is the diagnosis of hyperthyroidism made?

27. Name some signs and symptoms of hyperthyroidism.

28. What is the most common cause of hyperthyroidism?

29. What approximate percent of parturients become hyperthyroid?

30. How should patients with hyperthyroidism who are scheduled to undergo elective surgery be managed?

31. How should patients with hyperthyroidism who are scheduled to undergo emergent surgery be managed?

32. Why should special attention be paid to the preoperative airway examination in patients with hyperthyroidism?

33. How should the induction of anesthesia be achieved in patients with hyperthyroidism?

34. What consideration should be made before the administration of neuromuscular blocking drugs to facilitate intubation of the trachea in patients with hyperthyroidism?

35. Why might a traditional dose of neuromuscular blocking drug in patients with hyperthyroidism result in a prolonged response? How might the drug dose be altered for these patients?

36. What is the goal of maintenance anesthesia in patients with hyperthyroidism? What anesthetic agents may be used for this purpose?

37. How is the minimum alveolar concentration (MAC) of anesthesia for a patient altered by hyperthyroidism?

38. Why might there be a clinical impression of an increase in the MAC of anesthesia in patients with hyperthyroidism?

39. For patients with hyperthyroidism undergoing anesthesia, how might an increase in body temperature affect the MAC of anesthesia in these patients?

40. What is the concern with regard to the antagonism of nondepolarizing neuromuscular blocking drugs that have been administered to patients with hyperthyroidism?

41. What is a concern with regard to patients with exophthalmos undergoing general anesthesia?

42. Intraoperative monitoring of patients with hyperthyroidism should be directed toward the recognition of which potential complication?

43. How might hypotension be treated in hyperthyroid patients undergoing surgery?

44. What is the advantage of regional anesthesia in a patient with hyperthyroidism who is undergoing a surgical procedure?

45. What is the controversy regarding the addition of epinephrine to a regional anesthetic solution in patients with hyperthyroidism?

46. What is thyroid storm? How does it manifest clinically?

47. When is thyroid storm associated with surgery most likely to present relative to the surgical procedure?

48. How is perioperative thyroid storm treated?

49. What other hypermetabolic states must thyroid storm be distinguished from in the perioperative period?

50. What are some complications that can occur after a total or subtotal thyroidectomy?

51. What structures are innervated by the superior laryngeal nerve?

52. What structures are innervated by the recurrent laryngeal nerve?

53. What patient phonation exercise can be used to evaluate function of the vocal cords after thyroidectomy?

54. What is the most common nerve injury after a thyroidectomy? How does it manifest?

55. How does bilateral recurrent laryngeal nerve injury manifest clinically?

56. What can result from superior laryngeal nerve injury?

57. What are two reasons why compression of the trachea and airway obstruction may occur after a thyroidectomy?

58. What approximate percent of patients undergoing a total thyroidectomy may have accidental intraoperative removal of the parathyroid glands? How might this manifest clinically? In what time course?

HYPOTHYROIDISM

59. What is hypothyroidism?

60. What is the most common cause of hypothyroidism?

61. How is the diagnosis of hypothyroidism made?

62. Is the onset of hypothyroidism usually gradual or rapid?

63. Name some signs and symptoms of hypothyroidism.

64. What is subclinical hypothyroidism? What percent of the general population is estimated to have subclinical hypothyroidism? What percent of the elderly population is estimated to have subclinical hypothyroidism?

65. What is the anesthetic or surgical risk for patients with asymptomatic hypothyroidism?

66. How should patients with hypothyroidism who are scheduled to undergo elective surgery be managed? What is the risk of anesthesia in these patients?

67. How should patients with hypothyroidism who are scheduled to undergo emergent surgery be managed?

68. When might supplemental cortisol be considered for administration to patients with hypothyroidism?

69. How should the induction of anesthesia be achieved in patients with hypothyroidism?

70. What neuromuscular blocking drug should be used for neuromuscular blockade in patients with hypothyroidism?

71. Why might a traditional dose of neuromuscular blocking drug in patients with hypothyroidism result in a prolonged response?

72. What anesthetic agents may be used for maintenance anesthesia in patients with hypothyroidism? What is the potential problem with the administration of volatile anesthetics in patients who are hypothyroid?

73. How does the minimum alveolar concentration (MAC) of anesthesia change in patients with hypothyroidism?

74. How might the Pa_{CO_2} of hypothyroid patients be altered?

75. Is regional anesthesia in patients with hypothyroidism safe?

76. Intraoperative monitoring of patients with hypothyroidism should be directed toward the recognition of which potential complication? How would this complication present intraoperatively?

77. How might intraoperative hypotension be treated in patients with hypothyroidism?

78. What are some potential postoperative complications that can occur in patients with hypothyroidism?

79. When should extubation of the trachea take place in hypothyroid patients after undergoing a surgical procedure?

CORTICOSTEROID THERAPY BEFORE SURGERY

80. What is the rationale behind the perioperative administration of supplementary doses of corticosteroids to patients who are being chronically treated for adrenocortical insufficiency?

81. How does the chronic administration of daily corticosteroids for diseases unrelated to the anterior pituitary gland or adrenal cortex affect the pituitary-adrenal axis? What is the duration of this effect?

82. How might acute adrenal insufficiency present in the perioperative period?

83. What is the recommendation regarding the administration of supplementary doses of corticosteroids to patients at risk for adrenal insufficiency in the perioperative period?

84. What are some potential risks of the administration of supplementary doses of corticosteroids to patients in the perioperative period?

PHEOCHROMOCYTOMA

85. What is pheochromocytoma?

86. What is the hallmark sign of pheochromocytoma?

87. Name some signs and symptoms of pheochromocytoma.

88. What is the most common cause of pheochromocytoma?

89. From what other hypermetabolic disease states must pheochromocytoma be distinguished?

90. How is the diagnosis of pheochromocytoma made?

91. How does oral clonidine affect the plasma catecholamine concentration of patients with pheochromocytoma?

92. How must pheochromocytoma patients be managed preoperatively?

93. Why is it recommended that beta-adrenergic blockade only be instituted in the presence of alpha-adrenergic blockade in patients with pheochromocytoma?

94. What are the potential benefits of the preoperative institution of alpha-adrenergic blockade in patients with pheochromocytoma?

95. What additional medicine should be administered to patients undergoing surgical excision of a pheochromocytoma if a bilateral adrenalectomy is planned?

96. When might echocardiography be indicated preoperatively in patients with pheochromocytoma?

97. What is the goal of the anesthetic management of patients undergoing surgical excision of a pheochromocytoma?

98. What intraoperative monitor should be instituted before the induction of anesthesia in patients with pheochromocytoma?

99. What are three times during excision of a pheochromocytoma that the patient is at the greatest risk of activation of the sympathetic nervous system?

100. What agents may be used for the induction of anesthesia in patients with pheochromocytoma?

101. How is the maintenance of anesthesia most often achieved in patients with pheochromocytoma? What volatile anesthetics may be used for the maintenance of anesthesia in patients with pheochromocytoma?

102. What agents may be used for neuromuscular blockade in patients with pheochromocytoma?

103. Why must an adequate level of anesthesia be established before intubation of the trachea of a patient with pheochromocytoma?

104. What medicines can be administered to patients with pheochromocytoma to treat hypertension that accompanies intubation of the trachea?

105. How can intraoperative hypertension be treated in patients with pheochromocytoma?

106. How can intraoperative tachycardia be treated in patients with pheochromocytoma?

107. How can intraoperative cardiac dysrhythmias be treated in patients with pheochromocytoma?

108. What hemodynamic change may occur rapidly intraoperatively during ligation of the venous drainage of a pheochromocytoma? How can this hemodynamic change be treated?

109. What serum glucose abnormalities may be seen intraoperatively and postoperatively in patients with pheochromocytoma?

110. What are the benefits and disadvantages of regional anesthesia for patients undergoing open surgical excision of a pheochromocytoma?

111. What approximate percent of patients will remain hypertensive during the early postoperative period after surgical excision of a pheochromocytoma?

MORBID OBESITY

112. What is the definition of obesity? What is the approximate prevalence of obesity in the United States?

113. What is the definition of morbid obesity? What is the approximate prevalence of morbid obesity in the United States?

114. Name some adverse effects of obesity.

115. What is believed to be the cause of hypertension associated with obesity?

116. How much does cardiac output approximately increase with each 1 kg of weight gain of adipose tissue?

117. What is the appropriate size of blood pressure cuff for an obese person? What can result from an erroneously sized blood pressure cuff?

118. What is the cause of pulmonary hypertension associated with obesity?

119. What effects does obesity have on ventilatory mechanics?

120. How does the Pa_{O_2} of obese patients compare with that of patients at their ideal body weight?

121. How does the Pa_{CO_2} of obese patients compare with that of patients at their ideal body weight?

122. What is obesity-hypoventilation syndrome? What is another name for this syndrome? What approximate percent of obese patients have this syndrome?

123. What is believed to be the cause of obesity-hypoventilation syndrome?

124. Why are obese patients at a greater risk of the aspiration of gastric contents? How should intubation of the trachea of obese patients be achieved?

125. Why might endotracheal intubation be difficult in obese patients?

126. Why are obese patients at risk of rapid decreases in the Pa_{O_2} during periods of apnea? What consequence does this have for the anesthesiologist caring for the obese patient?

127. How does the rate of increase of alveolar concentrations of inhaled gases in obese patients compare with that of patients at their ideal body weight?

128. What is the benefit of controlled mechanical ventilation of the lungs of obese patients undergoing surgical procedures?

129. What should the dose of injected drugs be based on in obese patients? What is the risk of repeated injections of intravenous drugs in obese patients?

130. Does delayed awakening occur with a greater frequency in obese patients undergoing general anesthesia for surgical procedures?

131. What is the potential difficulty in administering spinal or epidural anesthesia in obese patients?

132. What is the benefit of placing obese patients in the semi-sitting position postoperatively?

133. When is the maximal decrease in the Pa_{O_2} likely to occur postoperatively relative to the surgical procedure?

134. What is the benefit of early postoperative ambulation in obese patients?

MALNUTRITION

135. How can caloric support be provided for patients with metabolic energy requirements not being fulfilled by oral intake?

136. What are some advantages of enteral feedings when compared with the parenteral route for nutrition?

137. What percent body weight loss warrants nutritional treatment before an elective surgical procedure?

138. After what time course postoperatively does the inability to eat or absorb food warrant nutritional treatment?

139. What are some complications of enteral feedings?

140. What is total parenteral nutrition? When is it indicated?

141. When is total parenteral nutrition able to be provided by a large peripheral vein?

142. Name some potential adverse effects of total parenteral nutrition.

143. Why might hypoglycemia accompany total parenteral nutrition?

144. What is the potential effect of increased carbon dioxide production that can accompany total parenteral nutrition?

145. Why is catheter-related sepsis a risk of total parenteral nutrition? What precautionary measures can be taken to minimize this risk?

146. Why can metabolic acidosis accompany total parenteral nutrition?

147. How should total parenteral nutrition infusions be managed perioperatively?

ENDOCRINE AND METABOLIC CHANGES IN THE PERIOPERATIVE PERIOD

148. Which produces a greater endocrine and metabolic response, surgical stimulation or anesthetic drugs?

149. What is the single anesthetic drug that has endocrine effects associated with its administration? What are its endocrine effects?

150. What effect does surgical stimulation have on circulating concentrations of cortisol?

151. What effect does surgical stimulation have on circulating concentrations of insulin?

152. How does surgical stimulation affect protein degradation?

153. How does surgical stimulation affect the release of antidiuretic hormone and aldosterone?

154. How is regional anesthesia believed to affect the endocrine response to surgery?

ANSWERS*

DIABETES MELLITUS

1. Approximately 2.4% of the population of the United States has diabetes. It commonly manifests as an increase in serum glucose concentration, with or without symptoms of an osmotic diuresis. Diabetes is usually diagnosed by elevated fasting plasma glucose concentrations or by an oral glucose tolerance test. (307; **905**)

2. The two major classifications of diabetes are insulin-dependent diabetes mellitus and non–insulin-dependent diabetes mellitus. Insulin-dependent diabetes mellitus, or type 1 diabetes, most often occurs in children and young adults. These patients are usually nonobese and are susceptible to ketoacidosis. Type 1 diabetes occurs as a result of immune-mediated destruction of insulin-producing cells in the pancreas. Non–insulin-dependent diabetes mellitus, or type 2 diabetes, usually occurs in obese patients after the age of 40 as a result of a resistance to the action of insulin. These patients are relatively resistant to ketoacidosis but may be prone to a hyperglycemic hyperosmolar nonketotic state. Over 90% of diabetics have type 2 diabetes mellitus. (307, Table 23–1; **906**)

---

*Numbers in parentheses: lightface numbers refer to pages, figures, or tables in Stoelting RK, Miller RD: Basics of Anesthesia, 4th ed. Philadelphia, Churchill Livingstone, 2000; **boldface numbers** refer to pages, figures, or tables in Miller RD: Anesthesia, 5th ed. Philadelphia, Churchill Livingstone, 2000.

3. Treatments for diabetes include a diabetic diet, oral hypoglycemic agents, and exogenous insulin. (307; **906–907**)

4. Acute or chronic complications that can occur as a result of diabetes mellitus include hyperglycemia, hypoglycemia, ketoacidosis, autonomic neuropathy, coronary artery disease, cerebral vascular disease, peripheral vascular disease, nephropathy, retinopathy, sensory neuropathy, and stiff joint syndrome. (307; **906–907**)

5. Patients with type 1 diabetes mellitus are predisposed to getting ketoacidosis. Ketoacidosis is a condition that occurs as a result of a severe insulin deficiency, usually in response to a precipitating stress. Patients with ketoacidosis may present with nausea and vomiting, lethargy, and abdominal pain. The diagnosis of ketoacidosis is made when hyperglycemia is accompanied by a severe metabolic acidosis leading to hyperventilation, an elevation in the anion gap, and the presence of ketones in the serum. (307; **908–909, 1598, 2475–2476**).

6. Causes of ketoacidosis include poor compliance with insulin therapy, infection, silent myocardial infarction, pregnancy, or some other physiologic stress. An underlying cause of ketoacidosis should be sought. Ketoacidosis is treated with intravascular fluid replacement; an insulin infusion to control the plasma glucose level; possible bicarbonate, potassium, and phosphate administration; and close monitoring of the urine output, serum glucose level, and electrolytes. (307; **908–909, 1598, 2475–2476**)

7. Autonomic neuropathy, a dysfunction of the autonomic nervous system, occurs as a result of damage of small nerve fibers. This results in the loss of vagally controlled heart rate, a decrease in peripheral sympathetic nervous system tone resulting in orthostatic hypotension, decreases in peripheral blood flow, and diminished sweating. It is estimated that 50% of patients with diabetes and hypertension have autonomic neuropathy. (307–308; **567, 911**)

8. Signs and symptoms that a patient with diabetes has autonomic neuropathy include orthostatic hypotension, resting tachycardia, absent variation in heart rate with deep breathing, gastroparesis, peripheral neuropathy, asymptomatic hypoglycemia, and impotence. The diagnosis of autonomic neuropathy has clinical importance for the anesthesiologist managing the patient in the perioperative period. Patients with diabetic autonomic neuropathy are at an increased risk of delayed gastric emptying, perioperative hemodynamic instability, cardiac arrhythmias, silent myocardial infarction, impaired respiration, and cardiopulmonary arrest. In addition, these patients have a blunted response to atropine, making the early treatment of bradycardia essential in these patients. (308; **567, 911**)

9. The risk of a peripheral neuropathy increases with the duration of diabetes in diabetic patients regardless of degree of glucose control. It has been estimated that 50% of patients with diabetes of 25 years' duration have a peripheral neuropathy. Chronic hyperglycemia appears to be associated with the loss of myelinated and unmyelinated fibers, whereas acute hyperglycemia acutely decreases peripheral nerve function. These patients are therefore susceptible to compressive peripheral nerve injuries in the perioperative period. (308; **911**)

10. The goals of the anesthetic management of patients with diabetes include the maintenance of serum glucose, electrolyte, and intravascular fluid volume status. These goals can be achieved through adequate rehydration, often with a glucose-containing maintenance solution as well as an insulin infusion, the perioperative monitoring of serum glucose and electrolyte levels, and close monitoring of the urine output. (308; **909–910**)

11. Considerations in the preoperative evaluation of the diabetic patient include the degree of glucose control; the patient's medical regimen for glucose control; evaluation of the serum electrolytes and other laboratory analysis; and any history or manifestations of cardiovascular disease, cerebral vascular disease, renal impairment, or autonomic or peripheral neuropathy. Indeed, diabetes itself may not be as predictive of perioperative morbidity as the end-organ effects of the diabetes. (308–309; **831, 905–906**)

12. Coronary artery disease, a frequent co-morbid condition in diabetic patients, accounts for the most common cause of perioperative morbidity in diabetic patients. These patients are susceptible to painless myocardial ischemia and cardiovascular instability in the perioperative period. (309; **911–912**)

13. A serum glycohemoglobin level provides an assessment of glycemic control. Glucosylation of hemoglobin occurs when blood glucose levels are elevated. The glucosylation persists for the lifetime of the red blood cell, making it a reliable reflection of blood glucose levels over the previous 7 to 21 days. (309; **906, 1597**)

14. Diabetic patients benefit from having surgery early in the day, preferably as the first case in the morning. This minimizes interruption of the patient's usual treatment routine as well as the duration of time in which fasted patients may be at risk of hypoglycemia. (308)

15. Diabetic patients may require admission to the hospital on the night before surgery if their diabetes is poorly controlled, if they are unable to provide a history or monitor their own glucose levels, if they have end-organ disease that requires special monitoring, if they need careful prehydration, or if they are pregnant. (308–309; **909–910**)

16. Diabetic patients undergoing surgery require insulin treatment in the perioperative period. There are multiple regimens by which insulin and glucose administration can be implemented. There are two general approaches. One is for the purpose of maintaining tightly controlled plasma glucose levels, within the range of 80 to 120 mg/dL. The other is to maintain plasma glucose levels and provide adequate hydration such that hypoglycemia, ketoacidosis, and hyperosmolar states are prevented. For the tightly controlled plasma glucose levels the patient has a maintenance infusion of 5% dextrose in water through a peripheral intravenous catheter. Via the same intravenous catheter an infusion of insulin is started at a rate equivalent to the plasma glucose (mg/dL)/150. The infusions should be started the night before surgery and the glucose monitored every 4 hours through the night. On the morning of surgery the same infusion can be continued but the serum glucose concentration should be monitored and the infusion adjusted every 1 to 2 hours throughout the surgery and postoperatively overnight.

    For the other approach to perioperative plasma glucose control, the aim is typically to keep serum glucose concentrations between 100 and 200 mg/dL. The night before surgery patients are placed on their normal insulin schedule. The morning of surgery patients are started on a maintenance infusion of intravascular fluids containing 5% dextrose, as well as one half of their usual subcutaneous dose of insulin. Intraoperatively, the 5% dextrose maintenance solution can be continued, as well as starting an insulin infusion. Serum glucose levels should be monitored every 1 to 2 hours in the perioperative period and supplemental insulin administered or the insulin infusion adjusted as needed. Indeed, the exact technique of insulin administration has been shown to be less important than frequent plasma glucose monitoring and adjustments. (309, Table 23–2; **909–910, 1596–1598**)

17. Patients who may benefit from tight glucose control in the perioperative period include pregnant patients, patients scheduled to undergo cardiopulmo-

nary bypass, or patients who are at risk for global central nervous system ischemia. Benefits of tight glucose control for these patients include possible improved wound healing, benefits to the offspring of the pregnant patient, improved neurologic outcome after focal or global central nervous system ischemia, and/or improved weaning from cardiopulmonary bypass. (309; **905, 909–910**)

18. Oral hypoglycemic therapy should be continued on its normal schedule through the night before surgery. On the morning of surgery it is recommended that the medicine be held to prevent hypoglycemia. The patient's plasma glucose can be checked, and elevated plasma glucose levels can be treated with a sliding scale of insulin if necessary. These patients are at risk of delayed hypoglycemia and lactic acidosis, however. One medicine of particular concern is metformin. Patients being treated with metformin can develop delayed hypoglycemia up to 48 hours after its last ingestion. These patients may benefit from discontinuing this medicine for 24 hours before surgery. If these patients are undergoing major surgery, it may be prudent to monitor intraoperative pH levels as well. (309; **909–910**)

19. All induction and maintenance anesthetic drugs can be used in patients with diabetes. The presiding concern specific to these patients intraoperatively is the management of serum glucose concentration and intravascular fluids. (309)

20. Volatile anesthetics impair insulin secretion in response to glucose. (309)

21. Any evidence of a peripheral sensory neuropathy is important to note before the administration of a regional anesthetic in diabetic patients to prevent the incorrect assumption that the sensory deficits occurred as a result of the anesthetic. Preoperative cardiac autonomic dysfunction in diabetic patients who are to undergo regional anesthesia may be an indication that they may not have the usual response to atropine should hypotension and bradycardia occur. (309–310; **567**)

HYPEROSMOLAR HYPERGLYCEMIC NONKETOTIC COMA

22. Signs and symptoms of hyperosmolar hyperglycemic nonketotic coma include plasma hyperosmolarity, hyperglycemia, a normal arterial pH, osmotic diuresis associated with hypokalemia, hypovolemia, the absence of serum ketones, and seizures and coma. (310)

23. Type 2 diabetic patients and elderly patients with an impaired thirst mechanism are vulnerable to hyperosmolar hyperglycemic nonketotic coma. Patients with type 2 diabetes undergoing cardiopulmonary bypass are especially vulnerable to the development hyperosmolar hyperglycemic nonketotic coma secondary to the insulin resistance and hyperglycemia associated with this procedure. Other precipitants of hyperosmolar hyperglycemic nonketotic coma include sepsis, hyperalimentation, and pancreatectomy procedures. (310; **917**)

24. Patients with hyperosmolar hyperglycemic nonketotic coma should be managed in a similar manner to patients with ketoacidosis. They can be treated with intravascular fluid replacement; an insulin infusion; possible bicarbonate, potassium, and phosphate administration; and close monitoring of the urine output, serum glucose, and electrolytes. Although insulin therapy for the treatment of hyperosmolar hyperglycemic nonketotic coma is beneficial, the majority of patients who were not on insulin previously do not require insulin therapy after they have recovered. (310; **908–909, 1598, 2475–2476**)

HYPERTHYROIDISM

25. Hyperthyroidism is a condition in which there is an excess of thyroid hormone circulating in the serum. The excess in thyroid hormone can be attributable to autonomous overproduction, excessive release by an injured gland, exogenous ingestion, or hypersecretion of thyroid stimulating hormone. (310; **927–928**)

26. The diagnosis of hyperthyroidism is made based on the clinical signs and symptoms as well as laboratory analysis. Hyperthyroidism is characterized by elevated thyroxine (T_4) or triiodothyronine (T_3) levels in the blood. In addition, there is usually a normal or decreased level of thyroid stimulating hormone in the blood of patients with hyperthyroidism. (310; **927–928**)

27. Signs and symptoms of hyperthyroidism include anxiety, fatigue, weight loss, diarrhea, heat intolerance, warm moist skin, skeletal muscle weakness, tachycardia, tachydysrhythmias, and exophthalmos. (310; **928**)

28. Graves' disease, or diffuse toxic goiter, is the most common cause of hyperthyroidism. Graves' disease typically occurs in women between 20 and 40 years old. (310; **928**)

29. Approximately 0.2% of parturients become hyperthyroid. (310; **928**)

30. Patients with hyperthyroidism who are scheduled to undergo elective surgery should have their surgical procedure postponed until they can be made pharmacologically euthyroid. This can be achieved through the administration of propranolol and iodides. Propranolol is beneficial not only for its effects of beta blockade, but also because it inhibits the peripheral conversion of T_4 to T_3. Other traditional treatments for hyperthyroidism include propylthiouracil or methimazole, both of which decrease the synthesis of thyroxine. Propylthiouracil, like propranolol, also inhibits the peripheral conversion of T_4 to T_3. The administration of medicines to treat hyperthyroidism usually requires 2 to 6 weeks before the patient is euthyroid. (310; **928**)

31. Patients with hyperthyroidism who are scheduled to undergo emergent surgery require aggressive management of the up-regulated sympathetic nervous system. This can be achieved with an intravenous esmolol infusion that is titrated to the desired cardiovascular effect. This should be done, if possible, before the induction of anesthesia to prevent a hyperreactive response to direct laryngoscopy with hypertension and tachycardia. In addition, the serum electrolytes should be measured and the intravascular fluid volume restored. Hyperthyroid patients may benefit from premedication in the preoperative period to help reduce anxiety. (310–311; **928**)

32. Hyperthyroid patients may have airway obstruction secondary to a large goiter or mass. These patients may benefit from a computed tomography scan of the neck to evaluate the extent of the compression, and their airway can then be managed accordingly. (310; **928, 2184**)

33. The intravenous induction of anesthesia in patients with hyperthyroidism can be achieved with any intravenous induction agent, with the exception of ketamine. The sympathetic nervous stimulation that is associated with ketamine administration makes it a poor choice as an induction agent in these patients. Alternatively, an inhaled induction of anesthesia may be administered, thereby preserving skeletal muscle tone and spontaneous ventilation when airway compression secondary to a large mass is feared. (310–311; **242–243, 928**)

34. Neuromuscular blocking drugs should probably not be administered to patients with hyperthyroidism before intubation of the trachea when they have airway obstruction from a mass. The extent of airway compression by a mass

should be evaluated preoperatively by computed tomography. Hyperthyroid patients in the absence of any potential for airway compromise may have succinylcholine or nondepolarizing neuromuscular blocking drugs administered. (311; **928**)

35. A traditional dose of neuromuscular blocking drug in patients with hyperthyroidism may result in a prolonged response if the patient has preoperative skeletal muscle weakness. The initial drug dose in these patients may be decreased, with monitoring of the neuromuscular junction with a peripheral nerve stimulator used as a guide for subsequent dosing requirements. (311)

36. The goal of the anesthetic maintenance of patients with hyperthyroidism is the avoidance of drugs and events that would result in sympathetic nervous system stimulation. In addition, adequate anesthesia should be administered to depress these sympathetically mediated responses if possible. Anesthetic agents that may be used for this purpose include volatile anesthetics, nitrous oxide, and opioids. (310–311; **928**)

37. The minimum alveolar concentration (MAC) of anesthesia for a patient is not altered by hyperthyroidism. (311; **1095–1098, Table 29–1**)

38. There may be a clinical impression of an increase in the MAC of anesthesia in patients with hyperthyroidism secondary to the increase in cardiac output that is associated with hyperthyroidism. The increase in cardiac output results in an increase in the rate of uptake of anesthetic agent and therefore a need to increase the inhaled concentration of anesthetic to achieve an effect. (311; **81**)

39. An increase in the body temperature of patients with hyperthyroidism does result in an increase in the MAC of anesthesia in these patients. In fact, the MAC of anesthesia increases by about 5% for each degree the temperature increases over 37°C. (311; **1095–1098, Table 29–1**)

40. There has been concern regarding the antagonism of nondepolarizing neuromuscular blocking drugs that have been administered to patients with hyperthyroidism secondary to the administration of an anticholinergic agent that could potentially cause a tachycardia. There has been no clinical adversity associated with this practice, however. Even so, the administration of glycopyrrolate instead of atropine for the antagonism of nondepolarizing neuromuscular blocking drugs may be prudent because it has less of a chronotropic effect on the heart. (311; **928**)

41. A concern with regard to patients with exophthalmos undergoing general anesthesia is for the increased risk that these patients have for sustaining an intraoperative corneal abrasion or drying. It is important to mechanically close the eyelids of these patients with tape after the induction of anesthesia and frequently check the eyes intraoperatively. (311; **2182**)

42. The intraoperative monitoring of patients with hyperthyroidism should be directed toward the recognition of any indications that thyroid gland activity is increasing. Intraoperative indications of an increase in thyroid gland activity might include hyperthermia, tachycardia, tachydysrhythmias, and hypertension. An esmolol infusion titrated to achieve the desired effect may be used to treat complications associated with increased activity of the thyroid gland intraoperatively. Hyperthermia can be treated by cooling the temperature in the room, the removal of blankets or covers from the patient, placement of a cooling blanket on the patient, the infusion of cool fluids, and the placement of ice packs on the patient. (311; **928, 1046–1047**)

43. Intraoperative hypotension in patients with hyperthyroidism can be treated with the administration of low doses of phenylephrine. It may be prudent to

avoid the use of an indirect-acting sympathomimetic such as ephedrine in these patients, because they could potentially have an exaggerated response to this drug. (311)

44. The advantage of regional anesthesia in a patient with hyperthyroidism who is undergoing a surgical procedure is that there is blockade of the sympathetic nervous system associated with this technique. An epidural may be the preferred regional anesthetic technique in these patients given the slower onset of sympathetic nervous system blockade. This may preclude an abrupt hypotensive response that can be seen with the administration of spinal anesthesia. Hyperthyroid patients with evidence of high output congestive heart failure are not candidates for regional anesthesia. (311–312)

45. The addition of epinephrine to a regional anesthetic solution could conceivably result in its systemic absorption and systemic sympathetic nervous system effects. In patients with hyperthyroidism, the systemic sympathetic nervous system effects resulting from the systemic absorption of epinephrine may be exaggerated. For this reason, it may be prudent to avoid the addition of epinephrine in regional anesthetic solutions in patients with hyperthyroidism. (312)

46. Thyroid storm, or thyrotoxicosis, is not a discrete syndrome but is a systemic response to sudden, excessive thyroid hormone release into the circulation. Clinically, it is manifest as hyperthermia, tachycardia, hypovolemia, congestive heart failure, and mental status abnormalities. (312; **929**)

47. Although thyroid storm associated with surgery can occur intraoperatively, it is most likely to present 6 to 18 hours after the surgical procedure. (312)

48. Perioperative thyroid storm treatment is aimed toward decreasing the amount of circulating thyroid hormone and toward decreasing the increase in sympathetic nervous system stimulation. An esmolol infusion can be started and titrated to the desired hemodynamic and cardiovascular effects. Dexamethasone may be administered to block the release of thyroid hormone from the thyroid gland as well as the peripheral conversion of T_4 to T_3. Propylthiouracil may be administered to block the uptake of iodine from the thyroid gland, after which iodine may be administered to inhibit the release of thyroid hormone from the thyroid gland. Treatment should also be supportive, with the monitoring and treatment of abnormalities in the patient's intravascular fluid status, electrolytes, glucose and body temperature. (312; **929**)

49. Other hypermetabolic states that may be difficult to distinguish from thyroid storm include malignant hyperthermia, pheochromocytoma, neuroleptic malignant syndrome, and sepsis. (312; **929**)

50. Complications that can occur after a total or subtotal thyroidectomy include injury to laryngeal nerves, tracheal compression, and accidental removal of the parathyroid glands resulting in hypocalcemia. (312; **928–929, 2184**)

51. The superior laryngeal nerves supply sensation above the level of the vocal cords and the motor supply to the cricothyroid muscles. (312; **1440, 1541–1542**)

52. The recurrent laryngeal nerves supply sensation below the level of the vocal cords. They also provide the motor supply to all the muscles of the larynx except the cricothyroid muscles. (312; **1440, 1541–1542**)

53. Evaluation of the function of the vocal cords after a thyroidectomy can be achieved by asking the patient to phonate the "e" sound. The production of this sound is impaired in patients who have unilateral vocal cord paralysis, causing the patient to sound hoarse. Bilateral vocal cord paralysis would result in aphonia. (312; **928–929**)

54. The most common nerve injury after a thyroidectomy is unilateral recurrent laryngeal nerve injury. It may go unnoticed because of compensatory overadduction of the unimpaired vocal cord. A unilateral recurrent laryngeal nerve injury may be detected by hearing hoarseness with phonation of the "e" sound. (312; **929**)

55. Bilateral recurrent laryngeal nerve injury manifests clinically as aphonia. (312; **928–929**)

56. Superior laryngeal nerve injury can result in a loss of sensation above the level of the vocal cords, making the patient vulnerable to the aspiration of contents in the pharynx. It also results in voice hoarseness. (312; **928–929**)

57. Compression of the trachea and airway obstruction may occur after a thyroidectomy procedure because of a hematoma or tracheomalacia. Tracheomalacia can occur from chronic compression of the tracheal rings by a goiter. (312; **928**)

58. Approximately 1% of patients undergoing a total thyroidectomy have accidental intraoperative removal of the parathyroid glands. Clinically, this can manifest as laryngospasm or inspiratory stridor secondary to the sensitivity of the laryngeal muscles to hypocalcemia. Signs of hypocalcemia after this complication do not usually manifest until 24 to 72 hours after the procedure. (312; **929, 932**)

HYPOTHYROIDISM

59. Hypothyroidism is a condition in which there is insufficient thyroid hormone circulating in the serum. The deficiency in thyroid hormone can be due to autonomous destruction, thyroidectomy, thyroiditis, radioactive iodine therapy, neck irradiation, or insufficient secretion of thyroid stimulating hormone. (312; **929**)

60. The most common cause of hypothyroidism is chronic thyroiditis, or Hashimoto's thyroiditis. Chronic thyroiditis is an autoimmune disease that results in destruction of the thyroid gland. (312; **929**)

61. The diagnosis of hypothyroidism is made by measuring decreased levels of thyroxine or triiodothyronine in the blood. In addition, there is usually an increased level of thyroid stimulating hormone in the blood of patients with hypothyroidism. (312; **929**)

62. The onset of hypothyroidism is usually gradual and insidious. (312; **929**)

63. Signs and symptoms of hypothyroidism include lethargy, dry skin, periorbital edema, cold intolerance, bradycardia, decreased cardiac output, slowed gastric emptying, peripheral vasoconstriction, hyponatremia, atrophy of the adrenal cortex, and slowed mental functioning. Because the onset of hypothyroidism is so gradual these signs and symptoms may go unnoticed. In severe cases patients may have cardiomegaly, pleural effusions, ascites, and peripheral edema. (313; **929**)

64. Subclinical hypothyroidism is an increased serum level of thyroid stimulating hormone that is not associated with any symptoms. It is estimated that about 5% of the general population and about 13.2% of the elderly population have subclinical hypothyroidism. (312; **929**)

65. There does not appear to be any increased anesthetic or surgical risk for patients with asymptomatic hypothyroidism. (312; **929**)

66. Although patients with mild to moderate hypothyroidism are not known to be at any increased risk of anesthesia or surgery, it is generally accepted that

all patients with hypothyroidism should have their elective surgery postponed until they can be made pharmacologically euthyroid. (313; **929**)

67. Patients with hypothyroidism who are to undergo emergent surgery should be evaluated for any evidence of myxedema coma, which occurs in severe hypothyroidism. Myxedema coma is characterized by hypothermia, hypotension, hypoventilation, hyponatremia, and bradycardia. Treatment of the thyroid disease can take place intraoperatively with the administration of intravenous triiodothyronine. The administration of triiodothyronine must be done with caution in patients with coronary artery disease or angina. All hypothyroid patients who are to undergo emergent surgery should have their electrolyte and fluid status evaluated preoperatively if possible. The induction and maintenance drugs should be administered to these patients with the understanding that they may have exaggerated effects of sedation postoperatively. (313; **929–930**)

68. Supplemental perioperative cortisol administration may be considered for patients with hypothyroidism who may have underlying adrenal dysfunction. (313; **930**)

69. The induction of anesthesia in patients with hypothyroidism can be achieved with the administration of any intravenous induction agent, including ketamine. (313; **929**)

70. Succinylcholine or any nondepolarizing neuromuscular blocking drug can be used for neuromuscular blockade in patients with hypothyroidism. (313)

71. Patients with hypothyroidism who have co-existing skeletal muscle weakness may have an exaggerated effect from a traditional dose of neuromuscular blocking drug. In addition, the incidence of myasthenia gravis is higher in patients with hypothyroidism. Once the initial dose of neuromuscular blocking drug is administered, monitoring of the neuromuscular junction with a peripheral nerve stimulator should be used as a guide for subsequent dosing requirements. (313; **930**)

72. All anesthetic agents may be used for the maintenance of anesthesia in patients with hypothyroidism, with the understanding that patients with severe hypothyroidism may not tolerate the myocardial depression that can be associated with the administration of volatile anesthetics. (313)

73. The MAC of anesthesia does not change in patients with hypothyroidism. (313; **929, 1095–1098, Table 29–1**)

74. The Pa_{CO_2} of hypothyroid patients may be decreased secondary to a decrease in the metabolic rate, making hypothyroid patients susceptible to hypocarbia during controlled ventilation of the lungs. (313; **930**)

75. There does not appear to be any increased risk of regional anesthesia in patients with hypothyroidism. (313)

76. The intraoperative monitoring of patients with hypothyroidism should be directed toward the recognition of congestive heart failure and hypothermia. Congestive heart failure may present as increased central venous or pulmonary capillary wedge pressures. Patients with congestive heart failure may also have decreases in their arterial blood pressure. Patients with severe hypothyroidism who are undergoing invasive surgical procedures may therefore benefit from the placement of an intra-arterial catheter as well as a central venous or pulmonary artery catheter. Hypothermia that presents intraoperatively can be treated by warming the room, warming inhaled gases, warming intravenous fluids, and placement of a warming blanket. (313; **929–930**)

77. Intraoperative hypotension in patients with hypothyroidism can be treated with the administration of intravenous fluids and sympathomimetics. If the patient is euvolemic, and the patient remains hypotensive despite the administration of sympathomimetics, consideration should be given to the possibility that the patient may have acute adrenal insufficiency. (313; **930**)

78. Potential postoperative complications that can occur in patients with hypothyroidism include hypothermia, delayed awakening, and a corresponding need for the prolonged mechanical ventilation of the lungs. These complications can be minimized by minimizing the dose of administered sedating drugs and anesthetics. (313; **929–930**)

79. Extubation of the trachea of a hypothyroid patient should occur when the patient is taking adequate tidal volumes, is maintaining his or her minute ventilation, is sufficiently awake and cooperative, and has intact laryngeal reflexes. (313; **929–930**)

CORTICOSTEROID THERAPY BEFORE SURGERY

80. Adrenocortical insufficiency can be due to the destruction of the adrenal cortex by cancer, tuberculosis, or hemorrhage; to deficiency in adrenocorticotropic hormone; or to the prolonged exogenous administration of corticosteroids. The adrenal cortex of the adrenal gland synthesizes glucocorticoids, mineralocorticoids, and androgens. Cortisol, a glucocorticoid, is essential for the maintenance of blood pressure and the conversion of norepinephrine to epinephrine in the adrenal medulla. Indeed, acute adrenocortical insufficiency can be life threatening. Cortisol also plays an important role in gluconeogenesis, sodium retention, and potassium excretion and has anti-inflammatory effects. Surgical stimulation normally results in an increase in the amount of circulating cortisol. Patients who are being chronically treated for adrenocortical insufficiency have impaired cortisol secretion and may have cardiovascular compromise because they are unable to respond to the physiologic stress of surgery with the secretion of cortisol. This is the basis for the perioperative administration of supplementary doses of corticosteroids to these patients. (313–314; **920–922**)

81. The chronic administration of daily corticosteroids for diseases unrelated to the anterior pituitary gland or adrenal cortex produces suppression of the pituitary-adrenal axis. The dose of corticosteroids that produces this effect and the duration of the effect are unknown. Even topical corticosteroids have been shown to suppress adrenal function for as long as 1 year. Laboratory tests of adrenal function are not readily available and are impractical before surgery. It is therefore generally recommended that if a patient has taken corticosteroids for a month or more at any time during the previous year he or she should be assumed to have potentially suppressed function of the pituitary-adrenal axis and may be at risk for acute adrenal insufficiency in the perioperative period. (314; **921–922, Table 25–8**)

82. Acute adrenal insufficiency, or addisonian crisis, presents as hypovolemia, hyponatremia, and hyperkalemia. Patients may also have hypotension, decreases in systemic vascular resistance, and decreases in left ventricular stroke index severe enough to lead to death. (314; **921–922**)

83. Patients at risk for adrenal insufficiency typically receive supplementary doses of corticosteroids in the perioperative period given they cannot respond to the increased stress of surgery with the secretion of cortisol. Perioperative acute adrenal insufficiency occurs rarely but can be severe and potentially fatal. In contrast, the administration of perioperative high-dose corticosteroids places the patient at minimal risk. The precise dose of corticosteroid supple-

mentation has not been studied. There has been a correlation established between the stress of surgery and the natural response of a healthy adrenal gland. Under perioperative conditions the adrenal gland secretes 120 to 185 mg of cortisol per day. Under maximum stressful conditions the adrenal gland may secrete 200 to 500 mg/d. One method of administering supplementary corticosteroids is to mimic the natural response of the adrenal gland. For more stressful surgical procedures hydrocortisone can be administered at a dose of 200 mg/d, while for minor surgical stresses a hydrocortisone dose of 100 mg/d should be adequate in the average-sized adult patient. The dose can be decreased by 25% each postoperative day until the patient is able to take the normal oral dose. (314; **921–922**)

84. The potential risks of the administration of supplementary doses of corticosteroids to patients in the perioperative period are few. In theory, patients may have aggravation of hypertension, fluid retention, stress ulcers, and psychiatric disturbances. Of concern are impaired wound healing and an increased rate of infections, because these have been seen to occur clinically. These events still occur rarely, however. It is generally recommended that supplementary corticosteroids are administered to patients at risk in the perioperative period because the potential risks are minimal and rare and are outweighed by its potential benefit. (314; **922–923**)

PHEOCHROMOCYTOMA

85. Pheochromocytoma is a tumor derived from chromaffin tissue that produces, stores, and secretes catecholamines. A pheochromocytoma is most often derived from the adrenal medulla but can develop anywhere. (314; **924**)

86. The hallmark sign of pheochromocytoma is paroxysmal or sustained hypertension. (314; **924**)

87. Signs and symptoms of pheochromocytoma include paroxysmal hypertension, diaphoresis, tachycardia, headache, tremulousness, weight loss, decreased intravascular fluid volume, orthostatic hypotension, a hematocrit greater than 45%, cardiomyopathy, and an intracerebral hemorrhage. The triad of diaphoresis, tachycardia, and headache in a hypertensive patient is highly suggestive for pheochromocytoma. (314; **924**)

88. The most common cause of pheochromocytoma is a unilateral solitary lesion. In approximately 5% of cases of pheochromocytoma it can be inherited as an autosomal dominant trait either alone or in combination with other abnormalities. When combined with other abnormalities it is often designated as multiple endocrine neoplasia, of which medullary thyroid carcinoma is often present. Bilateral pheochromocytomas are common in the familial syndromes. (314; **924**)

89. Pheochromocytoma must be distinguished from malignant hyperthermia, neuroleptic malignant syndrome, thyroid storm, and sepsis. (314; **928**)

90. The diagnosis of pheochromocytoma is made by confirming an excess of catecholamine release. This can be done by analyzing a 24-hour urine collection for catecholamine or catecholamine metabolite levels. (314; **924, Table 25–9**)

91. Oral clonidine does not suppress the plasma catecholamine concentration in patients with pheochromocytoma, although it will suppress plasma catecholamine concentrations in patients with essential hypertension. In some cases this can be used as an aid to the diagnosis of pheochromocytoma. The definitive treatment of pheochromocytoma is its surgical removal. (314)

92. The preoperative management of patients with pheochromocytoma should

include restoration of the intravascular fluid volume, the establishment of alpha-adrenergic blockade, and the treatment of cardiac dysrhythmias or tachycardia with beta-adrenergic antagonists. Most patients require 10 to 14 days of preoperative therapy to adequately stabilize the blood pressure and control symptoms. (314–315; **924–925**)

93. It is recommended that beta-adrenergic antagonists be administered in patients with pheochromocytoma only after alpha-adrenergic blockade has been established. The concern is that should the administration of beta antagonists precede the administration of alpha antagonists, there would be a resultant abrupt increase in systemic vascular resistance from unopposed alpha receptor stimulation by the catecholamines. The abrupt increase in systemic vascular resistance could lead to malignant hypertension and may decrease the ability of the heart to generate an adequate cardiac output. (314–315; **925**)

94. The preoperative institution of alpha-adrenergic blockade in patients with pheochromocytoma facilitates the restoration of the intravascular fluid volume. This occurs because the blockade of the alpha-adrenergic receptor opposes the actions of the catecholamines at the receptor and reverses the catecholamine-induced vasoconstriction. Hydration of the patient is facilitated with the reversal of the vasoconstriction. In addition, the preoperative institution of alpha-adrenergic blockade in patients with pheochromocytoma may help to decrease the risk of hyperglycemia in the perioperative period by stimulating the release of insulin. (314–315; **924–925**)

95. Patients undergoing bilateral adrenalectomy for the surgical excision of a pheochromocytoma should have supplemental cortisol administered in either the preoperative or early intraoperative period. (315)

96. Echocardiography might be indicated preoperatively in patients with pheochromocytoma when there is evidence of a cardiomyopathy. (315)

97. The goal of the anesthetic management of patients undergoing surgical excision of a pheochromocytoma is the avoidance of drugs or events that might result in stimulation of the sympathetic nervous system, as well as the administration of drugs to suppress this effect. The intraoperative mortality of patients with unsuspected pheochromocytoma was as high as 50% in the past. The mortality has decreased to 0% to 6% coincident with the institution of alpha-adrenergic blockade preoperatively. The administration of alpha- and beta-adrenergic blockade should be continued through the intraoperative period. (315; **925, Table 25–10**)

98. Intraoperative monitoring geared toward the early detection of catecholamine-induced changes of the cardiovascular system include monitoring of the intra-arterial blood pressure and central venous pressure. An intra-arterial blood pressure monitor should be instituted before the induction of anesthesia in patients with pheochromocytoma. Placement of the intra-arterial blood pressure monitor will enable the early detection of catecholamine-induced changes in blood pressure and heart rate that may occur with direct laryngoscopy and intubation of the trachea. For certain patients, monitoring of the pulmonary artery occlusion pressures or transesophageal echocardiography may be useful as well. (315; **925**)

99. A patient undergoing excision of a pheochromocytoma is at the greatest risk of hemodynamic instability during intubation of the trachea, during manipulation of the tumor, and during the time after ligation of the tumor's venous drainage. (315; **925**)

100. All intravenous induction agents may be used for the induction of anesthesia in patients with pheochromocytoma except for ketamine. The sympathetic nervous system stimulation associated with the administration of ketamine

precludes it from being used in patients undergoing resection of pheochromo-cytoma. (315; **925**)

101. The maintenance of anesthesia in patients with pheochromocytoma is most often achieved with the administration of a volatile anesthetic in combination with nitrous oxide and an opioid. Volatile anesthetics are useful for the maintenance of anesthesia in patients with pheochromocytoma because of their ability to decrease sympathetic nervous system activity. An exception to this is halothane, which is not recommended for administration to patients with pheochromocytoma. Halothane may have deleterious effects in that it sensitizes the myocardium to catecholamines, making the heart more likely to become dysrhythmic in its presence. Another possible exception is desflurane, owing to the catecholamine release associated with its administration. (315; **925, Table 25–11**)

102. Nondepolarizing neuromuscular blocking drugs with vagolytic or histamine-releasing effects are best avoided in patients with pheochromocytoma. (315)

103. Intubation of the trachea in patients with pheochromocytoma can result in excessive catecholamine release, and an exaggerated, malignant hypertension can result. To minimize this risk an adequate level of anesthesia, preferably with a volatile anesthetic, must be established before intubation of the trachea of a patient with pheochromocytoma. It may be useful to administer lidocaine as an intravenous bolus just before intubation of the trachea to attenuate catecholamine-induced responses, including cardiac dysrhythmias. Other use-ful adjuncts include an intravenous opioid and the rapid access to a short-acting vasodilator such as nitroprusside should it become necessary. (315; **925**)

104. Hypertension that accompanies intubation of the trachea in patients with pheochromocytoma can be treated with the administration of intravenous nitroglycerin, nitroprusside, and/or esmolol if it is accompanied by tachycar-dia. (315; **925**)

105. Intraoperative hypertension not controlled by volatile anesthetic in patients with pheochromocytoma can be treated with the administration of a nitroprus-side infusion. (315; **925**)

106. Intraoperative tachycardia in patients with pheochromocytoma can be treated with the administration of an esmolol infusion. Tachycardia can occur as a reflex in these patients as a result of nitroprusside-induced vasodilation. The anesthesiologist must be aware that beta-adrenergic antagonists may contrib-ute to myocardial dysfunction in these patients, and the patients must be monitored appropriately for the early detection of myocardial dysfunction should beta-adrenergic antagonists be used intraoperatively. (315; **925**)

107. Cardiac dysrhythmias in patients with pheochromocytoma can be treated intraoperatively with the administration of intravenous lidocaine or with a lidocaine infusion for persistent dysrhythmias. (315; **925**)

108. Ligation of the venous drainage of a pheochromocytoma can result in abrupt decreases in the amount of circulating catecholamines, reflected by an abrupt decrease in blood pressure. The decrease in blood pressure can be treated with the rapid administration of intravenous fluids and by decreasing the inspired concentration of volatile anesthetic. Typically, these two interventions in combination are sufficient. Hypotension that persists despite these interven-tions should be treated with the intravenous administration of phenylephrine. (315; **925**)

109. The serum glucose of a patient with pheochromocytoma may be initially increased at the onset of surgery, with hypoglycemia occurring after ligation

of the venous drainage of the tumor. Hyperglycemia under these circumstances results from the suppression of insulin release by stimulation of the alpha-adrenergic receptors by circulating catecholamines. Hypoglycemia can occur after this stimulation has been discontinued. These changes can be managed intraoperatively with frequent serum glucose measurements and treatment when appropriate. (315)

110. Regional anesthesia for patients undergoing open surgical excision of a pheochromocytoma may appear to be beneficial in that there is peripheral sympathetic nervous system blockade associated with regional anesthesia. There are some disadvantages of regional anesthesia for these patients, however. First, postsynaptic circulating catecholamines can still directly stimulate alpha receptors. Second, patients with pheochromocytoma who are anesthetized with a regional anesthetic may have a precipitous drop in blood pressure on ligation of the venous drainage of the tumor that cannot be subsequently treated with activation of the sympathetic nervous system. (316; **925**)

111. Approximately 50% of patients will remain hypertensive during the early postoperative period after surgical excision of a pheochromocytoma, making continued alpha-adrenergic blockade useful as well as vigilant monitoring. (316; **925**)

MORBID OBESITY

112. Obesity is defined as a body weight more than 20% above the ideal body weight for height, or a body mass index greater than 28 for men or 27 for women. The body mass index is equal to weight (kg) ÷ height^2 (meters). Approximately 33% of people in the United States are considered to be obese. (316; **913–914**)

113. Morbid obesity is defined as a body weight more than double the ideal body weight for their height, 45 kg above their ideal body weight, or a body mass index greater than 31. The body mass index is equal to weight (kg) ÷ height^2 (meters). It is estimated that 3% to 5% of people in the United States are morbidly obese. (316; **913–914**)

114. Adverse effects of obesity include systemic hypertension, cardiomegaly, congestive heart failure, coronary artery disease, pulmonary hypertension, decreased lung volumes and functional residual capacity, arterial hypoxemia, restrictive lung disease, sleep apnea, abnormal liver function test results, fatty liver infiltration, insulin resistance leading to diabetes, hypercholesterolemia, and osteoarthritis. (316; **914**)

115. Hypertension associated with obesity is correlated with the degree of weight gain as well as with cardiomegaly. There is a necessary increase in cardiac output and blood volume in obese patients in order to perfuse the adipose tissue. One kilogram of adipose tissue has about 3000 meters of blood vessels. It is therefore believed that the increase in blood pressure occurs as a result of this increase in blood volume and cardiac output, and together these result in associated cardiomegaly. (316; **914**)

116. Cardiac output increases by approximately 0.1 L/min with each 1 kg gain of weight due to adipose tissue. (316; **914**)

117. The appropriate size of blood pressure cuff for an obese person is a blood pressure cuff whose width is greater than one-third the arm circumference. An erroneously sized blood pressure cuff can lead to erroneous blood pressure measurements. A cuff that is too narrow or too loose will lead to blood pressures that are artificially high. (316; **1121**)

118. Pulmonary hypertension associated with obesity is believed to be due to an

increase in the blood volume and from chronic pulmonary vasoconstriction in response to chronic arterial hypoxemia. (316; **914**)

119. The increased weight on the chest and abdomen of obese patients has multiple effects on ventilatory mechanics. First, the increased weight causes a decrease in the expiratory reserve volume, vital capacity, and functional residual capacity of these patients. Second, the weight of the abdomen impedes diaphragmatic excursion. Finally, the infiltration of fat in the muscles used for breathing decreases their capacity. These combined result in a restrictive ventilatory defect in these patients and an increase in the work of breathing. This can be reflected in the rapid, shallow breathing pattern characteristic of obese patients. (316–317; **914**)

120. The PaO_2 of obese patients, when compared with that of patients at their ideal body weight, is decreased. This is believed to occur as a result of the increase in ventilation-to-perfusion mismatch in these patients. The ventilation-to-perfusion mismatch increases with decreases in lung volumes and capacities. (316; **914**)

121. The $PaCO_2$ of obese patients, when compared with that of patients at their ideal body weight, usually remains normal. This is due to the high diffusion capacity of carbon dioxide, but the reserve is limited. Obese patients may have an exaggerated ventilatory effect from the administration of opioids. Obese patients who begin to have elevations in their $PaCO_2$ are said to have obesity-hypoventilation syndrome. (316–317; **914**)

122. Obesity-hypoventilation syndrome, or pickwickian syndrome, is characterized by massive obesity, alveolar hypoventilation, an increase in the $PaCO_2$, arterial hypoxemia, respiratory acidosis, pulmonary hypertension, right-sided cardiac failure, and polycythemia. These patients may also complain of daytime somnolence as a result of frequently waking in the night from sleep apnea. Approximately 8% of obese patients have this syndrome. (317; **914**)

123. Obesity-hypoventilation syndrome is believed to occur secondary to an inability of the ventilatory muscles to respond to neural impulses, a failure of the regulation of ventilation in the central nervous system, or a combination of the two. (317; **914**)

124. Obese patients are at a greater risk of the aspiration of gastric contents for several reasons. In obese patients there is an increased incidence of gastroesophageal reflux and hiatal hernia. There is also an increase in the acidity of gastric fluids, an increase in the volume of gastric fluid, and an increase in the intragastric pressure. For these reasons, intubation of the trachea of obese patients should be achieved via a rapid sequence induction in the presence of continuous cricoid pressure after adequate preoxygenation. This is providing the preoperative airway examination of the obese patient does not lead the anesthesiologist to believe that intubation of the trachea via direct laryngoscopy may be difficult. In the event that the preoperative airway examination indicates a potentially difficult intubation of the trachea via direct laryngoscopy, other methods of intubating the trachea of these patients while minimizing the risk of the aspiration of gastric contents should be sought. (317; **914, Figs. 25–4, 25–5**)

125. Endotracheal intubation may be difficult in obese patients as a result of the alterations in anatomy caused by excess adipose tissue. Excess adipose tissue of the airway increases the amount of soft tissue in the pharynx, decreasing the amount of space in the oral cavity. In addition, excess adipose tissue can result in a decrease in the amount of cervical and mandibular mobility. Finally, excessive weight of the head, neck, and chest may physically hinder placement of the laryngoscope in obese patients. For these reasons, placement of an obese patient in the appropriate position for intubation of the trachea

via direct laryngoscopy with extra blankets under the shoulders and neck is essential. If the preoperative airway examination indicates a potentially difficult intubation of the trachea via direct laryngoscopy, other methods of intubating the trachea of these patients should be considered. (317; **914**)

126. The decrease in functional residual capacity associated with obesity places obese patients at risk of rapid decreases in the Pa_{O_2} during periods of apnea. The propensity of these patients to desaturate quickly with apnea can make direct laryngoscopy challenging. To minimize the risk of arterial hypoxemia during direct laryngoscopy, adequate preoxygenation should precede the induction of anesthesia. (317, Fig. 23–1; **914, Fig. 25–3**)

127. The rate of increase of alveolar concentrations of inhaled gases in obese patients is increased secondary to the decrease in functional residual capacity that is associated with obesity. (317)

128. Controlled mechanical ventilation of the lungs of obese patients undergoing surgical procedures allows for large tidal volumes to be delivered to the patient. This decreases the patient's risk of intraoperative arterial hypoxemia and hypercarbia and postoperative atelectasis. (317–318)

129. The dose of drugs injected in obese patients should be based on a weight closer to the patient's ideal body weight rather than their true body weight. The basis for this is the decreased relative blood flow through adipose tissue than through other tissues. For this reason, a dose of drug injected based on the patient's true body weight would result in plasma concentrations of drug greater than anticipated, depending on the degree of obesity. A more prudent approach would be to inject a dose of drug based on the patient's ideal body weight for height and then administer additional doses based on the patient's response to the original dose. The risk of repeated intravenous injections of drugs in obese patients could lead to cumulative effects of the drugs, especially in drugs that are lipid soluble and stored in adipose tissue. (317–318; **916**)

130. Delayed awakening in obese patients undergoing general anesthesia for surgical procedures has not been proven to occur at an increased frequency from patients at their ideal body weight, despite the theoretical possibility of lipid-soluble agents being taken up in adipose tissue and slowly released back into the circulation. (318, Fig. 23–2; **916**)

131. The administration of spinal or epidural anesthesia in obese patients is made potentially difficult by difficulty in positioning the patient and a decreased capacity to feel bony landmarks. (318; **1499**)

132. Placing obese patients in a semi-sitting position postoperatively may decrease the work of breathing, leading to better ventilation of the lungs and a decrease in the potential for arterial hypoxemia. (318; **914**)

133. The maximal decrease in the Pa_{O_2} postoperatively is likely to occur 2 to 3 days after the surgical procedure. (318; **914, 2309–2310**)

134. Early ambulation decreases the risk of pulmonary embolism from deep venous thrombosis and may decrease the risk of pulmonary complications in postoperative patients. Because obese patients are at an increased risk of these complications postoperatively, early ambulation may be particularly important in these patients. (318; **916**)

MALNUTRITION

135. Caloric support can be provided to patients with metabolic energy requirements that are not being fulfilled with oral food intake by means of enteral feedings via the gut or parenterally via a central or peripheral vein. (318; **917, 2519**)

136. Nutritional supplementation should be provided by enteral feedings whenever possible. This provides for a normal route of nutrition absorption, may have decreased risks of infection when compared with parenteral nutrition, and is less expensive. Enteral nutrition can be delivered by continuous infusion via a tube through the nose or mouth to the stomach or duodenum. (318; **2519–2520**)

137. A 20% body weight loss warrants nutritional treatment before an elective surgical procedure. (318; **917**)

138. After 1 week postoperatively the inability to eat or absorb food warrants nutritional treatment. (318; **917**)

139. Complications of enteral feedings include diarrhea, hypovolemia, and hyperglycemia leading to an osmotic diuresis. (318; **2519–2520**)

140. Total parenteral nutrition, or hyperalimentation, is the intravenous administration of nutritive supplements. It is indicated when a patient is unable to fulfill his or her metabolic energy requirements with oral intake and the gastrointestinal tract is not functioning. (318; **917, 2519–2520**)

141. Total parenteral nutrition may be provided by a large peripheral vein when the patient requires less than 2000 calories a day and the estimated need for total parenteral nutrition is less than 2 weeks. (318; **2519–2520**)

142. Potential adverse effects of total parenteral nutrition include hyperglycemia, hypoglycemia, nonketotic hyperosmolar hyperglycemic coma, fluid overload, increased carbon dioxide production, catheter-related sepsis, electrolyte abnormalities, hepatic dysfunction, renal dysfunction, and thrombosis of the central veins. The most common adverse effects of total parenteral nutrition are catheter-related sepsis and metabolic abnormalities. (318–319; **917, 2520–2525, Tables 74–7, 74–8**)

143. Total parenteral nutrition stimulates an increased secretion of insulin. Because of this, hypoglycemia may occur as a result of the abrupt intentional or unintentional discontinuation of the total parenteral nutrition infusion. The intentional discontinuation of total parenteral nutrition should be immediately followed by the administration of a 5% or 10% dextrose solution to prevent hypoglycemia. (318; **917–918, 2523**)

144. Increased carbon dioxide production associated with total parenteral nutrition may occur as a result of the metabolism of large amounts of glucose. The increase in carbon dioxide production leads to increased respiratory work in response to the increase in carbon dioxide and stimulated ventilatory drive. Patients being mechanically ventilated may have difficulty being weaned from the ventilator or may have metabolic acidosis as a result. (318; **2523**)

145. Catheter-related sepsis is a risk of total parenteral nutrition secondary to the rich medium for bacteria and fungi to grow that is provided by the parenteral nutrition solutions. Precautionary measures that can be taken to minimize the risk of catheter-related sepsis include placement and use of the catheter with strict aseptic technique, the avoidance of drawing blood samples from the catheter, the avoidance of using the catheter for the transduction of central venous pressures, and the avoidance of the administration of medicines via the catheter. (318–319; **917, 2520**)

146. Metabolic acidosis associated with total parenteral nutrition may occur as a result of the metabolism of amino acids or may be due to an increased production of carbon dioxide from the metabolism of glucose. (318; **917, 2523**)

147. Total parenteral nutrition can be continued throughout the perioperative period, thus avoiding the risk of hypoglycemia from its discontinuation. The

same infusion rate should be continued with an intravenous pump, and asepsis should be maintained. The access port should not be used for the infusion of any other medicines or for any other purpose. Alternatively, it may be discontinued gradually before surgery. The primary reason for gradually decreasing the infusion rate or discontinuing the total parenteral nutrition infusion before surgery is to avoid the risk of its accidental rapid infusion resulting in plasma hyperosmolarity intraoperatively. When discontinuing total parenteral nutrition preoperatively it can be done over the course of the night preceding surgery while starting replacement maintenance therapy with a 5% or 10% dextrose solution. (318; **917–918**)

ENDOCRINE AND METABOLIC CHANGES IN THE PERIOPERATIVE PERIOD

148. Surgical stimulation produces marked endocrine and metabolic responses, while the effects of anesthetic drugs are minimal. (319; **652, 2505**)

149. Etomidate is the single anesthetic drug known to have significant endocrine effects associated with its administration. Etomidate causes adrenal suppression, thus interfering with the synthesis of cortisol in the adrenal cortex. The effects of etomidate on the adrenal gland appear to be dose and time related. Its effects on the adrenal cortex have been documented to last for 24 hours after its administration. It may be prudent to treat hypotension and electrolyte abnormalities indicative of adrenal insufficiency that occur after the administration of etomidate with corticosteroids. (319; **922**)

150. Surgical stimulation results in an increase in the circulating concentrations of cortisol and catecholamines. (319; **652, 921, 2505**)

151. The increased circulating catecholamines associated with surgical stimulation result in an inhibition of insulin release, thereby decreasing circulating concentrations of insulin and contributing to hyperglycemia. (319; **652, 921, 2505**)

152. Surgical stimulation results in an increased rate of protein degradation. There is a corresponding increase in urinary nitrogen excretion and loss of lean body weight postoperatively. (319; **652, 2505**)

153. Surgical stimulation results in an increase in the release of antidiuretic hormone and aldosterone, which is evidenced by sodium and water retention and potassium excretion postoperatively. (319; **921**)

154. Regional anesthesia with its associated afferent neural blockade attenuates the endocrine and metabolic responses to surgery. It is believed, however, that the endocrine and metabolic responses to surgery are merely postponed under these circumstances. (319; **652, 921**)

Chapter 23

Central Nervous System Disease

INTRACRANIAL TUMORS

1. What are some of the presenting signs and symptoms of patients with an intracranial tumor?

2. What is the goal of the anesthetic management for patients undergoing surgical resection of an intracranial tumor?

3. Name some factors that influence cerebral blood flow.

4. What is normal cerebral blood flow?

5. For every 1°C decrease in temperature below normal body temperature, what is the corresponding decrease in cerebral blood flow?

6. How do changes in the Pa_{CO_2} result in changes in cerebral blood flow?

7. How much does cerebral blood flow change for every 1 mm Hg increase or decrease in Pa_{CO_2} from 40 mm Hg?

8. How does local acidosis surrounding an intracranial tumor influence the effect of changes in the Pa_{CO_2} on local cerebral blood flow?

9. What is the intracranial steal syndrome? What is reverse steal syndrome? What is the clinical importance of each of these syndromes?

10. Below what Pa_{O_2} will increases in cerebral blood flow be noted?

11. What is the cerebral perfusion pressure equal to? What is the cerebral perfusion pressure in cases of a high intracranial pressure?

12. Between what mean arterial pressures will cerebral blood flow remain relatively constant?

13. What are some things that impair the autoregulation of cerebral blood flow?

14. How do volatile anesthetics affect cerebral blood flow? Which volatile anesthetic has the least effect on cerebral blood flow?

15. How do volatile anesthetics affect the cerebral metabolic oxygen requirement?

16. How does nitrous oxide affect cerebral blood flow?

17. How does ketamine affect cerebral blood flow?

18. How does thiopental affect cerebral blood flow?

19. How does propofol affect cerebral blood flow?

20. How does etomidate affect cerebral blood flow?

21. How do benzodiazepines affect cerebral blood flow?

22. How do opioids affect cerebral blood flow?

23. Draw graphs depicting the impact of each of the following on cerebral blood flow: Pa_{O_2}, Pa_{CO_2}, cerebral perfusion pressure, and intracranial pressure.

24. Draw an intracranial pressure-volume compliance curve illustrating the impact of expanding intracranial tumors on intracranial pressure.

25. What is a normal intracranial pressure?

26. What are some effects of an increasing intracranial pressure?

27. How do drug-induced increases in cerebral blood flow affect the intracranial pressures of normal patients and of patients with intracranial tumors?

28. Name some methods used to decrease an elevated intracranial pressure.

29. Name some signs and symptoms that may be noted preoperatively that provide evidence that a patient may have an increased intracranial pressure.

30. Why is it important to limit drug-induced depression of ventilation with preoperative medicines in patients who are scheduled to undergo surgical resection of an intracranial tumor?

31. How is the induction of general anesthesia in patients undergoing surgical resection of an intracranial tumor achieved?

32. What is the neuromuscular blocking drug of choice in patients scheduled to undergo surgical resection of an intracranial tumor?

33. What measures can an anesthesiologist undertake to attenuate increases in arterial blood pressure and intracranial pressure during direct laryngoscopy?

34. How is maintenance anesthesia usually achieved in patients undergoing surgical resection of an intracranial tumor?

35. When using a volatile anesthetic for maintenance anesthesia in patients undergoing surgical resection of an intracranial tumor, which volatile anesthetic is usually chosen?

36. What MAC of volatile anesthetic should be administered when used for maintenance anesthesia in patients undergoing surgical resection of an intracranial tumor?

37. Within what range should the $Paco_2$ be maintained for the maximal benefit of decreased cerebral blood flow?

38. What is a potential problem of the administration of positive end-expiratory pressure during mechanical ventilation of the lungs in patients undergoing surgical resection of an intracranial tumor?

39. How do peripheral vasodilators affect cerebral blood flow? What is the recommendation regarding the use of these drugs intraoperatively in patients undergoing surgical resection of an intracranial tumor?

40. Why is neuromuscular blockade commonly maintained throughout intracranial surgical procedures?

41. How can cerebral swelling be treated intraoperatively?

42. How should intravenous fluid administration be managed intraoperatively in patients undergoing surgical resection of an intracranial tumor?

43. Which fluid solutions are acceptable for intravenous fluid administration intraoperatively in patients undergoing surgical resection of an intracranial tumor? Why should glucose-containing intravenous solutions be avoided in these patients?

44. What intraoperative monitoring is useful in patients undergoing surgical resection of an intracranial tumor?

45. Why should coughing and straining by patients awakening from anesthesia be avoided after intracranial surgery? What are some methods by which these responses by the patient can be avoided?

46. How should delayed recovery after intracranial surgery be evaluated? When should

tension pneumocephalus be considered as a possible cause of postoperative delayed recovery?

47. Why are patients undergoing surgical resection of an intracranial tumor at an increased risk for venous air embolism?

48. Describe what happens in the case of a venous air embolism. What percent of adult patients have a probe patent foramen ovale?

49. What are some methods by which a venous air embolism can be detected? Which of these is the most sensitive?

50. What are some signs of a clinically significant venous air embolism?

51. What is the treatment for a venous air embolism?

52. Why should nitrous oxide administration be discontinued in the presence of a venous air embolism?

53. What is the usefulness of a pulmonary artery catheter in the presence of a venous air embolism?

54. How efficacious is the use of positive end-expiratory pressure in the prevention of a venous air embolism?

55. When death occurs as a result of a venous air embolism, what is it usually due to?

CAROTID ENDARTERECTOMY

56. What are some indications for a carotid endarterectomy?

57. Why should patients undergoing a carotid endarterectomy have their cardiovascular and neurologic status closely evaluated preoperatively?

58. What is the goal of the intraoperative anesthetic management for patients undergoing a carotid endarterectomy? What is the critical period during this surgery?

59. What is the purpose of intraoperative neurologic monitoring? What are some methods of intraoperative neurologic monitoring?

60. When is an intraluminal shunt placed by the surgeons?

61. Does local anesthesia or general anesthesia for carotid endarterectomy have better outcomes?

62. How is local anesthesia for a carotid endarterectomy achieved? What is an advantage of local anesthesia for this procedure?

63. How is general anesthesia for a carotid endarterectomy usually achieved? What is an advantage of general anesthesia for this procedure?

64. How should the arterial blood pressure be managed during a carotid endarterectomy?

65. What are some potential problems with intraoperative hypertension during a carotid endarterectomy?

66. How should the $Paco_2$ be managed during a carotid endarterectomy?

67. What are some postoperative problems that may occur after a carotid endarterectomy?

68. Which postoperative problem is most common after a carotid endarterectomy: hypertension or hypotension? Explain why each may occur.

INTRACRANIAL ANEURYSMS

69. How do patients with ruptured intracranial aneurysms usually present?

70. How might the electrocardiogram of patients with a ruptured intracranial aneurysm appear?

71. What is the major cause of morbidity after rupture of an intracranial aneurysm? When is it most likely to occur? How is it treated?

72. What is the goal of the anesthetic management of a patient undergoing resection of an intracranial aneurysm?

73. What is the usefulness of controlled hypotension during resection of an intracranial aneurysm? What are some pharmacologic methods by which this may be accomplished?

74. What is a disadvantage of controlled hypotension during resection of an intracranial aneurysm?

75. When controlled hypotension is planned during resection of an intracranial aneurysm, why is it useful to place the transducer for the arterial blood pressure at the level of the brain when the head is elevated?

SPINAL CORD TRANSECTION

76. What is the most common cause of spinal cord transection?

77. What special precaution must be taken during the emergent intubation of the trachea of a patient in cervical spine precautions?

78. When is succinylcholine not recommended for neuromuscular blockade to facilitate intubation of the trachea after spinal cord injury?

79. Why are patients who have suffered spinal cord transection prone to hypotension?

80. Why are patients who have suffered spinal cord transection prone to hypothermia?

81. What is autonomic hyperreflexia? What is the mechanism by which it occurs? How can it be treated intraoperatively?

82. What level of spinal cord transection is most likely to be associated with autonomic hyperreflexia?

83. What surgical manipulations are most likely to trigger autonomic hyperreflexia?

84. Of general, epidural, or spinal anesthesia, which is most likely to prevent autonomic hyperreflexia?

SLEEP APNEA SYNDROME

85. What is sleep apnea syndrome?

86. What are two different causes of sleep apnea syndrome?

87. Name some of the manifestations of sleep apnea syndrome.

88. What are some surgical treatments of sleep apnea syndrome? What anesthetic considerations must be made for patients undergoing these surgical procedures?

ANSWERS*

INTRACRANIAL TUMORS

1. Presenting signs and symptoms of patients with an intracranial tumor are typically reflective of an elevated intracranial pressure due to a space-occupying mass. Seizures presenting in adulthood are worrisome for an intracranial tumor. Other manifestations of an elevated intracranial pressure include nausea and

*Numbers in parentheses: lightface numbers refer to pages, figures, or tables in Stoelting RK, Miller RD: Basics of Anesthesia, 4th ed. Philadelphia, Churchill Livingstone, 2000; **boldface numbers** refer to pages, figures, or tables in Miller RD: Anesthesia, 5th ed. Philadelphia, Churchill Livingstone, 2000.

vomiting, hypertension, bradycardia, personality changes, altered levels of consciousness, altered patterns of breathing, and papilledema. (321; **974, 1895**)

2. The anesthetic management for patients undergoing surgical resection of an intracranial tumor is geared toward the avoidance of drugs or events that will cause undesirable changes in cerebral blood flow or intracranial pressure. (321; **702, 1898–1899**)

3. Factors that influence cerebral blood flow include the Pa_{O_2}, the Pa_{CO_2}, level of arousal, body temperature, central venous pressure, mean arterial pressure, autoregulation, vasodilators, and anesthetic drugs. (321; **695–696, Table 19–3**)

4. Normal cerebral blood flow is 50 mL/100 g of brain tissue per minute. (321; **695, Table 19–2**)

5. For every 1°C decrease in temperature below normal body temperature there is a corresponding decrease in cerebral blood flow by about 7%. (321; **697–698, 718–719, 1376, Fig. 19–3**)

6. Cerebral blood flow is linearly related to the Pa_{CO_2}, such that increases in the Pa_{CO_2} result in increases in cerebral blood flow and vice versa. This effect of the Pa_{CO_2} occurs as a result of the effect of the arterial carbon dioxide tension on pH. An increase in Pa_{CO_2} leads to acidosis, which in turn leads to cerebral vascular vasodilation. The duration of this effect is 6 to 8 hours, after which cerebral blood flow normalizes through the transfer of bicarbonate out of the cerebrospinal fluid. This effect is only in response to respiratory acidosis. The cerebral vasculature is not affected by metabolic acidosis, owing to the blood-brain barrier protection against the diffusion of hydrogen ion from the vascular space. (321; **698, 1900, Figs. 19–4, 52–5**)

7. Cerebral blood flow increases by 1 mL/100 g of brain tissue per minute for every 1 mm Hg increase in the Pa_{CO_2} from 40 mm Hg. Conversely, cerebral blood flow decreases by 1 mL/100 g of brain tissue per minute for every 1 mm Hg decrease in the Pa_{CO_2} from 40 mm Hg. The impact of this can be marked, given that a decrease in the Pa_{CO_2} from 40 to 25 mm Hg can lead to approximately a 33% decrease in cerebral blood flow. (321; **698**)

8. Local acidosis surrounding an intracranial tumor caused by tumor metabolites results in maximally dilated vessels surrounding the tumor. This local acidosis leads to increased blood flow surrounding the tumor relative to the rest of the brain. This has been termed *luxury perfusion*. A decrease in the Pa_{CO_2} under these circumstances may not result in a decrease in cerebral blood flow surrounding the tumor. (321; **698**)

9. Intracranial steal syndrome refers to the shunting of blood flow away from the tumor. This might occur in situations when local acidosis surrounding the tumor leads to maximally dilated vessels surrounding the tumor. An increase in the Pa_{CO_2} at that time could potentially increase blood flow in other vessels in the brain but not the blood vessels surrounding the tumor that have been maximally dilated. This is the basis for the intracranial steal syndrome. The converse occurs in reverse steal syndrome. That is, local acidosis surrounding the tumor will result in the shunting of blood to the tumor during times of a decreased Pa_{CO_2} and vasoconstriction in other areas of the brain. It is not known whether these syndromes have any clinical importance. (321; **698**)

10. Cerebral blood flow increases dramatically when the Pa_{O_2} falls below 50 mm Hg. (322; **698**)

11. The cerebral perfusion pressure is the difference between mean arterial pressure and central venous pressure. When the intracranial pressure is higher than the central venous pressure, the cerebral perfusion pressure is the difference between mean arterial pressure and intracranial pressure. (321; **699, 1480**)

12. Cerebral blood flow remains relatively constant between mean arterial pressures of 60 to 150 mm Hg. Within this range of blood pressures the cerebral vasculature is able to vasodilate or vasoconstrict in response to changes in mean arterial blood pressure to maintain a constant cerebral blood flow. Below a mean arterial pressure of about 60 mm Hg cerebral blood flow decreases proportionally to mean arterial pressure, and above a mean arterial pressure of about 150 mm Hg cerebral blood flow increases proportionally to mean arterial pressure. (322; **699, 1480–1481, Fig. 41–6**)

13. The autoregulation of cerebral blood flow is impaired in the presence of an intracerebral tumor, head trauma, subarachnoid hemorrhage, or volatile anesthetics. Chronic arterial hypertension results in a shift of the autoregulatory curve to the right, such that cerebral blood flow is maintained between pressures higher than 60 to 150 mm Hg. This effect is believed to occur after 1 to 2 months of hypertension. (322; **699, 721–722, 1480–1481, Fig. 41–6**)

14. Volatile anesthetics at concentrations above 0.6 MAC increase cerebral blood flow in a dose-dependent manner, most likely through the direct relaxation of vascular smooth muscle leading to vasodilation. The effect of volatile anesthetics on cerebral blood flow is time dependent in animal studies, meaning that cerebral blood flow normalizes with time. This has not been shown to be true in humans. Isoflurane has the least effect on cerebral blood flow, such that the increase in cerebral blood flow seen with isoflurane is relatively less than the increase in cerebral blood flow seen with the other volatile anesthetics. (322, Fig. 24–2; **702–707, 1898, Figs. 19–5, 19–8, 19–9**)

15. Volatile anesthetics decrease the cerebral metabolic oxygen requirement. Volatile anesthetics also increase cerebral blood flow. Normally, cerebral blood flow parallels the cerebral metabolic oxygen requirement, such that as the cerebral metabolic oxygen requirement increases so does cerebral blood flow. Given that volatile anesthetics increase cerebral blood flow and decrease cerebral metabolic oxygen requirements, it has been said that volatile anesthetics uncouple these two physiologic characteristics. (322; **697, 702–703, 707–708, Fig. 19–8**)

16. Nitrous oxide increases cerebral blood flow through cerebral vasodilation. The effect of nitrous oxide appears to be blunted in the presence of intravenous anesthetics. Nitrous oxide has less of an effect on cerebral blood flow than volatile anesthetics. Limitation of the inspired concentration of nitrous oxide to less than 0.7 MAC minimizes its effect of cerebral vasodilation. (322; **710–711, 1898**)

17. Ketamine increases cerebral blood flow to a significant degree, limiting its use for patients with intracerebral tumors. (322; **702, 1898**)

18. Thiopental decreases cerebral blood flow via cerebral vasoconstriction. It also decreases cerebral metabolic oxygen requirements and reliably decreases the intracranial pressure. (322; **703, 719–720, 1898**)

19. Propofol decreases cerebral blood flow via cerebral vasoconstriction in a manner similar to thiopental. It also decreases cerebral metabolic oxygen requirements and reliably decreases the intracranial pressure. (322–323; **703, 720, 1898–1899**)

20. Etomidate decreases cerebral blood flow and cerebral metabolic oxygen requirements in the absence of myoclonus or seizure activity. (323; **703, 720, 1898**)

21. Benzodiazepines minimally decrease cerebral blood flow and do not appear to cause an increase in intracranial pressure. (323; **705, 1898**)

22. Studies evaluating the effects of opioids on cerebral blood flow have yielded inconsistent results. Opioids either very minimally decrease cerebral blood flow or produce no effect at all. (323; **703–705, 1898**)

23. (322, Fig. 24–1; **699, Fig. 19–4**)

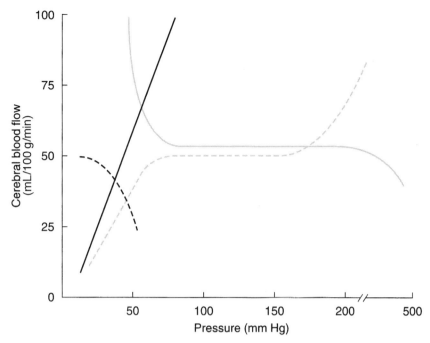

Figure 23–1. Schematic depiction of the impact of intracranial pressure (dashed black line), PaO_2 (solid gray line), $PaCO_2$ (solid black line), and cerebral perfusion pressure (mean arterial pressure minus intracranial pressure or right atrial pressure, whichever is greater) (dashed gray line) on cerebral blood flow. Cerebral perfusion pressures less than 50 mm Hg (mean arterial pressure 65 mm Hg assuming an intracranial pressure of 15 mm Hg) do not necessarily produce cerebral ischemia, but the physiologic reserve is decreased. In the presence of a decreased physiologic reserve, the addition of anemia may result in cerebral ischemia. (From Stoelting RK, Miller RD: Basics of Anesthesia, 4th ed. Philadelphia, Churchill Livingstone, 2000, p 322.)

24. (324, Fig. 24–4; **1896–1898, Fig. 52–2**)

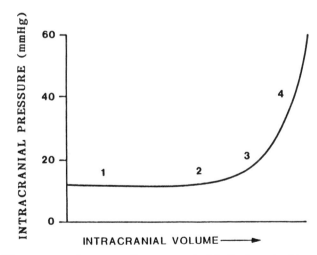

Figure 23–2. The pressure-volume compliance curve depicts the impact of increasing intracranial volume on intracranial pressure (ICP). As volume increases from point 1 to point 2 on the curve, the ICP does not increase because cerebrospinal fluid is shifted from the cranium into the spinal subarachnoid space. Patients with intracranial tumors and who are between point 1 and point 2 on the compliance curve are unlikely to manifest clinical symptoms of increased ICP. Patients who are on the rising portion of the pressure-volume curve (point 3) can no longer compensate for increases in intracranial volume, and ICP begins to increase. Clinical symptoms due to increased ICP are likely at this stage. Additional increases in volume at this point, as produced by increased CBF during anesthesia, can precipitate abrupt increases in ICP (point 4). (From Stoelting RK, Miller RD: Basics of Anesthesia, 4th ed. Philadelphia, Churchill Livingstone, 2000, p 324.)

25. A normal intracranial pressure is lower than 15 mm Hg. (323; **696, 1896–1897, Table 19–2**)

26. The intracranial pressure is determined by the intracranial contents occupying a fixed space. The intracranial components include brain tissue, intracerebral fluids, blood, and the cerebrospinal fluid. Increases in brain tissue or fluid, such as by brain tumor and edema, are space occupying and could potentially increase the intracranial pressure. Initially, the displacement of cerebrospinal fluid from the cranium compensates for increases in the space-occupying mass, but as the mass enlarges increases in the intracranial pressure become apparent clinically. The relationship between the intracranial volume and intracranial pressure is such that after compensatory mechanisms are exhausted small increases in the intracranial volume result in marked increases in the intracranial pressure. Marked increases in a patient's intracranial pressure can interfere with cerebral perfusion such that cerebral ischemia results. (323; **695–696, 708–709, 712–713, 1896–1898, Fig. 52–3**)

27. Although drug-induced increases in cerebral blood flow do not greatly affect the intracranial pressures of normal patients, patients with intracranial tumors are not able to compensate for the changes in cerebral blood flow. This may lead to an increase in intracranial pressures in these patients. (323; **708–709, 712–713, 1896–1899**)

28. Methods used to decrease an elevated intracranial pressure include positioning of the head to facilitate venous drainage, hyperventilation of the lungs, the drainage of cerebrospinal fluid, hypothermia, the administration of drugs, and surgical decompression. Drugs that may be administered to decrease the intracranial pressure include osmotic diuretics, renal tubular diuretics, corticosteroids, and barbiturates. (323; **1896–1902**)

29. Signs and symptoms of an increased intracranial pressure include nausea and vomiting, hypertension, bradycardia, personality changes, altered levels of consciousness, altered patterns of breathing, papilledema, and seizures. (323; **974, 1895**)

30. Preoperative medicines that result in drug-induced depression of ventilation in patients with an intracranial tumor could potentially lead to increases in the Pa_{CO_2}. This in turn could lead to an increase in cerebral blood flow and a corresponding increase in the intracranial pressure. (324; **696–698, 1898**)

31. The induction of general anesthesia in patients scheduled to undergo surgical resection of an intracranial tumor can be achieved with the administration of thiopental or propofol at a dose that is certain not to allow an increase in the intracranial pressure with direct laryngoscopy. Etomidate may be useful in situations in which patients have a suspected elevated intracranial pressure but are also hemodynamically unstable or hypovolemic, such as trauma patients. (324–325; **1898**)

32. Succinylcholine and all the nondepolarizing neuromuscular blocking drugs can be administered to patients undergoing surgical resection of an intracranial tumor. Succinylcholine is advantageous in circumstances in which rapid intubation of the trachea is desired. A drawback of succinylcholine is the mild increase in intracranial pressure that is associated with its administration. If succinylcholine were to be used, adequate doses of an intravenous induction agent should precede its administration, the Pa_{CO_2} should be controlled, and the blood pressure should be maintained to attenuate any increase in the intracranial pressure. The effects of nondepolarizing neuromuscular blocking drugs on cerebral blood flow and the intracranial pressure are limited to its effects of histamine release, if any. Histamine release causes an increase in cerebral blood flow through cerebral vasodilation, a possible increase in intracranial pressure,

and subsequent decrease in the cerebral perfusion pressure. Thus, in circumstances in which intracranial pressure control is critical, nondepolarizing neuromuscular blocking drugs not associated with histamine release may be preferred for administration. (324–325; **711–712, 1898**)

33. Before direct laryngoscopy and intubation of the trachea there are several measures that can be taken to attenuate increases in arterial blood pressure and intracranial pressure. Neuromuscular blockade should be confirmed with a peripheral nerve stimulator. This ensures that dangerous rises in intracranial pressure due to coughing or bucking in response to direct laryngoscopy do not occur. The administration of an additional dose of thiopental, an opioid, deeper levels of a volatile agent, a bolus of intravenous lidocaine, or a beta-adrenergic antagonist just before direct laryngoscopy are all methods that may be used to attenuate an increase in intracranial pressure. Finally, the duration of direct laryngoscopy should be minimized. (325; **708–709, 1898–1899, 1918**)

34. Maintenance anesthesia in patients undergoing surgical resection of an intracranial tumor is usually achieved with the administration of a low concentration of volatile anesthetic in conjunction with nitrous oxide and an opioid. The volatile anesthetic contributes to decreased awareness and the blunting of sympathetic nervous system responses. The disadvantage of volatile anesthetics during the resection of an intracranial tumor is its potential to increase cerebral blood flow. (325; **1898–1899**)

35. The volatile anesthetic traditionally chosen for maintenance anesthesia in patients undergoing surgical resection of an intracranial tumor is isoflurane. Isoflurane is chosen based on its relatively decreased effect on cerebral blood flow. That is, isoflurane increases cerebral blood flow less than the other volatile anesthetic agents. Recent studies of sevoflurane and desflurane have shown that their effects on cerebral blood flow are similar to isoflurane, suggesting that these may also be reasonable choices for maintenance anesthesia for patients with an intracranial tumor. (325, Figs. 24–2, 24–3; **708–709, 1898–1899, Figs. 19–7, 19–8**)

36. To limit the degree of increase in cerebral blood flow associated with its administration the MAC of volatile anesthetic administered should not exceed 0.6 MAC when administered for maintenance anesthesia in patients undergoing surgical resection of an intracranial tumor. It may be prudent to avoid the administration of volatile anesthetics altogether when even slight increases in cerebral blood flow and intracranial pressure are potentially harmful to the patient. Likewise, the administration of a volatile anesthetic should be discontinued intraoperatively if operating conditions are persistently difficult secondary to cerebral swelling. (325; **706–709, 1898**)

37. A Pa_{CO_2} maintained between 25 and 30 mm Hg provides the maximal benefit of decreased cerebral blood flow with minimal risk of cerebral ischemia. Below a Pa_{CO_2} of 25 mm Hg there is no evidence of any additional benefit. (325; **698, 1899–1900**)

38. Positive end-expiratory pressure during mechanical ventilation of the lungs in patients undergoing surgical resection of an intracranial tumor may lead to an increase in intracranial pressure by increasing the central venous pressure. (325; **698, 1919**)

39. Peripheral vasodilators increase cerebral blood flow by causing cerebral vascular vasodilation while simultaneously decreasing mean arterial blood pressure and the cerebral perfusion pressure. Among the agents that exert this effect are nitroglycerin, nitroprusside, adenosine, calcium channel blockers, and hydralazine. These drugs are not recommended for use in patients undergoing surgical

resection of an intracranial tumor during which increases in the intracranial pressure can be deleterious. (325; **700, 1900–1901, 1920–1921**)

40. Neuromuscular blockade is commonly maintained throughout intracranial surgical procedures to minimize the risk of patient movement, coughing, or bucking that may result in dangerous increases in intracranial pressure. Patient movement may also result in an increase in operative site bleeding and bulging of the brain into the operative site, making it difficult for the surgeons to operate. (325; **1898**)

41. Cerebral swelling occurring intraoperatively can be treated a number of ways. First, it should be confirmed that the maximal benefit is being derived from hyperventilation of the lungs with a $Paco_2$ between 25 and 30 mm Hg. Next, drugs that will cause cerebral dehydration may be administered. Mannitol at a dose of 0.25 to 1 g/kg or furosemide at a dose of 0.5 to 1 mg/kg are frequently used for this purpose. Intermittent injections of an intravenous anesthetic such as thiopental or propofol may also be administered. The administration of corticosteroids may be considered. Finally, the patient may benefit from hypothermia and being placed in a head-up position to facilitate jugular venous drainage. (325; **1898–1902**)

42. Intravenous fluid administration during surgical resection of an intracranial tumor should be given at maintenance doses to maintain an adequate intravascular fluid volume while minimizing increases in the water content of the brain. (325; **1910–1911**)

43. Fluid solutions that are isotonic or hypertonic relative to the serum are acceptable for intravenous fluid administration intraoperatively in patients undergoing surgical resection of an intracranial tumor. The basis for this is that fluid shifts across the blood-brain barrier are driven by differences in osmolarity across it, not by differences in oncotic pressure. Thus, a hyperosmolar solution will cause water to exit the brain, whereas the opposite may occur with a hypo-osmolar solution. As a point of reference, the osmolarity of normal plasma is about 285 mOsm, that of lactated Ringer's solution is about 272 mOsm/L, and that of normal saline is 308 mOsm/L. Normal saline is therefore probably a slightly better choice than lactated Ringer's solution, although clinically the administration of lactated Ringer's solution at maintenance rates has not been shown to have any detrimental results. Colloids are also acceptable solutions for administration intraoperatively. Glucose-containing intravenous solutions should be avoided in these patients secondary to the increase in brain swelling that can occur. Glucose distributes rapidly throughout total body water. If the concentration of glucose in the blood becomes less than that of the brain, the brain osmolarity becomes greater, attracting water. Water will then enter the brain and may cause cerebral edema. In addition, hyperglycemia can increase neurologic damage to ischemic neural cells. (325; **1910–1911**)

44. Intraoperative monitoring useful during surgical resection of an intracranial tumor includes an intra-arterial blood pressure monitor that also facilitates periodic arterial blood gas sampling. The exhaled carbon dioxide concentration measurements are useful to guide the minute ventilation of the lungs. A central venous catheter, an end-tidal nitrogen concentration measure, and a Doppler transducer placed to the right of the sternum are all monitors that may be useful in the detection and/or treatment of a venous air embolism. A bladder catheter can be used to monitor urine output, particularly if diuretics are to be administered. A peripheral nerve stimulator will assist in the titration of doses of neuromuscular blocking drugs. (325; **1909–1910, Table 52–8**)

45. Coughing and straining in patients awakening from anesthesia after intracranial surgery can result in dangerous increases in the intracranial pressure, increases in cerebral edema, and evoke postoperative bleeding. This can be avoided by

the administration of small doses of propofol or intravenous lidocaine at the conclusion of the procedure during reversal of neuromuscular blockade. The emergence from anesthesia is better timed to follow placement of the head dressings because movement of the head at the conclusion of surgery in the lightly anesthetized patient can stimulate bucking on the endotracheal tube. Alternatively, if the patient is an appropriate candidate for extubation while deeply anesthetized, this could prevent awakening with the noxious stimulus of the endotracheal tube. (325; **1911–1912**)

46. Delayed recovery as well as worsening neurologic function after intracranial surgery without an obvious cause warrant evaluation by computed tomography or magnetic resonance imaging. A tension pneumocephalus may be considered as a possible cause of postoperative delayed recovery when nitrous oxide was administered intraoperatively, particularly after posterior fossa surgeries in the sitting position. Tension pneumocephalus occurs as a result of air entering the subdural cavities. The treatment of a tension pneumocephalus is bur hole removal of the gas. Symptoms due to tension pneumocephalus resolve quickly after treatment. (325; **1905–1906, 1912**)

47. Patients undergoing surgical resection of an intracranial tumor are at an increased risk for a venous air embolism secondary to positioning of the patient's head above the level of the heart and because veins transected while cutting the skull stay tented open after transection. Patients undergoing posterior fossa craniotomies in the sitting position are at particular risk of an intraoperative venous air embolism. For this reason, many neurosurgeons prefer to do posterior fossa craniotomies with the patient in the prone position. (325–326; **1024–1026, 1900**)

48. A venous air embolism is the entry of air into the venous circulation, where it circulates with blood into the right side of the heart. After entry into the heart, the air may take three paths. First, it may stay in the right ventricle, interfering with blood flow into the pulmonary artery. Second, it may enter the pulmonary circulation. Once in the pulmonary circulation it can cause a pulmonary embolus or it could traverse the pulmonary circulation and enter the arterial circulation. Finally, from the right atrium it could enter the left atrium through a probe patent foramen ovale, which is present in approximately 25% of adults. Arterial emboli to the cerebral and coronary circulations can lead to neurologic and coronary infarctions, respectively. (325–326; **1027–1029, 1906–1909**)

49. Methods by which a venous air embolism can be detected include transesophageal echocardiography, Doppler transducer-assisted detection of air in the right side of the heart, a sudden decrease in the exhaled carbon dioxide concentrations due to a sudden increase in the ventilation of deadspace, increased end-tidal nitrogen concentrations, and what would appear to be sudden attempts by the patient to initiate spontaneous ventilation during controlled ventilation. In response to a pulmonary embolus, patients may have bronchoconstriction, pulmonary edema, elevated right atrial or pulmonary artery pressures, and elevated peak inspiratory pressures. The most sensitive method to detect a venous air embolism is through the use of transesophageal echocardiography. It is also beneficial in that it allows for the identification of right-to-left air shunting. The drawbacks of routine transesophageal echocardiography monitoring for venous air embolism are its invasiveness, bulk, and cost. An acceptable alternative to transesophageal echocardiography for monitoring is through the combined use of a Doppler transducer and monitoring exhaled concentrations of carbon dioxide. The transducer should be placed between the third and sixth intercostal spaces to the right of the sternum. The Doppler transducer is able to recognize small volumes of intracardiac air, but it is not able to distinguish between small volumes and large volumes of air. (326; **1026–1029, 1906–1907, Figs. 26–15, 52–9, 52–10**)

50. Signs of a clinically significant venous air embolism include hypotension, tachycardia, cardiac dysrhythmias, cyanosis, and a characteristic "mill wheel" murmur. (326; **1026–1029, 1906–1907**)

51. The treatment of a venous air embolism includes the prompt administration of 100% oxygen and the discontinuation of nitrous oxide administration. The surgeons should be asked to irrigate the operative field with fluid and to occlude the bone edges to prevent the further entry of air. Gentle compression of the jugular veins can be instituted. In addition, if a central venous catheter is in place, placement of the patient in the Trendelenburg position and aspiration on the catheter to retrieve the air may be attempted. Other treatment methods of a venous air embolus are supportive as needed for hypotension, decreased cardiac output, bronchoconstriction, or other manifestations. (326; **1026–1029, 1906–1909**)

52. Nitrous oxide administration should be discontinued in the presence of a venous air embolism. The diffusion of nitrous oxide into the air embolus could potentially increase its size and worsen its clinical effects. Some clinicians choose to avoid the administration of nitrous oxide in patients at risk for a venous air embolus. (326; **1909**)

53. Although a pulmonary artery catheter is not useful for aspirating a venous air embolism because of its small catheter size, it may be useful in detecting increases in the pulmonary artery pressures in the presence of a pulmonary embolus. (326; **1026–1028**)

54. Positive end-expiratory pressure has not been shown to be efficacious in the prevention of a venous air embolism. (326; **1908–1909**)

55. Death occurring as a result of a venous air embolism is usually due to an obstruction of forward flow from the right side of the heart. Acute cor pulmonale, cardiovascular collapse, and arterial hypoxemia result. (326; **1908–1909**)

CAROTID ENDARTERECTOMY

56. The indications for a carotid endarterectomy are not clearly defined and are still under investigation. It is generally believed that the procedure should be performed in patients with a history of transient ischemic attacks or when symptomatic with a stenosis greater than 70% of a carotid artery. The decision to operate on asymptomatic patients should be determined by the outcomes at a specific center. Patients who have suffered an acute stroke are not candidates for a carotid endarterectomy. (326; **1878**)

57. Patients undergoing a carotid endarterectomy often have co-existing cardiovascular and neurologic disease. Indeed the leading cause of perioperative mortality after carotid endarterectomy is myocardial infarction. The function of each of these systems should be closely evaluated preoperatively and medically optimized. The range of normal blood pressures for the patient should be determined. Neurologic symptoms and deficits should be documented preoperatively to prevent any dysfunction noted postoperatively from being incorrectly attributed to the surgical procedure or intraoperative events. (326; **1878–1879, 1882–1883**)

58. The primary goal of the anesthetic management for patients undergoing a carotid endarterectomy is the maintenance of cerebral blood flow and cerebral perfusion pressure on the side of the brain of the diseased coronary artery. The critical period of the procedure occurs while the carotid artery is clamped, during which time neurologic dysfunction and/or hemodynamic responses may occur. Other goals include protection of the myocardium from ischemia, control of the heart rate and blood pressure, and blunting of the sympathetic nervous

system responses to pain. Ideally, the patient should be able to follow commands shortly after surgery to facilitate neurologic evaluation. (326; **1879**)

59. The purpose of intraoperative neurologic monitoring is to identify patients in need of having an intraluminal shunt placed for perfusion to the ipsilateral brain while the diseased carotid artery is clamped. The stump pressure is the blood pressure in the diseased carotid artery distal to the placement of the surgical clamp. The stump pressure reflects the pressure that is transmitted from the opposite carotid artery via the circle of Willis. A stump pressure of 60 mm Hg or greater is considered to be adequate for cerebral perfusion ipsilateral to the clamped carotid artery. The stump pressure is easy to obtain, although its accuracy has come into question. Other methods of evaluating the adequacy of ipsilateral cerebral perfusion during clamping of the diseased carotid artery include the use of an electroencephalogram, somatosensory evoked potentials, direct measurement of cerebral blood flow, and transcranial Doppler ultrasonography. Alternatively, in some centers, an intraluminal shunt is routinely placed. (326; **1881–1882**)

60. An intraluminal shunt is placed by the surgeons when there is concern regarding the cerebral perfusion on the side of the diseased carotid artery. The intraluminal shunt provides continued blood flow through the clamped carotid artery. The shunt may be placed before clamping, may be placed in response to an inadequate stump pressure after clamping, or may be placed after clamping in response to neurologic changes in the monitored patient. In some centers intraluminal shunts are placed routinely. The placement of a shunt still requires a brief period of carotid clamping and potential ipsilateral cerebral ischemia. (326; **1881**)

61. The administration of either local or general anesthesia for carotid endarterectomy is acceptable. Neither has been shown to have better outcomes or reduced morbidity or mortality. (326; **1881, Table 51–10**)

62. Local anesthesia for a carotid endarterectomy is achieved with the administration of a deep cervical plexus block in combination with a superficial cervical plexus block through local anesthetic infiltration. A deep cervical plexus block provides anesthesia to the C1–C4 nerve distribution. The cervical plexus ends in four peripheral nerves that are subsequently blocked by this technique. These are the greater auricular, lesser occipital, transverse cervical, and supraclavicular nerves. The superficial cervical plexus block anesthetizes the cutaneous nerves. A distinct advantage of local anesthesia for this procedure is the ability to continually monitor the neurologic function of the patient, particularly during clamping of the carotid artery. Typically monitored during this time are the patient's contralateral grip strength, level of consciousness, and quality of prompted speech. (326; **1540–1541, 1880–1881, Figs. 43–21, 43–22**)

63. The induction of general anesthesia for a carotid endarterectomy is usually achieved with the administration of an intravenous induction agent and a neuromuscular blocking drug. The maintenance of anesthesia is typically with the administration of a volatile anesthetic in conjunction with nitrous oxide and an opioid. Neuromuscular blockade is usually maintained throughout the course of the procedure. Isoflurane provides the greatest decrease in cerebral metabolic oxygen requirement when compared with other volatile anesthetics as well as the least increase in cerebral blood flow. For these reasons isoflurane has been historically selected as the volatile anesthetic agent of choice during these procedures. Sevoflurane and desflurane likely have similar effects as isoflurane. An advantage of general anesthesia is the ability to manipulate cerebral blood flow and the cerebral metabolic oxygen requirement. In addition, with general anesthesia, airway protection is already provided and other interventions are easily accomplished when compared with patients under local anesthesia. Gen-

eral anesthesia may also be advantageous when patients are unable to communicate or when their neck anatomy appears difficult for the administration of local anesthesia. (327; **1879–1880**)

64. During a carotid endarterectomy procedure the arterial blood pressure should be maintained in a normal range or slightly elevated specific to that patient. It may be helpful to blunt sympathetic nervous system responses to direct laryngoscopy to avoid hypertension. A high-normal range of mean arterial pressures might be maintained during carotid artery clamping to increase collateral blood flow and prevent cerebral ischemia when there is no intraluminal shunt in place. Bradycardia and hypotension can occur abruptly with surgical manipulation of the carotid sinus and baroreceptors. Local infiltration of the carotid bifurcation with 3 to 5 mL of 1% lidocaine usually controls this. Intraoperative hypotension can be treated with phenylephrine. (327; **1880**)

65. Potential problems with intraoperative hypertension during a carotid endarterectomy are cerebral edema, increased cerebral metabolic oxygen requirements, and myocardial ischemia. (327; **1880**)

66. During a carotid endarterectomy the $Paco_2$ should be maintained near normal, at about 35 mm Hg. There does not seem to be any derived benefit from manipulating ventilation of the lungs to vasodilate or vasoconstrict cerebral vessels. (327; **1881**)

67. Postoperative problems that may occur after a carotid endarterectomy include recurrent laryngeal nerve injury, blood pressure lability, airway compression secondary to wound hematoma, loss of carotid body function, myocardial infarction, and neurologic dysfunction. Neurologic dysfunction after carotid endarterectomy is usually due to intraoperative embolization or hypoperfusion during carotid artery clamping. (327; **1882–1883**)

68. Postoperative hypertension is more common after a carotid endarterectomy. Chronic hypertension is present in 60% to 80% of patients undergoing a carotid endarterectomy. These patients are especially at risk of postoperative hypertension. Hypertension may also occur secondary to the loss of function of the carotid sinus or the loss of innervation to the carotid sinus during surgery. Hypotension occurs almost as frequently as hypertension after a carotid endarterectomy. Hypotension is thought to occur secondary to renewed activity of a carotid sinus that was previously blocked by an atheromatous plaque. It is frequently associated with bradycardia when it occurs. Typically, hypotension after carotid endarterectomy lasts for only 12 to 24 hours. (327; **1882–1883**)

INTRACRANIAL ANEURYSMS

69. Ruptured intracranial aneurysms have a mortality of 40% to 50%. Patients with ruptured intracranial aneurysms usually present with signs of an elevated intracranial pressure. These can include hypertension, headache, nausea, vomiting, nuchal rigidity, focal neurologic signs, and changes in the level of consciousness. The immediate management of patients with a ruptured intracranial aneurysm is to treat elevations in the intracranial pressure. The general consensus is that surgical intervention should take place within 72 hours of onset of a subarachnoid hemorrhage to minimize the risk of rebleeding. (327; **1913–1914, Table 52–10**)

70. The electrocardiogram of patients with a ruptured intracranial aneurysm often appears abnormal and may mimic myocardial ischemia. These changes are usually due to a neurologic mechanism and are not from injury to the myocardium. Changes frequently seen on the electrocardiogram of these patients include arrhythmias, sinus bradycardia, Q waves, deep inverted T waves, prolonged QT intervals, and ST segment elevation. (327; **1915–1916, Fig. 52–12**)

71. The major cause of morbidity after rupture of an intracranial aneurysm is vasospasm of the cerebral arteries. Vasospasm occurs in about 70% of patients after a ruptured intracranial aneurysm. Drowsiness is the most common clinical sign of vasospasm, and radiologic studies confirm its presence. Surgery previously scheduled may be delayed once vasospasm has occurred. Vasospasm is most likely to occur 5 to 7 days after rupture, but it can occur 4 to 12 days after rupture. Most episodes of vasospasm last for 2 to 3 weeks. Treatment of cerebral vasospasm is by increasing cardiac output; administering intravenous fluids to achieve hypertension, hypervolemia, and hemodilution; and administering the calcium channel blocker nimodipine. (327; **1914–1915**)

72. The goal of the anesthetic management of a patient undergoing resection of an intracranial aneurysm is the avoidance of drugs or events that will cause increases in arterial blood pressure or intracranial pressure and the facilitation of surgical exposure. Increases in the arterial blood pressure alone or concomitant with decreases in the intracranial pressure would result in increases in the transmural pressure in the aneurysm and place the patient at an increased risk of rupture of the aneurysm. For this reason exaggerated increases in arterial blood pressure during direct laryngoscopy must be attenuated. A volatile anesthetic such as isoflurane can be used in conjunction with nitrous oxide for maintenance anesthesia. In cases of elevated intracranial pressures or cerebral swelling an alternative to a volatile anesthetic may be chosen. (327; **1916**)

73. Controlled hypotension during surgery for resection of an intracranial aneurysm is used as a means to prevent re-rupture of the aneurysm during surgery and also facilitates surgical exposure. It may also facilitate the placement of a clamp on the afferent blood supply to achieve surgical control of the aneurysm. Hypotension may be accomplished with the administration of an intravenous infusion of nitroprusside or nitroglycerin in conjunction with esmolol to control reflex tachycardia. Resistance to controlled hypotension may be noted in younger patients, hypervolemic patients, or patients with a light level of anesthesia. (327–328; **1472–1476, 1916**)

74. A disadvantage of controlled hypotension during resection of an intracranial aneurysm is the loss of cerebral autoregulation that results from the administration of peripheral vasodilators. Controlled hypotension for intracranial aneurysms is no longer performed routinely because of the concern that decreases in mean arterial pressure may result in decreases in cerebral blood flow to areas that are only marginally perfused. Placement of a clamp on the aneurysm's afferent blood supply may obviate the need for controlled hypotension. (328; **1480–1482, 1485, 1916**)

75. When controlled hypotension is planned during resection of an intracranial aneurysm, placement of the transducer for the arterial blood pressure at the level of the brain when the head is elevated gives a more reliable indicator of the cerebral perfusion pressure. This is because the mean arterial blood pressure decreases by about 0.7 mm Hg for each centimeter above the level of the heart. For example, when the head is elevated 20 cm above the level of the heart the cerebral perfusion pressure is about 14 mm Hg less than the mean arterial blood pressure at the level of the heart. Therefore, a mean arterial blood pressure of 60 mm Hg at the heart level would actually correspond to a mean arterial blood pressure of 46 mm Hg at the level of the brain and a corresponding decrease in the actual calculated cerebral perfusion pressure. (328; **1485–1486**)

SPINAL CORD TRANSECTION

76. The most common cause of spinal cord transection is trauma. Spinal cord transection is only a figurative term. Injury to the spinal cord may result in dysfunction that resembles literal transection of the spinal cord. (328; **1919**)

77. In addition to the usual precautionary measures taken during emergent intubation of the trachea, emergent intubation of the trachea of a patient in cervical spine precautions is best achieved with cervical spine in-line manual stabilization or an awake intubation. (328; **1919, 2163–2165, Figs. 52–13, 62–2**)

78. Succinylcholine is not recommended for neuromuscular blockade to facilitate intubation of the trachea after 24 hours after spinal cord injury. The concern is for a hyperkalemic response caused by its administration secondary to the excessive release of potassium from extrajunctional receptors that proliferated as a result of denervation injury. The duration of the hyperkalemic response to the administration of succinylcholine in patients who have suffered a denervation injury is estimated to be 3 to 6 months after injury. There have been reports of hyperkalemic responses to succinylcholine administration greater than 6 months after injury, however. (328; **422–423, 926**)

79. Patients who have suffered a spinal cord transection are prone to hypotension because of the lack of sympathetic nervous system activity below the level of the injury. This is particularly true in the first month after spinal cord injury. Hypotension may be especially marked during times of changes in posture, blood loss, or with the institution of positive pressure ventilation of the lungs. (328; **568–569**)

80. Patients who have suffered a spinal cord transection are prone to hypothermia below the level of the injury because of the lack of cutaneous vasodilation or of an ability to shiver. (328; **568–569, 926**)

81. Autonomic hyperreflexia is characterized as a reflexive, abrupt, persistent arterial hypertension and an associated compensatory bradycardia in response to cutaneous or visceral stimulation below the level of the transection. Autonomic hyperreflexia coincides with the return of spinal reflexes after the acute shock stage of injury, typically 3 to 4 weeks after the initial injury. Autonomic hyperreflexia is believed to occur secondary to carotid sinus activation in response to a stimulus. The stimulus and response result in persistent vasoconstriction and decreased blood flow to the periphery manifesting as hypertension. Flushing and sweating above the level of the transection and bradycardia occur, owing to parasympathetic nervous system responses above the level of the transection. These manifestations persist secondary to the physical inability of parasympathetic-mediated vasodilatory impulses from the central nervous system to modulate the reflex below the level of spinal cord transection. Autonomic hyperreflexia that occurs intraoperatively can be treated with the intravenous administration of nitroprusside. (328–329, Fig. 24–5; **568–569, 926**)

82. Spinal cord transection above T6 is most likely to be associated with autonomic hyperreflexia. As many as 85% of patients with a T6 transection or higher are estimated to have this disorder. Patients with transection of the cord below T10 rarely have autonomic hyperreflexia. (328; **568–569, 925**)

83. Surgical distention of a hollow viscus, such as the bowel or bladder, are most likely to trigger autonomic hyperreflexia. Autonomic hyperreflexia is often noted during transurethral cystoscopy. (328; **568–569, 925**)

84. Spinal anesthesia is most likely to prevent autonomic hyperreflexia by effectively blocking the peripheral sympathetic nervous system stimulation. (328; **568–569**)

SLEEP APNEA SYNDROME

85. Sleep apnea syndrome is defined as the constellation of symptoms that arise from the recurrent cessation of air flow at the mouth for longer than 10 seconds. (329; **914–915, 2466**)

86. Causes of sleep apnea syndrome include mechanical upper airway obstruction or a loss of central nervous system control over ventilation. (329; **914–915, 2466**)

87. Manifestations of sleep apnea syndrome include daytime somnolence, a history of loud snoring, obesity, hypertension, arterial hypoxemia, polycythemia, hypercarbia, and cor pulmonale. (329; **914–915, 2466**)

88. Surgical treatments of sleep apnea syndrome include resection of nasal polyps or hypertrophied adenoids, uvulopalatopharyngoplasty, and radiofrequency ablation of the tongue or palate. Anesthetic considerations for patients undergoing these surgical procedures include the risk of depression of ventilation with preoperative medicines or as a delayed effect of intraoperative medicines. Patients may also develop soft tissue airway obstruction with the induction of anesthesia. Tracheal extubation after the procedure should be delayed until these patients are fully awake and cooperative. Postoperatively, these patients should be closely observed in a monitored setting for episodes of apnea and arterial hypoxemia. (329; **914–915, 2466**)

Chapter 24

Ophthalmology and Otolaryngology

OPHTHALMOLOGY

1. What is the normal intraocular pressure? How is this intraocular pressure maintained?

2. How much does intraocular pressure increase during coughing or vomiting?

3. What are some times of intraocular pressure increase in patients undergoing surgical procedures under general anesthesia?

4. What is the mechanism for the increase in intraocular pressure that is seen with the administration of succinylcholine?

5. How much does intraocular pressure increase with the intravenous administration of succinylcholine? What is the duration of this effect?

6. How much does intraocular pressure increase with the intramuscular administration of succinylcholine? What is the duration of this effect?

7. How does pretreatment with subparalyzing doses of a nondepolarizing neuromuscular blocking drug before the administration of succinylcholine affect the rise in intraocular pressure normally seen with the administration of succinylcholine?

8. How do paralyzing doses of nondepolarizing neuromuscular blocking drugs affect intraocular pressure?

9. How do inhaled anesthetics affect intraocular pressure?

10. Name some intravenous anesthetics and their effect on intraocular pressure.

11. How does ketamine affect intraocular pressure? What other actions of ketamine make it a poor choice for anesthesia in patients undergoing ophthalmologic procedures?

12. How do changes in arterial blood pressure affect intraocular pressure?

13. How do changes in the Pa_{CO_2} affect intraocular pressure?

14. How do carbonic anhydrase inhibitors affect intraocular pressure?

15. How do osmotic diuretics affect intraocular pressure?

16. What topical ophthalmic medicines may be absorbed sufficiently to exert systemic effects?

17. Why are beta antagonists, such as timolol, administered as a topical ophthalmic medicine? What systemic effects have been attributed to the topical ophthalmic application of this drug?

18. Why is the long-acting anticholinesterase echothiophate sometimes administered as a topical ophthalmic medicine? What systemic effects have been attributed to the topical ophthalmic application of this drug?

19. Why is phenylephrine administered as a topical ophthalmic medicine? What systemic effects have been attributed to the topical ophthalmic application of this drug?

20. What is the desired effect of the topical ophthalmic medicine cyclopentolate? What

systemic effects have been attributed to the topical ophthalmic application of this drug?

21. Why is epinephrine administered as a topical ophthalmic medicine? What systemic effects have been attributed to the topical ophthalmic application of this drug?

22. Why are carbonic anhydrase inhibitors, such as acetazolamide, administered as topical ophthalmic medicines? What systemic effects have been attributed to the topical ophthalmic application of this drug?

23. What is the oculocardiac reflex? When is it most likely to occur?

24. What cardiac rhythms are likely to result from the oculocardiac reflex?

25. How does hypercarbia affect the oculocardiac reflex? How does arterial hypoxemia affect the oculocardiac reflex?

26. What is the first line of treatment for the oculocardiac reflex? What other measures may be taken if the reflex persists?

27. Which patients may benefit from the prophylactic use of atropine when undergoing ophthalmic surgical procedures?

28. What are some of the goals for the anesthetic management of patients undergoing ophthalmic surgery?

29. Why is intubation of the trachea sometimes necessary in patients undergoing ophthalmic surgery?

30. What is the potential problem during surgery in which the globe is opened? How can this potential problem be minimized?

31. How safe has the retrobulbar block proved to have been in elderly patients undergoing ophthalmic procedures?

32. What does a retrobulbar block actually provide anesthesia to? How is akinesia of the eyelids achieved if necessary?

33. What are some complications of a retrobulbar block?

34. How can patient comfort be optimized during the performance of a retrobulbar block?

35. How can increases in intraocular pressure be minimized during the induction of general anesthesia and intubation of the trachea in patients undergoing ophthalmic procedures?

36. How can increases in intraocular pressure be minimized during the emergence from general anesthesia in patients undergoing ophthalmic procedures under general anesthesia?

37. Why are neuromuscular blocking drugs often administered intraoperatively to patients undergoing ophthalmic procedures?

38. How does the reversal of nondepolarizing neuromuscular blocking drugs with an anticholinesterase drug and an anticholinergic drug affect the intraocular pressure?

39. Why are antiemetics often administered to patients prophylactically at the conclusion of general anesthesia for ophthalmic surgery?

40. What are some special anesthetic considerations for children undergoing strabismus surgery?

41. What are the concerns regarding the use of succinylcholine in children scheduled to undergo strabismus surgery?

42. What are some special anesthetic considerations for patients with glaucoma undergoing surgery?

43. How should the perioperative administration of topical ophthalmic medicines used to treat glaucoma be managed?

44. What is the risk of the administration of anticholinergic drugs either alone as premedicants or in combination with anticholinesterase drugs for the reversal of neuromuscular blocking drugs in patients with glaucoma?

45. What is the risk of the transient increase in intraocular pressure seen with succinylcholine when administered to patients with glaucoma?

46. What is the risk of prolonged intraoperative hypotension in patients with glaucoma?

47. What are some special considerations for the anesthetic management of patients undergoing surgery for cataract extraction?

48. When general anesthesia is chosen for patients undergoing cataract surgery, what is the recommendation with regard to the administration of succinylcholine to facilitate intubation of the trachea?

49. What are the anesthetic considerations for patients undergoing surgery to repair a retinal detachment?

50. What are some intravenous medicines that can be used intraoperatively to decrease the intraocular pressure in patients undergoing surgery to repair a retinal detachment?

51. When must nitrous oxide be avoided as a maintenance anesthetic for patients undergoing surgery to repair a retinal detachment? What is the risk associated with this?

52. What are some special considerations for the anesthetic management of patients undergoing surgery for the emergent repair of an open eye injury?

53. What are some options for intubation of the trachea of patients who have had recent food ingestion and have an open globe?

54. What is the most common ocular complication associated with general anesthesia?

55. When corneal abrasions occur in patients who have undergone a surgical procedure under general anesthesia, what portion of the cornea is most likely to be affected?

56. Why are patients who are undergoing a surgical procedure under general anesthesia at risk for a corneal abrasion?

57. What are some methods by which the risk of corneal abrasions in patients undergoing a surgical procedure under general anesthesia can be minimized? What are some of the potential problems with the routine use of ophthalmic ointment?

58. When should a corneal abrasion be suspected? How should it be diagnosed?

59. How are corneal abrasions treated? How long do corneal abrasions normally take to heal?

60. What is the potential risk of retinal ischemia occurring in the perioperative period?

61. What are some possible causes of retinal ischemia in the perioperative period?

62. How can the risk of retinal ischemia in the perioperative period be minimized?

OTOLARYNGOLOGY

63. What are some special considerations for the anesthetic management of patients undergoing surgery on the ear?

64. How is surgical identification of the facial nerve done intraoperatively in patients undergoing surgery on the ear? How might this affect the anesthetic management of these patients?

65. What is the concern with regard to the administration of nitrous oxide as maintenance anesthesia to patients undergoing surgery on the middle ear?

66. What is the concern with regard to the administration of nitrous oxide as maintenance anesthesia to patients undergoing a tympanoplasty?

67. How can the rapid absorption of nitrous oxide after its discontinuation during surgery affect the middle ear of patients with abnormal eustachian tube function?

68. What are some special considerations for the anesthetic management of patients undergoing nasal and sinus surgery?

69. What can the systemic absorption of topical cocaine result in?

70. How can maintenance anesthesia be achieved in patients undergoing nasal and sinus surgery?

71. Given that nasal sinuses are air-filled cavities, is there a risk of administering nitrous oxide for maintenance anesthesia in patients undergoing nasal and sinus surgery?

72. What are some special considerations for the anesthetic management of patients undergoing airway endoscopy?

73. What type of endotracheal tube should be used for intubation of the trachea of patients undergoing laryngoscopy by the otolaryngologist?

74. How can neuromuscular blockade be achieved in patients undergoing laryngoscopy?

75. What is a laser? What are its advantages with regard to its use for surgical procedures?

76. Name some hazards that are associated with laser surgery.

77. What is the purpose of a smoke evacuator that is used during laser surgery?

78. What are the potential hazards of misdirected laser energy during laser surgery?

79. How might laser surgery result in eye injury? Who is at risk?

80. What are some measures that can be taken during laser surgery of the airway to minimize the risk of an endotracheal tube fire?

81. What is the concern regarding the delivery of volatile anesthetics during laser surgery of the airway?

82. What are the steps the anesthesiologist and surgeon should take in the event of an airway fire during laser surgery of the airway?

83. What type of endotracheal tube should be used for the intubation of the trachea of patients undergoing bronchoscopy?

84. What are some potential problems that can occur if a patient were to move during rigid bronchoscopy?

85. What are some considerations for the anesthetic management of patients undergoing head and neck surgery?

86. What are some methods by which intraoperative blood loss can be minimized during head and neck surgery?

87. What electrocardiographic changes might be noted in patients undergoing radical neck dissection on the right side? Why is this thought to occur?

88. What are some special considerations for the anesthetic management of patients undergoing adenotonsillectomy?

89. What is the potential for blood loss during an adenotonsillectomy? Why is the blood loss often underestimated?

90. What position are patients often placed in for recovery after having undergone an adenotonsillectomy?

91. When postoperative bleeding after an adenotonsillectomy is significant to require reoperation, what is the time course relative to the surgical procedure in which the bleeding is typically manifested?

92. What are some considerations for the anesthetic management of patients who return to surgery because of significant postoperative bleeding after an adenotonsillectomy?

93. What is the difference between a tracheostomy and a cricothyrotomy? When is it appropriate for each to be performed?

94. What are some early complications of a tracheostomy?

ANSWERS*

OPHTHALMOLOGY

1. Normal intraocular pressure is 10 to 22 mm Hg. This pressure is maintained through a dynamic balance between the production and elimination of aqueous humor, a watery, clear fluid. Aqueous humor is produced in the ciliary body and is eliminated into the venous system through the canal of Schlemm at the iridocorneal angle. (331; **2176–2177, Fig. 63–1**)

2. Intraocular pressure can increase to as much as 35 to 50 mm Hg with coughing or vomiting. This represents the greatest known increase in intraocular pressure. (331; **2176–2177**)

3. Patients undergoing surgical procedures under general anesthesia probably have the greatest potential for large increases in intraocular pressure during direct laryngoscopy or while awakening, especially if either of these is accompanied by coughing. (331; **423, 2178**)

4. The mechanism for the increase in intraocular pressure that is seen with the administration of succinylcholine is not definitively known. It is believed, however, that the prolonged tonic contraction of the extraocular muscles that is caused by succinylcholine contributes to the increase in intraocular pressure. Interestingly, sectioning the recti eye muscle does not prevent the increase in intraocular pressure produced by succinylcholine. (331; **423, 2177–2178**)

5. Intraocular pressure increases by about 8 mm Hg with the intravenous administration of succinylcholine. The peak of this effect of succinylcholine is within 1 to 4 minutes, and the duration of this effect is approximately 7 minutes. (331, Fig. 25–1; **423, 2178**)

6. Intraocular pressure increases by about 8 mm Hg with the intramuscular administration of succinylcholine as well. The duration of the increase in intraocular pressure after the administration of intramuscular succinylcholine is approximately 15 minutes. (331; **423, 2177**)

7. Pretreatment with subparalyzing doses of a nondepolarizing neuromuscular blocking drug before the administration of succinylcholine may attenuate the rise in intraocular pressure that is normally seen with the administration of succinylcholine. Pretreatment does not reliably prevent the increase in intraocular pressure, however. (331; **423, 2178**)

8. Paralyzing doses of nondepolarizing neuromuscular blocking drugs decrease

*Numbers in parentheses: lightface numbers refer to pages, figures, or tables in Stoelting RK, Miller RD: Basics of Anesthesia, 4th ed. Philadelphia, Churchill Livingstone, 2000; **boldface numbers** refer to pages, figures, or tables in Miller RD: Anesthesia, 5th ed. Philadelphia, Churchill Livingstone, 2000.

intraocular pressure. Although the mechanism for the decrease in intraocular pressure that is seen with the administration of nondepolarizing neuromuscular blocking drugs is not definitively known, it is thought to be due to relaxation of the extraocular muscles. (331; **2178**)

9. Inhaled anesthetics lower intraocular pressure. (331; **2177**)

10. Most intravenous anesthetics, including barbiturates, propofol, benzodiazepines, etomidate, and opioids, lower intraocular pressure. The exception to this is ketamine. (331; **2177**)

11. Ketamine appears to have variable effects on intraocular pressure. Although early studies have shown that ketamine increases intraocular pressure, more recent data have shown that with premedication the opposite may be true. Other effects of ketamine that continue to make it a poor choice for anesthesia in patients undergoing ophthalmic procedures include blepharospasm and nystagmus. (331; **244, 2177**)

12. Changes in arterial blood pressure have minimal effect on the intraocular pressure if the alterations in blood pressure are within the normal physiologic range and not sudden, extreme changes in blood pressure. (331; **2177**)

13. Changes in the Pa_{CO_2} without changes in the central venous pressure have minimal effects on the intraocular pressure. (331; **2177**)

14. Carbonic anhydrase inhibitors acutely decrease intraocular pressure by interfering with the secretion of aqueous humor. Acetazolamide is a carbonic anhydrase inhibitor that is frequently administered in the perioperative period for this purpose. (332; **2176**)

15. Osmotic diuretics acutely decrease intraocular pressure by interfering with the secretion of aqueous humor. Mannitol is an osmotic diuretic that may be administered for this purpose. (332)

16. All topical ophthalmic medicines may be absorbed sufficiently to exert systemic effects. (332; **2181–2182**)

17. Beta antagonists, such as timolol, are administered as a topical ophthalmic medicine to treat glaucoma. Systemic effects that have been attributed to the topical ophthalmic application of beta antagonists include bradycardia, hypotension, congestive heart failure, and exacerbation of asthma and myasthenia gravis. (332; **2182**)

18. The anticholinesterase echothiophate is sometimes administered as a topical ophthalmic medicine to treat glaucoma. A systemic side effect of this medicine is the prolongation of the effects of succinylcholine and mivacurium through its reduction in plasma cholinesterase activity. The duration of action of this side effect of echothiophate is 4 to 6 weeks. (332; **2182**)

19. Phenylephrine is administered as a topical ophthalmic medicine to produce capillary decongestion and mydriasis. Systemic effects that have been attributed to the topical ophthalmic application of phenylephrine include hypertension, arrhythmias, headache, tremulousness, and myocardial ischemia. (332; **2182**)

20. Cyclopentolate is administered as a topical ophthalmic medicine to produce mydriasis. Central nervous system toxicity has been attributed to the topical ophthalmic application of this drug, manifesting as disorientation, dysarthria, and seizures. (332; **2182**)

21. Epinephrine is administered as a topical ophthalmic medicine to produce mydriasis. Systemic effects that have been attributed to the topical ophthalmic application of epinephrine include tachyarrhythmias, premature ventricular contractions, angina, and nervousness. (332; **2182**)

22. Carbonic anhydrase inhibitors, such as acetazolamide, are administered as topical ophthalmic medicines to decrease intraocular pressure in patients with glaucoma. A systemic effect attributed to the chronic topical ophthalmic application of acetazolamide is the renal loss of bicarbonate ions and potassium, which has in turn led to metabolic acidosis and hypokalemia. (332)

23. The oculocardiac reflex is a cardiac reflex that can occur in response to pressure on the eyeball, traction on the extraocular muscles, an orbital hematoma, or ocular trauma. The medial rectus muscle is the extraocular muscle most likely to elicit this reflex. The reflex is mediated by a trigeminal reflex arc that typically results in bradycardia. A nodal rhythm, ectopic beats, and asystole have also occurred through this reflex. (332; **2175, 2181**)

24. The cardiac rhythms most likely to result from the oculocardiac reflex are bradycardia and a junctional ventricular rhythm. (332; **2175, 2181**)

25. Hypercarbia and arterial hypoxemia both increase the incidence and severity of the oculocardiac reflex. (332; **2181**)

26. The first line of treatment for the oculocardiac reflex is removal of the surgical stimulus, which is usually sufficient treatment. Other measures that may be taken if the reflex persists include the administration of atropine and the local injection of lidocaine into the eye muscle. (333; **2175, 2181**)

27. Pediatric patients undergoing strabismus surgery may benefit from the prophylactic use of atropine secondary to their propensity to have hyperreactive vagal reflexes. (333; **2181**)

28. Goals for the anesthetic management of patients undergoing ophthalmic surgery include control of the intraocular pressure, akinesia of the eye, avoidance and management of the oculocardiac reflex, awareness of potential drug interactions, and a smooth awakening from anesthesia without coughing, nausea, or vomiting. (333; **2174**)

29. Intubation of the trachea is sometimes necessary for patients undergoing ophthalmic surgery for two reasons. One is to allow for positive pressure ventilation of the lungs because neuromuscular blockade may be instituted to ensure patient immobility during a procedure in which the globe will be opened. The second is to secure the airway, which will be draped and inaccessible to the anesthesiologist during the surgery secondary to the proximity of the sterile surgical field to the airway. (333; **2173, 2178–2179**)

30. A potential problem during ophthalmic surgery in which the globe is opened is the extrusion of ocular contents, resulting in increases in ocular pressure and the subsequent loss of vision. (333; **2173, 2179**)

31. Retrobulbar blocks have proven to be extremely safe in elderly patients undergoing ophthalmic procedures. (333; **1543, 2175**)

32. Retrobulbar blocks produce akinesia and local anesthesia to the globe. Akinesia of the eyelids can be achieved with local anesthetic infiltration of the branches of the facial nerve that supply the orbicularis muscle if necessary. (333; **1543, 2175**)

33. Complications of a retrobulbar block include ocular hemorrhage, the oculocardiac reflex, local anesthetic intravascular injection resulting in local anesthetic toxicity, and local anesthetic direct spread into the central nervous system via the cerebrospinal fluid, resulting in unconsciousness and apnea. (333; **1543, 2175–2176**)

34. Patient comfort during the performance of a retrobulbar block can be optimized through the administration of a sedating drug just before the administration of

the block. Among the sedating medicines that have been used include thiopental, propofol, opioids, and benzodiazepines. (333; **2174**)

35. Increases in intraocular pressure during the induction of general anesthesia in patients undergoing ophthalmic procedures can be minimized by administering sufficient drug to produce an adequate depth of anesthesia. In addition, nondepolarizing neuromuscular blocking drugs should be administered before intubation of the trachea and their effect confirmed with a peripheral nerve stimulator in patients who have an open globe in whom coughing may lead to irreversible damage. A short duration of direct laryngoscopy in conjunction with the administration of intravenous lidocaine further serves to prevent increases in intraocular pressure associated with intubation of the trachea. (333; **2178–2179**)

36. Increases in intraocular pressure during the emergence from general anesthesia can be minimized by administering lidocaine intravenously before extubation of the trachea to minimize bucking in response to endotracheal intubation. Alternatively, in appropriate patients the endotracheal tube may be removed while the patient is still deeply anesthetized. (333; **2179**)

37. Neuromuscular blocking drugs are often administered intraoperatively to patients undergoing ophthalmic procedures under general anesthesia to minimize the risk of increases in intraocular pressure and irreversible damage to the patient's vision that could occur if the patient were to move during surgery. (333; **2179**)

38. The reversal of nondepolarizing neuromuscular blocking drugs with an anticholinesterase drug and an anticholinergic drug has minimal effect on intraocular pressure. (333; **2177**)

39. Antiemetics are often administered to patients prophylactically at the conclusion of general anesthesia for ophthalmic surgery to minimize the risk of nausea and vomiting. There is an increased incidence of nausea and vomiting after ophthalmic surgery. The sudden increases in intraocular pressure that are associated with nausea and vomiting can be detrimental to the surgical repair. (334; **2179**)

40. Anesthetic considerations specific to children undergoing strabismus surgery include debate over the practice of administering succinylcholine, the increased incidence of the oculocardiac reflex, the increased incidence of postoperative nausea and vomiting, and the possible susceptibility to malignant hyperthermia. (334; **2179–2181**)

41. Concerns regarding the use of succinylcholine in children scheduled to undergo strabismus surgery are based on the potential for succinylcholine to cause sustained contractions of the extraocular muscles, thereby interfering with the forced duction test for up to 20 to 30 minutes after its administration. In addition, children with strabismus may have a generalized skeletal muscle disturbance. This is reflected in the increased incidence of malignant hyperthermia in children undergoing strabismus surgery. Therefore, the routine administration of succinylcholine to these patients is debatable. (334; **2180**)

42. Anesthetic considerations specific to patients with glaucoma undergoing surgery include the maintenance of drug-induced miosis throughout the perioperative period, avoidance of venous congestion that may worsen glaucoma, and awareness of potential adverse interactions between anesthetic drugs and those used to treat glaucoma. (334; **998**)

43. The administration of topical ophthalmic medicines used to treat glaucoma should be continued throughout the perioperative period. (334)

44. The administration of anticholinergic drugs either alone as premedicants or in combination with anticholinesterase drugs for the reversal of neuromuscular

blockade in patients with glaucoma is associated with very little risk. Although theoretically hazardous, the amount of drug that actually reaches the eye is so little that the mydriatic effect that may be associated with these drugs does not occur. (334; **2177**)

45. There is no known risk associated with the transient increase in intraocular pressure seen with succinylcholine when it is administered to patients with glaucoma. (334)

46. Patients with glaucoma have an increased risk of retinal artery thrombosis associated with prolonged intraoperative hypotension. (334)

47. Considerations for the anesthetic management specific to patients undergoing surgery for cataract extraction include the likely presence of co-existing disease in these typically elderly patients, the need for immobility during the procedure, and the desire to minimize the occurrence of postoperative nausea and vomiting. (334; **2173**)

48. The administration of succinylcholine to facilitate intubation of the trachea in patients undergoing cataract surgery under general anesthesia is well accepted because the globe is not open and the increase in intraocular pressure does not provide any risk of damage. By the time of the surgical incision the effects of succinylcholine on intraocular pressure have subsided. (334)

49. Considerations for the anesthetic management of patients undergoing surgery to repair a retinal detachment include required reduction of the intraocular pressure intraoperatively, the potential for the oculocardiac reflex to be elicited, and the avoidance of nitrous oxide when the surgeon plans to do an intravitreal injection of sulfur hexafluoride and air. (335; **2178**)

50. Intravenous medicines that can be used intraoperatively to decrease the intraocular pressure in patients undergoing surgery to repair a retinal detachment include acetazolamide and mannitol, both of which act by interfering with the secretion of aqueous humor. (335; **2177**)

51. Nitrous oxide must be avoided as a maintenance anesthetic for patients undergoing surgery to repair a retinal detachment when the surgeon plans to do an intravitreal injection of sulfur hexafluoride and air. The bubble is injected by the surgeons with the intent of providing a long-acting bubble to hold the retina in place. The risk associated with nitrous oxide under these conditions is one of expansion of the intravitreal bubble with the diffusion of nitrous oxide into the bubble. Within 19 minutes the bubble can increase to three times its original size, and the intraocular pressure can increase to 30 mm Hg. Discontinuing nitrous oxide will cause the bubble to decrease to its original size in the same amount of time. These fluctuations in intraocular pressure can adversely affect the surgical outcome. To minimize this risk of nitrous oxide its administration should be discontinued at least 20 minutes before the injection of the bubble. (335; **2178**)

52. Considerations for the anesthetic management of patients undergoing emergent surgery for the repair of an open eye injury include the possibility of recent food ingestion and the need to secure the airway rapidly, coupled with the need to avoid any increases in intraocular pressure. (335; **2178–2179**)

53. One option for intubation of the trachea of patients who have had recent food ingestion and have an open globe is a standard rapid sequence induction including the administration of succinylcholine. If this method of intubation of the trachea is selected, pretreatment with a nondepolarizing neuromuscular blocking drug and adequate induction doses of thiopental to offset the potential increase in intraocular pressure from succinylcholine should be given. With this method of administering the medicines, no reports of adverse outcomes have

been reported. An alternative to this is using large doses of a nondepolarizing neuromuscular blocking drug such as rapacuronium or rocuronium. (335; **2178–2179**)

54. The most common ocular complication associated with general anesthesia is a corneal abrasion. (335; **2182**)

55. Corneal abrasions that occur in patients who have undergone a surgical procedure under general anesthesia are usually in the inferior one third portion of the cornea. This is the area that is exposed when the eyes are not mechanically closed. (335)

56. Patients who are undergoing a surgical procedure under general anesthesia are at risk for a corneal abrasion for two reasons. First, there is a loss of protective eye closure when the patient is anesthetized. Second, general anesthesia causes a reduction in tear production. (335; **2182**)

57. The risk of corneal abrasions in patients undergoing a surgical procedure under general anesthesia can be minimized by gentle mechanical closure of the eyelids and maintaining the eyelids in the closed position with the application of adhesive strips. Potential problems with the routine use of ophthalmic ointment include occasional allergic reactions, potential flammability, and blurred vision in the early postoperative period, which can lead to patient anxiety and disorientation. (335; **2182**)

58. A corneal abrasion should be suspected in any patient who postoperatively complains of a sensation of a foreign body in the eye, tearing, conjunctivitis, photophobia, and pain. The pain associated with corneal abrasions worsens with blinking. Diagnosis of a corneal abrasion is achieved by examination of the eye with fluorescein. (335; **2182**)

59. Corneal abrasions are treated by placing a prophylactic antibiotic in the eye and patching the eye. Corneal abrasions typically heal in 48 hours. (335; **2182**)

60. Loss of vision can result from retinal ischemia occurring in the perioperative period. (336; **1484**)

61. Causes of retinal ischemia in the perioperative period include positioning in which there is external compression on the eye and hypotension. The two combined increase the risk of retinal ischemia even further. Other causes of perioperative retinal ischemia include an improperly fitting anesthetic face mask, embolism during cardiac surgery, or the combination of sulfur hexafluoride and nitrous oxide leading to increases in intraocular pressure. (336; **1484**)

62. The risk of retinal ischemia in the perioperative period can be minimized through anesthesiologist awareness of the patient positions in which the eye may be externally compressed. For instance, when the patient is in the prone position the anesthesiologist should perform routine checks of the eyes to ensure there is no compression of the eyes. In addition, minimizing excessive hypotension, especially in hypertensive patients, and the avoidance of nitrous oxide administration with sulfur hexafluoride would minimize the risk as well. (336; **1484**)

OTOLARYNGOLOGY

63. Considerations for the anesthetic management of patients undergoing surgery on the ear include preservation of the facial nerve, the surgical use of epinephrine, and the effect of nitrous oxide on middle ear pressure. (336; **2193–2194**)

64. Surgery on the ear can result in facial nerve paralysis. Surgeons often seek to identify the facial nerve intraoperatively by electrically stimulating the tissues believed to be the nerve and monitoring for a response. This requires that the

patient have minimal effects of neuromuscular blocking drugs intraoperatively during these procedures. Often, no neuromuscular blocking drug is administered at all so as not to confound the results, although maintenance of only about 20% of the baseline ulnar nerve twitch height by a peripheral nerve stimulator is probably sufficient for facial nerve identification. (336; **2193**)

65. The administration of nitrous oxide as maintenance anesthesia to patients undergoing surgery on the middle ear can result in an increase in middle ear pressure through the diffusion of nitrous oxide into the middle ear. Under normal circumstances this increase in air pressure would be easily vented through the eustachian tube. Under surgical conditions, however, there may be narrowing of the eustachian tube by acute inflammation or in the presence of scar tissue preventing the air to be vented. Complications that have been attributed to this increase in middle ear pressure include tympanic membrane rupture and disruption of previous middle ear reconstructive surgery. These potential complications lead many anesthesiologists to avoid the administration of nitrous oxide during middle ear surgery. (337; **2193–2194**)

66. The increase in middle ear pressure that may result from the administration of nitrous oxide as maintenance anesthesia to patients undergoing a tympanoplasty has been implicated as causing displacement of the tympanic membrane graft. If nitrous oxide is initially administered during a tympanoplasty it should be discontinued about 15 minutes before the placement of the graft. (337; **2193–2194**)

67. The rapid absorption of nitrous oxide on its discontinuation in patients with abnormal eustachian tube function may lead to negative middle ear pressures. The negative pressure in the middle ear has been implicated in the development of serous otitis, disarticulation of the stapes, and impaired hearing. (337; **2193–2194**)

68. Considerations for the anesthetic management of patients undergoing nasal and sinus surgery include the intraoperative application of topical cocaine for vasoconstriction, use of a posterior pharyngeal pack, the possibility of large intraoperative blood losses, and the need for extubation of the trachea only on the return of protective airway reflexes. (337)

69. The systemic absorption of cocaine after topical administration can result in tachycardia, hypertension, restlessness, and myocardial ischemia. Rarely, systemic absorption has resulted in ventricular fibrillation and cardiac arrest. (337; **2192–2193**)

70. Maintenance anesthesia in patients undergoing nasal and sinus surgery can be achieved through the use of a volatile anesthetic in combination with nitrous oxide and/or opioids. The administration of a volatile anesthetic may facilitate better control of blood pressure, thus optimizing surgical conditions. (337)

71. Although the nasal sinuses are air-filled cavities, there is no risk associated with the administration of nitrous oxide for maintenance anesthesia to patients undergoing nasal and sinus surgery. There has been no evidence to show that there is a dangerous increase in air pressure in these spaces. (337)

72. Considerations for the anesthetic management of patients undergoing airway endoscopy include the possibility of a co-existing airway abnormality, management of an upper airway that is shared with the surgeon, the need to minimize oral secretions, the need for the suppression of coughing and laryngeal reflexes, the need for a relaxed mandible, protection of teeth with a dental guard, and the need for rapid awakening with the return of protective upper airway reflexes. (337; **2188**)

73. Intubation of the trachea of patients undergoing laryngoscopy by an otolaryn-

gologist should be performed with an endotracheal tube that is small. For an adult patient an endotracheal tube with a 5- to 6-mm internal diameter may be chosen. The smaller endotracheal tube allows the surgeon to be able to visualize the vocal cords and surrounding tissues while still maintaining control of the airway during the administration of neuromuscular blocking drugs. (337; **2185–2186**)

74. Neuromuscular blockade in patients undergoing laryngoscopy can be achieved through the use of a succinylcholine drip. This allows for sufficient neuromuscular blockade to prevent vocal cord movement for these short surgical procedures. Short-acting nondepolarizing neuromuscular blocking drugs may be used as well. (337; **2185–2186**)

75. Laser is an acronym for light amplification by stimulated emission of radiation. It produces an intense, focused light beam that allows for precisely controlled coagulation, incision, or vaporization of tissues. Advantages to the use of lasers for surgical procedures include their ability to access confined or difficult-to-reach sites and a small target area that allows for minimal resultant edema, rapid healing, and minimal damage to surrounding tissues. (337–338; **2186–2187, 2203–2204, Fig. 64–5**)

76. Hazards that are associated with laser surgery include atmospheric contamination by smoke and fine particles from vaporized tissues, misdirected laser energy, venous gas embolism, ocular injury to the cornea or retina, and endotracheal tube fire during airway surgery. (338; **2186–2187, 2204–2205, Figs. 64–6, 64–7, 64–9**)

77. Smoke evacuators that are used during laser surgery at the surgical site are intended to evacuate smoke and fine particles that are vaporized by the laser and that could potentially be inhaled by the personnel in the operating room. (338; **2186–2187, 2204–2205**)

78. Potential hazards of misdirected laser energy during laser surgery include perforation of a viscus or large blood vessel, ocular injury, and endotracheal tube fire. (338; **2186–2187, 2205**)

79. Misdirected energy from a carbon dioxide laser during surgery can result in eye injury for both the personnel in the room and the patient. The patient's lids should be taped closed, and all people in the room including the patient should wear protective eye goggles. (338; **2186–2187, 2205**)

80. Measures that can be taken during laser surgery of the airway to minimize the risk of an endotracheal tube fire include placing a metallic foil wrap around the tube to decrease its potential flammability, using a special endotracheal tube with a laser-resistant coating of aluminum powder in silicone incorporated into the tube, minimizing the delivered concentration of oxygen, and filling the endotracheal tube cuff with saline instead of air. (338; **2187, 2205–2208, Fig. 64–8**)

81. Volatile anesthetics are nonflammable and nonexplosive in the concentrations used in clinical practice. During a fire, however, volatile anesthetics may undergo pyrolysis to potentially toxic compounds. This is the basis for the concern for an endotracheal tube fire that develops during the delivery of volatile anesthetics during laser surgery of the airway. (338; **2206–2207**)

82. In the event of an airway fire during laser surgery of the airway, the anesthesiologist and surgeon should remove the ignition source, discontinue ventilation of the lungs to remove the oxygen source, extubate the trachea and extinguish the removed flaming material in water, ventilate the lungs by mask with 100% oxygen, assess the oropharynx and face, perform rigid bronchoscopy to survey damage and remove potential debris, and obtain a chest radiograph. If there is

any airway damage present during bronchoscopy, the patient's trachea should be re-intubated for airway protection should edema develop. (338; **2187, 2210**)

83. Intubation of the trachea of patients undergoing bronchoscopy should be done with an endotracheal tube that is appropriately sized to allow passage of the bronchoscope and concomitant ventilation of the lungs. Typically, the internal diameter of this tube is 8.0 mm or greater. (338)

84. Patient movement during rigid bronchoscopy can result in a tracheal tear or a pneumothorax. (338)

85. A consideration for the anesthetic management of patients undergoing head and neck surgery is the potential compromise of the native airway by tumor. This may necessitate the placement of a tracheostomy before initiating the procedure. Other considerations include the potential elicitation of vagal responses while working near the carotid sinus, the possibility for a venous air embolism, and the potential for excessive blood loss. (339; **2183–2184**)

86. Intraoperative blood loss can be minimized during head and neck surgery by maintaining the blood pressure in the low-normal range and by placing the patient in a 10- to 15-degree head-up position during the procedure. (339; **2183–2184**)

87. Patients undergoing radical neck dissection on the right side may have cardiac arrhythmias and a prolonged QT interval on the electrocardiogram. This is thought to result from trauma to the right stellate ganglion and cervical autonomic nervous system during the procedure. (339, Fig. 25–2; **2183–2184**)

88. Considerations for the anesthetic management of patients undergoing adenotonsillectomy include the preoperative evaluation of coagulation status, the preoperative determination of the presence of loose teeth, the provision of adequate mandibular and pharyngeal muscle relaxation, the suppression of laryngeal reflexes, and rapid awakening with the return of protective upper airway reflexes. (339; **2187–2188**)

89. The potential for blood loss during an adenotonsillectomy is quite significant. Blood loss estimates are often underestimated during these procedures secondary to blood that drains down into the stomach through the esophagus and is therefore not visible to the anesthesiologist or surgeons. (339; **2188**)

90. During recovery after adenotonsillectomy, patients are often placed in the lateral position with their head lower than their hips. This so-called tonsil position facilitates the drainage of blood out of the stomach and not back onto or through the vocal cords. (339; **2188**)

91. When postoperative bleeding after an adenotonsillectomy is significant to require reoperation, the time course in which the bleeding typically manifests is within 9 hours after surgery. (339; **2188**)

92. Considerations for the anesthetic management of patients who return to surgery because of significant postoperative bleeding after an adenotonsillectomy include the potential for the loss of large volumes of blood; the potential for hypovolemia; and the patient having a stomach full of blood, which necessitates rapid securement of the airway to minimize the risk of the pulmonary aspiration of the gastric contents. (339–340; **2188**)

93. A tracheostomy differs from a cricothyrotomy in that a cricothyrotomy is only a temporizing measure as a lifesaving procedure in which there is acute upper airway obstruction and translaryngeal intubation of the trachea is not possible. A tracheostomy, on the other hand, should be performed electively, usually in

the operating room, under controlled situations for long-term ventilation of the lungs. (340; **2191–2192**)

94. Early complications of a tracheostomy include tube displacement, hemorrhage, and a pneumothorax. (340; **2191–2192**)

Chapter 25

Obstetrics

PHYSIOLOGIC CHANGES IN THE PARTURIENT

1. Are the physiologic changes in pregnancy predictable or not predictable?

2. What are some aspects of the cardiovascular system that undergo physiologic change in the parturient?

3. How does the maternal intravascular fluid volume change? During which trimester does this change take place?

4. By what percent does the plasma volume change in the parturient? By what percent does the erythrocyte volume change?

5. What is the explanation for the relative anemia of pregnancy?

6. What is the coagulation status of the term parturient?

7. What is the average maternal blood loss during the vaginal delivery of a newborn? What is the average maternal blood loss during cesarean section?

8. How does the maternal total plasma protein concentration change during pregnancy?

9. How does the maternal cardiac output change from nonpregnant levels? At what week of gestation does this change take place?

10. Given that cardiac output equals stroke volume times heart rate, how much of the change in cardiac output can be attributed to a change in stroke volume? How much can be attributed to a change in heart rate?

11. How does cardiac output change with the onset of labor? When is the maximal change in cardiac output in the parturient?

12. How does a regional anesthetic affect the cardiac output of the parturient in labor? When might this effect be useful?

13. In what time course post partum does the cardiac output return to prepregnancy values?

14. In an uncomplicated pregnancy, what changes occur in the systolic blood pressure of the parturient?

15. In an uncomplicated pregnancy, what changes occur in the systemic vascular resistance of the parturient?

16. How does the central venous pressure change during pregnancy?

17. What is the supine hypotension syndrome? What symptoms accompany the syndrome? Approximately what percent of pregnant females have this syndrome?

18. What is the mechanism for the supine hypotension syndrome?

19. What compensatory mechanisms do most women have that prevents them from experiencing the supine hypotension syndrome? How are these compensatory mechanisms affected by regional anesthetic techniques?

20. What maternal symptoms result from compression of the aorta by the gravid uterus?

21. What is the major clinical significance of the supine hypotension syndrome? What maternal blood pressure is worrisome?

22. How can the supine hypotension syndrome be minimized?

23. What are some aspects of the pulmonary system that undergo physiologic change in the parturient?

24. Why is the need for gentleness emphasized when instrumenting the upper airway of a parturient? Why might it be prudent to select a smaller cuffed endotracheal tube for intubation of the trachea?

25. Why might insertion of the laryngoscope in the mouth of the parturient be difficult?

26. How is the minute ventilation changed from nonpregnant levels in the parturient? During which trimester does this change take place?

27. Given that minute ventilation equals tidal volume times respiratory rate, how much of the change in minute ventilation in parturients can be attributed to a change in tidal volume? How much can be attributed to a change in respiratory rate?

28. What is presumed to be the stimulus for the change in minute ventilation during pregnancy?

29. How does the resting maternal Pa_{CO_2} change as a result of the change in minute ventilation?

30. How does maternal arterial pH change as a result of the change in minute ventilation?

31. At what time during pregnancy do maternal lung volumes start to change? Why does this occur? What is the percent change in lung volumes? How is vital capacity affected?

32. How does the change in maternal pulmonary physiology affect induction, emergence, and changes in the depth of anesthesia in parturients?

33. How does maternal Pa_{O_2} change early in gestation? How does the Pa_{O_2} change later in gestation?

34. What are two possible explanations for the rapid decrease in Pa_{O_2} during apnea, as in during the induction of general anesthesia, in the parturient? What precautionary measure must be taken before the induction of general anesthesia in the parturient?

35. How is the minimum alveolar concentration (MAC) altered in the pregnant patient? Why is this thought to occur?

36. What is the important clinical consequence of the change in MAC in pregnant women?

37. How does the epidural space change in parturients? How does the change in the epidural space of parturients affect the dosing requirements for epidural anesthesia?

38. How does the subarachnoid space change in parturients? How does the change in the subarachnoid space of parturients affect the dosing requirements for spinal anesthesia?

39. How is the sensitivity to local anesthetics different in the pregnant versus nonpregnant patient?

40. How do renal blood flow and glomerular filtration rate change in pregnancy? At what gestational month of pregnancy is this effect at a maximum? How does this affect the normal upper limits of creatinine and blood urea nitrogen in parturients?

41. How is plasma cholinesterase activity altered by pregnancy? How does this manifest clinically?

42. What are four gastrointestinal changes in pregnancy that render the parturient vulnerable to the regurgitation of gastric contents? What other factors during labor can further retard gastric emptying? What clinical significance does this have?

43. What pharmacologic interventions are recommended in the parturient to help minimize the risk of pulmonary aspiration?

PHYSIOLOGY OF UTEROPLACENTAL CIRCULATION

44. What is the function of the placenta? How is maternal blood delivered to the placenta?

45. What is uterine blood flow at term? How much can uterine blood flow decrease before fetal distress is detected?

46. What are the determinants of uterine blood flow?

47. How does maternal hypotension affect uterine blood flow? How do anesthetics delivered to the mother during labor and delivery affect uterine blood flow? How do epidural and spinal anesthesia affect uterine blood flow?

48. How do alpha-adrenergic agonists affect uterine blood flow? How do endogenous catecholamines affect uterine blood flow?

49. How does ephedrine affect uterine blood flow?

50. How do uterine contractions affect uterine blood flow?

51. How does the placental exchange of substances occur? What are some factors that affect this exchange? What is the most reliable way to minimize fetal transfer of a drug?

52. Why is maternal protein binding of local anesthetics important? At typical clinical concentrations, what percent of lidocaine is bound to protein? What percent of bupivacaine?

53. How does the molecular weight of nondepolarizing neuromuscular blocking drugs affect their ability to transfer across the placenta? Does succinylcholine cross the placenta?

54. Do barbiturates cross the placenta? Do opioids cross the placenta?

FETAL UPTAKE AND DISTRIBUTION OF DRUGS

55. What pH of drug is facilitated in crossing the placenta?

56. What is ion trapping? What is the potential clinical consequence of this with respect to lidocaine administration to the mother?

57. How well do the neonatal enzyme systems metabolize most drugs? Which local anesthetic is a possible exception to this?

58. What are two ways in which the fetal circulation is protective against the distribution of large doses of drugs to vital organs?

MATERNAL MEDICATION DURING LABOR

59. What types of medications may be administered systemically to the mother during labor and delivery to help decrease pain and anxiety? What influences the degree of fetal depression that may result?

PROGRESS OF LABOR

60. What defines the beginning of the first stage of labor? What phases is this stage divided into?

61. What is the approximate duration of the first stage of labor in the typical primigravida? In the multigravida?

62. What defines the beginning of the second stage of labor?

63. What defines the beginning of the third stage of labor?

64. How predictable is the progress of labor? What factors may influence the progress of labor?

65. What is the most common cause of prolongation of the latent phase of labor?

66. What are the most common causes of prolongation of the active phase of labor?

67. How do volatile anesthetics affect uterine activity?

REGIONAL ANESTHESIA FOR LABOR AND DELIVERY

68. What are two advantages of regional analgesia over general analgesia for labor and delivery?

69. What regional anesthetic techniques are effective during the first stage of labor?

70. What regional anesthetic techniques are effective during the second stage of labor?

71. What type of pain predominates during the first stage of labor? What is the cause of the pain? What spinal cord level is involved in the transmission of pain impulses during the first stage of labor?

72. What type of pain predominates during the second stage of labor? What is the cause of the pain? What spinal cord level is involved in the transmission of pain impulses during the second stage of labor?

73. What are some advantages of lumbar epidural analgesia for labor and delivery?

74. How does lumbar epidural analgesia during labor and delivery influence the risk of the parturient undergoing a subsequent cesarean section for delivery of the newborn?

75. How does lumbar epidural analgesia during labor and delivery influence the duration of the first stage of labor?

76. How does lumbar epidural analgesia during labor and delivery influence the duration of the second stage of labor?

77. What are some variables related to epidural analgesia that may influence its effects on the progress of labor?

78. When is the institution of lumbar epidural analgesia for labor and delivery appropriate?

79. What are some issues related to the epidural test dose that are unique to labor and delivery? When should an epidural test dose be administered?

80. How might the epidural catheter be initially dosed to relieve the pain associated with the first stage of labor?

81. What is the advantage of the addition of low doses of an opioid to the local anesthetic to be administered for epidural analgesia?

82. What is a "walking epidural"?

83. How long should the parturient be observed after the initial administration of local anesthetic for lumbar epidural analgesia?

84. How should hypotension in the parturient after the administration of epidural analgesia be managed?

85. Where is local anesthetic injected to achieve a caudal analgesic block?

86. What is the advantage of caudal analgesia when compared with lumbar epidural analgesia?

87. What are some disadvantages of caudal analgesia in the parturient?

88. What are some potential indications for a spinal anesthetic during labor and delivery?

89. How is a saddle anesthetic block for labor and delivery achieved?

90. What is a disadvantage of a saddle anesthetic block?

91. How is the combined spinal and epidural technique for analgesia for labor and delivery usually performed? When might the combined spinal and epidural technique for analgesia be useful for labor and delivery?

92. What are some advantages of the combined spinal and epidural technique for analgesia for labor and delivery?

93. What are some disadvantages of the combined spinal and epidural technique for analgesia for labor and delivery?

94. When is the pudendal block done by obstetricians useful? What are the advantages of this type of block?

95. Where is local anesthetic injected to achieve a paracervical block? For which stage of labor is this block effective?

96. What is the major disadvantage of a paracervical block? In which patients should this block be avoided?

INHALATION ANALGESIA FOR VAGINAL DELIVERY

97. What is the goal of inhalation analgesia for the parturient during labor and delivery?

98. What are the risks of inhalation analgesia for the parturient? What effect can it have on the fetus?

99. How should inhaled anesthetics be administered for analgesia for labor and delivery? What inhaled anesthetics may be used?

GENERAL ANESTHESIA FOR VAGINAL DELIVERY

100. What situation may result in the need for general anesthesia for vaginal delivery?

ANESTHESIA FOR CESAREAN SECTION

101. What are some indications for cesarean section?

102. What is the incidence of backache in the parturient after the administration of a spinal anesthetic?

103. How frequently does venous air embolism occur in patients undergoing cesarean section?

104. What are some benefits of regional anesthesia over general anesthesia for cesarean section?

105. What are some advantages and disadvantages of spinal anesthesia for cesarean section?

106. What dermatome level of spinal anesthesia ensures patient comfort adequate for cesarean section? How can this be achieved?

107. What are the potential benefits of the addition of an opioid to the local anesthetic when administering a spinal anesthetic for cesarean section?

108. What is the likelihood of maternal hypotension after the administration of a spinal anesthetic for cesarean section? How should it be managed?

109. What is the most common neurologic dysfunction seen in the parturient in the postpartum period? How does it present?

110. What are some advantages and disadvantages of epidural anesthesia for cesarean section?

111. What local anesthetics and at what doses can they be administered to achieve an adequate dermatomal level of epidural anesthesia for cesarean section?

112. What is the advantage of the administration of morphine into the epidural space for cesarean section? What are some of the negative side effects that may accompany this route of administration of morphine to the parturient?

113. What are some indications for general anesthesia for cesarean section?

114. What are some benefits of general anesthesia for cesarean section?

115. What are some preoperative medicines that may be administered to the parturient before the induction of general anesthesia?

116. How is the induction of general anesthesia for the parturient accomplished?

117. What is the level of exposure of the fetal brain to thiopental after the administration of induction doses of thiopental to the parturient?

118. How should difficulty with endotracheal intubation be managed by the anesthesiologist?

119. What are some of the considerations for the anesthetic maintenance of the parturient undergoing cesarean section? How might maintenance anesthesia be achieved?

120. What is an effect of mechanical hyperventilation in the parturient?

121. Why is the time from uterine incision to delivery of the newborn important? At what approximate time delay between uterine incision and delivery of the newborn do Apgar scores become decreased?

122. When should the cuffed endotracheal tube be removed from the mother's trachea?

ABNORMAL PRESENTATIONS AND MULTIPLE BIRTHS

123. What is the most common fetal presentation?

124. What fetal presentations are considered abnormal?

125. When does the fetus assume the occiput anterior position?

126. What are the disadvantages to the mother when the fetus presents in the persistent occiput posterior position? What implications does this have with regard to regional anesthesia for the parturient?

127. What maternal morbidities are associated with breech deliveries of the newborn?

128. What neonatal morbidities are associated with breech deliveries of the newborn?

129. When breech presentations are delivered by elective cesarean section, what type of anesthetic may be chosen?

130. What difficulties may the obstetrician encounter when delivering the breech neonate through a uterine incision? How can this be managed?

131. When breech presentations are delivered vaginally, what type of anesthetic may be chosen?

132. What difficulties may the obstetrician encounter when delivering the breech neonate vaginally? How can this be managed?

133. What factors should be considered when choosing an anesthetic for the delivery of multiple gestation fetuses?

PREGNANCY AND HEART DISEASE

134. For the parturient with preexisting heart disease, what is the general concern with regard to labor and delivery?

135. Does the type of heart disease a parturient has mandate a specific type of anesthetic?

136. What advantages does a continuous lumbar epidural anesthesia have for the parturient with preexisting heart disease?

137. What advantages does general anesthesia have over regional anesthesia in the parturient with heart disease?

PREGNANCY-ASSOCIATED HYPERTENSION

138. What is pregnancy-associated hypertension? How frequently does it occur?

139. What is the cause of preeclampsia?

140. What effects does preeclampsia have on the major organ systems?

141. What are the diagnostic criteria for mild preeclampsia?

142. What are the diagnostic criteria for severe preeclampsia?

143. What are the diagnostic criteria for eclampsia? What percent of parturients with preeclampsia get eclampsia?

144. What is the approximate percent maternal mortality of parturients with eclampsia? What are some causes of maternal mortality from eclampsia?

145. How should eclampsia be managed?

146. What is the definitive treatment for pregnancy-associated hypertension?

147. When do the manifestations of preeclampsia resolve?

148. What are the goals of the pharmacologic management of preeclampsia?

149. What are some of the effects of magnesium on the parturient when administered for pregnancy-associated hypertension? What is the anesthetic implication of this?

150. What is the therapeutic level of magnesium when administered for pregnancy-associated hypertension? How can the levels of magnesium be monitored clinically?

151. What are some signs of increasing magnesium toxicity? What is the antidote for magnesium toxicity?

152. How is magnesium cleared from the body?

153. What antihypertensives are commonly used to treat maternal hypertension?

154. What is the concern regarding the administration of nitroprusside to parturients?

155. Why is it important to continuously monitor fetal heart rate while administering antihypertensives?

156. What is the role of regional anesthesia in parturients with pregnancy-associated hypertension?

157. What is the advantage of continuous lumbar epidural analgesia for the labor and delivery of the preeclamptic parturient?

158. What are some concerns regarding the administration of epidural analgesia for the labor and delivery of the preeclamptic parturient? How should epidural analgesia be administered?

159. What laboratory studies should be obtained before the administration of a regional anesthetic in the preeclamptic parturient?

160. When is cesarean section necessary in the preeclamptic parturient?

161. What is the advantage of general anesthesia in the preeclamptic parturient undergoing cesarean section for fetal distress? What monitors would be useful in these cases?

162. How should general anesthesia be induced in the preeclamptic parturient?

163. What special concerns are there for the preeclamptic parturient undergoing cesarean section with general anesthesia?

HEMORRHAGE IN THE PARTURIENT

164. What are some causes of hemorrhage in the parturient? When do these typically manifest?

165. What is placenta previa? How does it present? How can the diagnosis be confirmed?

166. What are some risk factors for placenta previa?

167. How should examination of the cervical os of a woman suspected of having placenta previa be undertaken?

168. What is abruptio placentae? What are the possible clinical presentations of abruptio placentae?

169. What are some risk factors for abruptio placentae?

170. What is the definitive treatment of abruptio placentae?

171. How should the parturient with abruptio placentae be managed?

172. What are some risk factors for uterine rupture? What percent of patients with uterine rupture have an identifiable risk?

173. What approximate percent of vaginal deliveries are associated with some amount of retained placenta? What is the treatment?

174. What are some options for the anesthetic management of patients with retained placenta?

175. What is uterine atony? When does it present?

176. What are some risk factors for uterine atony?

177. How should uterine atony be managed?

178. What is the risk of the rapid administration of synthetic oxytocin? How can this risk be avoided?

179. Why is it important that the synthetically made oxytocin drugs do not contain vasopressin?

AMNIOTIC FLUID EMBOLISM

180. What is the clinical presentation of an amniotic fluid embolism? What are some conditions that may mimic amniotic fluid embolism and must therefore be ruled out?

181. What patients are most at risk for an amniotic fluid embolism?

182. How is the definitive diagnosis of an amniotic fluid embolism made?

183. What is the treatment of an amniotic fluid embolism?

ANESTHESIA FOR NONOBSTETRIC SURGERY DURING PREGNANCY

184. What are some anesthetic goals specific to the pregnant patient undergoing nonobstetric surgery?

185. What is the critical gestational period for organogenesis? Why is this important?

186. Are anesthetics teratogenic?

187. What inhaled anesthetic is cautiously administered to parturients during the first trimester?

188. How can intrauterine fetal hypoxia and acidosis be prevented?

189. What is retrolental fibroplasia? Is retrolental fibroplasia at risk of developing in the fetus in utero?

190. What is the definition of premature labor in the parturient?

191. What is the usual etiology of premature labor that presents in the parturient after having undergone nonobstetric surgery? What monitors should be used in these circumstances?

192. How can premature labor be treated?

193. When should elective nonobstetric surgery be performed in the parturient?

194. What is the preferred trimester for surgery to take place when surgery in the parturient is not elective? What type of anesthetic is preferred if possible?

195. After what gestational age is fetal heart rate monitoring intraoperatively helpful?

SUBSTANCE ABUSE

196. How might cocaine and/or heroin abuse affect the outcome of the newborn?

197. What is the preferred method of anesthesia during labor and delivery in the parturient who has been known to abuse drugs?

DIAGNOSIS AND MANAGEMENT OF FETAL DISTRESS

198. How is fetal well-being best evaluated?

199. How are fetal electrocardiograms obtained?

200. What is the normal fetal heart rate?

201. What is the normal fetal heart rate variability per minute?

202. What types of fetal distress may be reflected as a decrease in the fetal heart rate beat-to-beat variability?

203. What types of drugs often administered by an anesthesiologist may result in a decrease in the fetal heart rate beat-to-beat variability? What is the clinical implication of this?

204. What are early decelerations in fetal heart rate? What are they thought to be due to?

205. What are late decelerations in fetal heart rate? What are they thought to be due to? What further diagnostic intervention can be made in this circumstance?

206. What are variable decelerations in fetal heart rate? What are they thought to be due to?

EVALUATION OF THE NEONATE AND NEONATAL RESUSCITATION

207. What is the value of the Apgar score? What is its use?

208. Complete the following table indicating the five characteristics of the newborn for each Apgar score:

CHARACTERISTIC	SCORE = ZERO	SCORE = ONE	SCORE = TWO

209. What type of intervention is usually sufficient for infants with an Apgar score of 8 to 10?

210. What type of neonatal injury is most likely to be associated with Apgar scores between 5 and 7? What type of intervention is usually necessary for these infants? When should ventilation of the newborn's lungs be instituted under these circumstances?

211. How does the newborn with Apgar scores between 3 and 6 appear? What intervention may be necessary for this newborn?

212. What type of neonatal injury is most likely to be associated with Apgar scores between 0 and 2? What type of intervention is usually necessary for these infants?

213. At what rate should the lungs of a neonate be ventilated? How should the adequacy of ventilation be evaluated?

214. What is the peak airway pressure that should be delivered to a neonate during ventilation of the lungs?

215. At what heart rate should external cardiac compression be instituted in the neonate?

216. What is the appropriate dose of epinephrine for the severely hypotensive and bradycardic neonate?

217. Why should glucose administration be considered in the neonate with Apgar scores less than 2?

218. What is the risk of meconium-stained amniotic fluid for the neonate? How should it be managed?

219. What is the advantage to having an umbilical artery catheter? Describe the procedure for cannulation of the artery.

220. Which newborns are at risk of being hypovolemic at birth?

221. What is the appearance of a hypovolemic newborn? How should these newborns be managed?

NEUROBEHAVIORAL TESTING

222. What is neurobehavioral testing useful for? What does it test specifically?

223. What have studies evaluating neurobehavioral scores of neonates exposed to local anesthetics shown when compared with neonates not exposed to local anesthetics?

224. What have studies evaluating neurobehavioral scores of neonates exposed to general anesthesia shown when compared with neonates not exposed to general anesthesia?

POSTPARTUM TUBAL LIGATION

225. What sensory dermatomal level must be achieved for patient comfort during a postpartum tubal ligation under regional anesthesia?

226. Why is it common to wait 8 to 12 hours post partum before performing a tubal ligation?

ANSWERS*

PHYSIOLOGIC CHANGES IN THE PARTURIENT

1. The physiologic changes seen in pregnancy are predictable. By knowing these, the anesthesiologist is better able to care for the pregnant patient. In general, the changes the parturient undergoes in the cardiovascular system are teleologically advantageous for two reasons. First, the needs of the developing fetus are provided for. Second, the mother is better equipped to handle the stresses she will face during labor and delivery. (341)

2. Aspects of the cardiovascular system that undergo physiologic change in the parturient include the intravascular fluid volume, the constituents of the intravascular fluid volume, the cardiac output, and the peripheral circulation. (341, Table 26–1; **2025–2027, Table 57–3**)

3. The maternal intravascular fluid volume increases from its prepregnancy volume. The increase in intravascular volume begins in the first trimester of pregnancy. By term the total increase in intravascular fluid volume is approximately 1000 mL. (341; **2025–2027, Fig. 57–5**)

4. Plasma volume in the parturient patient increases by approximately 45%. The erythrocyte volume in the parturient patient increases by approximately 20%. (341; **2026, Fig. 57–5**)

---

*Numbers in parentheses: lightface numbers refer to pages, figures, or tables in Stoelting RK, Miller RD: Basics of Anesthesia, 4th ed. Philadelphia, Churchill Livingstone, 2000; **boldface numbers** refer to pages, figures, or tables in Miller RD: Anesthesia, 5th ed. Philadelphia, Churchill Livingstone, 2000.

5. Because the plasma volume increases by over twice as much as the erythro-cyte volume, the parturient has a relative physiologic anemia. That is, the hematocrit of the parturient patient is relatively less than her prepregnancy state. This is termed the *physiologic anemia of pregnancy*. (341; **2026, Fig. 57–5**)

6. The term parturient is in a hypercoagulable state secondary to increases in factors VII, VIII, X, and plasma fibrinogen. (**2029**)

7. The average maternal blood loss during the vaginal delivery of a newborn is 400 to 600 mL. The average maternal blood loss during the delivery of a newborn by cesarean section is 1000 mL, but blood loss during a cesarean section is greatly variable. The increase in intravascular fluid volume and the hypercoagulable state of the mother help to counter the blood losses incurred during this time. (341; **2029**)

8. The maternal total plasma protein concentration decreases during pregnancy. This is secondary to a dilutional effect of the increased intravascular fluid volume. (341; **2029**)

9. The maternal cardiac output during pregnancy increases by approximately 40% of its prepregnancy value. This increase has taken place by the tenth week of gestation. (341; **2025–2026**)

10. The cardiac output, which increases by about 40% in pregnancy, is equal to stroke volume times heart rate. The 40% increase in cardiac output is primarily due to an increase in stroke volume. The increase in heart rate during pregnancy is minimal and is therefore only a minimal contributor to the increase in cardiac output. The augmentation and maintenance of cardiac output in the pregnant patient is believed to be due to circulating placental and ovarian steroids released during pregnancy. (341; **2025–2026, Figs. 57–3, 57–4**)

11. With the onset of labor, cardiac output increases to approximately 45% above prelabor values. The cardiac output increases further just after delivery, to about 60% above prelabor values. This is the maximal change in cardiac output in the parturient. (341–342; **2027**)

12. Regional anesthesia may attenuate the increase in cardiac output normally seen in the laboring parturient. This effect may be useful in parturients during the peripartum period who have a compromised cardiovascular system. (342)

13. Cardiac output returns to prepregnancy values by about 2 weeks post partum. (342)

14. The systolic blood pressure of the parturient having an uncomplicated pregnancy does not exceed her prepregnancy blood pressure. (342; **2025**)

15. The systolic blood pressure does not increase during pregnancy and usually stays about the same as prepregnancy values in an uncomplicated pregnancy. Cardiac output, however, increases by approximately 40%. Given that, the systemic vascular resistance must decrease to maintain an equal systolic blood pressure. Systemic vascular resistance does decrease, by approximately 20%. (342; **2025**)

16. Central venous pressure does not change during pregnancy. In the presence of increased intravascular fluid volume, the lack of change of central venous pressure presumably reflects a decrease in the resistance of the systemic and pulmonary vasculature. (342)

17. The supine hypotension syndrome, as the name implies, is the decrease in blood pressure seen in the parturient when she lies in the supine position at or near term. Symptoms that accompany the hypotension include diaphoresis,

nausea, vomiting, and possible changes in cerebration. This syndrome occurs in approximately 10% of pregnant women. Symptoms must be present for the patient to considered susceptible to the supine hypotension syndrome. (342; **2026–2029, Figs. 57–3, 57–6, 57–7, 57–8**)

18. The supine hypotension syndrome occurs because of a decrease in cardiac output. When the term or near-term parturient lies in the supine position, the gravid uterus compresses the inferior vena cava, resulting in decreased venous return. The decreased venous return to the heart leads to a decreased preload for the heart. The cardiac output subsequently decreases. (342, Fig. 26–1; **2027, Fig. 57–7**)

19. Most pregnant women, when lying in the supine position, are able to compensate for the possible decrease in blood pressure that results from the compression of the inferior vena cava by the gravid uterus. One compensatory mechanism includes maintaining venous return by diverting blood flow from the inferior vena cava to the paravertebral venous plexus. The blood then goes to the azygos vein and returns to the heart via the superior vena cava. Another compensatory mechanism is an increase in peripheral sympathetic nervous system activity. This increases peripheral vascular tone and helps to maintain venous return to the heart. Because of these compensatory mechanisms only about 10% of pregnant women at or near term suffer from the supine hypotension syndrome. Regional anesthesia, however, can interfere with these compensatory mechanisms by causing sympathetic nervous system blockade, rendering the pregnant woman at term more susceptible to decreases in blood pressure. (342; **2027–2028**)

20. Compression of the aorta by the gravid uterus does not typically lead to any symptoms in the pregnant woman. The blood pressure in the lower extremities may decrease, whereas the blood pressure measured from the upper extremities remains unchanged. (342; **2027**)

21. The major clinical significance of the supine hypotension syndrome is the decrease in placental and uterine blood flow that results. The decrease in blood flow through the uteroplacental unit leads to a decrease in blood flow to the fetus. Indeed, progressive fetal distress and bradycardia may result from decreases in systolic blood pressure to below 100 mm Hg for longer than 10 to 15 minutes. (342–343; **2027–2028**)

22. The supine hypotension syndrome can be minimized by having the parturient lie in the lateral position. Uterine displacement can also be used, typically with displacement being to the left because the inferior vena cava sits just to the right of and anterior to the spine. Left uterine displacement is easily accomplished by the placement of a foam rubber wedge or folded blanket under the right hip, elevating the hip by 10 to 15 cm. (343, Fig. 26–2; **2029**)

23. Aspects of the pulmonary system that undergo physiologic change in the parturient include the upper airway, minute ventilation, lung volumes, and arterial oxygenation. (343, Table 26–2; **2024–2025, Table 57–1**)

24. Instrumentation of the upper airway of the parturient, whether by laryngoscope, nasal airway, oral airway, or suctioning, must be done gently. Capillary engorgement of the mucosal layer of the upper airways in these patients makes them susceptible to trauma and bleeding. In addition, because the vocal cords and arytenoids are often edematous, smaller-sized cuffed endotracheal tubes may be a better selection for intubation of the trachea for these patients. Endotracheal tubes with internal diameters of 6.5 to 7.0 mm may be appropriate. (343; **2025**)

25. Insertion of the laryngoscope into the parturient's mouth may be made

physically difficult because of a short neck and large breasts. (343; **2049–2053**)

26. The minute ventilation of the parturient increases to about 50% above prepregnancy levels. This change occurs in the first trimester of pregnancy and remains elevated for the duration of the pregnancy. (343; **2024**)

27. Minute ventilation is a factor of tidal volume and respiratory rate. Minute ventilation increases in the parturient by about 50%. An increase in tidal volume is the main contributor to the increase in minute ventilation seen. The respiratory rate of the parturient does not change significantly from the prepregnancy rate. (343; **2024**)

28. The stimulus for the change in minute ventilation that is observed during pregnancy is thought to be the increased levels of progesterone circulating in the mother's blood. (343)

29. During the first trimester, as a result of the increase in minute ventilation, the resting maternal Pa_{CO_2} decreases from 40 mm Hg to about 30 mm Hg. (343; **2024**)

30. As a result of the change in minute ventilation, the maternal Pa_{CO_2} decreases to about 30 mm Hg. A respiratory alkalosis is not seen in the parturient, however, because of increased renal excretion of bicarbonate ions. This allows for maintenance of a normal arterial pH in the parturient. (343; **2024, Fig. 57–1**)

31. Maternal lung volumes start to change in the fifth month of pregnancy. This is a result of mechanical compression by the gravid uterus as it enlarges and forces the diaphragm cephalad. This leads to a decrease in the parturient's functional residual capacity by approximately 20% at term. There is no significant change in vital capacity seen in the parturient. (343; **2024**)

32. The rates of induction of anesthesia, emergence from anesthesia, and changes in depth of anesthesia are influenced by the pulmonary physiologic changes in the parturient during pregnancy. The rate of each is increased secondary to the increase in minute ventilation and decrease in functional residual capacity. (343; **2025**)

33. Maternal Pa_{O_2} changes during the progression from early gestation to term. Early in gestation the Pa_{O_2} in the mother is slightly increased over prepregnancy values to over 100 mm Hg breathing room air. This is secondary to maternal hyperventilation during this time. As the pregnancy progresses the Pa_{O_2} is normal or even slightly decreased. The decrease in Pa_{O_2} during the course of pregnancy results from airway closure. (344; **2024–2025**)

34. Apnea in the parturient rapidly leads to arterial hypoxemia. There are at least two explanations for this. First, a decreased functional residual capacity and subsequent decreased oxygen reserve are contributors. Second, aortocaval compression and decreased venous return leading to decreases in cardiac output may also contribute. The decrease in cardiac output would lead to an increase in oxygen extraction and therefore decrease the level of oxygenation of blood returning to the heart. Because of the rapid decrease in maternal Pa_{O_2} with apnea or hypoventilation, supplemental oxygen should be administered to the parturient during a regional anesthetic. In addition, before the induction of general anesthesia preoxygenation with 100% O_2 for 3 minutes or for eight deep breaths over 60 seconds is recommended. (344; **2032**)

35. The minimum alveolar concentration (MAC) is decreased in the parturient. This is thought to be due at least in part to the sedative effects of progesterone. (358; **2037–2038, Table 61–4**)

36. The important clinical consequence of the change in MAC in the pregnant woman is that concentrations of inhaled anesthetics that would not produce unconsciousness in a woman before pregnancy may be sufficient to do so during pregnancy. The change in MAC is compounded by the increased rate of induction of anesthesia with inhaled agents secondary to a decreased functional residual capacity. These together can quickly lead to dangers to the ability of the parturient to protect her airway and render her subject to the consequences of pulmonary aspiration. (344; **2030**)

37. The epidural space of parturients is decreased from its prepregnancy state. This occurs because of both the engorgement of epidural veins and the increased intra-abdominal pressure resulting from the progressive enlargement of the uterus. The decrease in the epidural space decreases the required volume of local anesthetic necessary to achieve a particular level of anesthesia by facilitating its spread in the epidural space. The decrease in the dose of local anesthetic required is estimated to be 30% to 50%. (344; **2030**)

38. The subarachnoid space of parturients is decreased from its prepregnancy state. Just as the epidural space decreases as a result of the progressive enlargement of the uterus increasing intra-abdominal pressure, so does the subarachnoid space decrease. The decreased space facilitates the spread of local anesthetic and decreases the dose required by 30% to 50% from prepregnancy values. (344; **504–505, 2030**)

39. There appears to be an increased sensitivity to local anesthetics by women who are pregnant. The decreased local anesthetic requirement in parturients appears to have a biochemical component to it as well as a mechanical one. (344; **504–505, 2030**)

40. Renal blood flow and glomerular filtration rate in the parturient are both increased. By the fourth month of pregnancy the increase is 40%. This results in a decrease in what is considered the normal upper limit of both the blood urea nitrogen and serum creatinine concentrations in parturients to about 50% of what it was in the prepregnancy state. (344; **2030**)

41. Plasma cholinesterase, or pseudocholinesterase, decreases in activity by about 25% during pregnancy. This decrease in activity is first noted by about the tenth week of gestation and persists for as long as 6 weeks post partum. There is no clinical manifestation of this change in plasma cholinesterase activity. There is unlikely to be a significant change in the duration of action of succinylcholine or mivacurium, for instance. (344; **2029**)

42. There are at least four gastrointestinal changes in pregnancy that render the parturient vulnerable to the regurgitation of gastric contents. Two of these result from the enlarged uterus, which acts to displace the pylorus upward and backward from its usual position. First, this retards gastric emptying. Second, it also leads to a change in the angle of gastroesophageal junction, leading to relative incompetence of the physiologic gastroesophageal sphincter. Gastroesophageal reflux and subsequent esophagitis are common in parturients. A third cause is from circulating progesterone, which decreases gastrointestinal motility. Gastric fluid volume tends to be increased as a result, even in the fasting state. Finally, gastrin secreted by the placenta stimulates gastric hydrogen ion secretion. The pH of the parturient's gastric fluid is predictably low as a result. During labor, anxiety, pain, and the administration of opioids can further decrease gastric emptying. Clinically, this means that the parturient must always be treated as if she has a full stomach. In one study in which ultrasound was used to evaluate gastric emptying in parturients, solid food was found in the stomachs of 41% of parturients whose last ingestion of solids was 8 to 24 hours previously. Regardless of what amount of time has

elapsed since her last ingestion of solids, she is at increased risk of regurgitation and aspiration of gastric contents. (344–345; **2029**)

43. Pharmacologic interventions that are recommended in the parturient to help minimize the risks of pulmonary aspiration are aimed at decreasing the severity of acid pneumonitis should aspiration occur. The administration of antacids to the parturients before the induction of anesthesia is common practice. This is as an attempt to increase the pH of gastric contents. Sodium citrate is the antacid commonly used. A single administration is recommended, because repeated doses of antacid have not been proven to provide any additional benefit. Of note, the antacid must be nonparticulate, because aspiration of particulate matter contained in some antacids is in itself a hazard. Histamine-2 receptor antagonists can increase the pH of gastric fluid. They do not increase the pH of gastric contents already present, unlike antacids. Some reports indicate that combining histamine-2 receptor antagonists with antacids may work better than antacids alone in maintaining the increase in pH of gastric contents. Metoclopramide may also be useful in decreasing the gastric fluid volume in parturients, although it is usually reserved for those patients who are considered to be at high risk for increased gastric fluid volumes. When opioids have caused hypomobility of the stomach, metoclopramide may not be as effective. (344–345; **2029, 2221–2222**)

PHYSIOLOGY OF UTEROPLACENTAL CIRCULATION

44. The function of the placenta is to unite maternal and fetal circulations. The union allows for the physiologic exchange of nutrients and waste. Maternal blood is delivered to the placenta by the uterine arteries. Fetal blood is delivered to the placenta by the two umbilical arteries. The two most important determinants of placental function are uterine blood flow and the characteristics of the substances to be exchanged across the placenta. (345; **2031–2032**)

45. Uterine blood flow at term is 500 to 700 mL/min. Uterine blood flow must be maintained to ensure placental circulation is adequate and therefore guarantee fetal well-being. In a normal placenta, uterine blood flow can decrease by about 50% before fetal distress, diagnosed by the presence of fetal acidosis, is detected. (345; **2030, Fig. 57–10**)

46. Uterine blood flow is not autoregulated. Uterine blood flow is proportional to the mean blood pressure of the blood supplying the uterus and inversely proportional to the resistance of the uterine vasculature. Drugs that alter either of these, such as drugs that decrease systemic blood pressure, affect uterine blood flow. (345; **2030**)

47. Maternal hypotension, of any cause, results in a decrease in uterine blood flow. Uterine blood flow is decreased by a decrease in the perfusion pressure of blood supplying the uterus. Anesthetics delivered to the parturient during labor and delivery that decrease maternal blood pressure could decrease uterine blood flow. Epidural and spinal anesthesia do not, in and of themselves, decrease uterine blood flow in the absence of maternal hypotension. (345; **2030–2031, 2043**)

48. Alpha-adrenergic agonists, such as phenylephrine, increase uterine vascular resistance and therefore decrease uterine blood flow. Endogenous catecholamines, as with maternal pain or anxiety, also increase uterine vascular resistance and decrease uterine blood flow. (345, Figs. 26–3, 26–4; **2030–2031, Fig. 57–9**)

49. Ephedrine administration does not result in any change in uterine blood flow. Ephedrine is therefore useful for increasing blood pressure when the parturient is hypotensive. (345, Fig. 26–3; **2031, Fig. 57–9**)

50. Uterine contractions increase uterine venous pressure, thereby decreasing uterine blood flow. (345)

51. Diffusion from the maternal circulation to the fetal circulation and vice versa is the primary way in which the placental exchange of substances occurs. Some factors that affect the exchange of substances from the maternal circulation to the fetus include the concentration gradient of the substance across the placenta, maternal protein binding, molecular weight, lipid solubility, and degree of ionization of the substance. The most reliable way to minimize the amount of drug that reaches the fetus is by minimizing the concentration of the drug in the maternal blood. (345–346, Table 26–3; **2031–2032**)

52. Protein binding of local anesthetics in the parturient is important because only the free form, or unbound portion, of the drug is available for diffusion across the placenta to the fetus. At typical clinical concentrations, lidocaine is 50% to 70% protein bound. This compares with bupivacaine, which is 95% protein bound. This means that at typical clinical concentrations the decreased bound fraction of lidocaine results in more local anesthetic being available to diffuse across the placenta. (346; **2032**)

53. Nondepolarizing neuromuscular blocking drugs, such as vecuronium, have a high molecular weight and low lipid solubility. These two characteristics together limit the ability of nondepolarizing neuromuscular blocking drugs to cross the placenta. Succinylcholine is highly ionized, preventing it from diffusing across the placenta despite its low molecular weight. (346; **2032, 2052**)

54. Barbiturates and opioids both readily diffuse across the placenta, owing to their relatively low molecular weights. (346; **308–309, 2032, 2051–2052**)

FETAL UPTAKE AND DISTRIBUTION OF DRUGS

55. Fetal blood is slightly more acidic than maternal blood, with a pH about 0.1 unit less than maternal blood pH. The lower pH of fetal blood facilitates the fetal uptake of drugs that are basic. (347; **2032**)

56. Weakly basic drugs, such as local anesthetics and opioids, that cross the placenta in the nonionized state become ionized in the fetal circulation. This results in an accumulated concentration of drug in the fetus for two reasons. First, once the drug becomes ionized it cannot readily diffuse back across the placenta. This is known as *ion trapping*. Second, a concentration gradient of nonionized drug is maintained between the mother and the fetus. In the case of lidocaine administration, this may mean that if the fetus was distressed and acidotic and lidocaine was given in sufficient doses to the parturient, lidocaine may accumulate in the fetus. (347, Fig. 26–5; **2032**)

57. Neonatal enzyme activity is decreased in comparison to the enzyme activity of an adult. Despite the decreased activity, however, neonatal enzyme systems are sufficiently developed for the metabolism of most drugs delivered to the mother. A possible exception to this is mepivacaine. (347; **2032**)

58. There are two ways in which the fetal circulation inherently provides some protection to vital organs against large doses of drugs. First, about 75% of the blood that is coming to the fetus via the umbilical vein passes through the liver. This allows for a significant amount of metabolism of the drug to

take place before going to the fetal arterial circulation and delivery to the heart and brain. Second, blood with drug in it from the umbilical vein enters the inferior vena cava via the ductus venosus. This blood is diluted by drug-free blood returning from the lower extremities and pelvic viscera of the fetus, resulting in a decrease in the concentration of the drug that is in the inferior vena cava. (347; **2032–2033, 2051, Fig. 57–11**)

MATERNAL MEDICATION DURING LABOR

59. Systemic medications that are most often administered to the parturient to help decrease pain and anxiety during labor include opioids, benzodiazepines, and ketamine. Although different drugs will produce varied levels of depression in the fetus, the administration of any systemic medication to a parturient will result in the transfer of drug to the fetus to some extent. Other factors that influence the degree of fetal depression include the dose of the drug administered, the route of administration, and the time of administration before delivery. (347–348; **308–309, 2041–2044**)

PROGRESS OF LABOR

60. The *progress of labor* is a term used to describe the progression of increasing cervical dilation, effacement, and descent of the fetus in the birth canal with time. The onset of the first stage of labor is defined by the onset of regular contractions. The first stage of labor is divided into the latent and active phases of labor. The woman enters her active phase of the first stage of labor at 3- to 4-cm dilation of the cervix. (348, Fig. 26–6; **2033, Fig. 57–12**)

61. The first stage of labor in the typical primigravida lasts 7 to 13 hours. In the multigravida the first stage of labor lasts 4 to 5 hours. (348; **2033, Table 57–5**)

62. The second stage of labor begins with complete dilation of the cervix. (348; **2033**)

63. The third stage of labor begins with delivery of the newborn and ends with delivery of the placenta. (348; **2033**)

64. The progress of labor is not very well predicted. Factors that may influence the progress of labor include maternal pain, parity, size and presentation of the fetus, and drugs and techniques that were used to provide the mother with analgesia during her labor and delivery. (348; **2033–2034, Table 57–5**)

65. The most common cause for prolongation of the latent stage of labor is excessive sedation or early initiation of a regional anesthetic. (348; **2033–2034**)

66. The most common causes for prolongation of the active stage of labor are cephalopelvic disproportion, fetal malposition, and fetal malpresentation. (348; **2033–2034**)

67. Volatile anesthetics decrease uterine activity in a dose-dependent fashion. This is most useful clinically when rapid uterine relaxation is required, as in a tetanic contraction. In higher doses during a cesarean section it may also contribute uterine atony and unwanted bleeding after delivery of the fetus. (348–349; **2046, 2052**)

REGIONAL ANESTHESIA FOR LABOR AND DELIVERY

68. Two advantages of regional anesthesia over general anesthesia for labor and vaginal delivery include decreased risk of pulmonary aspiration in the parturient and a decreased likelihood of fetal drug depression. (349; **2046**)

69. Regional anesthetic techniques that are effective during the first stage of labor include paracervical blocks, lumbar epidural analgesia, and caudal analgesia. (349, Table 26–4; **2037–2038, 2042, 2045–2046**)

70. Regional anesthetic techniques that are effective during the second stage of labor include lumbar epidural analgesia, caudal analgesia, spinal analgesia, and pudendal nerve blocks. (349, Table 26–4; **2037–2038, 2042, 2046**)

71. During the first stage of labor the pain experienced by the parturient is primarily visceral in origin. The pain results from contractions of the uterus and dilation of the cervix. During this stage of labor visceral pain impulses from the uterus and cervix enter the spinal cord at a T10–L1 level for transmission to the cortex. (349, Fig. 26–7; **2034**)

72. During the second stage of labor the pain experienced by the parturient is primarily somatic. The pain results from stretching of the vagina and perineum by the descending fetus. During the second stage of labor the somatic pain impulses originating from the vagina and perineum enter the spinal cord at a S2–S4 level via the pudendal nerves for transmission to the cortex. (349–350, Fig. 26–7; **2039**)

73. There are several advantages of using a well-placed epidural catheter for continuous lumbar epidural analgesia during labor and delivery. First, the ability to maintain a segmental band of analgesia during the first stage of labor is easily achieved. The analgesic band can be extended to the sacral roots during the second stage of labor. Second, minimal local anesthetic doses are required to maintain analgesia, and the doses can increase as the parturient's labor progresses and her pain increases. Third, pelvic muscle tone is easily maintained, which facilitates rotation of the fetal head in utero. Finally, it provides a means for surgical anesthesia should it become necessary. (350; **2037–2038**)

74. In multiple studies, lumbar epidural analgesia during labor and delivery does not appear to influence the risk of the parturient undergoing a subsequent cesarean section for delivery of the newborn. This has been shown to be true even when epidural analgesia is administered in the early latent phase of the first stage of labor, when cervical dilation is 2 to 4 cm. What appears to have a greater influence on the risk of subsequent cesarean section is the obstetrician's practice style. This issue remains controversial, however, because other studies have not corroborated these results. (350; **2034**)

75. Lumbar epidural analgesia during labor and delivery does not typically cause any prolongation of the active stage of labor provided hypotension is avoided. (348, 350; **2033–2034**)

76. Lumbar epidural analgesia during labor and delivery may decrease the reflexive urge to bear down that women experience in the second stage of labor. Because of this, prolongation of the second stage of labor by 20 to 40 minutes may result from the administration of epidural analgesia. (348, 350; **2033–2034**)

77. There are several variables under the control of the anesthesiologist that may influence the effects of epidural analgesia on the progress of labor. These include the timing of the administration of epidural analgesia, the extent of analgesia, the choice of local anesthetic, the addition of other additives such as an opioid or epinephrine to the local anesthetic solution, and the avoidance of or prompt treatment of maternal hypotension. Many of these variables influence the degree of subsequent motor blockade. The local anesthetics most often chosen for lumbar epidural analgesia are bupivacaine and ropivacaine. The advantage these two local anesthetics have over other local anesthetics is that they tend to preferentially block sensory nerve fibers over

motor nerve fibers, thus being more likely to provide adequate analgesia while still maintaining motor tone. An advantage of ropivacaine compared with bupivacaine is its decreased potential for cardiotoxicity. (350; **2040**)

78. The appropriate time for the institution of lumbar epidural analgesia for labor and delivery should be judged on an individual basis. However, it is usually instituted with the establishment of the active phase of the first stage of labor. This would be confirmed with dilation of the cervix by about 5 cm in a primigravida or 4 cm in a multigravida woman. (350; **2033–2034**)

79. After the placement of an epidural catheter an epidural test dose should always be administered to confirm the catheter was not placed in an epidural vein or in the intrathecal space. A negative aspiration of the catheter does not ensure that this is the case. The usual test dose is 45 mg of lidocaine with 15 μg of epinephrine. There are some unique issues related to the epidural test dose in labor and delivery, however. First, the elevation in heart rate associated with uterine contractions may falsely mimic the effects of a test dose that is positive for the intravenous administration of epinephrine. Furthermore, because of elevated levels of circulating catecholamines, the laboring parturient may have an attenuated response to the intravascular administration of 15 μg of epinephrine. Epinephrine may also have deleterious effects on uterine blood flow, particularly in preeclamptic patients. Finally, parturients with elevated systemic blood pressures may have an exaggerated response to intravascular epinephrine. In any case, it is prudent to initially dose the epidural catheter with local anesthetic in fractionated doses in the event the catheter is misplaced. (350; **2038**)

80. During the first stage of labor the epidural catheter can be dosed with a dilute local anesthetic solution sufficient to provide a T10–L1 segmental band of analgesia. This can usually be accomplished with 5 to 10 mL of 0.125% bupivacaine. (350; **2039–2040**)

81. The onset of analgesia for the laboring parturient may be accelerated by the addition of low doses of an opioid to the local anesthetic being administered for epidural analgesia. In addition to accelerating the onset of analgesia, the addition of an opioid to the local anesthetic appears to provide a more complete analgesic block. The addition of an opioid to a low-dose continuous infusion of local anesthetic for epidural analgesia provides the added benefit of not only a more complete analgesic block but also of increased analgesia while preserving skeletal muscle tone. The opioids typically administered are fentanyl and sufentanil. As an initial bolus, the doses are fentanyl, 50 to 100 μg, and sufentanil, 5 to 10 μg. For administration as a continuous infusion the doses are fentanyl, 1 to 2 μg/mL, or sufentanil, 0.1 to 0.3 μg/mL. (350; **2038–2041**)

82. A *walking epidural* is a term used to describe the analgesia that results when a very dilute local anesthetic, usually with an opioid, is administered for labor and delivery. The local anesthetic solution, while providing analgesia, has minimal effects on sympathetic or motor nerves. This allows the parturient to ambulate after tests for motor blockade indicate that she is not at risk of falling. Even so, the parturient should be closely monitored and ideally should only ambulate when accompanied because proprioception and balance may be impaired. (350; **2040–2041**)

83. After the initial bolus administration of local anesthetic in the epidural space, the parturient must be carefully monitored by the anesthesiologist for the following 10 to 20 minutes. This also holds true after any additional boluses are administered via the epidural catheter on subsequent occasions. The purpose of the vigilant monitoring is to have prompt recognition and treatment of maternal hypotension. The risk of maternal hypotension after the adminis-

tration of epidural analgesia can be decreased by the prophylactic administration of 500 to 1000 mL of intravenous crystalloid. (350; **2041**)

84. When maternal hypotension follows dosing of an epidural catheter in the parturient, several measures can be taken to re-institute the blood pressure. First, left uterine displacement must be confirmed. The rapid infusion of intravenous fluids should be started. The parturient should be placed in the Trendelenburg position to increase venous return to the heart, and supplementary oxygen should be administered. If within 1 to 2 minutes conservative measures of treating the hypotension have not resulted in reversal of the hypotension, pharmacologic management of the blood pressure is indicated. Pharmacologic management of hypotension in the parturient is best done with 5 to 10 mg of ephedrine initially, followed by 5 to 10 mg every 1 minute for continued hypotension. Ephedrine's benefit in the parturient population arises from the preservation of uterine blood flow with its administration. Hypotension that should be managed pharmacologically in the parturient is a systolic blood pressure equal to or less than 100 mm Hg, or more than a 20% decrease in the systolic blood pressure. Fetal heart tones should be continuously monitored. After resolution of the hypotension the parturient should be encouraged to remain in a position that allows for uterine displacement to the left or right, as in the lateral position. (350; **2041**)

85. Local anesthetic is injected in the epidural space at the sacral level to achieve a caudal analgesic block. Ten to 12 mL of local anesthetic is typically used for a caudal block. (**2042**)

86. The advantages of caudal analgesia over lumbar epidural analgesia are twofold. First, there is a decreased risk of an accidental dural puncture and subsequent headache. Second, there is better analgesia provided to areas supplied by the sacral spinal roots, such as the perineum. (**2042**)

87. There are several disadvantages of the performance of caudal analgesia for labor and delivery. First, a caudal block is technically difficult to perform because of difficulties in identification of the sacral hiatus in adults and also because it is difficult to keep the sacral area clean for the procedure. Second, more local anesthetic drug is necessary in the earlier stages of labor to provide adequate analgesia to the T10 dermatome. This would necessarily result in greater blockade of the fibers of the sacrum; and if pelvic tone is not retained, spontaneous rotation of the fetal head may be impaired. A further disadvantage is the potential complication of the accidental injection of local anesthetic into the fetal head. Finally, should cesarean section become necessary a caudal anesthetic does not provide a sufficient level of anesthesia. (**2042**)

88. Potential indications for a spinal anesthetic block for labor and delivery include the need for vacuum-assisted or forceps-assisted vaginal delivery, and for the repair of perineal lacerations after delivery. A spinal anesthetic block may be administered to a laboring patient when pain is inadequately controlled and delivery is expected to occur reasonably soon. In all these cases the sacral roots are primarily targeted for analgesia. (351; **2043**)

89. A saddle anesthetic block is achieved by a subarachnoid injection of small doses of a dilute, hyperbaric local anesthetic, such as 5 to 6 mg of bupivacaine, with the parturient in a seated upright position. The parturient should remain seated upright for 1 to 2 minutes after injection to ensure that the sacral roots are well anesthetized, thus resulting in a saddle area distribution of anesthesia. After the administration of a true saddle block the parturient has good relief from pain conducted from the perineal area via the sacral roots. Unfortunately, the pain of uterine contractions persists. The saddle block can be modified to help alleviate the pain associated with uterine

contractions by increasing the injected dose of local anesthetic to 7 to 8 mg of dilute, hyperbaric bupivacaine intrathecally and having the parturient remain seated upright for only 30 seconds. This modification of the saddle block increases the level of anesthetic to approximately a T10 level to provide analgesia for uterine contractions. (351; **2043**)

90. A disadvantage of a saddle anesthetic block is the potential for postspinal headache that follows dural puncture. Fortunately, the risk of headache decreases with the newly designed, smaller-gauged pencil-point Sprotte, Whitacre, and Gerdie Marx spinal needles. (351)

91. The combined spinal and epidural technique for analgesia for labor and delivery is performed by first locating the epidural space as one would for epidural catheter placement. Once the epidural space has been located, a spinal needle can be passed through the epidural needle to locate the intrathecal space. On location of the intrathecal space, the spinal anesthetic solution can be deposited, the spinal needle removed, and an epidural catheter threaded through the epidural needle and secured in the epidural space. The spinal anesthetic solution may be opioid alone, local anesthetic alone, or a combination of both. This technique may be useful to provide for analgesia in the early stages of labor or during precipitous, rapidly progressing labor. (351; **2043**)

92. Advantages of the combined spinal and epidural technique for analgesia for labor and delivery include more rapid onset and more reliable analgesia. For rapidly progressing labor the pain associated with labor may be rapidly controlled to allow for the threading of the epidural catheter and the slower onset of epidural analgesia. (351; **2043**)

93. Disadvantages of the combined spinal and epidural technique for analgesia for labor and delivery include its relatively greater invasiveness and the associated risks of infection and trauma, the risk of a postdural puncture headache, and the greater difficulty associated with the added steps required for the spinal portion of the block. (351; **2043**)

94. Pudendal nerve block is useful when perineal analgesia is needed for delivery, as with an episiotomy or low forceps delivery. The pudendal nerve block needs supplementation for a mid-forceps delivery. The obstetrician typically performs this block, which is done transvaginally with the parturient in the lithotomy position. The advantages of a pudendal block are that the urge to bear down is preserved, it is not associated with sympathetic nervous system blockade of the periphery, and labor is not prolonged. (351; **2046**)

95. For achievement of a paracervical block, local anesthetic must be injected in the vagina, lateral to the cervix and into the fornix bilaterally. Sensory fibers that come from the uterus, cervix, and upper vagina travel through this area. Therefore, this block is most effective to help provide analgesia during the first stage of labor and is usually not effective for the second stage of labor. (**2045–2046, Fig. 57–21**)

96. The major disadvantage of a paracervical block is potential fetal bradycardia. In 8% to 40% of parturients who receive this block fetal bradycardia develops 2 to 10 minutes after the local anesthetic solution is injected. It is believed that the bradycardia results from decreased uterine blood flow secondary to uterine vasoconstriction. This may occur because the injection of local anesthetic in a paracervical block is very close to the uterine arteries, and absorption into the uterine arteries may take place. An additional cause of the bradycardia may be a bolus dose of local anesthetic to the fetal heart, causing direct cardiac toxicity. Although the definitive cause of the bradycardia is not known, it is often associated with fetal acidosis. A paracervical

block is best avoided in patients with known uteroplacental insufficiency or fetal distress. (**2045–2046, Fig. 57–21**)

INHALATION ANALGESIA FOR VAGINAL DELIVERY

97. The goal of inhalation analgesia during labor and delivery is to provide some analgesia and comfort to the parturient during the first and second stages of labor. (351; **2037**)

98. Aspiration is the main risk for the parturient receiving inhalation analgesia. This is especially true given the parturient's decreased functional residual capacity and decreased minimum alveolar concentration (MAC). The patient must be awake with intact laryngeal reflexes maintained for her airway protection. Inhaled anesthetics readily cross the placenta. The effects on the neonate, however, are minimal when the inhaled anesthetic is being administered at a concentration of 0.3 to 0.4 MAC for analgesic purposes. (351; **2037**)

99. The inhaled anesthetic that is most often used for analgesia in the parturient is nitrous oxide in concentrations of 30% to 50%. It is usually administered in a blend with oxygen. The other inhaled anesthetics are rarely used for this purpose. The inhalation of nitrous oxide for analgesia during labor and delivery should only be self-administered or administered by an anesthesiologist. The anesthesiologist should remain in verbal contact with the patient to ensure that the level of consciousness and the protective airway reflexes are maintained. Optimal results from the administration of nitrous oxide for the parturient are obtained by having the parturient inhale the nitrous oxide between contractions, so that an effective concentration of nitrous oxide is achieved for the uterine contraction. About 50 seconds of continuous breathing of the nitrous oxide are necessary before the concentration is optimal. (351–352; **2037**)

GENERAL ANESTHESIA FOR VAGINAL DELIVERY

100. General anesthesia may be necessary for vaginal delivery when the immediate delivery of a fetus in distress prohibits the time necessary to administer a regional anesthetic or if regional anesthesia is contraindicated. In addition, high levels of volatile anesthetic in conjunction with intravenous nitroglycerin can be used for profound uterine relaxation, as might be needed for complete breech extraction, the manual retrieval of retained placenta, or for the replacement of an inverted uterus. General anesthesia should be administered with precautions taken to minimize the risk of the aspiration of gastric contents. Once uterine relaxation becomes unnecessary, the dose of volatile agent should be decreased to decrease bleeding due to uterine atony. Oxytocin may also be administered intravenously to facilitate uterine contraction. (352; **2046**)

ANESTHESIA FOR CESAREAN SECTION

101. Some indications for cesarean section include fetal distress, cephalopelvic disproportion, malpresentation, and failure of the progression of labor. A cesarean section may also be indicated if the parturient had a previous cesarean section with a uterine incision other than a lower segment transverse uterine incision or if the current fetus is not in the vertex position. (352; **2049**)

102. Backache frequently accompanies pregnancy, labor, and delivery. The incidence of backache does not increase after regional anesthesia. (352)

103. Venous air embolism is estimated to occur in 20% to 50% of patients undergoing cesarean section. In most cases a venous air embolus is not of a magnitude to produce clinical symptoms. The incidence of venous air emboli during cesarean section can be decreased by keeping the patient in a head-up position of approximately 5 degrees or more during the procedure. (352)

104. Benefits of regional anesthesia over general anesthesia for cesarean section include avoidance of the risks of general anesthesia, including a decreased risk of pulmonary aspiration, decreased fetal depression from anesthetic agents, and the maintenance of maternal awareness. No differences in neonatal outcome after cesarean section with regional anesthesia or general anesthesia have been shown. (352; **2046**)

105. Advantages of spinal anesthesia for cesarean section include its technical ease of administration, the low levels of systemic medicines that potentially reach the fetus, its low failure rate, and its rapid onset time. Disadvantages of spinal anesthesia for cesarean section include the finite time of anesthesia provided, its higher incidence of hypotension, and the risk of a postdural puncture headache. (352; **2046–2047**)

106. Spinal anesthesia with a sensory level of T4 is usually sufficient for patient comfort during cesarean section. Exteriorization of the uterus or traction of the abdominal viscera may still lead to discomfort in the parturient. A T4 sensory level can be achieved with the administration of bupivacaine 12 to 15 mg. The parturient's height has been used as a guide to judge the appropriate dose necessary to provide a sufficient dermatome level of spinal anesthesia, although there are conflicting data to show that dermatome level and height are unrelated. (352, Table 26–5; **2047, Fig. 57–22**)

107. The addition of fentanyl or sufentanil to the local anesthetic administered for spinal anesthesia for cesarean section may benefit the patient by providing for a more dense anesthetic block for surgery. The administration of preservative-free morphine to the local anesthetic solution administered for spinal anesthesia provides for postoperative pain relief for approximately 24 hours. The intrathecal dose of preservative-free morphine used for this purpose is 0.1 to 0.25 mg. Epinephrine, 0.2 mg, administered intrathecally may also augment the anesthetic block. (352; **2047, 2330, Tables 57–2, 69–4**)

108. After the administration of a spinal anesthetic for cesarean section there is a significant risk of hypotension, given the peripheral sympathetic nervous system blockade that accompanies a T4 sensory level of spinal anesthesia. The risk of hypotension can be minimized by prehydrating the parturient with 500 to 1000 mL of lactated Ringer's solution before the administration of the spinal anesthetic and placing the parturient in a position of continuous left uterine displacement. Some anesthesiologists may also wish to inject ephedrine, 25 to 50 mg, intramuscularly 15 minutes before administering spinal anesthesia. When the parturient's systolic blood pressure falls to lower than 100 mm Hg or by more than 20% after the administration of spinal anesthesia, 5 to 15 mg of ephedrine should be administered intravenously and repeated as necessary until the blood pressure is restored. Neo-Synephrine may also be administered in 100 μg increments if necessary. (352–353; **2046**)

109. Nerve damage resulting from spinal anesthesia is extremely rare. The most common neurologic dysfunction in the postpartum period results from compression of the lumbosacral trunk between the descending head of the fetus and the sacrum that can occur with prolonged bearing down in the lithotomy position. This nerve injury presents as footdrop combined with a sensory deficit. Recovery from lumbosacral injury may require 12 to 16 weeks. (353; **2044, Fig. 57–19**)

110. Advantages of epidural anesthesia for cesarean section include the ability to extend the duration of anesthesia if necessary, to control block height, to slowly titrate the dose to avoid precipitous maternal hypotension, and the decreased risk of postdural puncture headache. Disadvantages of epidural anesthesia for cesarean section include the potential for intravascular injection of toxic levels of local anesthetic and its technical difficulty, longer onset time, and less reliability. (353; **2047–2048**)

111. An approximate volume of 15 to 20 mL of local anesthetic solution must be delivered in the epidural space to achieve the T4 sensory level of anesthesia necessary for cesarean section. Before the administration of such high volumes of local anesthetics a test dose for epidural catheter placement should be administered. Local anesthetics that can be administered for cesarean section by epidural catheter placement include 2% lidocaine, 0.5% bupivacaine, 0.5% ropivacaine, and 3% 2-chloroprocaine. Each of these should be administered in increments to further minimize the risk of accidental intravenous administration of toxic levels of local anesthetic. The cardiotoxic effects of bupivacaine are minimized by limiting the administered dose of bupivacaine to 0.5%. Ropivacaine is less cardiotoxic than bupivacaine at equipotent doses. For the rapid onset of analgesia with a lumbar epidural catheter, as in an urgent cesarean section, 2-chloroprocaine 3% can be used. The anesthesiologist must be certain that subarachnoid injection of the chloroprocaine has not occurred, because permanent neurologic damage has resulted from some formulations of this local anesthetic when it was injected intrathecally. (353; **2047–2049, Table 57–8**)

112. The administration of preservative-free morphine into the epidural space during cesarean section extends the duration of analgesia by 12 to 24 hours into the postoperative period. The dose of morphine administered is 3 to 5 mg. Some negative effects of morphine that may accompany this route of administration include pruritus, nausea and vomiting, and, on rare occasions, delayed respiratory depression. The risk of respiratory depression in one study of patients receiving 5 mg epidural morphine was 0.1%. Patients recovering from cesarean section may be at a decreased risk for respiratory depression from a single bolus of epidural morphine when compared with other postoperative patients for several reasons. First, a postoperative infusion of epidural morphine is not typically started. Second, progesterone is a respiratory stimulant. Finally, most cesarean section patients are young and healthy. (353; **2048, 2330, Table 57–8, Table 69–5**)

113. Indications for general anesthesia for cesarean section include fetal distress and required emergent delivery to prevent poor fetal outcome, maternal hemorrhage, and contraindications to regional anesthesia such as maternal coagulopathy. (353; **2049**)

114. Benefits of general anesthesia for cesarean section include more rapid onset of anesthesia, less hypotension and hemodynamic instability than regional anesthesia, and control of the airway and ventilation. (353; **2049**)

115. Preoperative medicines that may be administered to the parturient before the induction of anesthesia to decrease the risk of pulmonary aspiration include a nonparticulate antacid, histamine-2 receptor antagonists, and metoclopramide. The intervention most utilized by the anesthesiologist is the administration of a nonparticulate antacid such as sodium citrate. These are useful just before the induction of anesthesia because they increase the pH of the gastric fluid already present in the stomach. Histamine-2 receptor antagonists also increase the gastric fluid pH but require more time to take effect. Metoclopramide facilitates gastric emptying by increasing gastric motility, although its usefulness in the parturient undergoing cesarean section is not proven. A

benzodiazepine can be administered to the parturient before an elective cesarean section if the parturient is particularly apprehensive or anxious. (353; **2049, Table 57–9**)

116. When the parturient is brought to the operating room for cesarean section under general anesthesia she should be positioned with left uterine displacement and placed in an appropriate sniff position. The induction of general anesthesia should be preceded by preoxygenation with a well-fitting face mask for 3 to 5 minutes. Cricoid pressure should be applied before the induction of general anesthesia. The induction of general anesthesia should be rapidly followed by the administration of a neuromuscular blocking drug with rapid onset such as succinylcholine or rapacuronium. Intubation of the trachea with a cuffed endotracheal tube should be confirmed before the release of cricoid pressure. (353–354; **2049, Table 57–9**)

117. The level of exposure of the fetal brain to thiopental after the administration of thiopental to the parturient for the induction of general anesthesia is generally low as long as the dose administered to the parturient is less than 5 mg/kg. There are two reasons for this. First, the drug is partially cleared as it passes through the liver of the fetus before reaching the fetal heart. Second, the blood reaching the fetal heart from the placenta is diluted by the blood from the fetal viscera and lower extremities. (354; **2051, Fig. 61–25**)

118. A major cause of morbidity and mortality for the parturient with regard to general anesthesia is failed or difficult intubation of the trachea. The possibility of difficult endotracheal intubation is higher among parturients than general surgical patients. Contributing factors include inadequate time for preoperative evaluation of the airway, unpredicted airway edema, and emergency situations. If a difficult airway is suspected preoperatively, an awake fiberoptic intubation of the trachea should be considered. The anesthesiologist must have a management plan to follow should he or she be confronted with a difficult or failed intubation. There should be equipment immediately available for the difficult airway, such as a variety of functioning laryngoscope blades, several sizes of endotracheal tubes, laryngeal mask airways, a fiberoptic bronchoscope, and the means to perform a cricothyrotomy. Extra help should be solicited. Multiple attempts at laryngoscopy should be avoided to prevent increasing airway edema and bleeding. If hypoxia should occur during attempted laryngoscopy, the patient should be hand ventilated with bag and mask while cricoid pressure is maintained. Difficulty with mask ventilation may warrant an attempt at ventilation without cricoid pressure, although alternative methods for reversing the patient's arterial hypoxemia should be sought. Options may include allowing the patient to resume spontaneous ventilation, waking the patient and doing an awake fiberoptic intubation of the trachea, or, in dire circumstances of hypoxemia, proceeding to a surgical airway. (354; **2049–2051, Fig. 57–24**)

119. Some considerations for anesthetic maintenance specific to the parturient undergoing cesarean section under general anesthesia include the potential transfer of medicines to the fetus, uterine blood flow before delivery, and uterine tone after delivery. Before delivery, uterine blood flow should be maintained by maintaining maternal blood pressure and minimizing autonomic nervous system responses to surgical stimulation by circulating catecholamines. Agents that may be used for the maintenance of anesthesia in the parturient undergoing cesarean section include 50% inspired nitrous oxide and a low concentration of a volatile anesthetic. The addition of the volatile anesthetic helps to decrease parturient awareness during the procedure. A neuromuscular blocking drug may be administered if necessary. Uterine tone after delivery is maintained when the concentration of volatile anesthetic used is approximately 0.5 minimum alveolar concentration (MAC). When this low

concentration of volatile anesthetic is used for cesarean section, maternal blood loss is minimized, the uterine response to oxytocin is not altered, and little neonatal depression is seen. After delivery the inhaled concentration of nitrous oxide may also be increased, intravenous opioid may be administered, and any other indicated intravenous agents may be administered. (354; **2052**)

120. Mechanical hyperventilation of the parturient under general anesthesia can result in decreases in uterine blood flow through the effects of positive pressure ventilation and also possibly by decreased umbilical blood flow secondary to hypocarbia. Maternal hyperventilation also causes a leftward shift in the oxygen-hemoglobin dissociation curve, decreasing the availability of oxygen to the fetus. (354; **2051**)

121. Impairments in uteroplacental blood flow may result from uterine incision, making the time from uterine incision to delivery of the newborn important in neonatal outcome. When the uterine incision-to-delivery time is more than 180 seconds Apgar scores are often decreased. (354; **2051**)

122. The cuffed endotracheal tube in the mother's trachea should be removed at the conclusion of surgery when it is certain that the laryngeal reflexes of the parturient have returned and she is able to protect her airway. (354)

ABNORMAL PRESENTATIONS AND MULTIPLE BIRTHS

123. The fetal position is described by its head, chin, or sacrum in relation to the parturient's right or left. The most common fetal presentation is in the occiput transverse or occiput anterior position, with approximately 90% of fetuses presenting in this position. (354)

124. Any fetal presentation that is not occiput transverse or occiput anterior is considered an abnormal presentation. (354)

125. The fetus undergoes spontaneous internal rotation to the occiput anterior position during active labor. The fetus remains in a persistent occiput posterior position when spontaneous internal rotation does not occur. (354)

126. When the fetus presents in the persistent occiput posterior position the parturient experiences a prolonged and painful labor. The fetal occiput presses against the posterior sacral nerves resulting in severe back pain. With regard to regional anesthesia, when the fetus is in the persistent occiput posterior position anesthetic techniques that result in relaxation of the maternal perineal muscles may be avoided until the spontaneous internal rotation of the fetal head has occurred. If vaginal delivery is difficult, the obstetrician may elect to rotate the occiput with forceps or forceps-assisted delivery may be necessary. (354)

127. Maternal morbidities associated with breech deliveries of the newborn include cervical lacerations, retained placenta, and hemorrhage. (354)

128. Neonatal morbidities associated with breech deliveries of the newborn include intracranial hemorrhage and prolapse of the umbilical cord. A prolapsed umbilical cord may necessitate emergent delivery of the neonate. (354)

129. When the fetus is in the breech presentation and will be delivered by elective cesarean section, anesthesia may be either general or regional. (354; **2055**)

130. Difficulty in delivering the breech neonate through a uterine incision during regional anesthesia may result from the uterus being insufficiently relaxed. In the acute situation in which there is difficulty delivering the breech neonate through a uterine incision, nitroglycerin may be administered to relax the uterus. Alternatively, general anesthesia may be induced and the trachea

intubated to allow the administration of a volatile anesthetic to relax the uterus. (354; **2055**)

131. For the vaginal delivery of the breech-presenting neonate a continuous lumbar epidural anesthetic may be chosen for anesthesia. A continuous lumbar epidural anesthetic provides for analgesia and relaxation in the perineal area that may be necessary to facilitate the delivery of the breech neonate. (354–355; **2055**)

132. The obstetrician may encounter difficulty in delivering the breech neonate for reasons of either insufficient uterine relaxation or inadequate perineal relaxation. A contraction of the lower uterine segment may also trap the head of the fetus, requiring immediate intervention, although this is rare. In the acute situation in which there is difficulty delivering the breech neonate vaginally, nitroglycerin may be administered or general anesthesia may be induced and the trachea intubated to allow the administration of a volatile anesthetic to relax the uterus. (354; **2055**)

133. Factors that should be considered when choosing an anesthetic for the delivery of multiple gestation fetuses are the frequent occurrence of prematurity, breech presentation, and assisted delivery. The large uterus may make maternal supine hypotension syndrome more likely. Uterine atony is also more likely to occur after delivery. A lumbar epidural catheter is often placed in parturients with multiple gestation to provide flexibility in their management. Because the presentation of the second fetus may change after the delivery of the first, vaginal delivery should take place in a setting where emergent cesarean section can be performed. (355; **2056**)

PREGNANCY AND HEART DISEASE

134. The parturient with preexisting heart disease is at significant risk for congestive heart failure during labor and delivery due to increases in cardiac output. With each contraction of the uterus the central blood volume increases by 10% to 25%. The risk of congestive heart failure increases further after the delivery of the fetus, because compression on the inferior vena cava and aorta is relieved, allowing marked increases in blood volume. Indeed, after delivery of the fetus the autotransfusion that results causes an increase in stroke volume and cardiac output up to 80% of prelabor values. (355)

135. For most types of heart disease there is no single best anesthetic plan. It may be prudent to monitor central venous pressures or pulmonary capillary wedge pressures in some patients to guide fluid and anesthetic management. (355)

136. For the parturient with preexisting heart disease a continuous lumbar epidural anesthetic offers the advantage of decreased pain and anxiety and decreased cardiac output. The decrease in systemic vascular resistance and venous return that may accompany an epidural anesthetic may be deleterious in parturients with aortic stenosis, right-to-left shunts, and pulmonary hypertension. (355)

137. General anesthesia offers advantages over regional anesthesia in the parturient with preexisting heart disease by allowing more control of the blood pressure. This is in contrast to regional anesthesia, in which the sudden decrease in systemic vascular resistance can result in sudden drops in arterial blood pressure. (355)

PREGNANCY-ASSOCIATED HYPERTENSION

138. *Pregnancy-associated hypertension* is a term used to describe a range of disorders that present in pregnancy and have in common the clinical presenta-

tion of hypertension. It includes disorders such as gestational proteinuric hypertension, preeclampsia, and eclampsia. Pregnancy-associated hypertension was formerly known as toxemia of pregnancy. It occurs in 5% to 15% of all pregnancies. Understanding the pathophysiology of pregnancy-associated hypertension is important for the appropriate management of the parturient. (355; **2053**)

139. The exact cause of preeclampsia is still unknown. It is believed that preeclampsia may involve damage to endothelial cells that triggers vasoconstriction, platelet activation, and an imbalance between prostacyclin and thromboxane. The endothelial cell damage also results in a loss of capillary integrity, leading to generalized edema. (355; **2053**)

140. Preeclampsia is a major cause of morbidity and mortality for both the parturient and the neonate. Preeclampsia has the following potential effects on the major organ systems (355; **2061**):

Cardiovascular system: generalized vasoconstriction, increased vascular responsiveness to sympathetic nervous system stimulation, and decreased uteroplacental perfusion

Hepatorenal system: decreased hepatic blood flow, decreased glomerular filtration rate, decreased renal blood flow, and retention of sodium and water

Pulmonary system: interstitial fluid accumulation, decreased PaO_2, exaggerated edema of upper airway and larynx

Central nervous system: hyperreflexia, cerebral edema, and seizure activity

Intravascular fluid volume: hypovolemia

Coagulation: decreased platelet count, increased fibrin split products

Uterus: hyperactive, premature labor

141. Preeclampsia can be diagnosed after the twentieth week of gestation. The criteria that must be met to diagnose mild preeclampsia include hypertension with a blood pressure higher than 140/90 mm Hg, proteinuria of over 0.3 g/day, and generalized edema. (355; **2053, Table 57–10**)

142. The parturient with preeclampsia is said to have severe preeclampsia if she has any one of the following: a blood pressure >160/110 mm Hg, proteinuria >5 g/day, cerebral involvement such as headaches or visual disturbances, oliguria <500 mL/24 hr, an increased serum creatinine level, pulmonary edema, epigastric pain, right upper quadrant pain, or HELLP syndrome, thrombocytopenia, or disseminated intravascular dissemination. The HELLP syndrome is characterized by hemolysis, elevated liver enzymes, and a low platelet count. (355; **2053, Table 57–10**)

143. When a parturient with preeclampsia has a seizure her disease has progressed to eclampsia. The exact mechanism for eclamptic seizures is unknown, but they may occur from vasospasm, hypertensive encephalopathy, or cerebral edema. Approximately 5% of parturients with preeclampsia develop eclampsia. (355; **2054**)

144. The approximate maternal mortality of parturients with eclampsia is 10%. Some causes of maternal mortality from eclampsia include congestive heart failure and cerebral hemorrhage. (356)

145. Eclampsia should be managed supportively by first ensuring adequate oxygenation and circulation. Supplemental oxygen should be applied and the parturient positioned with left uterine displacement. Magnesium can be administered to control the seizures. In the event that seizures persist, oxygenation is

inadequate, or the airway is unprotected, intubation of the trachea may be necessary. Delivery of the fetus may be indicated if the fetus becomes distressed. (356; **2054**)

146. The definitive treatment for pregnancy-associated hypertension is delivery of the fetus and placenta. (356; **2053**)

147. The manifestations of preeclampsia usually resolve within 48 hours of delivery of the fetus. (356; **2053**)

148. The goals of the pharmacologic management of preeclampsia include blood pressure control and seizure prophylaxis. (356; **2054**)

149. The goal of the administration of magnesium in parturients with pregnancy-associated hypertension is to decrease central nervous system irritability, which in turn decreases the likelihood of seizures. Magnesium also relaxes uterine and vascular smooth muscle tone, resulting in increases in uterine blood flow. There are several other effects of magnesium that require understanding by the anesthesiologist for the appropriate management of anesthesia. First, magnesium decreases activity at the neuromuscular junction, possibly by decreasing the presynaptic release of acetylcholine as well as by decreasing postjunctional membrane sensitivity to acetylcholine. Clinically, this can enhance the neuromuscular blockade produced by nondepolarizing neuromuscular blocking drugs. Second, magnesium-induced relaxation of uterine and vascular smooth muscle tone may contribute to uterine atony and increased bleeding after delivery. Third, magnesium can enhance the effects of opioids and sedatives. Finally, magnesium readily crosses the placenta. Neonatal muscle tone may be decreased at birth as a result of magnesium administration to the mother. (356; **2054–2056**)

150. The therapeutic serum level of magnesium when administered for pregnancy-associated hypertension is 4 to 6 mEq/L. Clinical monitoring of the magnesium level can be achieved by evaluating the parturient's deep tendon reflex response. Marked depression of the deep tendon reflexes gives evidence for impending magnesium toxicity. (356; **2054**)

151. When toxic levels of serum magnesium are reached the parturient may experience severe skeletal muscle weakness, hypoventilation, and cardiac arrest. The therapeutic serum level of magnesium is 4 to 6 mEq/L. A prolonged PQ interval and QRS complex widening on the electrocardiogram indicate that serum levels of magnesium are 5.0 to 10 mEq/L. The loss of the parturient's deep tendon reflex response occurs when serum levels are about 10 mEq/L. Sinoatrial and atrioventricular block and respiratory paralysis may become evident when serum magnesium levels reach about 15 mEq/L, and at serum levels of 25 mEq/L cardiac arrest may occur. The antidote for magnesium in the event of magnesium toxicity is the intravenous administration of calcium. (356; **2054–2055, Table 57–11**)

152. Magnesium is cleared by renal excretion. The parturient with pregnancy-associated hypertension who also has renal dysfunction should have her serum magnesium levels closely monitored. (356)

153. Antihypertensive therapy for the parturient with pregnancy-associated hypertension is likely to be initiated when the maternal diastolic blood pressure is more than 110 mm Hg. Antihypertensives that are commonly used to treat pregnancy-associated hypertension include hydralazine and a beta-adrenergic antagonist such as labetalol. Hydralazine is often chosen because of its rapid onset and its preservation of renal blood flow. Labetalol is often chosen because of its ability to block a reflex tachycardia. (356; **2054–2055**)

154. Nitroprusside is generally avoided in parturients because of the concern with

cyanide accumulation in the fetus. Cyanide results from the degradation of nitroprusside, which can cross the placenta and may have detrimental effects on the fetus. (356)

155. The continuous monitoring of fetal heart rate during the administration of antihypertensives gives information about the well-being of the fetus while changes in the maternal blood pressure are being made. The concern is that decreases in maternal blood pressure may result in decreases in the uterine perfusion pressure. The effect on uteroplacental circulation could manifest as changes in fetal heart rate. (356; **2055**)

156. The role of regional anesthesia in parturients with pregnancy-associated hypertension is for pain control and the reduction of sympathetically mediated effects of pain during labor. Regional anesthesia should not be used as an attempt to lower the blood pressure. (356; **2055**)

157. The advantage of continuous lumbar epidural analgesia for labor and delivery for the preeclamptic parturient is the management of pain and anxiety and the associated decreases in circulating catecholamines. This also helps to ensure that increases in the parturient's blood pressure during labor and delivery are minimized. In addition, the fetus of preeclamptic patients is frequently delivered prematurely. Continuous lumbar epidural analgesia precludes the need for parenteral opioids for pain control and the possible effects on the fetus that opioids may have. (356; **2055**)

158. Sympathetic nervous system blockade and maternal hypotension may lead to decreases in the uterine perfusion pressure, leading some to be concerned with the administration of epidural analgesia to parturients with preeclampsia. An additional concern is the administration of intravenous fluids leading to pulmonary edema or cerebral edema. Epidural analgesia can still be safely administered to the parturient with preeclampsia, however. First, because the preeclamptic parturient is frequently intravascularly volume depleted, prehydration with 200 to 500 mL of lactated Ringer's solution before the administration of a continuous lumbar epidural analgesia helps to avoid significant decreases in maternal blood pressure that may result from the peripheral sympathetic nervous system blockade associated with epidural analgesia. Hydration may be guided by central venous pressure monitoring in difficult cases. A dilute local anesthetic solution may be used initially and administered slowly in fractionated doses. Should hypotension occur, only small doses of ephedrine (2.5 mg) should be administered to restore the blood pressure because the maternal vasculature may be hypersensitive to vasopressors. (356; **2055**)

159. A progressively decreasing platelet level is commonly seen in preeclampsia, which may place the parturient at risk of an epidural hematoma with the administration of a regional anesthetic. Coagulation studies and platelet levels should be assessed before the administration of regional anesthesia. (356; **2055**)

160. In addition to the usual indications, cesarean section becomes necessary in the preeclamptic parturient when the parturient becomes eclamptic, or when fetal distress occurs. Fetal distress in this situation is often secondary to decreases in the function of the uteroplacental circulation. (356; **2055**)

161. For the parturient undergoing cesarean section for fetal distress, general anesthesia is usually chosen as the form of anesthesia because it allows for better hemodynamic control. The rapid onset of regional anesthesia required under these conditions is associated with extensive peripheral sympathetic nervous system blockade and hypotension in these parturients. Monitoring that may be useful in the preeclamptic parturient undergoing cesarean section

under general anesthesia includes intra-arterial blood pressure, central venous pressure, urine output, and fetal heart rate. In some cases it may also be beneficial to monitor cardiac filling pressures. (357; **2055**)

162. The induction of general anesthesia in the preeclamptic parturient is typically accomplished by the administration of thiopental and succinylcholine or rapacuronium. Just as in other parturients, concerns for pulmonary aspiration warrant premedication with an antacid, adequate preoxygenation, cricoid pressure, and a rapid sequence induction of general anesthesia with the parturient in a position of leftward displacement of the uterus. The risk of difficult tracheal intubation is increased in parturients with preeclampsia. If there are concerns of difficulty intubating the trachea after the preoperative airway examination, alternative methods of inducing general anesthesia should be considered. (357; **2055**)

163. There are several special concerns for the preeclamptic parturient undergoing cesarean section with general anesthesia. First, there are exaggerated sympathetically mediated responses to direct laryngoscopy in these patients, making minimizing this time important. The prophylactic administration of hydralazine 10 to 15 minutes before or nitroglycerin 1 to 2 minutes before laryngoscopy may be useful to attenuate these responses. Once endotracheal intubation has been accomplished and confirmed, volatile anesthetics may be used to help control hypertension in the intraoperative period. A second concern for preeclamptic parturients is the enhancement of neuromuscular blockade and potential for uterine atony when the parturient has had magnesium treatment for seizure prophylaxis. Methylergonovine administration should be avoided because it may result in a hypertensive crisis to parturients with preeclampsia. Finally, hemodynamic monitoring of the parturient may need to be continued in the postpartum period. (357; **2055**)

HEMORRHAGE IN THE PARTURIENT

164. Causes of hemorrhage in the parturient include placenta previa, abruptio placentae, uterine rupture, retained placenta, cervical or vaginal lacerations, and uterine atony. Abruptio placentae and placenta previa are major causes of bleeding in the third trimester. Uterine rupture occurs during labor and is associated with uncontrolled hemorrhage. Retained placenta, uterine atony, and cervical or vaginal lacerations are all causes of bleeding in the postpartum period. Three to 5% of all vaginal deliveries have some postpartum hemorrhage. (357; **2056–2058**)

165. Placenta previa is the implantation of the placenta in the uterus in an abnormally low position. Placenta previa classically presents as painless vaginal bleeding. This usually occurs around the thirty-second week of gestation when the lower uterine segment is beginning to form. The diagnosis of placenta previa can be made by ultrasound examination of the placenta. If ultrasound is not satisfactory for a diagnosis of placenta previa, diagnosis can be made by direct examination of the os. The anesthesiologist may better manage the parturient for labor and delivery with knowledge of the position of the placenta. For example, in cases of cesarean delivery there may be excessive intraoperative blood loss if the position of the placenta requires that the obstetrician cut through the placenta to access the fetus. (357; **2056, Fig. 57–26**)

166. Risk factors for placenta previa include advanced age, multiparity, previous cesarean section, and a history of prior placenta previa. (**2056**)

167. The direct examination of the cervical os of a woman suspected of having a placenta previa should only be undertaken in the operating room while

prepared to proceed with an emergent cesarean section with acute blood loss because of the risk of inducing hemorrhage with the cervical examination. This is termed a *double set-up,* in which the obstetrician and anesthesiologist are present and prepared to proceed with emergent cesarean delivery of the newborn. Two large-bore peripheral intravenous catheters should be in place, and blood typed and crossed with the parturient's blood should be available in the operating room. Double set-up examinations of the cervical os have become less common as ultrasound techniques have improved. (357; **2056**)

168. Abruptio placentae is the separation of a normally implanted placenta leading to bleeding behind the placenta after the twentieth week of gestation. The parturient often has painful, frequent uterine contractions. The separation can involve only the placental margin, presenting as vaginal bleeding. Abruptio placentae can also occur without vaginal bleeding. In these cases, blood can accumulate in large volumes and be entirely sequestered within the uterus. Therefore, the degree of vaginal bleeding may not reflect the total amount of blood loss from the placenta. In cases of severe abruption, the parturient may have clotting abnormalities and disseminated intravascular coagulation, uterine hypertonicity and pain, and hypotension in addition to fetal distress or death. (358; **2056–2057**)

169. Risk factors for abruptio placentae include chronic hypertension, advanced maternal age, multiparity, abdominal trauma, cocaine use, and a history of prior abruption. (**2057**)

170. The definitive treatment of abruptio placentae is delivery of the fetus and emptying the uterus of the placenta. (358; **2056–2057**)

171. The management of the parturient with abruptio placentae is guided by the degree of abruption of the placenta. In cases in which labor and vaginal delivery will proceed, continuous epidural analgesia can be instituted, provided there are no signs of maternal hypovolemia, clotting abnormalities, or fetal distress. An emergent cesarean section should be performed in the parturient with abruptio placentae in circumstances in which there is severe hemorrhage. The induction of general anesthesia may be accomplished with ketamine or low doses of thiopental. When neonates are born under circumstances of severe maternal hemorrhage they are predictably acidotic and hypovolemic. (358; **2056–2057**)

172. Uterine rupture is rare. Risk factors for uterine rupture include a previous uterine scar, rapid spontaneous delivery, trauma, aggressive uterine manipulation with forceps or curettage, or excessive oxytocin stimulation. These risks being stated, only about 20% of uterine ruptures are associated with an identifiable risk. The remaining 80% of uterine ruptures occur spontaneously. The treatment of uterine rupture associated with hemorrhage is emergent laparotomy. (358; **2057–2058**)

173. Retained placenta occurs when some portion of the placenta has not been spontaneously delivered within 1 hour of delivery of the fetus. Uterine bleeding continues due to the inability of the uterus to contract around adherent placenta. Approximately 1% of all vaginal deliveries are associated with some retained placenta. The treatment involves manual exploration of the uterus for the removal of retained placental parts. (358; **2058**)

174. The anesthetic management of patients with retained placenta has as its goal uterine relaxation as well as decreasing the pain and anxiety of the patient. Anesthetic methods that may be used to accomplish this include intravenous sedation, epidural anesthesia, spinal anesthesia, and general anesthesia. The patient's protective airway reflexes must be retained when intravenous sedation is administered. (358; **2058**)

175. Uterine atony is the most common cause of postpartum hemorrhage. It occurs when inadequate contraction of the uterus after delivery of the placenta leads to ongoing blood loss from the uterus. It can present immediately after delivery or can occur several hours after delivery. (358; **2058**)

176. Risk factors for uterine atony include prolonged labor, multiple gestations, grand multiparity, and the administration of tocolytics to the parturient. Tocolytics include beta-2-adrenergic agonists, magnesium, and inhaled anesthetics. (358; **2058**)

177. The treatment of uterine atony is by the administration of agents that increase uterine tone. Such agents include synthetic oxytocins, methylergonovine, and/or Hemabate, an analog of prostaglandin $F_{2\alpha}$. (358; **2058**)

178. Rapid intravenous administration of synthetic oxytocin can result in vasodilation, hypotension, and tachycardia in the patient. This risk can be avoided by administering synthetic oxytocin in a continuous infusion of 10 to 15 units in 500 mL of crystalloid. (358)

179. It is important that synthetically made oxytocin does not contain vasopressin. If it did, parturients who had been previously treated with sympathomimetics may have responded to its administration with exaggerated increases in blood pressure. (358)

AMNIOTIC FLUID EMBOLISM

180. The clinical presentation of an amniotic fluid embolism that is sufficiently large to cause symptoms is the sudden onset of respiratory distress, hypotension, and arterial hypoxemia. Amniotic fluid embolisms may obstruct pulmonary blood flow leading to pulmonary hypertension and decreased cardiac output. Hemorrhage often develops due to disseminated intravascular coagulation. Some conditions that may mimic an amniotic fluid embolism include the inhalation of gastric contents, air embolism, pulmonary embolism, and local anesthetic toxicity. (358)

181. Patients most at risk for an amniotic fluid embolus are multiparous parturients who experience a tumultuous labor. (358)

182. The definitive diagnosis of an amniotic fluid embolus is made by recovering amniotic fluid from the parturient's blood when aspirating from a central venous catheter. (358)

183. The treatment of an amniotic fluid embolus is supportive, including cardiopulmonary resuscitation and the correction of arterial hypoxemia. (358)

ANESTHESIA FOR NONOBSTETRIC SURGERY DURING PREGNANCY

184. Anesthetic goals specific to the pregnant patient undergoing nonobstetric surgery include the avoidance of teratogenic drugs, the avoidance of intrauterine fetal asphyxia, and the prevention of preterm labor. (358–359; **2059**)

185. The critical gestational period for organogenesis occurs between 15 and 56 days of gestation. This is important because drugs that are teratogenic will exert their most disastrous effects when they are administered to the parturient during this period. (358; **2088**)

186. Most data regarding the administration of anesthetics to pregnant women in the first trimester are retrospective. In most cases the anesthetic was administered before the knowledge that the patient was pregnant. After retrospective analysis, there is no evidence to support a teratogenic effect of inhaled or

regional anesthetics administered during pregnancy, nor is there evidence to support an adverse effect on the later mental and neurologic development of neonates. (359; **2059**)

187. Caution with the administration of nitrous oxide has been the practice of many anesthesiologists for circumstantial reasons. Nitrous oxide is the only inhaled anesthetic that has been shown to be teratogenic to experimental animals, although this was at high concentrations for prolonged periods. It appears that nitrous oxide may inhibit DNA synthesis through its effects of the inhibition of methionine synthase. (359; **165, 2060**)

188. Intrauterine fetal hypoxia and acidosis has been associated with maternal hypotension, arterial hypoxemia, and excessive changes in the $Paco_2$. Avoidance of these will help to minimize intrauterine fetal hypoxia and acidosis. It is recommended that the maternal inhaled concentration of oxygen should be at least 50%. (359; **2060**)

189. *Retrolental fibroplasia* is a term used to describe the pathology afflicting the retina of neonates exposed to high concentrations of inspired Pao_2. Retrolental fibroplasia is not at risk of developing in the fetus in utero even with high inspired levels of Pao_2 in the parturient. This is because of the high oxygen consumption of the placenta combined with the uneven distribution of maternal and fetal blood flow through the placenta. For these reasons, the fetal Pao_2 is prevented from exceeding more than 45 mm Hg. (359; **2179**)

190. Premature labor is defined as being at least eight uterine contractions every hour combined with cervical effacement greater than 75% in a parturient between 20 and 35 weeks of gestation. (359)

191. The usual cause of premature labor that presents in the parturient after having nonobstetric surgery is the underlying pathologic process that led to the need for surgery and not the anesthetic technique. Monitoring that should be done in these circumstances, in addition to the routine monitoring, includes continuous fetal heart rate monitoring and monitoring of maternal uterine activity. (359; **2059**)

192. Premature labor can be treated through the administration of tocolytics. Beta-2 agonists such as terbutaline or ritodrine are commonly used for this purpose. Beta-2 agonists relax uterine smooth muscle and thereby inhibit uterine contractions while improving uteroplacental blood flow. Side effects of the treatment of premature labor with beta-2 agonists include maternal hypokalemia and cardiac dysrhythmias. Side effects for the fetus include fetal tachycardia and hypoglycemia. (359; **2059**)

193. Elective nonobstetric surgery in the parturient should be performed some time after the delivery of the fetus. (359; **2059**)

194. If surgery is necessary during the course of a woman's pregnancy, the preferred time for the surgery to take place is during the second or third trimester. Spinal anesthesia limits the amount of anesthetic a fetus is exposed to, making spinal anesthesia the preferred method of anesthesia if possible in parturients undergoing surgical procedures. (359; **2059**)

195. Continuous fetal heart rate monitoring intraoperatively is helpful after approximately the sixteenth week of gestation. Fetal distress can be detected by continuous fetal heart rate monitoring intraoperatively, including distress that may result from impaired uteroplacental perfusion. If fetal heart rate monitoring is technically impossible intraoperatively, as with some abdominal procedures, it may be prudent to have monitoring done immediately before induc-

tion and before awakening to confirm a reassuring fetal status. (359; **2059–2060**)

SUBSTANCE ABUSE

196. Cocaine and/or heroin abuse in the parturient often leads to a neonate who is delivered prematurely and who is depressed at delivery. (359)

197. Regional anesthesia may be the preferred method for providing anesthesia to the parturient who has been known to abuse drugs, to minimize possible interactions with unknown drugs the parturient may have ingested. (359)

DIAGNOSIS AND MANAGEMENT OF FETAL DISTRESS

198. Fetal well-being is best evaluated by monitoring the fetal heart rate with particular interest in the number and type of fetal heart rate decelerations and in the beat-to-beat variability. The beat-to-beat variability is computed from R wave intervals on a fetal electrocardiogram. (359)

199. Fetal electrocardiograms are obtained directly and indirectly. Direct measurement is obtained by placing an electrode directly on the fetal presenting part. Indirect measurement is obtained by placing a sensor on the maternal abdomen and measuring the electrocardiogram via ultrasound. (359)

200. The normal fetal heart rate is between 120 and 160 beats per minute. (359)

201. The normal fetal heart rate variability is between 5 to 20 beats per minute. (359)

202. Types of fetal distress that may be reflected as a decrease in the fetal heart rate beat-to-beat variability include distress due to arterial hypoxemia, acidosis, or central nervous system damage. (359)

203. Fetal heart rate beat-to-beat variability may be decreased by the administration of drugs to the mother, such as local anesthetics and opioids used for continuous lumbar epidural analgesia, and intravenous opioids, benzodiazepines, beta-adrenergic blockers, and anticholinergics. Clinically, the administration of these drugs may produce effects on the fetus that may be confused with fetal distress. Conversely, true fetal distress may be masked by the administration of these drugs. (359–360)

204. Decelerations in fetal heart rate are defined by their timing with the uterine contraction. An early deceleration in fetal heart rate is a slowing of the fetal heart rate whose onset begins with the onset of the uterine contraction. Early decelerations are thought to be due to compression of the fetal head and a resultant reflexive vagal stimulation. Early decelerations are not considered to be an indication of fetal distress. (360, Fig. 26–8)

205. Decelerations in fetal heart rate are defined by their timing with the uterine contraction. A late deceleration in fetal heart rate is a slowing of the fetal heart rate whose onset begins 10 to 30 seconds after the onset of the uterine contraction. Late decelerations are thought to be due to arterial hypoxemia and/or uteroplacental insufficiency, as may result from maternal hypotension. Late decelerations are indicative of fetal distress, and under these circumstances the fetal scalp pH may be obtained for further evaluation of fetal well-being. (360, Fig. 26–9)

206. Variable decelerations in fetal heart rate are decelerations in the fetal heart

rate whose timing, magnitude, and duration vary with respect to the timing of the onset of the uterine contraction. Umbilical cord compression is believed to be a cause of variable decelerations in fetal heart rate. Prolongation of the fetal heart rate deceleration to more than 30 seconds or fetal bradycardia that is slower than 70 beats per minute are both factors that make variable decelerations worrisome. Under these conditions changing maternal position alone is often sufficient treatment for the deceleration. (360–361, Fig. 26–10)

EVALUATION OF THE NEONATE AND NEONATAL RESUSCITATION

207. The Apgar score is an assigned numerical value to the status of a newborn at various intervals after the time of delivery. The Apgar score is useful as a guide in identifying infants who require intervention or resuscitation at birth, although one should not wait until the 1-minute Apgar score to begin necessary resuscitation. (361; **2072**)

208. (361, Table 26–6; **2072–2073, Table 58–1**)

CHARACTERISTIC	SCORE = ZERO	SCORE = ONE	SCORE = TWO
Heart rate	Absent	<100	>100
Breathing	Absent	Slow	Irregular, crying
Reflex irritability	No response	Grimace	Cry
Muscle tone	Limp	Flexion of extremities	Active
Color	Cyanotic	Extremities cyanotic	Pink

209. Most newborns have an Apgar score between 8 and 10. These infants require only suctioning of the mouth and nose and placement on a heated bed. (361; **2075–2076**)

210. Newborns with Apgar scores between 5 and 7 have most likely suffered from some mild asphyxia before birth. The only intervention usually required for these infants is external stimulation and the delivery of supplemental oxygen. Ventilation of the lungs of the newborn should be instituted only if the newborn does not respond within 1 to 2 minutes or if the heart rate is less than 100 beats/min. (361; **2076**)

211. Newborns with Apgar scores between 3 and 6 appear cyanotic and have poor breathing efforts. Hand ventilation of the lungs with bag and mask must usually be instituted, although increased airway resistance may make this difficult. If this is the case, intubation of the trachea may become necessary. (361; **2076**)

212. Newborns with Apgar scores between 0 and 2 have suffered from severe asphyxia. Prompt, aggressive resuscitative measures must be taken, including intubation of the trachea, ventilation, and support of the cardiovascular system as necessary. (361; **2076**)

213. The lungs of a neonate should be ventilated at a rate of 30 to 60 breaths/min. The maintenance of 3 to 5 cm H_2O positive end-expiratory pressure may also be useful. The adequacy of ventilation of the lungs of the neonate is best evaluated by physical examination and arterial blood gas analysis. (361–362; **2076–2077**)

214. The lungs of a neonate should be ventilated with peak airway pressures no

greater than 25 cm H_2O. Ventilating the neonate's lungs with higher peak airway pressures may result in pulmonary leaks and barotrauma. (362; **2077**)

215. External cardiac compression in the neonate should be instituted if the heart rate is less than 60 beats per minute or is 60 to 80 beats per minute and is not increasing despite ventilation with 100% oxygen. (362; **2083–2084, Fig. 58–12**)

216. The appropriate dose of epinephrine to be administered to the severely hypotensive and bradycardic neonate is 5 μg/kg intravenously or via the endotracheal tube. (362; **2084, Table 58–5**)

217. Hypoglycemia contributes to central nervous system damage in hypoxic neonates. Glucose administration should be considered in the neonate whose Apgar score is less than 2, because these neonates are often hypoglycemic. (362; **2084**)

218. The risk of meconium-stained amniotic fluid for the neonate is meconium aspiration and respiratory compromise at birth. These neonates should have their tracheas intubated and suctioned at birth before ventilation occurs, in an attempt to minimize the meconium reaching the distal airways. Further management of the neonate should be guided by the cardiopulmonary status. (362; **2077–2078**)

219. The advantages to having an umbilical artery catheter are that it provides for vascular access for arterial blood gases, pH analysis, expansion of blood volume, and a means for drug administration. The procedure for cannulation of the umbilical artery begins with sterilely prepping and draping the umbilical stump, dilating the artery with a curved forceps, and then advancing a 3.5 to 5.0 French umbilical artery catheter. (362; **2079–2080**)

220. Hypovolemia may occur in neonates born prematurely secondary to early clamping of the umbilical cord to begin resuscitation. Term infants may be hypovolemic due to intrauterine asphyxia, a nuchal cord that required cutting to free the infant, placental abruption, or disruption of placental integrity while delivering the infant during cesarean section. (362; **2081–2082**)

221. The hypovolemic newborn appears pale with poor capillary filling, cold extremities, weak or absent distal pulses, and hypotension. Resuscitation of the hypovolemic newborn should include the expansion of blood volume, which can be accomplished with either blood, plasma, or crystalloid solutions. (362; **2081–2082**)

NEUROBEHAVIORAL TESTING

222. Neurobehavioral testing is useful for, among other things, the detection of subtle effects of drugs on the neonate that were administered during labor and delivery. It evaluates the neonate's state of wakefulness, reflex responses, skeletal muscle tone, and responses to sound. (362)

223. Studies evaluating the neurobehavioral scores of neonates exposed to local anesthetics have shown no differences when compared to the scores of neonates who had not been exposed. (362)

224. Studies evaluating the neurobehavioral scores of neonates exposed to general anesthetics have shown mild depression when compared with the scores of neonates who had not been exposed. There is no evidence of prolonged adverse effects under these circumstances. (362)

POSTPARTUM TUBAL LIGATION

225. Postpartum tubal ligation performed under regional anesthesia requires a sensory dermatomal level of T5 anesthesia to ensure patient comfort. (362)

226. Studies have shown that parturients have little change in their gastric fluid volume and pH in the first 8 hours after vaginal delivery. Despite this, it is common to wait 8 to 12 hours postpartum before performing a tubal ligation in an effort to allow for increased gastric emptying and thereby minimize the risk of the pulmonary aspiration of gastric contents. (362)

Chapter 26

Pediatrics

1. What age defines newborns?

2. What age defines neonates?

3. What age defines infants?

4. What age defines children?

PHYSIOLOGIC DIFFERENCES

5. How does the oxygen consumption of a neonate compare with that of an adult?

6. How does the cardiac output of a neonate compare with that of an adult?

7. Are changes of the cardiac output of a neonate more dependent on changes in the heart rate or stroke volume?

8. How does the position of the oxyhemoglobin dissociation curve in a neonate compare with that of an adult? Describe how this affects the affinity of oxygen for hemoglobin. At what age does the curve approximate that of an adult?

9. How does the hemoglobin level of a neonate compare with that of an adult? How does the hemoglobin level change as the infant progresses to 1 year old?

10. What hemoglobin level is worrisome in the newborn? What hemoglobin level is worrisome in infants older than 6 months of age?

11. At what age does the foramen ovale close? What percent of adults have a probe patent foramen ovale?

12. How well do neonates reflexively respond to hemorrhage as compared with adults?

13. How does alveolar ventilation in neonates compare with that of adults?

14. How does the tidal volume per weight in neonates compare with that of adults?

15. How does the respiratory rate in neonates compare with that of adults?

16. How does carbon dioxide production in neonates compare with that of adults? How does the Pa_{CO_2} in neonates compare with that of adults?

17. How does the Pa_{O_2} change in the first few days of life?

18. How predictable is the neonate's response to hypoxia?

19. What percent body weight in neonates is contributed by the extracellular fluid volume? How does this compare with an adult?

20. What are some ways in which infants and children maintain normal body temperature? Why is maintenance of normal body temperature more difficult in neonates and children than in an adult?

21. How effective is kidney function at birth? When does kidney function become approximately equivalent to that of an adult?

22. After fluid restriction, what is the maximum urine osmolarity possible for term neonates at birth? At what age are adult levels of urine concentrating abilities achieved?

PHARMACOLOGIC RESPONSE DIFFERENCES

23. What are some physiologic characteristics of neonates that explain the pharmacologic differences between pediatric and adult responses to drugs?

24. How is the uptake and distribution of inhaled anesthetics different in neonates and infants when compared with adults?

25. How does the minimum alveolar concentration (MAC) of inhaled anesthetics change from birth to puberty?

26. What physiologic factors increase the sensitivity of neonates to the effects of intravenous anesthetics?

27. How does the dose of thiopental change between neonates and adults?

28. How does the rate of plasma clearance of opioids differ between neonates and adults?

29. Are neonates more or less sensitive to nondepolarizing neuromuscular blocking drugs than adults? How does the initial drug dose differ between these two groups?

30. How does the duration of action of nondepolarizing neuromuscular blocking drugs differ between neonates and adults?

31. How does the dose of neostigmine necessary to antagonize neuromuscular blockade in the neonate compare with the dose necessary in the adult? How does this affect clinical practice?

32. How does the dose of succinylcholine necessary to produce neuromuscular blockade in the infant and neonate compare with the dose necessary in the adult?

PREANESTHETIC EVALUATION AND PREPARATION

33. What history should be obtained from a preoperative evaluation of a pediatric patient? What are some considerations that are specific to the pediatric population with regard to the history and physical?

34. What preoperative laboratory data may be important in the neonate to pediatric population?

35. What are the recommendations for the preoperative ingestion of solids and clear liquids for pediatric patients?

36. What are some considerations regarding the choice of premedicant in the pediatric patient? What are some drugs and their routes of administration for preoperative medication in the pediatric population?

INDUCTION AND MAINTENANCE OF ANESTHESIA

37. How can the induction of anesthesia be achieved in pediatric patients without an intravenous catheter in place?

38. What are some risks of an inhaled induction of anesthesia?

39. What is the indication for the placement of an intravenous catheter in the pediatric patient undergoing a surgical procedure?

40. How can the anesthesiologist regulate the intravenous fluids to be administered in the pediatric patient?

41. How can the induction of anesthesia be achieved in pediatric patients with an intravenous catheter in place?

42. How can the induction of anesthesia be achieved in pediatric patients without an intravenous catheter in place and in whom an inhalation induction is not possible?

43. What is the concern regarding the use of succinylcholine in pediatric patients? What are some alternatives that may be used?

44. Under what circumstances is succinylcholine accepted for use for neuromuscular blockade in the pediatric population?

45. What are some physiologic characteristics of the pediatric airway that differ from the adult airway?

46. Why are uncuffed endotracheal tubes frequently used for intubating the trachea of pediatric patients?

47. What is the benefit of the administration of heated and humidified gases in children undergoing prolonged operations?

48. What are some signs the clinician may use to determine the adequacy of the depth of anesthesia for surgery in the pediatric population?

49. When hypotension accompanies the administration of volatile anesthetics to neonates, what is it likely to be indicative of?

50. How does intraoperative monitoring in the pediatric population differ from intraoperative monitoring in the adult population?

51. What problem may be encountered with the monitoring of end-tidal carbon dioxide concentrations in pediatric patients?

52. How should the size of blood pressure cuff be selected? What errors in blood pressure measurement may be encountered with an erroneously sized cuff?

53. What veins may be used to monitor the central venous pressure in the neonate? In infants? In children?

54. What is the recommendation for fluid maintenance and replacement in the pediatric population?

55. What are the goals for urine output and specific gravity when using these methods to monitor the volume status of children intraoperatively?

56. When should glucose administration be considered in the pediatric population?

57. What formula can be used to help guide the anesthesiologist with blood loss replacement?

58. What are some regional anesthetic blocks that can be administered in the pediatric population?

59. What local anesthetic and what dose is commonly used in a caudal anesthetic? What is the approximate duration of the postoperative pain relief obtained from this caudal anesthetic? How is the length of the dural sac different in children and adults?

MEDICAL AND SURGICAL DISEASES THAT AFFECT PEDIATRIC PATIENTS

60. What is respiratory distress syndrome?

61. What are some physiologic complications that result from respiratory distress syndrome?

62. How should neonates with respiratory distress syndrome be managed intraoperatively?

63. What is bronchopulmonary dysplasia? What are some characteristic findings in these patients?

64. What is retinopathy of prematurity? What is another name for this pathologic finding?

65. What is a risk factor for retinopathy of prematurity? At what age does the risk of retinopathy of prematurity become negligible?

66. What Pa_{O_2} should be maintained during anesthesia in the premature neonate to minimize the risk of retinopathy of prematurity?

67. What age of patients are at risk of apnea spells in the postoperative period? What is the recommendation for these patients in the postoperative period?

68. Which pediatric patients are at risk of hypoglycemia?

69. What are some manifestations of hypoglycemia in this population? How do these manifestations change with general anesthesia? What is the immediate treatment of hypoglycemia in these patients?

70. Which pediatric patients are at risk of hypocalcemia?

71. When might hypocalcemia occur intraoperatively? How might intraoperative hypocalcemia manifest?

72. What and how specific are the signs of sepsis in neonates?

73. Trisomy 21 occurs in approximately what percentage of all live births? What are some congenital anomalies associated with trisomy 21?

74. What are some preoperative considerations specific to the child with trisomy 21?

75. Why might hand ventilation with bag and mask be difficult in the child with trisomy 21?

76. What is the risk of movement of the head and neck during direct laryngoscopy in the child with trisomy 21?

77. How does epiglottitis usually present? In what age group?

78. What bacterium is most likely to be the cause of epiglottitis?

79. What tissues are primarily involved in epiglottitis? What is the overwhelming concern for patients with epiglottitis?

80. How should patients with epiglottitis be managed?

81. What is the time course for epiglottitis? Under what circumstances should extubation of the trachea take place?

82. What is another name for croup? Compare and contrast epiglottitis with croup by completing the following table:

	EPIGLOTTITIS (SUPRAGLOTTITIS)	LARYNGOTRACHEO-BRONCHITIS
Age		
Incidence		
Cause		
Onset		
Signs and symptoms		
Lateral radiograph of the neck		
Treatment		

83. What is the incidence of malignant hyperthermia in the pediatric population? What is the incidence in the adult population?

84. What is the association between malignant hyperthermia and the calcium ion channel?

85. What are some anesthetic triggering drugs for malignant hyperthermia?

86. What is the relationship between trismus and malignant hyperthermia? How should patients with trismus be managed after the administration of succinylcholine?

87. What are some clinical signs of malignant hyperthermia?

88. What is the treatment of malignant hyperthermia?

89. How can the patient at risk for malignant hyperthermia be identified preoperatively?

90. Which anesthetic regimen is reliably safe for patients susceptible to malignant hyperthermia? Name some drugs used in anesthesia that have not been shown to trigger malignant hyperthermia.

91. What preparations must take place before the administration of anesthesia to patients susceptible to malignant hyperthermia?

92. Is regional anesthesia considered safe for patients at risk for malignant hyperthermia?

93. What is a diaphragmatic hernia? How are diaphragmatic hernias manifest in the neonate at birth?

94. What are some co-morbid conditions associated with diaphragmatic hernias?

95. How is the diagnosis of a diaphragmatic hernia made?

96. What is the immediate treatment for the neonate with a diaphragmatic hernia? What is the risk of hand ventilation with bag and mask in these neonates?

97. What is the risk of positive pressure ventilation of the lungs of the neonate with a diaphragmatic hernia?

98. What inhaled anesthetics can be used for the anesthetic maintenance of neonates with a diaphragmatic hernia?

99. What clinical circumstance leads to suspicion of a tracheoesophageal fistula in a neonate?

100. What are some other congenital anomalies associated with a tracheoesophageal fistula?

101. How should neonates with a tracheoesophageal fistula be managed?

102. What is pyloric stenosis? What is the incidence of pyloric stenosis per live birth?

103. How does the neonate with pyloric stenosis typically present?

104. What electrolyte imbalances are seen in infants with pyloric stenosis?

105. Is the surgical correction of pyloric stenosis in infants an elective or emergent procedure?

106. How should the induction of anesthesia in infants with pyloric stenosis proceed?

ANSWERS*

1. Newborns are defined as being 0 to 24 hours old. (364)

2. Neonates are defined as being between 1 and 28 days of age. (364)

*Numbers in parentheses: lightface numbers refer to pages, figures, or tables in Stoelting RK, Miller RD: Basics of Anesthesia, 4th ed. Philadelphia, Churchill Livingstone, 2000; **boldface numbers** refer to pages, figures, or tables in Miller RD: Anesthesia, 5th ed. Philadelphia, Churchill Livingstone, 2000.

3. Infants are defined as being between 28 days and 1 year of age. (364)

4. Children are defined as being 1 year of age to puberty. (364)

PHYSIOLOGIC DIFFERENCES

5. The oxygen consumption of a neonate is about twice that of an adult. In neonates the oxygen consumption increases from 5 mL/kg per minute at birth to about 7 mL/kg per minute at 10 days of life and 8 mL/kg per minute at 4 weeks of life. Oxygen consumption gradually declines over the subsequent months. (364, Table 27–1; **2445, 2456, Table 73–1**)

6. The cardiac output of a neonate is 30% to 60% higher than that of adults. This helps to meet the increase in oxygen demand neonates have as compared with adults. (364; **2089, 2444**)

7. Changes in the cardiac output of a neonate or infant are dependent on changes in the heart rate, because stroke volume is relatively fixed by the lack of distensibility of the left ventricle in this age group. (364, Table 27–1; **1806, 2089, 2444, Table 73–1**)

8. In neonates, the oxyhemoglobin dissociation curve is shifted to the left. This reflects a P_{50} lower than 26 mm Hg, meaning that less of a P_{O_2} is required for a 50% saturation of hemoglobin. Conversely, the oxygen is more tightly bound to hemoglobin in neonates, necessitating a lower Pa_{O_2} for release of oxygen to the tissues. This occurs as a result of fetal hemoglobin. The position of the oxyhemoglobin dissociation curve becomes equal to that of adults by 4 to 6 months of age. (364; **2456**)

9. The hemoglobin level of a neonate is approximately 17 g/dL. This, along with the increase in cardiac output, helps to offset the increase in oxygen requirements characteristic of neonates. At 2 to 3 months of age the hemoglobin of infants decreases to about 11 g/dL during the time period when fetal hemoglobin is being replaced by adult hemoglobin. This is termed the *physiologic anemia of infancy,* which may persist for a few months. During the remainder of the first year of life the hemoglobin level gradually increases and continues to do so until puberty, when hemoglobin levels approach adult hemoglobin levels. (364, Table 27–1; **Table 73–1**)

10. A hemoglobin level of 13 g/dL or less is worrisome in the newborn. In infants older than 6 months of age, a hemoglobin level less than 10 g/dL is worrisome. (364)

11. The foramen ovale closes between 3 and 12 months of age. Twenty to 30% of adults have a probe patent foramen ovale. (364; **2070, 2089**)

12. Because of the decreased ability of neonates to vasoconstrict in response to hypovolemia, neonates are less able to tolerate hemorrhage with vasoconstrictive responses. (364)

13. Alveolar ventilation in neonates is double that of adults. (364, Table 27–2; **2454, Table 73–7**)

14. Tidal volume per weight in neonates is similar to that of adults. (364, Table 27–2; **2454, Table 73–7**)

15. The respiratory rate in neonates is double that of adults. (364, Table 27–2; **2454, Table 73–7**)

16. Carbon dioxide production in neonates is higher than that of adults. The Pa_{CO_2} in neonates is similar to that of adults, despite the increase in production. This is due to the increase in alveolar ventilation in neonates when compared with adults. (364, Table 27–2; **2090, 2454, Table 73–7**)

17. The Pa_{O_2} in the first few days after birth increases rapidly. The initially low Pa_{O_2} is due to a decrease in the functional residual capacity and to the perfusion of alveoli filled with fluid. The functional residual capacity of neonates increases over the first few days of life until it reaches adult levels at about 4 days of age. (364)

18. The neonate's response to hypoxia is somewhat unpredictable, owing to the immaturity of the central nervous system regulatory centers for ventilation in this age group. Neonates have decreased ventilatory responses to hypoxemia and hypercarbia. (364; **2090, 2456**)

19. Extracellular fluid volume accounts for approximately 40% of the body weight of the neonate at birth. This compares with approximately 20% of body weight in adults being accounted for by extracellular fluid volume. The proportion of extracellular fluid volume to body weight in neonates approaches the adult proportion by 18 to 24 months of age. (364–365; **2092, Fig. 59–5**)

20. Some ways in which infants and children maintain normal body temperature include the metabolism of brown fat, crying, and vigorous movements. The metabolism of brown fat is stimulated by circulating norepinephrine. Children and infants, unlike adults, do not shiver to maintain their body temperature. Maintenance of normal body temperature is more difficult in neonates and infants than in adults because of their larger body surface area-to-volume ratio, as well as the relative lack of fat for insulation. (365; **2092**)

21. Kidney function at birth is immature. There is a decreased glomerular filtration rate, decreased sodium excretion, and decreased concentrating ability relative to that of an adult. Kidney function progressively matures over the first 2 years of life. Initially, in the first 3 months of life, kidney function increases rapidly to double or triple the glomerular filtration rate possible at birth. Kidney function then matures more slowly from 3 months to 24 months, when adult levels of kidney function are reached. (365; **2091, Fig. 59–4**)

22. After fluid restriction, the term neonate at birth can only concentrate urine to a maximum osmolarity of about 525 mOsm/kg. After 15 to 30 days of age neonates are able to concentrate their urine to a maximum osmolarity of about 950 mOsm/kg. Adult levels of urine concentrating ability are achieved by 6 to 12 months of age. (365; **2091, 2104**)

PHARMACOLOGIC RESPONSE DIFFERENCES

23. Some physiologic characteristics of neonates that explain the pharmacologic differences between pediatric and adult responses to drugs include an increased extracellular fluid volume, increased metabolic rate, decreased renal function, and decreased receptor maturity. (365; **2092–2093, Fig. 59–5**)

24. The uptake and distribution of inhaled anesthetics is more rapid in neonates than in adults. This is most likely due to a smaller functional residual capacity per body weight in neonates, as well as to greater tissue blood flow to the vessel-rich group. The vessel-rich group of tissues includes the brain, heart, kidneys, and liver. This group comprises approximately 22% of total body volume in neonates, as compared with the 10% of total body volume in adults. (365; **2092–2093**)

25. The minimum alveolar concentration (MAC) of inhaled anesthetics changes from birth to puberty. Preterm neonates have a lower MAC than term neonates, whose MAC is approximately 0.87% MAC of adults. The MAC increases until 2 to 3 months of age, peaking then at approximately 1.20% MAC of adults. After 3 months of age, the MAC of inhaled anesthetics

progressively decreases with age. (365–366, Figs. 27–1, 27–2; **2093, Fig. 59–6**)

26. Physiologic factors that make the neonate more sensitive to the effects of intravenous anesthetics include an immature blood-brain barrier and a decreased ability to metabolize drugs. In many cases the increased extracellular fluid volume and volume of distribution present in neonates offsets the increased sensitivity to intravenous drugs when compared with adults, thereby approximately equalizing the dose of initial intravenous injection of drug to achieve a given result. (366; **2092**)

27. The dose of thiopental required to produce loss of lid reflex is similar in neonates, children, and adults. (366, Table 27–3; **2095**)

28. The rate of plasma clearance of opioids is decreased in neonates when compared with adults. (366; **2096–2097**)

29. Neonates are more sensitive than adults to nondepolarizing neuromuscular blocking drugs. This means that a lower plasma concentration of drug is required to produce similar pharmacologic results. Because of an increased extracellular fluid volume and increased volume of distribution in neonates when compared with adults, the initial dose of nondepolarizing neuromuscular blocking drug in these two age groups is similar. This is true despite the increased sensitivity to the drug for neonates. (366–367; **454–456, 2097–2098**)

30. The duration of action of nondepolarizing neuromuscular blocking drugs in neonates may be prolonged while the mechanisms for clearance are still immature in the neonate. For example, the clearance of *d*-tubocurarine parallels glomerular filtration rate at various ages. There exists a great deal of variability among pediatric patients with regard to the duration of effect of nondepolarizing neuromuscular blocking drugs. Monitoring of the neuromuscular junction with a peripheral nerve stimulator is recommended when nondepolarizing neuromuscular blocking drugs are administered to this population. (367; **454–456, 2097–2098**)

31. The dose of neostigmine necessary to antagonize neuromuscular blocking drugs in the neonate is less than that of adults, although clinically the same dose may be used. (367; **454–456**)

32. The dose of succinylcholine per body weight necessary to produce neuromuscular blockade in the neonate and infant is increased from the adult dose. This is presumed to be due to the increase in extracellular fluid volume and increase in volume of distribution in neonates and infants. (367; **2097**)

PREANESTHETIC EVALUATION AND PREPARATION

33. The preoperative history in the pediatric patient often comes from a parent. The history obtained should include such things as congenital anomalies, allergies, bleeding tendencies, and any recent exposure to communicable diseases. A special consideration for the pediatric population is whether the patient has had any recent upper respiratory tract infection, which makes it more likely that the patient will have increased secretions and airway hyperreactivity with anesthesia. Elective surgeries may be delayed in the presence of an upper airway infection. With regard to the airway examination, the presence of loose teeth should be evaluated, and removal of the loose tooth or teeth before surgery should be considered. (367; **2099**)

34. Laboratory data are typically unnecessary in the routine pediatric patient. Laboratory data that may be important in the prenatal population are a

glucose level, calcium level, or the presence of clotting disorders. Other laboratory data should be ordered based on the history and physical examination. For example, if the child has any history of nausea, vomiting, or diarrhea, serum electrolytes and possibly a pH should be evaluated. (367)

35. The recommendations for the preoperative consumption of solids and clear liquids vary between institutions. In general, the recommendations allow for the ingestion of clear fluids up to 2 to 3 hours before anesthesia. The ingestion of milk and solids, including breast milk, is usually allowed 4 to 6 hours before anesthesia in infants younger than age 6 months. After 6 months of age pediatric patients should have fasted from milk or solids between 6 and 8 hours before the procedure. (368, Table 10–7; **1099–2100, Table 59–3**)

36. Premedication of the pediatric patient should take into consideration the age of the patient, the patient's underlying medical condition, the length of surgery, the mode of induction of anesthesia, and whether the patient will be staying in the hospital after the procedure. Infants younger than 6 months old typically do not require premedication, whereas infants between 9 and 18 months old may benefit from premedication before separation from their parents. Premedicants may be administered orally, intravenously, intramuscularly, rectally, sublingually, transmucosally, or intranasally. One drug available and commonly used for premedication in the pediatric population is midazolam. Midazolam can be administered intravenously, orally, or intranasally. When administered orally, midazolam can be given in a flavored syrup diluent for easier ingestion by the patient. The peak effect of midazolam after oral administration usually takes about 30 minutes after ingestion. The intranasal route of administration is irritating but has a rapid onset time. Fentanyl can also be used as a premedicant and can be given transmucosally. Sufentanil can also be administered intranasally for premedication. (367–368; **2095–2096, 2098–2099**)

INDUCTION AND MAINTENANCE OF ANESTHESIA

37. In the pediatric patient without an intravenous catheter anesthesia can be induced by an inhalation induction. An inhalation induction can be achieved by initially having the child breathe 70% nitrous oxide and 30% oxygen, followed by incremental increases in the concentration of a volatile anesthetic. The volatile anesthetics usually chosen for an inhalation induction are halothane and sevoflurane because they are relatively less pungent than the other volatile anesthetics. Other adjuncts that may be used to decrease patient anxiety and facilitate the induction of anesthesia under these circumstances include having the parents present during the time of induction, flavoring the anesthesia mask with flavored scents, and maintaining a constant monotone conversation with the patient. A story can be told by the anesthesiologist to distract the patient during induction. (368; **2100–2101**)

38. An inhaled induction of anesthesia has some inherent risks. First, while the pediatric patient is being induced the anesthesiologist often increases concentrations of the volatile anesthetic to dangerous inspired concentrations of volatile anesthetic if maintained. Once anesthesia is induced it is important to reduce the inspired concentrations of volatile anesthetic to routine maintenance levels. This is especially true just before intubating the trachea, because connection of the circuit and ventilating the intubated patient with high inspired concentrations of volatile anesthetic while potentially distracted with endotracheal tube positioning is a risk. High inspired concentrations of volatile anesthetic, if continued, can lead to myocardial depression that is difficult to reverse. Another risk of an inhaled induction of anesthesia is that of laryngospasm. Laryngospasm is accompanied by a rocking-boat motion of

the chest and abdomen as the patient attempts to inspire against a closed glottis. Laryngospasm should be treated by closing off the pop-off valve and creating positive pressure of about 10 cm H_2O against the glottis. If necessary, positive pressure ventilation can be attempted. In most circumstances these will reverse the laryngospasm and the patient will spontaneously ventilate. Should these two interventions not reverse the laryngospasm, succinylcholine can be administered intravenously or intramuscularly. Succinylcholine is the neuromuscular blocking drug of choice under these circumstances. (368; **2100–2101**)

39. The placement of an intravenous catheter should be done in every pediatric patient undergoing a surgical procedure other than for very short surgical procedures. (368; **2100**)

40. The administration of intravenous fluids in these patients can be regulated by the use of a calibrated drip chamber, so as to minimize the risk that excessive amounts of fluid are accidentally administered. (368)

41. In the pediatric patient with an intravenous catheter the induction of anesthesia can be achieved by the intravenous administration of an induction agent such as thiopental or propofol. This is the induction method of choice in patients at risk for the aspiration of gastric contents. (368; **2102**)

42. Another method of induction in the pediatric patient without an intravenous catheter and in whom an inhalation induction is not possible is by the intramuscular administration of ketamine. For infants a rectal induction of anesthesia is another alternative. Agents that can be administered by the rectal route for the induction of anesthesia include thiopental, methohexital, ketamine, and midazolam. (368; **2102**)

43. There are multiple concerns regarding the use of succinylcholine in pediatric patients. First, the administration of succinylcholine can result in cardiac arrhythmias, including bradycardia and, rarely, cardiac sinus arrest. The pretreatment of pediatric patients with atropine may reduce succinylcholine-induced bradycardia. Second, it is believed that in patients who have been administered succinylcholine and have subsequent masseter muscle rigidity there may be impending malignant hyperthermia. Finally, there have been reports of pediatric patients who were otherwise healthy and went into irreversible cardiac arrest after the administration of succinylcholine. Many of these patients had hyperkalemia, rhabdomyolysis, and acidosis. It is postulated that these pediatric patients may have had undiagnosed myopathies. Postmortem muscle biopsies have shown many of them to have muscular dystrophy. The group at highest risk of this catastrophic event are males 8 years of age or younger. Because of these concerns, many clinicians feel that the routine use of succinylcholine in pediatric patients should be abandoned. Some alternatives that may be used are the nondepolarizing neuromuscular blocking drugs, such as rapacuronium or rocuronium. (368; **422–423, 2097**)

44. Succinylcholine is accepted for use for rapid onset neuromuscular blockade in pediatric patients for the treatment of laryngospasm and in patients in whom the risk of aspiration is such that a rapid sequence induction for rapid intubation of the trachea is indicated. (368; **2097**)

45. There are multiple physiologic differences between the pediatric airway and the adult airway. Pediatric patients tend to have a larger tongue relative to the size of their mouths. Particularly true in neonates is that the occiput is larger, so that placing the head in the neutral position naturally places the head in a position favorable for direct laryngoscopy. Extending the head can make direct laryngoscopy difficult. The larynx is more cephalad in pediatric patients, with the cricoid cartilage opposing the C4 vertebra rather than the

C6 vertebra as in adults. The larynx is also more anterior. The epiglottis is longer, stiffer, and U shaped and has more of a horizontal lie. The narrowest point of the airway is at the level of the cricoid cartilage. These differences between the pediatric airway and the adult airway are present until about the age of 8 years, after which the difference between the pediatric airway and the adult airway is mainly just a difference in size. (368; **1444, 2455**)

46. Because the narrowest point of the pediatric airway is at the level of the cricoid cartilage, an endotracheal tube that passes easily through the larynx may cause ischemia or damage to the trachea distally. To decrease the risk of postintubation tracheal edema in the pediatric population, an uncuffed endotracheal tube is generally selected for children younger than 10 years of age. In addition, an air leak test is performed with positive airway pressure. The endotracheal tube should be small enough so that air will leak out of the trachea around the endotracheal tube audibly with airway pressures between 15 and 25 cm H_2O. The risk of postintubation tracheal edema is greatest in children between 1 and 4 years of age. Postintubation tracheal edema can be treated with humidified gases and aerosolized racemic epinephrine. Dexamethasone has also been administered intravenously for the treatment of postintubation tracheal edema. (368; **2103, 2455, 2460**)

47. The administration of heated and humidified gases in children undergoing prolonged operations is useful in decreasing intraoperative heat loss and in avoiding decreases in body temperature. (368; **2108**)

48. Signs for the adequacy of depth of anesthesia for surgery are the same for neonates, infants, and children as they are in adults. Those signs include blood pressure, heart rate, and skeletal muscle movement. (368; **1098–1100, 2109**)

49. Hypotension in the neonate that accompanies the administration of volatile anesthetics is likely to be indicative of hypovolemia. (368)

50. Intraoperative monitoring in the pediatric population is not any different from intraoperative monitoring in the adult population undergoing comparable surgical procedures. Routine monitors should include blood pressure, heart rate, electrocardiogram, peripheral oxygen saturation, and temperature monitoring. (369; **2107**)

51. The monitoring of end-tidal carbon dioxide concentrations in small children, infants, and neonates may be difficult because of the high inspired gas flows relative to the small volume of exhaled carbon dioxide. (369; **2107**)

52. An appropriately sized blood pressure cuff is one that is greater than one third of the circumference of the limb. A blood pressure cuff that is too small will result in artificially high blood pressures. The opposite is also true, that a blood pressure cuff that is too large will result in artificially low blood pressures. (369; **1121**)

53. Central venous pressure can be monitored in the neonate via an umbilical vein catheter. The external jugular vein, internal jugular vein, or subclavian vein can be used for central venous pressure monitoring in infants and children. (369; **2107**)

54. Fluid maintenance and replacement in the pediatric population is based on the patient's age and metabolic rate, underlying disease process, type and extent of surgery, and anticipated fluid translocation. The maintenance rate of pediatric patients is related to their metabolic demand, which in turn is related to the ratio of body surface to weight. Hourly fluid requirements are estimated to be 4 mL/kg for children up to 10 kg, an additional 2 mL/kg for each kilogram of body weight between 10 kg and 20 kg, and an additional 1 mL/kg for each kilogram of body weight above 20 kg. Additional fluid replace-

ment may be required for the patient's initial fluid deficit, third-space losses, or other losses. Fluid replacement can be guided by the patient's systemic blood pressure, tissue perfusion, and urine output. (369–370, Table 27–4; **2103–2104, Table 59–5**)

55. A goal for urine output intraoperatively in the pediatric patient is 0.5 mg/kg per hour. A goal for the urine specific gravity intraoperatively in pediatric patients is maintenance of a specific gravity lower than 1.010. (369)

56. Glucose administration in the pediatric patient can be considered in patients who are at a high risk for hypoglycemia. Pediatric patients at a high risk for hypoglycemia include newborns of diabetic mothers or neonates whose hyperalimentation has been discontinued. Maintenance fluids of 5% dextrose in 0.45 normal saline can be administered to these patients intraoperatively as a piggy-back infusion by pump with care not to bolus glucose-containing solutions. (369–370; **2104**)

57. A formula that may be used by the anesthesiologist to help guide blood loss replacement is:

$$\text{ABL (mL)} = \text{body weight (kg)} \times \text{EBV (mL/kg)} \times (H_0 - H_i/H_{avg})$$

ABL, allowable blood loss; EBV, estimated blood volume; H_0, starting hematocrit; H_i, lowest acceptable hematocrit; H_{avg}, average of starting and lowest acceptable hematocrit. The estimated blood volume is between 70 mL/kg at about 5 years of age to 100 mL/kg in the premature newborn. (370, Table 27–5; **2104–2105**)

58. There are several procedures in which regional anesthetic techniques can be considered in the pediatric population. For circumcision or hypospadias repair a penile block may be used. For inguinal hernia repair an ilioinguinal and iliohypogastric block may be used. For femur surgery a fascia iliaca compartment block may be used. For arm and wrist surgery a brachial plexus block may be used. Intravenous regional anesthesia may also be used in the pediatric patient for tendon laceration repairs or extremity fractures. Caudal anesthesia is a common form of anesthesia and is used for postoperative pain relief in the pediatric population in whom the surgical site is below the level of the diaphragm. Conversely, a lumbar epidural anesthetic may also be used in the pediatric patient. (369; **1560–1579, 2112, Table 44–2**)

59. For caudal anesthesia, the local anesthetic most commonly used is bupivacaine at a concentration of 0.17% to 0.25%. The volume is 1 mL/kg, up to a maximum of 25 mL. The duration of pain relief provided by this dose of bupivacaine in the caudal epidural space is 6 to 8 hours, therefore possibly providing some postoperative pain relief. The dural sac extends more caudad in children than in adults, making inadvertent intrathecal injection a possibility. The risks of caudal anesthesia are minimal. (369; **1560–1561, Fig. 44–2**)

MEDICAL AND SURGICAL DISEASES THAT AFFECT PEDIATRIC PATIENTS

60. Respiratory distress syndrome, also referred to as hyaline membrane disease, is a syndrome affecting preterm neonates who at birth have a deficiency of surfactant. Surfactant is necessary to maintain alveolar stability, so that without it alveoli collapse. Surfactant is a surface active phospholipid in the alveoli that can now be administered into the lungs of neonates for the treatment or prevention of respiratory distress syndrome. The compliance of the lung and arterial oxygenation often improve rapidly after its administration. The administration of surfactant has decreased the morbidity and mortality that resulted from this syndrome. (370; **2079**)

61. With the alveolar collapse associated with respiratory distress syndrome there is resultant right-to-left intrapulmonary shunting, arterial hypoxemia, and metabolic acidosis. (370; **2079**)

62. Neonates with respiratory distress syndrome should have their arterial oxygenation closely monitored intraoperatively. The PaO_2 the anesthesiologist should try to maintain in these patients is the PaO_2 level the patient had before surgery. This may require high inspired concentrations of oxygen and positive end-expiratory pressure. The PaO_2 should ideally be monitored from a preductal artery. If the surgical procedure is short and intra-arterial monitoring is not feasible, oxygenation may be monitored by pulse oximetry. These neonates are at an increased risk for pneumothorax with positive pressure ventilation. Neonates with respiratory distress syndrome should be well hydrated. It may be prudent to maintain the hematocrit near 40% to optimize the delivery of oxygen to the tissues. (370–371)

63. Bronchopulmonary dysplasia is a chronic pulmonary disorder in infants and children who had prolonged respiratory disease at birth. It is thought to result from the required high inspired concentrations of oxygen and mechanical ventilation with high peak airway pressures for a prolonged period of time as treatment for the respiratory disease. Some characteristic findings in patients with bronchopulmonary dysplasia are increased airway resistance, increased airway reactivity, decreased arterial oxygenation due to ventilation-to-perfusion mismatch, and recurrent pulmonary infections. Chest radiograph in these patients may show large lung volumes, fibrosis, and atelectasis. These patients may have chronic hypercarbia as well. The incidence of bronchopulmonary dysplasia has decreased since the advent of surfactant therapy in neonates at risk. (371; **2466**)

64. Retinopathy of prematurity, also referred to as retrolental fibroplasia, is a condition in which the retinal vasculature becomes neovascularized and scarred. Permanent visual impairment can result. (371; **2077, 2179**)

65. A risk factor for retinopathy of prematurity is a PaO_2 greater than 80 mm Hg or an oxygen saturation greater than 94% in the presence of prematurity. Retinopathy of prematurity has occurred in neonates whose PaO_2 was maintained at about 150 mm Hg for 2 to 4 hours. Neonates whose birth weights are lower than 1500 g are especially at risk. The risk of retinopathy of prematurity becomes negligible after 44 weeks after conception. (371; **2108, 2179**)

66. A PaO_2 between 60 and 80 mm Hg or an oxygen saturation between 87% and 94% should be maintained during anesthesia in the premature neonate to minimize the risk of retinopathy of prematurity. (371; **2077, 2108, 2179**)

67. Apnea spells that result in the cessation of breathing for 20 seconds or longer can lead to cyanosis and bradycardia. Especially at risk are preterm infants younger than 60 weeks post conception. It is estimated that 20% to 30% of preterm infants have apnea spells during their first month of life. Apnea spells may be increased in the neonate in the postoperative period secondary to the residual effects of inhaled and injected anesthetics that affect the control of breathing. The recommendation for these patients is that apnea and bradycardia monitors be used after surgery that will sound an alarm if apnea or bradycardia is detected in the patient. These patients are not candidates for outpatient surgery because of the risk of apnea occurring at home where health care providers are not available to respond. An alternative is to postpone nonessential surgery until infants are older than 60 weeks post conception. (**2110–2112**)

68. Neonates are at risk of developing hypoglycemia, particularly neonates of diabetic mothers. Hypoglycemia is defined by a plasma glucose concentration

less than 25 mg/dL in the preterm neonate, less than 35 mg/dL for the term neonate younger than 3 days old, and less than 45 mg/dL in the term neonate older than 3 days of age. Neonates are at risk of hypoglycemia secondary to their poorly developed system for the maintenance of adequate plasma glucose concentrations. (371–372; **2104**)

69. Manifestations of hypoglycemia in neonates include irritability, seizures, bradycardia, hypotension, and apnea. These clinical manifestations may be masked by general anesthesia, making anesthesiologist vigilance very important. The immediate treatment of hypoglycemia in neonates is the intravenous administration of 0.5 to 1 g/kg glucose. (371–372; **2083, 2104**)

70. Preterm neonates are at risk of developing hypocalcemia. Hypocalcemia in the neonate is defined by a plasma calcium concentration less than 7 mg/dL. Fetuses develop their calcium stores during the third trimester, so that the preterm neonate has inadequate calcium stores at birth. (372; **2451**)

71. Hypocalcemia might occur intraoperatively as a result of citrated blood transfusions or during an exchange transfusion. The rapid infusion of citrate that occurs with citrated blood or fresh frozen plasma transfusions can result in hypotension secondary to hypocalcemia. The hypotension can be minimized by the administration of calcium gluconate, 1 to 2 mg intravenously for every 1 mL of blood transfused. (372; **2083, 2105, 2451**)

72. The signs of sepsis in the neonate include tachypnea, hypoglycemia, decreased skeletal muscle tone, and lethargy. Unlike adults, fever and leukocytosis may not be present. The signs of sepsis in the neonate are not very specific. (372; **2484**)

73. Trisomy 21, or Down syndrome, occurs in approximately 0.15% of all live births. These patients may present for surgery for correction of an associated anomaly or for a dental procedure. Anomalies associated with trisomy 21 include atrial and ventricular septal defects, patent ductus arteriosus, tetralogy of Fallot, decreased thyroid function, and duodenal atresia. (372; **974**)

74. Some preoperative considerations specific to the child with trisomy 21 include the evaluation of associated anomalies, the choice of premedication of a possibly uncooperative child, the possible need to decrease airway secretions, and a thorough airway examination. (372; **974**)

75. Hand ventilation with bag and mask may become difficult with the onset of unconsciousness in the trisomy 21 child secondary to the child's anatomic airway. Children with trisomy 21 tend to be of short stature, with a short neck, small mouth, and large tongue. Although hand ventilation with bag and mask of the trisomy 21 child may be difficult, intubation of the trachea is usually not difficult. (372; **974, 1417, Table 39–2**)

76. About 15% of children with trisomy 21 have asymptomatic atlantoaxial instability. Although spinal cord compression rarely occurs, head and neck movement during the intubation of the trachea of the trisomy 21 patient must be done with caution. (372; **974**)

77. Epiglottitis usually presents as an acute onset in difficulty swallowing, high fever, and inspiratory stridor in children aged 2 to 6 years. The children affected are characteristically sitting upright, leaning forward, drooling, have a muffled voice, and appear toxic. (372; **2465**)

78. The causative bacterium for epiglottitis is most often *Haemophilus influenzae*. (372; **2465**)

79. The supraglottic tissues are primarily involved in epiglottitis. These tissues

are inflamed and edematous. The overwhelming risk of epiglottitis is sudden, fatal total airway obstruction that can occur at any time. (372; **2465**)

80. Epiglottitis management is geared toward airway management. The concern is that inflammation and edema of the supraglottis and epiglottitis can progress rapidly to total airway obstruction. Should this occur, subsequent manual ventilation of the lungs might be difficult, as may visualization during laryngoscopy for endotracheal intubation. Children who appear to be in respiratory distress should be quickly taken to the operating room for airway management without delay for chest radiograph or other interventions. Neither the airway examination nor intubation of the trachea should proceed unless the child is in the operating room and anesthesiologists or surgeons in the operating room are prepared to proceed with an emergency tracheostomy should intubation of the trachea prove to be difficult. Intubation of the trachea is usually done under general anesthesia. Ideally, an intravenous catheter is inserted before the induction of anesthesia. The induction of anesthesia for the child with epiglottitis is usually achieved by an inhalation induction with a nonpungent volatile anesthetic such as halothane or sevoflurane in oxygen. Neuromuscular blocking drugs should not be administered until the airway is secured, because the patency of the airway may be lost with relaxation of airway muscles. Finally, epiglottitis should be treated with the appropriate antibiotics. (372–373; **2465**)

81. Epiglottitis usually resolves in 2 to 4 days. Extubation of the trachea should proceed only after resolution of the supraglottic inflammation associated with epiglottitis has been confirmed by direct laryngoscopy in the operating room. (373; **2465**)

82. Another name for croup is laryngotracheobronchitis. (372, Table 27–7; **2465**)

	EPIGLOTTITIS (SUPRAGLOTTITIS)	LARYNGOTRACHEO-BRONCHITIS
Age	2–6 years	2 years or younger
Incidence	Accounts for 5% of children with stridor	Accounts for ~80% of children with stridor
Cause	Bacterial	Viral
Onset	Rapid over 24 hours	Gradual over 24–72 hours
Signs and symptoms	Inspiratory stridor Pharyngitis Drooling Fever >39°C Lethargic to restless Tachypnea Insistent on sitting up and leaning forward	Inspiratory stridor Croupy cough Rhinorrhea Fever >39°
Lateral radiograph of the neck	Swollen epiglottis	Narrowing of the subglottic area
Treatment	Oxygen Urgent intubation of the trachea Antibiotics	Oxygen Aerosolized racemic epinephrine Humidity

83. The incidence of malignant hyperthermia in the pediatric population is approximately 1 in 12,000 pediatric anesthetics. The incidence of malignant hyperthermia in the adult population is approximately 1 in 40,000 adult anesthetics. (373; **973–974, 1033**)

84. The calcium channel is thought to be important in the pathophysiology of

malignant hyperthermia. It is believed that there is a defect in the calcium release channel in the sarcoplasmic reticulum of the skeletal muscle. This defect allows for higher concentrations of calcium to be sustained in the mycoplasm, resulting in persistent skeletal muscle contractions when a patient at risk for developing malignant hyperthermia is exposed to inciting anesthetic agents or drugs. The genetic coding site for malignant hyperthermia and the calcium release channel of skeletal muscle sarcoplasmic reticulum is the same, lending biological evidence that an association exists between them. (373; **852, 1034–1040, Figs. 27–1, 27–2**)

85. Anesthetic triggering drugs for malignant hyperthermia include succinylcholine and volatile anesthetics. (373; **1044–1045, Table 27–2**)

86. A patient who develops trismus after the administration of succinylcholine may be at risk for developing malignant hyperthermia. The trismus that develops is masseter muscle spasm and jaw rigidity associated with limb muscle paralysis. The more exaggerated and prolonged the jaw muscle rigidity, the greater is the risk of malignant hyperthermia. If rigidity of other muscles becomes apparent, anesthesia should be discontinued and the treatment for malignant hyperthermia instituted. If, however, other muscles remain flaccid, the patient should be continually monitored and possibly laboratory analysis sent. The decision of whether to continue with anesthesia under these circumstances is dictated by the urgency of the surgical procedure and the degree of jaw muscle rigidity. Alternatively, anesthesia may be continued with nontriggering agents. (373; **1043, Fig. 27–4**)

87. Clinical signs of malignant hyperthermia are related to some of the consequences of sustained skeletal muscle contraction. These include tachycardia, arterial hypoxemia, metabolic acidosis, respiratory acidosis, and increases in body temperature. Early signs of malignant hyperthermia include tachycardia and an increase in the exhaled concentration of carbon dioxide that are otherwise unexplained. A late sign of malignant hyperthermia is the increase in body temperature. (373; **1045**)

88. The primary treatment for malignant hyperthermia is dantrolene. Dantrolene inhibits the release of calcium from the sarcoplasmic reticulum. The dose of dantrolene to be administered is 2 to 3 mg/kg intravenously and repeated every 5 to 10 minutes until the symptoms are controlled. Other treatment interventions for malignant hyperthermia are directed toward supportive management. First, the inhaled anesthetic being administered should be immediately discontinued. The lungs should be hyperventilated with oxygen. For the hyperthermia, active cooling should be initiated. Active cooling may include cold saline, 15 mL/kg intravenously every 10 minutes. Gastric lavage with cold saline and surface cooling may also be used. For the severely acidotic patient, sodium bicarbonate may be administered at a dose of 1 to 2 mEq/kg intravenously, and guided by arterial pH. Diuresis of the patient should also be considered, either by hydration, mannitol, or furosemide. (373; **1046–1047**)

89. The patient at risk for malignant hyperthermia may be identified preoperatively by a detailed preoperative medical history and by a family history that especially notes any problems with anesthesia. Preoperative testing of the level of creatinine kinase is not always useful, because only about 70% of patients who are susceptible to malignant hyperthermia have increased resting levels of creatinine kinase. The definitive diagnosis of a patient's susceptibility to malignant hyperthermia requires a skeletal muscle biopsy. The skeletal muscle is then tested in vitro for isometric contracture in response to exposure to caffeine or halothane or both. (373; **852, 973–974, 1048–1049**)

90. No anesthetic regimen is known to be reliably safe for administration to patients who are susceptible to malignant hyperthermia. Some drugs that are

used in anesthesia that have not been shown to trigger malignant hyperthermia include barbiturates, opioids, benzodiazepines, propofol, etomidate, nitrous oxide, local anesthetics, and nondepolarizing neuromuscular blocking drugs. (373; **1047–1048, Table 27–2**)

91. Prophylaxis against malignant hyperthermia in a susceptible patient undergoing a surgical procedure may be achieved by the administration of dantrolene preoperatively. Dantrolene prophylaxis can be administered by the intravenous administration of 1 to 2 mg/kg before the induction of anesthesia. It is now the consensus of many that preoperative dantrolene is not necessary in susceptible patients because general anesthesia with nontriggering agents has proven to be mostly uneventful. There are multiple preparations for the operating room before anesthetizing a patient at risk for malignant hyperthermia. The vaporizers may be removed or sealed. The soda lime should be changed, and the fresh gas outlet hose may be changed. High fresh gas flows should be maintained for at least 20 minutes prior to the induction of anesthesia, and an expired gas analyzer should be utilized to confirm that traces of anesthetic gases have been purged. (373–374; **973–974, 1047–1048**)

92. Regional anesthesia is considered safe for patients at risk for malignant hyperthermia. (373; **1048**)

93. A diaphragmatic hernia is a congenital anomaly that presents as having intestinal contents occupying the chest. Almost all the abdominal viscera can be in the chest, including the liver and spleen. It results from the incomplete closure of the diaphragm in an embryological stage of development of the fetus. The defect in the diaphragm is usually on the left through the foramen of Bochdalek. In the presence of a diaphragmatic hernia there is an associated hypoplasia of the lung on the ipsilateral side. The degree of hypoplasia depends on the gestational age at which the herniation occurred. Manifestations of diaphragmatic hernias at birth include a scaphoid abdomen, respiratory distress, acidosis, and profound arterial hypoxemia. The incidence of diaphragmatic hernias is about 1 in every 5000 live births. (375; **2079, 2110**)

94. Some co-morbid conditions associated with diaphragmatic hernias include polyhydramnios, congenital heart disease, and pulmonary hypertension. (375; **2079**)

95. The diagnosis of a diaphragmatic hernia can be made in utero during ultrasonography of the fetus. The diagnosis at birth is confirmed by the clinical manifestations of the anomaly, by auscultation of intestines and decreased breath sounds over the affected lung area, and by chest radiograph. On the chest radiograph loops of intestine are seen in the affected thorax as well as a shift of the mediastinum to the opposite side. (375)

96. The immediate treatment of a diaphragmatic hernia in a neonate involves decompression of the stomach with a nasogastric tube, an awake intubation without hand ventilation of the lungs, and the administration of oxygen. Positive pressure of the lung when ventilating by hand with bag and mask can increase the volume of the gastrointestinal tract with air, further compromising pulmonary function by direct mechanical compression. This can lead to hypotension as well as worsening hypoxemia. The lungs should be ventilated with small tidal volumes at a rate of 60 to 150 breaths per minute. Hyperventilation of the lungs with oxygen can improve pulmonary blood flow by reversing the hypoxia and acidosis. The neonate with a diaphragmatic hernia in whom arterial oxygenation is difficult may require extracorporeal membrane oxygenation for stabilization before surgical intervention. Extracorporeal membrane oxygenation of these neonates has led to a decrease in the mortality of neonates with a diaphragmatic hernia. Intrauterine fetal surgery

is also being performed to treat diaphragmatic hernias earlier to allow for greater ipsilateral lung maturity. (375; **2079, 2110**)

97. Positive pressure ventilation of the lungs of a neonate with a diaphragmatic hernia can result in a pneumothorax on the contralateral side of the affected lung if peak airway pressures exceed 25 to 30 cm H_2O. Expansion of the hypoplastic lung after surgical correction of the diaphragmatic hernia should not be attempted, owing to the risk of pneumothorax or other damage to the normal lung. (375; **2079, 2110**)

98. The anesthetic management of neonates with a diaphragmatic hernia undergoing a surgical procedure should include monitoring of arterial oxygenation and the avoidance of nitrous oxide. Nitrous oxide should be avoided because it can diffuse into the loops of intestine in the chest and expand the intestines further, leading to more pulmonary compromise. (375; **2079, 2110**)

99. A tracheoesophageal fistula should be suspected when soon after birth a neonate develops cyanosis and coughing during oral feedings. The clinician should also suspect the presence of a tracheoesophageal fistula when an oral catheter cannot be passed into the stomach. (374; **2078–2079, 2109–2110**)

100. Twenty percent of neonates with a tracheoesophageal fistula have associated congenital heart disease, including ventricular septal defect, tetralogy of Fallot, and coarctation of the aorta. Tracheoesophageal fistula is also a component of the VATER (vertebral defects, imperforate anus, tracheoesophageal fistula, and radial and renal anomalies) syndrome. Prematurity accompanies tracheoesophageal fistulas about 40% of the time. (374; **2109–2110**)

101. Neonates with a tracheoesophageal fistula are at risk for pulmonary aspiration, gastric distention, and difficulty with ventilation. These neonates should have a catheter placed in the esophagus to drain secretions and prevent the accumulation of fluids in the esophageal pouch. Manual positive pressure ventilation of the lungs with a mask should be kept at a minimum to lessen the risk of gastric distention and pulmonary aspiration. When intubating the trachea of an infant with a tracheoesophageal fistula the anesthesiologist must be careful to place the endotracheal tube distal to the level of the fistula. This can be confirmed through the auscultation of decreased breath sounds over the stomach. Care should be taken to avoid endobronchial intubation as well. Attention to breath sounds, chest movement with ventilation, peak inspiratory pressures, and oxygen saturation should continue throughout the surgical procedure because small movements in the endotracheal tube can lead to its malposition. (374–375; **2078–2079, 2109–2110**)

102. Pyloric stenosis occurs as a result of hypertrophy of the pyloric smooth muscle. The hypertrophy in combination with edema of the pyloric mucosa result in progressive obstruction of the pylorus. The incidence of pyloric stenosis is 1 in every 500 live births. (374; **2109**)

103. The usual clinical scenario of an infant with pyloric stenosis is one of persistent vomiting in a male infant at 2 to 5 weeks of age. (374; **2109**)

104. The electrolyte imbalances that are commonly seen in infants with pyloric stenosis occur as a result of the loss of hydrogen ions that is associated with persistent vomiting. These electrolyte imbalances include hyponatremia, hypokalemia, hypochloremia, and metabolic alkalosis. There is often a compensatory respiratory acidosis. (374; **2109**)

105. Concerns for the anesthesiologist caring for the patient with pyloric stenosis include the metabolic abnormalities, severe dehydration, and full stomach, often with barium after a radiologic study. These all place the infant at an increased risk for morbidity perioperatively. Although pyloric stenosis is a

medical emergency, surgical correction of pyloric stenosis is an elective procedure. The corrective procedure for these infants can be done after 24 to 48 hours of intravenous fluid rehydration, the correction of their electrolyte abnormalities, and suctioning on a catheter placed in the stomach. (374; **2109**)

106. The induction of anesthesia in infants with pyloric stenosis should be preceded by the emptying of stomach contents with a catheter to minimize the risk of the pulmonary aspiration of gastric contents. Induction should then be done in a rapid sequence fashion with cricoid pressure. Alternatively, an awake intubation may be performed. Extubation of the trachea after the procedure should only be performed when the infant is awake and vigorous because postoperative depression of ventilation is frequently seen in these infants. (374; **2109**)

Chapter 27

Elderly Patients

1. Why are elderly patients at a greater risk of perioperative complications?

2. Why is the risk of perioperative complications in the elderly increased in emergency surgery?

PSYCHOLOGICAL FACTORS

3. What psychological concerns might elderly patients face preoperatively that are specific to their age group?

4. How might chronic endogenous depression be distinguished from an acute short-term reactive depression in the elderly patient scheduled to undergo a surgical procedure?

PHYSIOLOGY

5. How is organ function in general affected by aging? How might this affect the elderly patient in the perioperative period?

6. Name some age-related diseases seen in elderly patients.

7. What age-related changes in the central and peripheral nervous systems occur in the elderly? How does this affect the minimum alveolar concentration (MAC) of anesthesia in the elderly patient?

8. What age-related changes in systolic blood pressure, heart rate, cardiac output, stroke volume, and cardiac conduction occur in the elderly?

9. How do drug-induced heart rate changes in the elderly compare with the heart rate response seen in younger patients administered the same drugs?

10. How do reflex-mediated heart rate increases in response to hypotension differ between elderly and younger patients?

11. What age-related changes in gas exchange, Pao_2, $A - aDo_2$, and the ventilation-to-perfusion ratio occur in the elderly?

12. What age-related changes in vital capacity, forced exhaled volume in 1 second, residual volume, and functional residual capacity occur in the elderly?

13. How do ventilatory responses to hypoxia and hypercapnia change with age? Why is this particularly important to the anesthesiologist?

14. Why does pneumonia occur at an increased frequency in elderly patients?

15. What age-related changes in renal blood flow, glomerular filtration rate, and urine-concentrating ability occur in the elderly? What clinical implications does this have?

16. How do plasma concentrations of creatinine change with age?

17. What age-related change in hepatic blood flow occurs in the elderly? What clinical implication does this have?

18. How does the production of albumin change with age? What clinical implication does this have?

19. What age-related changes in esophageal and intestinal motility and gastroesophageal sphincter tone occur in the elderly? What clinical implications do these have?

20. What are some diseases of the endocrine system that occur more frequently in the elderly?

21. What is subclinical hypothyroidism? What is its prevalence in the elderly population?

22. What clinical relevance do the age-related loss of collagen and decreases in skin elasticity have for the anesthesiologist caring for the elderly patient?

23. What clinical relevance do osteoporosis, osteoarthritis, and rheumatoid arthritis have for the anesthesiologist caring for the elderly patient?

PHARMACODYNAMICS

24. How are pharmacodynamic changes in the elderly reflected with regard to inhaled anesthetics? With regard to opioids?

25. How are pharmacodynamic changes in the elderly reflected with regard to nondepolarizing neuromuscular blocking drugs?

26. How are pharmacodynamic changes in the elderly reflected with regard to thiopental?

PHARMACOLOGY

27. What pharmacokinetic changes in the elderly make them susceptible to cumulative drug effects and adverse drug reactions?

28. What age-related changes in the elderly result in a decreased clearance of drugs? Give some examples of drugs whose elimination times may be affected by these.

29. What age-related changes in the elderly result in changes in the volume of distribution? Give some examples of drugs whose pharmacokinetic properties may be altered by these changes.

MANAGEMENT OF ANESTHESIA

30. What are some elements of the preoperative evaluation that are of particular relevance to elderly patients?

31. In an awake, elderly patient, what can orthostatic hypotension without an associated increase in heart rate be indicative of?

32. What might changes in mental status that occur with extension and rotation of the head be a reflection of?

33. Why should preoperative anxiolytics be used sparingly in the elderly population? What can be used as a substitute?

34. Why might electrolyte abnormalities be present in preoperative laboratory tests?

35. Why might hand ventilation by bag and mask be difficult in the edentulous patient?

36. Why might intubation be difficult in a patient with poor dentition or cervical arthritis?

37. How should the induction dose of anesthetic be altered in the elderly patient?

38. Are there any unique risks to the elderly with the reversal of nondepolarizing neuromuscular blocking drugs with anticholinesterase drugs?

39. What are some postoperative risks that elderly patients are more prone to than younger patients?

40. What types of procedures that elderly patients are likely to undergo might warrant regional anesthesia as an alternative to general anesthesia?

41. What is the advantage to maintaining consciousness in the elderly patient during a regional anesthetic for a surgical procedure?

42. What is an advantage that regional anesthesia may have over general anesthesia for hip surgery in elderly patients?

43. What are some reasons why elderly patients may be more sensitive than younger patients to regional anesthesia?

44. How might the hypotensive effects of a sympathectomy resulting from regional anesthesia be attenuated?

45. What advantage does epidural anesthesia have over spinal anesthesia that can be of particular benefit in the elderly population?

POSTOPERATIVE MENTAL DYSFUNCTION (DELIRIUM)

46. How frequently is postoperative delirium thought to occur in elderly patients?

47. When is postoperative delirium in the elderly patient most likely to present?

48. What are some possible clinical manifestations of postoperative delirium in the elderly patient?

49. How can postoperative delirium be distinguished from dementia in the elderly patient?

50. What are some causes of postoperative delirium?

51. What surgical procedures are most commonly associated with postoperative delirium in the elderly?

52. How is the risk of postoperative delirium in elderly patients altered by whether the surgical procedure was done under general anesthesia or regional anesthesia?

ANSWERS*

1. Elderly patients who require surgery are at a greater risk of perioperative complications than their younger counterparts. This is due to diseases and generalized decreases in organ function that are age related and are thus more likely to be present in the elderly. Some examples include a generalized decrease in maximal breathing capacity, vital capacity, cardiac index, glomerular filtration rate, and basal metabolic rate. In addition, decreases in the elderly patient's level of activity may lead to an inability of the cardiovascular system to respond to perioperative stressors. Age-related diseases are the most likely cause of perioperative complications or perioperative death, rather than the age of the patient itself. (376, Fig. 28–2; **2152, Fig. 61–10**)

2. Elderly patients are particularly at risk for perioperative complications in cases of emergency surgery for many reasons. The cause of the emergency itself may be compromising the patient's physiologic status, such as by hemorrhage or dehydration. In addition, emergency cases preclude the preoperative time necessary to control co-existing diseases and maximize organ function. (376; **2152**)

PSYCHOLOGICAL FACTORS

3. Elderly patients may be experiencing a number of psychological concerns before surgery in addition to the concerns that are common to all individuals facing

---

*Numbers in parentheses: lightface numbers refer to pages, figures, or tables in Stoelting RK, Miller RD: Basics of Anesthesia, 4th ed. Philadelphia, Churchill Livingstone, 2000; **boldface numbers** refer to pages, figures, or tables in Miller RD: Anesthesia, 5th ed. Philadelphia, Churchill Livingstone, 2000.

surgery. Psychological concerns that are more specific to the elderly patient include the concern for the potential loss of function and independence, concern about the possibility of death, and fear that the potential disability resulting from the current illness will lead to long-term institutionalization and disability postoperatively. A further compounding factor for the elderly is the sensory and social isolation that may occur perioperatively. (376; **2150–2151**)

4. Chronic endogenous depression may be distinguished from an acute short-term reactive depression in the elderly patient by a careful history and physical examination elicited by an aware anesthesiologist. Chronic endogenous depression is more likely to have the hallmark features associated with it, such as poor appetite resulting in weight loss, agitation, anhedonia, lethargy, and suicidal ideation. (376; **2150–2151**)

PHYSIOLOGY

5. Organ function, in general, declines with age. The decline in organ function associated with aging in the elderly has been characterized as a decline in the ability of the elderly patient's organs to adapt, or compensate, in response to acute stressors. The perioperative period is associated with stressors on numerous organs, making elderly patients at risk for organ dysfunction during this time. (376; **2140–2142, Fig. 61–1, Table 61–1**)

6. Age-related diseases seen in elderly patients include systemic hypertension, coronary artery disease, congestive heart failure, peripheral vascular disease, chronic obstructive pulmonary disease, anemia, renal disease, diabetes mellitus, subclinical hypothyroidism, arthritis, and dementia. (376, Fig. 28–2, **2141, Table 61–1**)

7. Age-related changes occur in both the central and peripheral nervous systems of elderly people. In the central nervous system there is a progressive decline in central nervous system activity and a loss of neurons. This is especially marked in the cerebral cortex and is reflected as a reduction of brain size in radiographic studies. Cerebral blood flow decreases in proportion to decreases in cerebral mass. The autoregulation of cerebral blood flow remains intact. In the peripheral nervous system there is a decrease in the conduction velocity of peripheral nerves and possibly a decrease in the number of fibers in spinal cord tracts as well. This is reflected in the increase in the thresholds for the perception of stimuli from virtually all the senses, including pain. The decrease in the number of motor nerves is offset by the increase in the number of cholinergic receptors at the neuromuscular junction. These physiologic changes in the central and peripheral nervous systems of elderly people result in a decrease in the minimum alveolar concentration (MAC) by as much as 30% from young adult values. This corresponds to a decreased dose of volatile anesthetic required to achieve a given physiologic central nervous system response in elderly patients. (377, Fig. 28–5; **2144–2148, Figs. 61–4, 61–5, Tables 61–1, 61–2**)

8. Age-related changes in the cardiovascular system of elderly people include an increase in blood pressure, a decrease in heart rate, a decrease in cardiac output, no significant change in stroke volume, and possible aberrance in cardiac conduction. Systemic blood pressure is thought to increase with age as a result of the decrease in compliance of arterial walls. Heart rate is thought to decrease as a result of a predominance of parasympathetic nervous system activity. Cardiac output is thought to decrease as a result of the decrease in tissue mass and perfusion requirements in elderly patients. Cardiac output further decreases with the sedentary lifestyle and decrease in physical conditioning that is frequently seen in elderly people. The decrease in cardiac output does not appear to occur in elderly patients who have maintained physical fitness. An aberrant cardiac conduction system may result from the unavoidable degenerative changes associated with age. (377, Fig. 28–3; **2148–2149, Table 61–1**)

9. The plasma concentration of adrenergic agents required to produce a specific cardiovascular response is increased in the elderly. When drugs such as isoproterenol or propranolol are administered to elderly patients their change in heart rate is less prominent than the changes in heart rate seen when the same drugs are administered to younger patients. This is believed to be due to a decrease in the elderly patient's responsiveness at the beta-adrenergic receptor. Although this was believed to be due to a decrease in the number of beta-adrenergic receptors in elderly patients, this has not been demonstrated. The decrease in responsiveness may occur secondary to a reduced affinity of beta-adrenergic agents for the receptor and/or the impairment of adenylate cyclase activation. This same effect of decreased cardiovascular response has also been noted with the administration of atropine and alpha-adrenergic agonists. (377; **2146–2147**)

10. When hypotension occurs in younger patients, there is a reflex-mediated increase in heart rate that occurs to help offset the physiologic effects of the hypotension. In the elderly patient the reflex-mediated increase in heart rate in response to hypotension is much less pronounced. (377–378; **2146–2147, Table 61–1**)

11. There is an age-related decrease in gas exchange in the elderly patient. The most significant age-related change in the lung of the elderly patient is a deterioration of lung elastin. As a result of the degenerative changes in the lungs, there is a breakdown of alveolar septa. This is accompanied by an increase in both anatomic and alveolar deadspace and an increase in ventilation-to-perfusion mismatch. These are reflected by an increase in the $A - aDo_2$ and a decrease in the Pao_2 by about 0.5 mm Hg per year after 20 years of age. There are no age-related changes in the $Paco_2$. (378, Fig. 28–4; **2149–2150, Figs. 61–6, 61–7, Table 61–1**)

12. Age-related changes in the pulmonary system of elderly people include a decrease in vital capacity, a decrease in the forced exhaled volume in 1 second, an increase in residual volume, and an increase in functional residual capacity. These occur as a result of the decreased elasticity of the lungs and increased stiffness of the thorax. (378–379; **2149–2150, Table 61–1**)

13. Elderly patients have a decreased ventilatory response to hypercapnia and hypoxia. When compared with younger patients this response can be decreased by about one half. It is important that the anesthesiologist be cognizant of this, because this response is further decreased by the administration of opioids and inhaled anesthetics. (378; **2149–2150**)

14. Elderly patients have decreases in pulmonary reserves; a decreased level of laryngeal, pharyngeal, and airway cough reflexes; and an increased propensity to aspirate pharyngeal secretions. Elderly patients also have depressed immune function, probably due to involution of the thymus gland and altered function of T lymphocytes. Together these may explain the increased risk of pulmonary aspiration and an increased incidence of pneumonia in elderly patients when compared with younger patients. (379; **2154**)

15. Decreases in renal blood flow, glomerular filtration rates, and urine-concentrating abilities accompany aging. These changes are due to alterations in the renal vasculature and may be at least partially due to the age-related decrease in cardiac output. There are also progressive decreases in the total number of nephrons and glomeruli units with age. Clinically, this has some implications for the anesthesiologist caring for the elderly patient. First, elderly patients may be more sensitive to and less able to adapt to fluid deprivation or fluid overload. Second, the elderly may be at an increased risk for renal ischemia in the perioperative period. Finally, drugs that are cleared renally may have a prolonged duration of effect, thereby decreasing the dose requirements of these drugs in the elderly patient. (379; **2143–2144, Table 61–1**)

16. Plasma creatinine concentrations do not change with age. Although renal function decreases with age, the increase in creatinine that would subsequently be expected in the elderly population is offset by the decrease in creatinine levels that results from decreases in muscle mass often seen in this population. There is a decreased production of creatinine secondary to this decrease in muscle mass. (379; **2144, Fig. 61–3**)

17. Decreases in hepatic blood flow are seen in the elderly as a direct result of decreases in hepatic tissue mass and decreases in cardiac output. Clinically, a delayed clearance of hepatically cleared drugs may result from the decrease in hepatic blood flow in elderly patients. Drugs that may be affected include opiates, barbiturates, benzodiazepines, propofol, etomidate, and most nondepolarizing neuromuscular blocking drugs. (379; **2143, 2147, Tables 61–1 and 61–2**)

18. The production of albumin is decreased in the elderly. Clinically, this may result in a decrease in the binding of drugs administered to elderly patients, and an increase in the free, active portion of the drug. (379; **2143**)

19. Esophageal and intestinal motility decrease with age, as does gastroesophageal sphincter tone. Clinically, these age-related changes in gastrointestinal function may lead to an increased risk of pulmonary aspiration in elderly patients undergoing general anesthesia. (379; **2154**)

20. Diabetes mellitus and hypothyroidism occur with an increased frequency in the elderly. Adrenal gland mass and associated cortisol secretion decrease with age. (379; **2146**)

21. Subclinical hypothyroidism is hypothyroidism that is detected by increased levels of plasma thyroid stimulating hormone, without any obvious clinical signs of hypothyroidism. It is believed that subclinical hypothyroidism is present in as many as 13% of elderly patients who are otherwise healthy. Elderly females are especially at risk of subclinical hypothyroidism. (379; **929–930**)

22. A loss of collagen and decreases in the elasticity of the skin of elderly people put them at an increased risk of sustaining injury to their skin during surgical procedures, particularly during prolonged procedures. Elderly patients are vulnerable to sustaining decubitus ulcers and injury during the removal of adhesive electrocardiogram pads or tape. (379; **2154**)

23. Osteoporosis, osteoarthritis, and rheumatoid arthritis occur most frequently in elderly people. These diseases must be considered while positioning the patient for a surgical procedure, as well as while positioning the head and neck for intubation of the trachea. Intubation of the trachea may be more difficult as a result of these diseases. (379; **2154**)

PHARMACODYNAMICS

24. Pharmacodynamic changes in the elderly are reflected by the plasma concentration of a drug required to produce a specific effect. In the case of inhaled anesthetics, opioids, and benzodiazepines the plasma concentration of these drugs required to produce a specific effect in an elderly person is decreased from that of younger counterparts. The dose of fentanyl and alfentanil required to achieve a given effect in elderly patients may be decreased by as much as 50% of the dose required for the same effect in young adults. The increased sensitivity to anesthetics seen in elderly patients parallels the decrease in cerebral cortex tissue mass and cerebral metabolic rate. This is subsequently reflected as a decrease in the MAC of anesthesia in elderly patients. (379, 381–382; **2147–2148, Table 61–2**)

25. The plasma concentration of nondepolarizing neuromuscular blocking drugs

required to produce a specific twitch response effect is similar in both elderly people and younger people. This implies that the sensitivity of elderly patients to nondepolarizing neuromuscular blocking drugs does not change with age. (380, 382; **456–457, 2146, Table 61–2**)

26. The plasma concentrations of thiopental, propofol, and etomidate required to produce a specific response is similar in both elderly people and younger people. (380–381; **211–214, 2147, 2153, Table 61–2**)

PHARMACOLOGY

27. Pharmacokinetic variables explain the concentration of the drug at the site of action in relation to the dose of drug administered. Pharmacokinetic changes in the elderly that make them susceptible to cumulative drug effects and adverse drug reactions include decreases in drug clearance and changes in the volume of distribution. (380–381; **2147, Table 61–2**)

28. A decreased clearance of drugs in the elderly can be attributed to decreases in renal blood flow, decreases in the glomerular filtration rate, decreases in hepatic blood flow, and decreases in hepatic microsomal enzyme activity. Decreases in renal blood flow and decreases in glomerular filtration rate together may result in the prolongation of the effects of pancuronium, digoxin, and several antibiotics in elderly patients who have been administered these drugs. Likewise, decreases in hepatic blood flow and decreases in hepatic microsomal enzyme activity together may result in the prolongation of the effects of vecuronium, lidocaine, propofol, and propranolol in elderly patients. (381; **2147, Table 61–2**)

29. The volume of distribution can be divided into the central volume of distribution and the peripheral volume of distribution. The central volume of distribution refers to the volume of the heart and great vessels and the venous volume. A decreased central volume of distribution in the elderly refers to an increased initial concentration of drug in the plasma after a bolus injection. The decrease in the central volume of distribution has been thought to be due to decreases in total body water in elderly patients. More recently, this theory has come under scrutiny. Nevertheless, higher initial plasma concentrations of drug after the initial bolus of conventional doses of the drug are seen in elderly patients. Drugs that are affected in this manner include thiopental, propofol, and etomidate when administered for the induction of anesthesia, as well as the initial bolus of opioids. In fact, it has been estimated that elderly patients require about 15% less of a drug dose of thiopental or propofol as a bolus for the induction of anesthesia. The peripheral volume of distribution includes additional volumes of distribution attached to the central volume. The peripheral volume of distribution in elderly patients is increased due to a relative increase in body fat and a decrease in the amount of drug bound by protein. The increased peripheral volume of distribution may also be reflected as a delay in the rate of elimination of lipid-soluble drugs that are stored in fat, such as opioids and the volatile anesthetics. (381–382; **16–17, 211–214, 2147, Table 61–2**)

MANAGEMENT OF ANESTHESIA

30. The preoperative evaluation of the elderly patient scheduled to undergo a surgical procedure should include the routine preoperative elements for any other patients. Specific to the elderly patient, emphasis should be placed on the presence of any co-existing diseases and their effects on organ function. Included is the patient's level of mentation, or any recent change in mental function. Additionally, the drugs and their doses taken by elderly patients must be thoroughly evaluated, possibly even by having the patient bring the vials to the hospital on the day of surgery or admission. Elderly patients are more likely

to be taking several medicines together, which may have an effect on them intraoperatively. Finally, drug and alcohol dependence must also be considered in the elderly patient scheduled for surgery. (382, Table 28–2; **2151–2152**)

31. In an awake, elderly patient being evaluated for orthostatic hypotension, the lack of an increase in heart rate on assuming the upright position in the presence of hypotension may be reflective of a sympathetic nervous system that is not appropriately functioning. The cause of the sympathetic nervous system dysfunction may be secondary to aging, co-existing disease, or drugs. (382; **2147**)

32. The elderly patient who experiences changes in mental status with extension and rotation of the head may have vertebrobasilar insufficiency or cervical osteoarthritis. (383)

33. Preoperative anxiolytics should be used sparingly in the elderly population, because they can cause undesirable levels of sedation and confusion in these patients. In addition, the residual effects of these medicines may persist even after the surgical case has been completed. In lieu of the preoperative anxiolytic medicines, a detailed explanation of the events that will occur before and after the surgical procedure may be a useful anxiolytic substitute. (382; **2153**)

34. Electrolyte abnormalities present in preoperative laboratory tests of elderly patients may occur as a result of medicines taken by the elderly patient, as well as of decreases in organ function. (383; **2151–2153**)

35. Hand ventilation by bag and mask may be difficult in the edentulous patient secondary to a poor mask-to-face fit. It is often easier to hand ventilate by bag and mask when the edentulous patient's dentures are left in place. (383; **1420**)

36. Patients with poor dentition may be difficult to intubate because of the need to avoid loose teeth during direct laryngoscopy to avoid dislodgment of the teeth. Patients with cervical arthritis may be difficult to intubate because of the decreased range of motion, especially extension, of the neck. (383; **1417, 2127**)

37. The induction dose of anesthetic in the elderly patient is generally decreased from the induction dose for a younger counterpart. This is for pharmacokinetic reasons. This means that less drug is necessary because the elderly patient's clearance of the drug and the central volume of distribution are decreased. The net result of this is that the drug administered for induction exerts its pharmacologic effects in the circulation for a longer amount of time. The induction dose of anesthetic in the elderly patient is not decreased for pharmacodynamic reasons, because the plasma concentration of induction drug required to produce a desired effect is equal in elderly and younger patients. (381, 383–384; **211–214, 2147, 2153, Table 61–2**)

38. The reversal of nondepolarizing neuromuscular blocking drugs in the elderly patient does not warrant any special considerations for the anesthesiologist, because there are not any unique risks of this in the elderly patient population. The incidence of cardiac dysrhythmias after the administration of neostigmine may be increased in elderly patients who have cardiovascular disease, however. (384; **2153**)

39. Some postoperative risks that elderly patients are more prone to than younger patients are generally those of organ dysfunction. Organ dysfunction of the cardiovascular system may manifest as myocardial ischemia or angina. Elderly patients are also more likely to develop pneumonia postoperatively than younger patients. Organ dysfunction of the pulmonary system may manifest as arterial hypoxemia. Elderly patients may also experience central nervous system changes perioperatively, such as confusion or memory loss. Early ambulation

may minimize the risk of pulmonary dysfunction in the perioperative period. It decreases the risk of a deep venous thrombosis as well. (384; **2151–2154**)

40. Regional anesthesia is an alternative to general anesthesia for elderly patients undergoing surgical procedures such as transurethral resection of the prostate, gynecologic procedures, inguinal hernia repair, or the treatment of hip fractures. (384; **2153**)

41. An advantage to maintaining consciousness in the elderly patient during a regional anesthetic for a surgical procedure is that the anesthesiologist is able to communicate with the patient during the procedure. This may allow for an earlier detection of changes in mentation or of myocardial ischemia presenting as angina. Additionally, there may be decreased immediate postoperative confusion in elderly patients after having received a regional anesthetic as compared with a general anesthetic. (384; **2153**)

42. Regional anesthesia for hip surgery may be associated with decreases in perioperative blood loss and decreases in the incidence of deep venous thrombosis in elderly patients. (384; **2132–2133**)

43. Elderly patients may be more sensitive than younger patients to regional anesthesia, especially spinal anesthesia. Possible reasons why this may be true include decreased vascular absorption from the spinal space, decreases in vertebral column length, and a decreased reflex compensatory sympathetic nervous system response. Together, these may manifest as a prolonged duration of action and exaggerated decreases in blood pressure. (384; **1505, 2147, 2153, Table 42–5**)

44. Attenuation of the hypotensive effects of a regional anesthetic may be achieved by the prophylactic administration of an intramuscular dose of ephedrine before administering the spinal anesthetic. Adequate hydration minimizes the effects of a sympathectomy on blood pressure. (384; **1496–1497**)

45. Epidural anesthesia may be administered more slowly than a spinal anesthetic, with the onset of the resulting sympathectomy being more gradual. This may result in a more gradual decrease in the elderly patient's blood pressure than that seen with a spinal anesthetic. (384; **1496–1497, 2153**)

POSTOPERATIVE MENTAL DYSFUNCTION (DELIRIUM)

46. Postoperative delirium has been estimated to occur in 10% to 15% of elderly patients undergoing surgical procedures. Postoperative delirium is thus one of the most common postoperative complications in the elderly. (384; **2154, 2341**)

47. Postoperative delirium is most likely to present one or more days after surgery. This type of delirium is termed *interval delirium*. This is in contrast to *emergence delirium* commonly seen in pediatric patients that occurs within minutes after the emergence from anesthesia. (384; **2154, 2341**)

48. Clinical manifestations of postoperative delirium may include alterations in attention, cognition, and sleep-wake cycles; a reduced level of consciousness; and increases or decreases in psychomotor behavior. These patients are often disoriented to time, place, and person. Close monitoring of these patients is essential to prevent patients from harming themselves by attempting to get out of bed or by pulling out catheters. (384; **2154, 2341**)

49. In the elderly patient it is important to distinguish postoperative delirium, a potentially reversible state, from dementia, a chronic, progressive state. Delirium is characterized as being acute in onset and often transient and most often occurring in the evening hours before bedtime. Dementia, on the other hand, is a chronic state that likely was present before surgery. It is characterized by

global cognitive impairment. A common cause of dementia in the elderly is Alzheimer's disease. (384; **2150, 2154**)

50. Causes of postoperative delirium include drug toxicity, fluid and electrolyte imbalances, and underlying medical problems such as myocardial ischemia, congestive heart failure, or infection. Antiparkinsonian drugs, antihypertensives, and psychotropic medications tend to increase the risk of drug interactions with anesthetics and postoperative analgesics to produce postoperative delirium. A deficiency of neurotransmitters such as acetylcholine and dopamine is hypothesized to be the underlying physiologic cause of postoperative delirium. (384–385; **2341, 2154**)

51. Surgical procedures of the hip are most commonly associated with postoperative delirium in the elderly, particularly femoral neck fractures. Other surgical procedures associated with postoperative delirium in the elderly include ophthalmologic and cardiac procedures. Delirium associated with cardiac surgery may be due to cerebral hypoperfusion or air microemboli occurring during cardiopulmonary bypass. (385; **2341, 2154**)

52. The risk of postoperative delirium in elderly patients is not altered by whether the surgical procedure was done under general anesthesia or regional anesthesia. (384–385; **2154**)

Chapter 28

Organ Transplantation

1. What organs may be transplanted?

2. How is the diagnosis of brain death made?

3. What are some goals of the anesthetic management of organ harvest procedures?

4. How are donor organs generally preserved after harvest?

5. What are some immunosuppressive agents commonly taken by transplant recipients? What are some side effects of these agents?

6. What is the most common cause of death in organ transplant recipients?

RENAL TRANSPLANTATION

7. Who is a candidate for renal transplantation?

8. How long can kidneys from cadaver donors be preserved before transplantation?

9. Where is the donor kidney transplanted in the recipient patient? From where does it derive its vascular supply? Where is the ureter anastomosed?

10. What are the preoperative considerations for the patient scheduled to undergo renal transplantation?

11. Why is general anesthesia preferred for renal transplantation over regional anesthesia?

12. What is the usual general anesthetic regimen administered for renal transplantation?

13. What consideration must be made when selecting a neuromuscular blocking drug for patients undergoing renal transplantation?

14. How well does a newly transplanted kidney clear drugs eliminated renally?

15. Why is optimal hydration necessary in renal transplant procedures? What type of crystalloid solution should be used for hydration? What monitoring method may be used to help guide hydration intraoperatively for renal transplantation?

16. Why is dopamine often administered intraoperatively during renal transplant procedures?

17. Why is mannitol administered intraoperatively during renal transplant procedures?

18. Cardiac arrest after completion of the renal artery anastomosis is thought to be secondary to what?

19. What hemodynamic change may be noted after unclamping of the iliac vessels?

20. How does an acute immunologic reaction to the newly transplanted kidney manifest? What is the treatment?

21. How might a postoperative hematoma present after renal transplantation?

LIVER TRANSPLANTATION

22. Who is a candidate for liver transplantation?

23. How well can cadaver livers be maintained before transplantation? How urgent are liver transplant procedures?

24. What physiologic disturbances are often present in patients before urgent liver transplantation?

25. What types of monitoring may be used intraoperatively during liver transplantation?

26. What types of intravenous access are typically established preoperatively for liver transplant procedures? Why should placement be supradiaphragmatic?

27. Why are cell-saver devices used intraoperatively for liver transplantation?

28. Why is calcium administration often required during liver transplantation?

29. What are the three stages of liver transplant procedures?

30. What are the characteristic physiologic derangements of the preanhepatic stage of liver transplant procedures?

31. What are the characteristic physiologic derangements of the anhepatic stage of liver transplant procedures?

32. What are the characteristic physiologic derangements of the neohepatic stage of liver transplant procedures?

33. What are some types of coagulopathies that can occur during a liver transplant procedure?

34. What can result from the metabolic acidosis that occurs in patients undergoing a liver transplant procedure?

35. What is the clinical significance of the prolongation of action of succinylcholine when used for intubation of the trachea?

36. Why is nitrous oxide avoided for maintenance anesthesia during liver transplantation?

37. Why is cisatracurium often selected as the nondepolarizing neuromuscular blocking drug of choice for liver transplant procedures?

38. When is extubation of the trachea after liver transplant surgery performed?

39. How does an acute immunologic reaction to the newly transplanted liver manifest? What other complications must be ruled out before making the diagnosis?

HEART TRANSPLANTATION

40. Who is a candidate for heart transplantation? What ejection fraction is commonly seen in patients undergoing heart transplantation?

41. How long can cadaver hearts be preserved before transplantation?

42. How might the induction and maintenance of anesthesia be achieved for heart transplantation?

43. Why is nitrous oxide often avoided for maintenance anesthesia during heart transplantation?

44. What vessels are transected and anastomosed during cardiac surgery? What does this mean with regard to a central venous or pulmonary artery catheter?

45. When the left internal jugular vein is catheterized for intravenous access, what might the right internal jugular vein be used for in the postoperative period?

46. Why might isoproterenol be indicated for administration during heart transplantation?

47. Does the transplanted heart react better to catecholamines that are direct or indirect acting?

48. Approximately what percentage of patients get coronary artery disease within 3 years of heart transplantation?

LUNG TRANSPLANTATION

49. Who is a candidate for single-lung transplantation? Who is a candidate for double-lung transplantation?

50. How urgent are lung transplant procedures?

51. What type of endotracheal tube is used in lung transplant procedures?

52. What are some intraoperative problems the anesthesiologist may encounter during lung transplant procedures?

53. When is extubation of the trachea performed after a lung transplant procedure?

54. Why are lung transplant patients predisposed to developing pneumonia in the transplanted lung?

PANCREAS TRANSPLANTATION

55. Who is a candidate for pancreas transplantation?

56. How is the success of a pancreas transplant measured postoperatively?

BONE MARROW TRANSPLANTATION

57. Who is a candidate for bone marrow transplantation?

58. How is bone marrow ablation achieved in the bone marrow recipient?

59. How is bone marrow harvested from a bone marrow donor?

60. Is general anesthesia or regional anesthesia used for bone marrow harvest procedures?

61. Why may nitrous oxide administration be avoided during bone marrow harvest procedures? What is the evidence for this?

62. How is intraoperative blood loss estimated during bone marrow harvest surgery?

ANSWERS*

1. Organs that may be transplanted in selected humans include the heart, kidneys, liver, lungs, and pancreas. The bone marrow may also be transplanted for certain forms of cancer. (386; **1977–1978**)

2. The diagnosis of brain death is based on the loss of cerebral cortical function, the loss of brain stem function, and supporting evidence from clinical studies. The loss of cerebral cortical function is implied from unconsciousness, the lack of spontaneous movement, and unresponsiveness to external stimuli. The loss of brain stem function is implied from apnea and absent cranial nerve reflexes. Clinical studies that may be performed to provide supporting evidence include an electroencephalogram or cerebral blood flow studies. Irreversibility of the diagnosis of brain death should also be established. This is usually achieved by the lack of any improvement in 12 to 24 hours after the diagnosis. Other derangements that must be excluded include central drug effects, postictal states, cardiovascular or metabolic instability, or hypothermia. The diagnosis of brain

---

*Numbers in parentheses: lightface numbers refer to pages, figures, or tables in Stoelting RK, Miller RD: Basics of Anesthesia, 4th ed. Philadelphia, Churchill Livingstone, 2000; **boldface numbers** refer to pages, figures, or tables in Miller RD: Anesthesia, 5th ed. Philadelphia, Churchill Livingstone, 2000.

death is always made before a donor procedure and never in the operating room. (386; **1979–1980, 2560–2570, Table 53–3**)

3. Goals of the anesthetic management of organ harvest procedures are to maintain physiologic stability and thus organ viability until the organs are harvested. Arterial oxygenation, systemic blood pressure, cardiac dysrhythmias, and hypothermia must all be controlled by the anesthesiologist. In many cases these treatments were instituted before arrival in the operating room and must be continued throughout the procedure. Hypotension is frequently present due to the loss of control from central vasomotor centers compounded by diuresis. Dopamine is preferred over phenylephrine for the treatment of hypotension because dopamine better preserves splanchnic perfusion. Reflex hypertension may accompany surgery. The surgical goal of the procedure is to minimize the time of warm ischemia and surgical trauma to the organs. (386; **1979–1980, 2561–2564**)

4. After harvest, donor organs need to be protected from ischemia. Donor organs are generally preserved through hypothermia and the use of preservative solutions. Hypothermia decreases cellular metabolism. The preservative solutions often contain electrolytes and chemical additives that provide energy, prevent vasospasm, and prevent the accumulation of toxic metabolites. (386; **1977–1978**)

5. Immunosuppressive agents commonly taken by transplant recipients include cyclosporine, azathioprine, corticosteroids, and antilymphocyte globulin. Cyclosporine can cause hypertension, nephrotoxicity through glomerulosclerosis, hepatocellular damage and elevated liver function test results, tremors, seizures, and confusion. Azathioprine can cause anemia, thrombocytopenia, leukopenia, hepatocellular damage, pancreatic damage, and decreased requirements for nondepolarizing neuromuscular blocking drugs. Corticosteroids can cause glucose intolerance, adrenal suppression, osteonecrosis, and peptic ulcer disease. Antilymphocyte globulin can cause leukopenia and thrombocytopenia. (386–387; **1975–1976, Table 55–2**)

6. The most common cause of death in patients who have received a transplant and are on chronic immunosuppressive agents is infection, most commonly a bacterial infection. This is an important point for the anesthesiologist caring for the patient during the transplant procedure as well as on subsequent occasions, because strict asepsis is of extreme importance in these patients. (386)

RENAL TRANSPLANTATION

7. Kidneys are the most commonly transplanted major organ. Patients who have end-stage renal disease and are chronically on dialysis are candidates for renal transplantation. Transplantation has led to lower overall morbidity and mortality than dialysis and to longer survival. The most common cause of end-stage renal disease leading to chronic dialysis dependence is diabetes mellitus. (387; **1981, Table 55–1**)

8. Kidneys from cadaver donors can be preserved for 24 to 72 hours after harvest for transplantation into the recipient. Living-related renal transplantation procedures are elective procedures. (387; **1982**)

9. The kidney is transplanted on one side of the recipient's lower abdomen. The vascular supply for the transplanted kidney is derived from the iliac vessels. The ureter of the transplanted kidney is anastomosed directly to the recipient patient's bladder. (387; **1983**)

10. Preoperative considerations for the patient scheduled to undergo a renal transplant are similar to any other surgical procedure in which the patient has chronic renal failure. This includes scheduling of hemodialysis directly before surgery

to optimize the patient's status with regard to coagulation capacity, hydration, electrolytes, and acid-base balance. The serum glucose levels of the patient with diabetes mellitus should also be evaluated before and during kidney transplant procedures. (387; **1982–1983**)

11. General anesthesia is the usual preferred method for anesthetizing patients undergoing renal transplantation. This is because of the disadvantages of regional anesthesia. First, with regional anesthesia the blockade of the peripheral sympathetic nervous system leads to unpredictable control of the patient's blood pressure as well as unpredictable perfusion of the transplanted kidney. Second, renal transplant procedures are of such a duration that extensive supplementary injected or inhaled anesthetics may be necessary. Third, the level of anesthesia required for regional anesthesia, surgical retractors in the abdomen, and intravenous sedation combined may lead to decreased tidal volumes and hypoventilation. Finally, regional anesthesia may place the patient with chronic renal failure at an increased risk of an epidural hematoma secondary to a potentially abnormal coagulation status. (387; **1983**)

12. The usual general anesthetic regimen for renal transplant procedures is that of a volatile anesthetic in combination with a short-acting opioid. Nitrous oxide may be avoided, owing to its potential to distend the bowel. (387; **1983**)

13. When selecting a neuromuscular blocking drug for the patient undergoing renal transplantation, consideration should be given to the method of clearance of the various neuromuscular blocking drugs. A neuromuscular blocking drug that does not rely primarily on renal clearance should be selected. Cisatracurium, for example, is among the possible neuromuscular blocking drugs that may be selected. (387–388; **1983**)

14. A newly transplanted kidney that is functioning well is able to clear drugs that are eliminated by glomerular filtration. Evaluation of the function of the newly transplanted kidney is most easily accomplished by monitoring urine output. (388; **1983**)

15. Optimal hydration is necessary during renal transplant procedures to improve the early function of the newly transplanted kidney. The crystalloid solution used for hydration intraoperatively should not contain potassium. Monitoring the patient's central venous pressure intraoperatively may be a useful guide for the anesthesiologist to hydrate the patient optimally. (388; **1983**)

16. Dopamine is often administered intraoperatively during renal transplant in an effort to increase renal blood flow and perfusion of the newly transplanted kidney. When dopamine is administered for this purpose it is administered at renal doses, or at 3 to 5 μg/kg per minute. Other methods of ensuring adequate renal perfusion are the maintenance of systemic blood pressure near normal and the provision of adequate hydration. (388; **1983**)

17. Mannitol is often administered intraoperatively during renal transplant procedures because the osmotic diuresis it produces facilitates the formation of urine in the newly transplanted kidney. (388; **1983**)

18. Cardiac arrest that occurs after completion of the renal artery anastomosis to the newly transplanted kidney is thought to be secondary to hyperkalemia. A potassium-containing solution is used to preserve the kidney before transplantation. The washout of this solution and accumulated acid metabolites is believed to be the cause of the hyperkalemia. Hyperkalemia sufficient to cause cardiac arrest is more likely to occur in pediatric patients. (388; **1983**)

19. After completion of the renal artery anastomosis to the newly transplanted kidney, unclamping of the common iliac vessels may result in hypotension. The

hypotension is most appropriately treated with the rapid intravenous infusion of fluids. (388; **1983**)

20. An acute immunologic reaction to the newly transplanted kidney manifests as microvascular thrombosis and possible necrosis of the graft. The only method of treatment of an acute immunologic reaction to a newly transplanted kidney is removal of the kidney. (388; **1983**)

21. A postoperative hematoma after renal transplantation may present as vascular or ureteral obstruction. (388)

LIVER TRANSPLANTATION

22. Patients in hepatic failure, patients with nonmalignant hepatomas or biliary tract tumors, and patients with genetically transmitted metabolic abnormalities affecting their liver are all candidates for liver transplantation. (388; **1984–1985**)

23. Cadaver livers are not easily maintained before surgery secondary to the vulnerability of procured livers to ischemia. A cadaver liver is vulnerable to ischemia due to its high metabolic rate as well as its large bulk, making cooling difficult. There are perfusion techniques for the liver, however, that allow for its procurement, its preservation for up to 24 hours, and its subsequent transfer over long distances. Liver transplant procedures are usually urgent because of the cadaver liver's vulnerability to ischemia. (388; **1978**)

24. Physiologic disturbances that are often present before liver transplantation affect virtually every organ system. The patient may have an encephalopathy that ranges from mild confusion to coma. Patients with liver failure frequently have a hyperdynamic circulation with decreased systemic vascular resistance, increased cardiac output, and a low normal blood pressure with a decreased plasma volume and ascites. Arterial hypoxemia may be due to pulmonary effusions or atelectasis. Renal dysfunction and oliguria may also be present. Patients may have anemia, thrombocytopenia, or coagulopathies. Electrolyte abnormalities that may be present include hypokalemia, hypocalcemia, and hyponatremia. Finally, these patients may have a glucose intolerance. (388; **1984–1985**)

25. Monitors that may be used intraoperatively to facilitate the anesthetic management of patients undergoing liver transplant procedures include invasive arterial blood pressure monitoring and monitoring of cardiac filling pressures using a pulmonary artery catheter. These monitors are useful because major shifts in the intravascular volume and hemodynamic instability almost always occur. Arterial blood pressure should be monitored from an artery above the level of the diaphragm because the aorta may be cross-clamped during the portion of the procedure in which anastomosis of the hepatic artery takes place. Transesophageal echocardiograms are being used to monitor the fluid volume status and cardiac function and for the early recognition of emboli. A Foley catheter allows for the measurement of urine output. (388; **1985–1986**)

26. Peripheral intravenous access should be established preoperatively using several large-bore catheters to allow for the ability to transfuse blood products rapidly. Placement of the intravenous catheters should be supradiaphragmatic, because the inferior vena cava will likely be cross-clamped above the level of the liver during the liver transplant procedure. (388; **1986**)

27. Cell-saver devices are often used intraoperatively during liver transplant procedures because of the massive amounts of blood loss and massive fluid requirements during the procedure. (388; **1988**)

28. Calcium administration is often required during liver transplantation because of the frequency with which hypocalcemia occurs and the potential for associated

myocardial depression that can result. Hypocalcemia occurs as a result of the binding of calcium with citrate that is infused with blood transfusion products. In addition, the liver is frequently unable to metabolize citrate, particularly during the anhepatic phase. This causes a decrease in the amount of free calcium in the patient's blood. (388–389; **1987–1988**)

29. The three stages of liver transplant procedures are the preanhepatic stage, the anhepatic stage, and the posthepatic stage. The preanhepatic stage involves the dissection of the portal venous structures and mobilization for removal of the native liver. The anhepatic stage begins when the native liver's blood supply is transected and the suprahepatic and infrahepatic inferior vena cava are occluded. The anhepatic stage ends and the neohepatic stage begins with the anastomosis of the major hepatic vessels. (388–389; **1987–1988**)

30. The preanhepatic stage of liver transplant procedures is characterized by cardio-vascular instability due to sudden decreases in the intra-abdominal pressure, venous pooling, the exacerbation of chronic hypovolemia, and impaired venous return. Metabolic and electrolyte abnormalities also occur during this stage, including metabolic acidosis, hyperkalemia, and hypocalcemia. Hemorrhage occurs frequently during this stage, often requiring the rapid infusion of fluids and blood products. (388–389; **1987–1988**)

31. The anhepatic stage of liver transplant procedures is characterized by precipitous decreases in venous return and cardiac output. For this reason, cardiac inotropic drugs and sympathomimetic drugs are often administered during this portion of the liver transplant procedure to maintain cardiac output. Venovenous bypass is also often utilized during this time. Retractors near the diaphragm may result in high peak inspiratory pressures with mechanical ventilation. The addition of positive end-expiratory pressure may become necessary. Hypocalcemia and metabolic acidosis also commonly occur during this stage. (389; **1988**)

32. The neohepatic stage of liver transplant procedures is characterized by the potential for hyperkalemia and air emboli with the perfusion of the allograft. Hyperkalemia may occur as a result of the washout of the potassium-containing solution used to preserve the liver and the unclamping of vessels that were clamped during a portion of the procedure. Hypotension, arrhythmias, and cardiac arrest may potentially occur during this time. Gradually, urine output improves, and the patient becomes metabolically and hemodynamically stable. (389; **1988**)

33. Coagulopathies that can occur during a liver transplant procedure include thrombocytopenia, decreased levels of multiple coagulation factors, and fibrinolysis. (389; **1987–1989**)

34. Metabolic acidosis predictably occurs during liver transplant procedures. The metabolic acidosis, particularly in the presence of hypothermia and electrolyte abnormalities, may result in cardiac dysrhythmias. (389; **1986–1988**)

35. Patients undergoing liver transplantation may have a deficiency of cholinesterase enzymes, resulting in a prolongation of the duration of action of succinylcholine. There is little clinical significance of the prolongation of action of succinylcholine when it is used to facilitate intubation of the trachea for two reasons. First, the prolongation of the duration of action is offset by the much longer duration of the surgical procedure. Second, cholinesterase enzyme is present in blood transfused during liver transplantation procedures. (388–389; **1986**)

36. Nitrous oxide is often avoided for maintenance anesthesia during liver transplantation for three reasons. First, nitrous oxide administration may result in bowel distention during the procedure. Second, there is a risk of venous air embolism during liver transplant procedures. When the transplanted liver is first perfused, air that has been trapped in the liver can be released into the circulation

of the patient and cause a venous air embolism. The administration of nitrous oxide may increase the size of the air bubble, increasing the risk associated with a venous air embolus. Third, the administration of nitrous oxide may increase pulmonary vascular resistance. Patients undergoing liver transplant procedures may have co-existing pulmonary hypertension. (388; **1986**)

37. Cisatracurium is often selected as the nondepolarizing neuromuscular blocking drug of choice in patients undergoing liver transplantation because its elimination is by spontaneous Hofmann elimination and ester hydrolysis. (388; **459–461**)

38. Patients generally remain intubated at the conclusion of a liver transplant procedure as a result of the massive amounts of fluids that are administered during the procedure. In about 20% of patients, in some centers, the trachea may be extubated at the end of the surgical procedure. The criteria for extubation at the end of the procedure requires that the patient be hemodynamically stable, pulmonary function is good, bleeding and coagulopathy are controlled, and the graft appears to be functioning well. Extubation of the trachea otherwise occurs early in the postoperative period. (388–389; **1988–1989**)

39. An acute immunologic reaction to the newly transplanted liver manifests as abnormalities in liver function test results. Other complications that may present as abnormalities in liver function and must be ruled out include mechanical factors during the procedure itself, infection, and effects of hepatotoxic drugs. The hepatotoxic drug most suspect during this time is cyclosporine. (389; **1988**)

HEART TRANSPLANTATION

40. Patients with end-stage heart disease in the absence of pulmonary hypertension are candidates for heart transplantation. Patients with pulmonary hypertension and end-stage heart disease are candidates for heart-lung transplant procedures. Patients undergoing a heart transplant procedure usually have heart disease secondary to coronary artery disease or a cardiomyopathy. The ejection fraction generally seen in these patients is less than 20%. (389; **1989**)

41. Cadaver hearts have a very short ischemic time. The donor heart may be preserved for only 4 to 6 hours before transplantation. (389; **1978**)

42. The induction of anesthesia for cardiac transplantation may include a benzodiazepine and an opioid. The maintenance of anesthesia may be opioid based as well. The goal of the anesthetic induction and maintenance is to provide good intubating and operating conditions while maintaining maximal cardiac function. The potential risk of using a high dose of a volatile anesthetic during a heart transplant procedure is that volatile anesthetics in high doses can produce excessive amounts of myocardial depression or vasodilation or both. (389; **1990**)

43. Nitrous oxide is often avoided for maintenance anesthesia during a heart transplant procedure because of the increased risk of a venous air embolus should one occur in the presence of nitrous oxide. There is a risk of venous air embolus during heart transplant procedures because of the opening of large blood vessels. Nitrous oxide may increase the size of the air bubble causing the embolus. Finally, the administration of nitrous oxide necessarily limits the inhaled concentration of the oxygen that may be delivered to the patient. (389)

44. Vessels that are transected and anastomosed during heart transplant procedures include the aorta, pulmonary artery, and left and right atria. These are done during cardiopulmonary bypass. A central venous or pulmonary artery catheter that is in place at the onset of surgery must be pulled back into the internal jugular vein when the patient's heart is removed. (389; **1990**)

45. Catheterization of the left internal jugular vein for intravenous access during a

heart transplant procedure leaves the right internal jugular vein available. The right internal jugular vein may then be used for access to the heart for the performance of endomyocardial biopsies in the postoperative period. Endomyocardial biopsies are performed to evaluate the heart for evidence of an acute allograft rejection. (389; **1991**)

46. Isoproterenol may be indicated for administration during a heart transplant procedure. The indication for isoproterenol is for the maintenance of myocardial contractility and heart rate in the denervated donor heart during the anastomosis of the vessels. Isoproterenol is also useful in decreasing pulmonary vasculature resistance should it become necessary. (389; **1991**)

47. The transplanted heart reacts better to direct-acting catecholamines. For example, the transplanted heart will not increase its heart rate in response to atropine. This is as a result of denervation of the autonomic fibers to the heart. (389; **1991–1993**)

48. Patients who have had a heart transplant have an accelerated rate of atherosclerosis in the denervated heart. Approximately 40% of patients get coronary artery disease within 3 years of having a heart transplant. (389; **1992, Fig. 55–9**)

LUNG TRANSPLANTATION

49. Patients with end-stage respiratory failure are candidates for lung transplantation. Patients with end-stage respiratory failure secondary to chronic interstitial pulmonary fibrosis most commonly undergo single-lung transplants. Patients with end-stage respiratory failure secondary to chronic obstructive pulmonary disease or cystic fibrosis most commonly undergo double-lung transplants. (389–390; **1993**)

50. Lung transplant procedures are relatively urgent secondary to the brief ischemic time of the lung. The maximum ischemic time of the lung is 6 to 8 hours. (390; **1978**)

51. Double-lumen endotracheal tubes are used for intubation of the trachea for lung transplant surgery. Double-lumen endotracheal tubes allow for isolated ventilation of the left and right lungs, such that one lung may be ventilated while the other lung is being transplanted. (390; **1994**)

52. Some intraoperative problems the anesthesiologist may encounter during lung transplant procedures include arterial hypoxemia and pulmonary hypertension. Arterial hypoxemia may occur during one-lung ventilation while the opposite lung is being transplanted. Pulmonary hypertension may occur when the pulmonary artery is clamped. (390; **1994**)

53. Extubation of the trachea of the patient who has undergone a lung transplant procedure usually takes place in the postoperative period. (390; **1995**)

54. Lung transplant patients are predisposed to developing pneumonia in the transplanted lung for multiple reasons. The lung transplant procedure disrupts lymphatic drainage, there is poor mucociliary function, suture lines are present across the airway, and there is a loss of the cough reflex in that lung. The patient is unable to clear the lower airways via the normal cough reflex as a result of the denervation of the lung. Lung infection may be confused with lung rejection in the postoperative period. (390; **1995**)

PANCREAS TRANSPLANTATION

55. Patients with severe diabetes mellitus, or brittle diabetics, are candidates for pancreas transplantation. (**1996**)

56. Evaluation of the success of a pancreas transplant is measured by monitoring

blood glucose levels after surgery. The return of blood glucose concentrations to a normal level, often within hours, is the marker for a successful pancreas transplant. Blood glucose levels should also be monitored intraoperatively during pancreas transplant procedures. (**1996**)

BONE MARROW TRANSPLANTATION

57. Patients with otherwise fatal leukemias are candidates for bone marrow transplantation. (390)

58. Bone marrow ablation in the bone marrow recipient is achieved by a combination of chemotherapy and whole-body irradiation. (390)

59. Bone marrow from a bone marrow donor is harvested from the superior iliac spines and iliac crests. The marrow is harvested by multiple aspirations from these areas with the patient in the prone position. (390)

60. Bone marrow harvest procedures may be done with the donor under either general or regional anesthesia. (390)

61. The purported potential of nitrous oxide administration causing bone marrow depression has resulted in the avoidance of this inhaled anesthetic during bone marrow harvest procedures by some anesthesiologists. Bone marrow engraftment and subsequent function have not been shown to be adversely affected by the administration of nitrous oxide for anesthesia, however. (390)

62. Intraoperative blood losses during bone marrow harvest procedures are easily estimated, because they parallel directly the volume of bone marrow that is harvested. It is important to realize that rapid, substantial blood losses may accompany this procedure, making fluid hydration important. (390)

Chapter *29*

Outpatient Surgery

1. What are some advantages of performing elective surgery as an outpatient procedure?

2. What special advantages are there for children to undergo elective surgery as an outpatient procedure?

3. What is the advantage of performing an elective procedure as an *AM admit* in which the patient stays in the hospital overnight after the procedure?

OFFICE-BASED ANESTHESIA

4. What is office-based anesthesia?

5. What types of surgical procedures are typically performed in the office?

FACILITIES

6. How should operating rooms, monitors, anesthetic equipment, and postoperative recovery room facilities in an outpatient surgery center differ from those used for inpatient surgery?

7. Who should be responsible for deciding whether a given procedure should be performed on an outpatient basis?

PATIENT SELECTION

8. What are some patient characteristics that make a patient a good candidate for having surgery performed on an outpatient basis?

9. Why might immunosuppressed patients and infants benefit from having their surgical procedure performed on an outpatient basis?

10. What is a potential risk of having premature neonates have surgery performed as outpatients? What other infants are at an increased risk of having surgery performed as outpatients?

11. What types of operative procedures are considered acceptable to be performed on an outpatient basis?

12. What types of operative procedures are not considered acceptable to be performed on an outpatient basis?

13. Does the need for a blood transfusion contraindicate outpatient surgery?

PREOPERATIVE PREPARATION AND INSTRUCTIONS TO THE PATIENT

14. What are the preoperative responsibilities of the surgeon scheduling an outpatient surgical procedure?

15. What are the advantages to having an outpatient anesthesia clinic for the patient undergoing an outpatient surgical procedure at a later date?

16. What laboratory tests should be ordered preoperatively for the patient scheduled to undergo an outpatient surgical procedure?

17. What should be included in the written instructions provided to the patient by the surgeon before undergoing an outpatient surgical procedure?

ARRIVAL ON THE DAY OF SURGERY

18. What history must be confirmed on the day of outpatient surgery when the patient arrives at the surgery clinic or hospital?

PREOPERATIVE MEDICATION

19. What are some reasons to administer preoperative medications to the outpatient surgical patient?

20. Why might preoperative anxiolytics be avoided in the outpatient setting? What other method might be used to help decrease preoperative anxiety?

21. Which patients may benefit from the preoperative administration of an anticholinergic drug?

22. Which patients should receive antiemetics preoperatively in the outpatient surgical setting?

TECHNIQUE OF ANESTHESIA

23. What additional goal must be considered by the anesthesiologist when selecting the anesthetic plan for a patient scheduled to undergo an outpatient surgical procedure?

24. Why should an intravenous catheter be placed in patients scheduled to undergo outpatient surgery?

25. What induction agent is commonly used for patients who undergo outpatient surgical procedures under general anesthesia? What are some other options?

26. What are some of the general methods by which the induction of anesthesia can be achieved in the pediatric patient scheduled to undergo an outpatient surgical procedure? What is a disadvantage to using rectal methohexital as an induction agent in the pediatric population?

27. What is the disadvantage to using succinylcholine to facilitate intubation of the trachea in an outpatient surgical procedure?

28. How can laryngeal trauma and edema be minimized for the patient undergoing general anesthesia for an outpatient surgical procedure?

29. What are some advantages to using a laryngeal mask airway for patients undergoing outpatient surgical procedures?

30. How might the maintenance of anesthesia be achieved in an outpatient setting? Which inhaled anesthetics result in more rapid awakening after their discontinuation?

31. What is the benefit of infiltration of the incision with local anesthetic at the onset of surgery?

32. What are some of the options for the treatment of postoperative pain after an outpatient surgical procedure?

33. What are some of the options for the treatment of postoperative nausea and vomiting after an outpatient surgical procedure?

REGIONAL ANESTHESIA

34. What are some disadvantages to regional anesthesia and peripheral nerve blocks in the outpatient setting?

SEDATION AND/OR ANALGESIA

35. What are some advantages to monitored anesthesia care for patients undergoing outpatient surgical procedures?

36. What drugs can be administered to patients undergoing monitored anesthesia care in the outpatient setting?

DISCHARGE FROM THE OUTPATIENT FACILITY

37. What are some criteria for discharge from an outpatient surgical facility?

38. Who should decide when the patient is able to be discharged from the outpatient surgical facility?

39. What written and verbal instructions should be given to a patient who has undergone an outpatient surgical procedure and is being discharged home?

40. What are some indications for unanticipated admission to the hospital after an outpatient surgical procedure has been performed?

ANSWERS*

1. There are several advantages for both the patient and the institution when procedures are performed on an outpatient basis. Advantages for the patient include the least amount of disruption from daily personal and family activities, decreases in medical costs, and decreases in the risk of becoming infected with hospital-acquired infections. Advantages for the institution also include a decrease in the medical cost and an increased availability of hospital beds for patients who require hospitalization. (391; **2213–2214**)

2. Children who undergo elective surgery as an outpatient rather than an inpatient procedure are able to return to their familiar surroundings sooner. In addition, outpatient elective surgery results in a shorter time of separation from family members. Together, these may lead to a decrease in short-term and potentially long-term psychological disturbances that can result from the stressors of a hospitalization and separation from family members. (391; **2213–2214**)

3. An elective procedure performed as an *AM admit* still maintains preservation of the patient's daily personal and familial activities up until the day of surgery. After surgery the planned admission to the hospital allows for closer observation for, and better management of, potential postoperative surgical or anesthetic complications. (391; **2214**)

OFFICE-BASED ANESTHESIA

4. Office-based anesthesia refers to anesthesia provided to patients undergoing procedures in the physician's office. The operating suites are typically managed in conjunction with the surgeon's offices. It is estimated that office-based anesthesia will account for more than 15% of anesthetics by the end of 2000. Office-based procedures have gained popularity among some surgeons because they have more control over costs. (391; **2214, 2231**)

5. Office-based surgical procedures include cosmetic surgery such as breast augmentation, facial surgery, and liposuction; laparoscopy; tubal ligation; colonoscopy; orthopedic surgery such as arthroscopy and hardware removal; and oral surgery. (391–392; **2215**)

---

*Numbers in parentheses: lightface numbers refer to pages, figures, or tables in Stoelting RK, Miller RD: Basics of Anesthesia, 4th ed. Philadelphia, Churchill Livingstone, 2000; **boldface numbers** refer to pages, figures, or tables in Miller RD: Anesthesia, 5th ed. Philadelphia, Churchill Livingstone, 2000.

FACILITIES

6. Operating rooms, monitors, anesthetic equipment, and postoperative recovery room facilities in an outpatient surgery center should be of the same caliber as those at a hospital used for inpatient surgery. There should be a portable crash cart and suction device in the event of the need for advanced cardiac life support. A malignant hyperthermia kit should also be available anywhere where general anesthesia is being administered. The postanesthesia care unit should be able to allow patients to stay several hours after surgery if necessary. (392; **2214–2215**)

7. The physician director of an outpatient surgery center, usually an anesthesiologist, should have the ultimate responsibility of deciding whether a given procedure should be performed on an outpatient basis. The decision not to perform a surgical procedure as an outpatient should be discussed with the surgeon. (392; **2215–2216**)

PATIENT SELECTION

8. Characteristics of patients that make them good candidates for having their surgery performed on an outpatient basis include those with good medical control of systemic diseases or otherwise in good health, those who do not require extended postoperative or postanesthesia monitoring, and those with dependable care providers at home who are of sound judgment. Patients in whom previous anesthetics have resulted in postanesthetic complications such as difficulty with pain control or postoperative nausea and vomiting are probably not good candidates for outpatient surgical procedures. Finally, patients must live within close proximity to the surgery center, preferably within 1 hour of travel time, in the event that postoperative complications require the rapid return to the facility for evaluation. (392; **2214–2215**)

9. Immunosuppressed patients and infants may benefit from having their surgical procedure performed on an outpatient basis because they are more prone to infection by hospital-acquired microorganisms. (392; **2216**)

10. Premature neonates have immature ventilatory control centers. These neonates are therefore at risk of apnea spells in the postoperative period, especially after the administration of medicines during anesthesia that further decrease the neonate's ventilatory drive. The recommendation is that premature neonates aged younger than 60 weeks post conception have their elective surgical procedures postponed until they reach that age. When younger than age 60 weeks post conception, only necessary surgical procedures should be performed. Premature infants having undergone a general anesthetic should remain in the hospital postoperatively for close observation, possibly with an apnea and bradycardia monitor. Infants who are also at an increased risk for having surgery performed as an outpatient are infants who have a family history of sudden infant death syndrome and infants who had been treated for respiratory distress syndrome after birth. Infants who had been treated for respiratory distress syndrome after birth are at an increased risk of developing bronchopulmonary dysplasia in the first 6 to 12 months after the cessation of ventilator management of the syndrome. (392; **2126, 2215, 2466**)

11. Operative procedures considered acceptable to be performed on an outpatient basis include those in which there is minimal bleeding expected, in which there is minimal postoperative pain, and procedures with minimal alterations in the patient's normal physiology. (392–393; **2215, Table 65–2**)

12. Operative procedures that interfere with a patient's normal physiology or that require major intervention into the cranium, thorax, or abdomen are not consid-

ered appropriate to be done on an outpatient basis. Procedures that interfere with a patient's normal airway anatomy, that are associated with postoperative airway obstruction, or that may interfere with a patient's early postoperative ambulation are also best not performed on an outpatient basis. Patients in whom the surgical procedure is not considered clean, or that is infected, should remain an inpatient after the surgical procedure. Emergency surgical procedures should be done on an inpatient basis. (393; **2215**)

13. In general, the need for a blood transfusion is not in and of itself a contraindication to performing a procedure as an outpatient. (393; **2215**)

PREOPERATIVE PREPARATION AND INSTRUCTIONS TO THE PATIENT

14. Preoperative responsibilities of the surgeon scheduling an outpatient surgical procedure include obtaining a medical history, performing a physical examination, obtaining the necessary laboratory tests, and providing the patient or the individual responsible for the patient with instructions and information. (393; **2217**)

15. An outpatient anesthesia clinic is advantageous in that it allows for the evaluation of the surgical patient by an anesthesiologist before the day scheduled for the procedure. It also provides the patient with an opportunity to get answers to questions they may have regarding the anesthetic they will receive. A preoperative telephone interview will also allow for the exchange of information between the anesthesiologist and the patient. A preoperative evaluation by the anesthesiologist on the day of the procedure may be the only alternative and is acceptable practice, however. (393; **2217–2218**)

16. Laboratory tests for outpatient surgical procedures, just as in inpatient surgical procedures, should be ordered preoperatively on an individual basis depending on the patient's age, medical condition, and the surgical procedure. (393; **2217**)

17. The written instructions provided to the patient scheduled to undergo an outpatient surgical procedure should include guidelines for the preoperative ingestion of solids and clear liquids; where and when to arrive on the day of the procedure; recommendations for not operating heavy machinery, making important decisions, consuming alcohol, or driving a car for 24 to 48 hours after surgery; the rule for the accompaniment by a responsible adult; and a phone number to contact a physician should there be a change in the patient's medical condition or for any further questions. (393–394; **2218**)

ARRIVAL ON THE DAY OF SURGERY

18. Confirmation of the patient's current medical condition, confirmation of the adherence to the recommendations regarding the ingestion of solids and clear liquids, a review of laboratory data, and confirmation of the patient's understanding of the events that will follow should occur on the day of outpatient surgery when the patient arrives at the surgery clinic or hospital. (394)

PREOPERATIVE MEDICATION

19. Some reasons to administer preoperative medications to the outpatient surgical patient include to control anxiety, for the antisialagogue effect, to decrease the risk of nausea and vomiting, to decrease the risk of the aspiration of gastric contents, and for the control of pain. Preoperative medicines given to outpatient surgical patients should not delay recovery from anesthesia or produce prolonged amnesia. (394; **2218–2222**)

20. Preoperative anxiolytics might be avoided in the outpatient setting. Preoperative anxiolytics may extend the time to wakefulness through interactions with other medications or if the duration of surgery is shorter than the duration of the anxiolytic. This may extend the recovery time after the procedure. An alternative method of reducing a patient's anxiety is by reassurance by the surgeon or the anesthesiologist preoperatively. (394; **2218–2219, 222–2229, Fig. 65–2**)

21. Patients who are scheduled for oral procedures, such as oral endoscopy or dental procedures, may benefit from the preoperative administration of an anticholinergic drug. The anticholinergic drug will decrease oral secretions and facilitate the procedure. (394; **2221**)

22. Patients at a high risk for nausea and vomiting either based on their medical condition or the surgical procedure they are scheduled to undergo may benefit from the administration of antiemetics preoperatively. These patients may also benefit from limiting the dose of opioid administered prophylactically for pain. In fact, postoperative nausea is a common cause for unanticipated admission to the hospital after outpatient surgery. The routine administration of antiemetics to patients is not considered cost effective because many patients do not experience nausea after surgery. (394–395; **2220–2221, Figs. 65–3, 65–4, Table 65–6**)

TECHNIQUE OF ANESTHESIA

23. The anesthetic plan for the patient scheduled to undergo an outpatient surgical procedure and then return home must include the additional goal of providing for a rapid, complete wake-up and recovery with the minimal amount of possible side effects. (395; **2223**)

24. A peripheral intravenous catheter should almost always be placed in a patient scheduled to undergo any surgical procedure. The peripheral intravenous catheter not only provides for the administration of intravenous fluids for the patient who has not consumed anything for hours, but it also allows for the administration of anesthetic and emergency drugs as indicated. An exception to this may be pediatric patients undergoing brief surgical procedures such as myringotomy or eye examination under anesthesia. (395; **2223**)

25. Propofol is commonly used as the induction agent in patients undergoing outpatient surgical procedures under general anesthesia. This is because of the relative lack of side effects and more rapid recovery associated with the administration of propofol. Propofol is also associated with a euphoric effect in patients emerging from anesthesia. Other options include thiopental and methohexital. (395, Fig. 30–3; **2224, Fig. 65–6, Table 65–8**)

26. Methods by which the induction of anesthesia can be achieved in the pediatric patient scheduled to undergo an outpatient surgical procedure include an inhalation induction, an intravenous induction, or by the administration of rectal methohexital. The disadvantage of the rectal administration of methohexital for the induction of anesthesia is the potential for delayed awakening. (395; **2226, 2229**)

27. A disadvantage to using succinylcholine to facilitate intubation of the trachea in an outpatient surgical procedure is the potential for associated postoperative myalgia. Another option includes using succinylcholine after pretreatment with a subparalyzing dose of a nondepolarizing neuromuscular blocking drug, such as *d*-tubocurarine, to prevent the fasciculations and possibly the myalgia associated with succinylcholine administration. The short-acting nondepolarizing neuromuscular blocking drug rapacuronium is an alternative for use to facilitate intubation of the trachea for outpatient surgical procedures. (395–396; **2228**)

28. Laryngeal trauma and edema can be minimized after intubation of the trachea

for an outpatient surgical procedure by selecting a small-diameter endotracheal tube with which to intubate the trachea. (396; **2226–2227**)

29. Benefits of the laryngeal mask airway for patients undergoing outpatient surgical procedures include the following: an airway can be maintained while allowing the anesthesiologist's hands to remain free, it is better tolerated by the patient at a lighter level of anesthesia, it has less of a cardiovascular response associated with its insertion, patients can breathe spontaneously, it does not require the administration of neuromuscular blocking drugs, and it decreases the risk of a sore throat or potential laryngeal edema postoperatively. The laryngeal mask airway does not protect the airway and cannot be used in patients at risk of the aspiration of gastric contents. When positive pressure is applied to the laryngeal mask airway for ventilation, gastric distention with air and aspiration or postoperative nausea and vomiting may result. (396; **2223–2224**)

30. The maintenance of anesthesia may be achieved with the administration of nitrous oxide in conjunction with a short-acting opioid, with a continuous infusion of propofol, or with a volatile anesthetic. The volatile anesthetics that result in the most rapid awakening after their discontinuation are desflurane and sevoflurane, secondary to their low blood and tissue solubilities. (396; **2225–2227, Tables 65–9, 65–10**)

31. Infiltration of the incision with a local anesthetic at the onset of surgery provides the patient with some postoperative incisional pain relief. It may also act to decrease the amount of subsequent pain associated with the surgical procedure by providing some preemptive pain control. This would decrease the amount of subsequent opioid required for pain control and possibly the associated side effects of the opioid as well. The local anesthetic most commonly used for this purpose is bupivacaine. (396; **2230**)

32. Options for the treatment of postoperative pain after an outpatient surgical procedure include the administration of oral analgesics and, for more severe pain, the administration of short-acting opioids. It is important that the patient have the pain controlled with an outpatient regimen before being discharged home. (396; **2227–2228, 2233, Table 65–11**)

33. Options for the treatment of postoperative nausea and vomiting after an outpatient surgical procedure are limited to the administration of antiemetics such as ondansetron, dolasetron, prochlorperazine (Compazine), or droperidol. It is important that the patient be able to tolerate oral liquids before being discharged home. (396; **2233–2234**)

REGIONAL ANESTHESIA

34. Disadvantages to regional anesthesia and peripheral nerve blocks in the outpatient setting include the potentially prolonged time required for the performance of the block, the possibility of block failure, and the potentially prolonged duration of blockade. Residual sympathetic nervous system blockade can result in persistent orthostatic hypotension after surgery, making ambulation difficult. Residual motor nervous system blockade can further impair the patient's ability to ambulate postoperatively. The risk of postspinal headache may also make regional anesthesia disadvantageous for outpatient surgical procedures. (396; **2230–2231**)

SEDATION AND/OR ANALGESIA

35. Advantages to monitored anesthesia care for patients undergoing outpatient surgical procedures include quicker recovery and fewer side effects than with general anesthesia and better tolerance during the procedure than if it were done with local anesthesia without sedation. (397; **2231**)

36. Drugs that can be administered to patients undergoing monitored anesthesia care in the outpatient setting include opioids, benzodiazepines, and propofol. Propofol is advantageous in that it is easily titratable to the desired level of sedation while still allowing for a rapid recovery. (397; **2225, 2230**)

DISCHARGE FROM THE OUTPATIENT FACILITY

37. Discharge from the outpatient surgical facility should occur when the patient has recovered from the surgical procedure and the anesthesia. Recovery should be evidenced by stable vital signs, the return of consciousness and orientation, and the ability to ambulate without assistance. Sensation and motor function should also have returned after the administration of a regional anesthetic. Patients should also have controlled pain, minimal postoperative nausea and vomiting, and minimal bleeding at the surgical site. It may not be necessary for the patient to void before discharge. (397; **2232–2234, 2240, Table 65–12**)

38. The decision to discharge a patient from the recovery room to home is usually made by an anesthesiologist, often in consultation with the surgeon. Most patients are able to be discharged from the outpatient surgical facility with a responsible adult escort about 1½ hours after their arrival at the recovery room. (397; **2232–2234**)

39. Written and verbal instructions must be given to the patient and the responsible adult on discharge from an outpatient surgical facility. These should include recommendations to avoid alcohol or important decision making in the first 24 to 48 hours postoperatively, despite feeling well. It should also include the recommendations for the resumption of a normal diet beginning with liquids and gradually introducing solid food. Patients should be provided with a prescription of oral analgesics and instructions for their use. Patients should also be provided with a phone number of a physician they may contact should any symptoms or problems arise. A list of symptoms for which the patient should contact the physician may also be useful to the patient. (397–398; **2240**)

40. The approximate unanticipated admission rates to the hospital after outpatient surgery have been cited to be lower than 1%. Severe postoperative pain, persistent postoperative nausea and vomiting, and postoperative bleeding are all indications for unanticipated admission to the hospital after an outpatient surgical procedure. Unanticipated admissions to the hospital after surgery warrant that free-standing surgery clinics not in a hospital have an agreement with a local hospital for transfer and admission to the hospital in the event of unexpected required hospitalization. (397; **2232–2234**)

Chapter *30*

Procedures Performed Outside the Operating Room

1. What are some fundamental capabilities available in the operating room that must also be available for the delivery of anesthesia in remote locations?

2. What are some special challenges facing the anesthesiologist when delivering anesthesia and at the conclusion of anesthesia in remote locations?

3. What are some safety concerns facing the anesthesiologist delivering anesthesia in remote locations?

DIAGNOSTIC AND THERAPEUTIC RADIOLOGY

4. Why might patients require anesthesia for diagnostic and therapeutic radiologic procedures?

5. How might the anesthesiologist limit his or her exposure to radiation during diagnostic and therapeutic radiologic procedures?

6. What are some side effects associated with intravenously administered contrast agent? What prophylaxis may be administered to patients at risk of a serious adverse reaction to intravenously administered contrast agent?

7. What is magnetic resonance imaging (MRI)? What is it useful for the evaluation of?

8. What are some contraindications to undergoing MRI?

9. What are some features of MRI that make it difficult for the patient to tolerate?

10. How should the patient be monitored when undergoing an anesthetic for MRI?

11. How must anesthetic equipment and monitors in the MRI center be altered for MRI compatibility? What are the risks of using standard operating room monitors?

12. How must accidental extubation of the trachea during MRI be managed?

13. Why is there an increased risk of hypothermia for patients in the MR imager?

14. What is computed tomography?

15. How does the management of anesthesia for patients undergoing computed tomography compare with the management of anesthesia for patients undergoing MRI?

16. Why might patients require anesthesia for radiation therapy?

17. Why must remote monitoring devices be used for patients undergoing radiation therapy under anesthesia?

18. Why might patients require anesthesia for cardiac catheterization? What effects should the anesthetic have on cardiac function during these procedures?

19. What Pa_{CO_2} should be maintained during anesthesia for cardiac catheterization?

20. What are complications that can occur as a result of cardiac catheterization procedures?

21. How might anxiety be allayed during cardiac catheterization procedures?

22. Why might the onset of action of inhaled or injected anesthetics be altered in patients undergoing cardiac catheterization procedures?

CARDIOVERSION

23. Why does a patient undergoing elective cardioversion require sedation and amnesia? How might this be accomplished?

24. How can the patient's airway be maintained during anesthesia for cardioversion?

25. What monitors should be used during anesthesia for a patient undergoing cardioversion?

ELECTROCONVULSIVE THERAPY

26. What patients are candidates for electroconvulsive therapy (ECT)? How is ECT accomplished?

27. What are some cardiopulmonary effects of ECT? In what sequence might these effects occur?

28. What are the most common causes of mortality after ECT?

29. How is cerebral blood flow affected by ECT?

30. How is intragastric pressure affected by ECT?

31. What are some contraindications and relative contraindications to ECT?

32. What are some post-ECT manifestations in the patient?

33. What is the recommendation for the ingestion of solids and liquids before the performance of ECT?

34. Why is preoperative medication not recommended for the patient who is to undergo ECT?

35. What agents might be used for the induction of anesthesia in a patient undergoing ECT?

36. After unconsciousness results from the induction of anesthesia, why might succinylcholine be administered to the patient? Before this is done, why might a tourniquet be applied to an extremity of the patient?

37. How can the airway of the patient undergoing ECT be managed? What equipment should be available to the anesthesiologist?

38. What monitors should be used during the administration of an anesthetic for ECT?

DENTAL SURGERY

39. What patients might require anesthesia for a dental procedure?

40. Why might an anticholinergic be administered to a patient before a dental procedure?

41. What agents can be used for the induction of anesthesia in patients requiring anesthesia for a dental procedure? What agent can be used in uncooperative patients when there is no intravenous access before the induction of anesthesia?

42. How is tracheal intubation usually accomplished to facilitate the dentist's ability to perform dental procedures in patients requiring general anesthesia for the procedure?

43. What are some special concerns for the patient during emergence and in the recovery period after having undergone a dental procedure under general anesthesia?

EXTRACORPOREAL SHOCK WAVE LITHOTRIPSY

44. What is extracorporeal shock wave lithotripsy (ESWL)?

45. What are the shock waves timed with during ESWL to avoid cardiac dysrhythmias?

46. Why is anesthesia required for patients undergoing ESWL?

47. What are some advantages of general anesthesia for patients undergoing ESWL?

48. What sensory level of regional anesthesia is recommended for patients undergoing ESWL with this anesthetic technique?

49. Why is intravenous fluid administration important during ESWL?

50. What are some contraindications to ESWL?

ANSWERS*

1. Fundamental capabilities for monitoring, the delivery of supplemental oxygen, mechanical ventilation of the lungs, the delivery of inhaled anesthetics, anesthesia equipment, and the availability of suction must all be available for the delivery of anesthesia in remote locations. (399; **2241–2242**)

2. Special challenges facing the anesthesiologist when delivering anesthesia in remote locations include the limited access to the patient's airway, poor availability of accessory help, and the potential difficulty in quickly obtaining emergency equipment. Special challenges facing the anesthesiologist at the conclusion of anesthesia in remote locations are based on the greater amount of distance the anesthesiologist must transport the patient before reaching the postanesthesia care unit. These may include a greater need for a supplemental oxygen supply and continuous monitoring. (399, Fig. 31–1; **2241–2242, 2244, Figs. 76–1, 66–2, 66–3,**)

3. Some safety concerns that may face the anesthesiologist delivering anesthesia in remote locations include the possibility of exposure to increased radiation and the scavenging of waste anesthetic gases. (399; **2241–2242**)

DIAGNOSTIC AND THERAPEUTIC RADIOLOGY

4. Patients, usually children, who cannot remain still or who cannot cooperate with instructions are most likely to require general anesthesia or sedation for diagnostic and therapeutic radiologic procedures. Adults may also require sedation or general anesthesia for radiologic procedures, especially patients who are developmentally delayed or have sustained trauma. (399; **2244**)

5. The anesthesiologist should attempt to limit his or her exposure to radiation by wearing a lead apron and thyroid shield, through the use of movable lead glass screens, and by remaining as far away as possible from the radiation source, preferably at least 1 to 2 meters. (399; **2245**)

6. Common side effects associated with the administration of intravenous contrast agents are nausea and vomiting, a perception of warmth, headache, and mild urticaria. Severe reactions may include vomiting, rigors, feeling faint, bronchospasm, chest pain, arrhythmias, and renal failure. Life-threatening reactions include severe bronchospasm, glottic edema, pulmonary edema, arrhythmias,

seizures, and cardiac arrest. The newer nonionic contrast dyes of lower osmolarity tend to be associated with fewer incidences of allergic reactions. Even so, patients at risk of an adverse reaction to a contrast agent should be pretreated with medicines to minimize the reaction to the contrast agent. Prednisolone can be administered at a dose of 50 to 100 mg intravenously both the night before and the morning of the procedure. Diphenhydramine, 50 mg, should also be given intravenously just before the procedure. Adequate hydration is necessary in these patients to maintain their intravascular volume because the intravenous contrast medium also acts as an osmotic load for the patient, inducing diuresis. (399–400; **2246–2247, Tables 66–3**)

7. Magnetic resonance imaging (MRI) is a radiologic study that provides digitalized tomographic images of the body by exposing the body to high-strength magnetic fields. MRI does not produce any ionizing radiation. These studies are useful for the evaluation of neurologic and soft tissues, because they can distinguish between fat, vessels, and tumor. (400; **1462, 2241, Figs. 66–4, 66–5**)

8. MRI is contraindicated in patients who have any implanted metals that are attracted to a magnetic force. Examples of such metals include artificial cardiac pacemakers, aneurysm clips, some intravascular clips, and some biologic pumps. (400–401; **2248–2249**)

9. MRI is difficult for the patient to tolerate based on the positioning of the patient during the study. The patient must lie on a long thin table and then be moved into a long thin tube that is close to the face of the patient. Patients during MRI may become claustrophobic. In addition, the MR imager has a loud booming noise that may augment a patient's discomfort. (400; **2249–2250, Fig. 66–6**)

10. The patient undergoing an anesthetic during MRI should have his or her blood pressure, pulse oximetry, and cardiac rhythm continually monitored. Capnograph monitors may also be used to detect end-tidal carbon dioxide, especially when monitoring from a distance. Extensions must be placed on all monitoring equipment because the patient moves into the MR imager during the study. (400; **1462, 2250–2251**)

11. Standard operating room monitors and anesthetic equipment must be altered for use in the MRI center. No ferromagnetic components are allowed for use near the scanner, because any ferromagnetic material will be forcefully attracted by the magnet and may cause injury to individuals in or near the scanner. Plastic, nonmagnetic steel, and aluminum components replace metal ones for anesthetic machines, equipment, and ventilators specially made for compatibility with the MR imager. In addition, traditional pulse oximeters must not be used in the MR imager, because they can cause burns to the patient. (400–401; **1462, 2249–2251, Fig. 66–8**)

12. Accidental extubation of the patient's trachea during MRI must be managed by immediate discontinuation of the imager, removing the patient from the imager, and rapidly controlling the patient's airway. In the event that resuscitative equipment is necessary in an emergency the patient must be moved far enough away from the MR imager to prevent metal components of the resuscitative equipment to become attracted to the magnet. (401; **2250**)

13. The air flow through the MR imager increases the amount of heat loss from the patient, placing the patient at an increased risk of hypothermia. This risk is of particular concern for pediatric patients undergoing MRI. (401)

14. Computed tomography (CT) is a radiologic imaging study that produces a two-dimensional image by a rotating x-ray beam around the subject for imaging. CT scanners emit ionizing radiation. (400; **2251**)

15. Anesthesia for CT scanning is similar to that for MRI. That is, access to the

patient is limited and monitoring is remote. Unlike with the MR imager nonferrous equipment is not necessary. (400; **2251**)

16. Patients undergoing radiation therapy may require anesthesia for immobilization during the procedure. Immobilization during radiation therapy is important because large doses of radiation are focused on specific target sites, and movement during the procedure can result in tissue damage to areas inadvertently radiated. The duration of the procedure is very brief, requiring that the patient must remain immobile for only a brief amount of time. (401; **2261–2262**)

17. Remote monitoring devices must be used for patients being sedated or anesthetized while undergoing radiation therapy because high doses of radiation require that all individuals must leave the area during the treatment period. (401; **2261–2262, Fig. 66–13**)

18. Children undergoing cardiac catheterization for the diagnosis of congenital cardiac lesions might require anesthesia for the procedure. The anesthetic employed must not have any significant effect on existing cardiac shunts so as not to interfere with the results of the study. The administration of anesthesia may cause myocardial depression or a decrease in preload by decreasing venous return, so care must be taken by the anesthesiologist to minimize these cardiovascular changes. (401; **2257–2258**)

19. The Pa_{CO_2} that should be maintained during anesthesia for children undergoing cardiac catheterization should be equal to the patient's resting Pa_{CO_2} so as not to influence myocardial activity or pulmonary pressures. (401; **2257–2258**)

20. Complications that can occur as a result of cardiac catheterization include bleeding at the vascular access site, perforation of the heart wall or great vessels, embolism, cardiac dysrhythmias, and heart block. In addition, thrombosis may occur in patients with a high hematocrit. (401; **2257–2258**)

21. Anxiety during cardiac catheterization procedures may be allayed by the administration of a benzodiazepine possibly in combination with a short-acting opioid. This may be important in patients with co-existing cardiopulmonary problems because of the potential for the exacerbation of their underlying disease by the anxiety. (401; **2257–2258**)

22. The onset of action of inhaled or injected anesthetics may be altered in patients undergoing cardiac catheterization secondary to the influence of left-to-right or right-to-left shunts that may be present in this patient population. A left-to-right shunt causes the arterial partial pressure of an inhaled anesthetic to be higher than it otherwise would be because the blood that has passed ventilated alveoli does not pass through tissues before returning to the heart. The clinical effect of a left-to-right shunt is negligible, however. A right-to-left shunt has the opposite effect. A right-to-left shunt causes the arterial partial pressure of an inhaled anesthetic to be lower than it otherwise would be secondary to the dilutional effect of the blood that enters the systemic circulation without passing by ventilated alveoli after returning from the tissues. The rate of induction, and subsequent onset of action, of inhaled anesthetics may therefore be slowed in the presence of a right-to-left shunt. (401)

CARDIOVERSION

23. Elective cardioversion can be painful during the electric shock, requiring the patient to have sedation and amnesia for a brief period during the administration of the shock. This can be accomplished by the intravenous injection of an induction drug such as thiopental, methohexital, or propofol after preoxygenation and just before the administration of the electric shock. (401; **2259–2260**)

24. The patient's airway can be maintained during anesthesia before and after the

cardioversion by hand with a mask provided the patient has fasted before the procedure. Equipment that should be available to the anesthesiologist providing anesthesia for cardioversion include a bag and mask for the support of ventilation, a supplemental oxygen source, suction, and the appropriate equipment for emergent intubation of the trachea. (401; **2259–2260**)

25. Monitoring of blood pressure, pulse oximetry, and the electrocardiogram should be the standard during anesthesia for cardioversion. (401; **2259**)

ELECTROCONVULSIVE THERAPY

26. Patients who have severe clinical depression that is refractory to medicines, patients who have become acutely suicidal, patients who are acutely psychotic or schizophrenic, and patients with acute mania are all candidates for electroconvulsive therapy (ECT). ECT is accomplished by administering an electric stimulus to the patient that is sufficient to induce a grand mal seizure. The mechanism for the benefit derived from ECT is unknown. (401; **2263**)

27. Cardiopulmonary effects of ECT are reflected as stimulation of the parasympathetic nervous system followed by stimulation of the sympathetic nervous system. Initially, the anesthesiologist may see bradycardia and hypotension, followed by an increase in heart rate, an increase in blood pressure, and cardiac dysrhythmias. Apnea may also be seen during ECT. (402; **2263**)

28. The most common causes of mortality after ECT are myocardial infarction and cardiac dysrhythmias. (402; **2263**)

29. Dramatic increases in cerebral blood flow occur during ECT. (402; **2263**)

30. Intragastric pressure is increased during ECT. (402; **2263**)

31. Contraindications and relative contraindications to ECT include pheochromocytoma, increased intracranial pressure, recent cerebrovascular accident, cardiovascular conduction defects, high-risk intrauterine pregnancy, and aortic or cerebral aneurysms. (402; **2263**)

32. After ECT, and the resultant grand mal seizure, the patient is likely to be postictal. Headache, confusion, agitation, cognitive impairment, and apnea may all be present after the procedure. (402; **2263–2264**)

33. Before the performance of ECT the patient must have fasted from solids and liquids just as a patient would before general anesthesia. This is to minimize the risk of the pulmonary aspiration of gastric contents, because protective airway reflexes will be lost with the induction of anesthesia and potentially during the seizure activity. (402; **2264**)

34. Preoperative medication is not recommended before an ECT procedure because the duration of the preoperative medicine would likely be longer than the duration of the procedure itself. This may cause a delay in the awakening of the patient and a delay in the recovery of the patient from the procedure. An intravenous anticholinergic drug may be administered to a patient undergoing ECT before the administration of anesthesia to prevent the parasympathetic nervous system–mediated bradycardia that is frequently seen early in ECT. The anticholinergic drug would therefore have to be given 1 to 2 minutes before the induction of anesthesia. The routine administration of an anticholinergic is not recommended, however, because the duration of the bradycardia is typically brief. (402; **2264**)

35. Most induction agents for general anesthesia may be used to induce anesthesia in patients undergoing ECT. These include propofol (1 to 1.5 mg/kg intravenously [IV]), thiopental (1.5 to 3 mg/kg IV), and methohexital (0.5 to 1 mg/kg IV). Careful hemodynamic monitoring must accompany the induction of anes-

thesia for ECT and continue throughout the entire procedure. (402, Fig. 31–2; **2264**)

36. After the induction of anesthesia and the onset of unconsciousness, succinylcholine is often administered in subclinical doses (0.3 to 1.0 mg/kg IV) to the patient undergoing ECT. The goal of succinylcholine administration is to attenuate the effects of seizure activity on skeletal muscle, mainly the tonic-clonic muscular contractions, that may cause some harm to the patient. Because the administration of succinylcholine before ECT may mask the seizure activity that results from ECT, isolation of an extremity with a tourniquet is often done before succinylcholine administration. Physiologically, this prevents the administered succinylcholine from reaching the neuromuscular junctions in the isolated extremity distal to the tourniquet. Clinically, this allows for the physician to confirm that seizure activity has resulted from the ECT by observing the muscular contractions in the isolated extremity. (402; **2264**)

37. The airway of the patient undergoing ECT can be managed by hand with a mask provided the patient is not at risk for the aspiration of gastric contents. Before the induction of anesthesia the patient must be well preoxygenated. The anesthesiologist must be prepared to ventilate by hand with bag and mask using supplemental oxygen before the onset of seizure activity and also in the postseizure period, given that apnea may follow seizure activity even after the termination of the effects of succinylcholine. The anesthesiologist must have all equipment needed to intubate the trachea of the patient should it become necessary. Suction must also be available, in the event that the regurgitation of gastric contents or excessive oral secretions should occur. (402; **2264**)

38. Routine monitors must be used during an ECT procedure, including pulse oximetry, blood pressure monitoring, and a continuous electrocardiogram. In addition to these, a peripheral nerve stimulator may be useful to confirm neuromuscular blockade and the recovery of skeletal muscle from neuromuscular blockade. An electroencephalogram may also be used to confirm grand mal seizure activity during ECT. (402–403; **2264**)

DENTAL SURGERY

39. Anesthesia for a dental procedure is usually required for patients who are very young or developmentally delayed and unable to tolerate the procedure. (403)

40. An anticholinergic may be administered to a patient before a dental procedure for its antisialagogue effect. (403; **1438**)

41. Any of the induction agents used to induce general anesthesia may be used for patients undergoing dental procedures, including methohexital, thiopental, propofol, and etomidate. When there is no intravenous access available, and the patient is uncooperative, the anesthesiologist may use intramuscular ketamine for the induction of anesthesia. (403–404)

42. Tracheal intubation is usually accomplished nasally to facilitate the dentist's ability to perform dental procedures on those patients requiring general anesthesia for the procedure. (404; **1432–1433**)

43. During the emergence from general anesthesia for dental procedures the anesthesiologist must exercise caution with regard to the patient's airway. The patient must have intact laryngeal reflexes for the safe extubation of the trachea. Oral bleeding and secretions that occurred intraoperatively may have led to gastric distention and irritation. Ongoing oozing and secretions may also place the patient at a greater risk for laryngospasm. The removal of oropharyngeal packing must be confirmed. In the recovery area the patient's airway must be closely observed by personnel with the appropriate equipment for airway management, including suction. (404)

EXTRACORPOREAL SHOCK WAVE LITHOTRIPSY

44. Extracorporeal shock wave lithotripsy (ESWL) is a noninvasive method using shock waves for the disintegration of renal stones. All lithotripters have an energy source, a system to focus the shock wave, and a system to visualize and localize the renal stone. The first lithotripters required that patients be immersed in a water bath supported in a seated position. The immersion itself altered the patient's physiology. For instance, the central venous pressure often increased and the patient often became hypotensive after being immersed in warm water. Newer lithotripters do not require a water bath, are on multifunctional tables where cystoscopy and ureteral stent placement may also take place, and provide more focused shock waves to minimize pain at the entry site. (404; **1950–1952**)

45. Shock waves in ESWL are timed with the patient's heart rate and are triggered by the R wave on the patient's electrocardiogram. The shock waves are subsequently delivered during the refractory period of the heart muscle, thus minimizing the risk of cardiac dysrhythmias. Despite this, atrial and ventricular premature complexes, atrial fibrillation, and supraventricular tachycardia have all been reported. (404; **1951**)

46. Anesthesia is required for patients undergoing ESWL for two reasons. First, the impact of the shock waves on the patient can be painful, especially in the immersion bath model of shock wave lithotripters. Second, immobilization of the patient is important for the success of the procedure. The shock waves are focused on the renal stones, and any movement of the patient can displace the focus of the shock wave so that it is no longer effectively targeting the renal stones. (404; **1463, 1950–1952**)

47. Advantages of general anesthesia for patients undergoing ESWL include rapid onset, better patient immobilization, and the control of ventilatory parameters to minimize stone movement with respiration. (404; **1951–1952**)

48. For a patient undergoing ESWL with a regional anesthetic, a T6 sensory level is necessary to ensure patient comfort during the procedure. Unfortunately this high level of anesthesia and sympathetic nervous system blockade may be associated with hypotension. This may be exacerbated by the sitting position necessary for some lithotripters. (405)

49. Intravenous fluid administration is important during ESWL for the maintenance of an adequate urine output. This helps facilitate the passage of stones that have been disintegrated by the shock waves. (405)

50. Contraindications to ESWL include pregnancy, coagulopathy, morbid obesity, and aortic aneurysms. Patients with pacemakers may undergo ESWL provided the pacemaker is placed above the diaphragm and not in the abdomen. (404; **1952**)

Chapter 31

Postanesthesia Care Unit

1. What is the postanesthesia care unit (PACU)?

2. What personnel should staff a PACU?

3. What are the advantages to having the PACU near the operating rooms?

4. About how many beds should there be in a PACU relative to the number of operating rooms? What type of equipment should be available in a PACU?

LEVELS OF POSTOPERATIVE OBSERVATION

5. What are some factors that influence what level of immediate postanesthesia care is needed for postoperative patients?

RECOVERY FROM ANESTHESIA

6. Where does extubation of the trachea usually occur at the conclusion of an anesthetic procedure?

7. On what is the rate of decrease in the alveolar concentration of an inhaled anesthetic dependent?

8. On what is the rate of recovery from injected anesthetic drugs dependent?

ADMISSION TO THE PACU

9. What information should the anesthesiologist provide the nurse on the arrival of a patient to the PACU?

10. What are some aspects of a patient recovering from anesthesia that should be closely observed?

11. How frequently should the patient's vital signs be recorded while in the PACU?

DISCHARGE CRITERIA FROM THE PACU

12. Who should evaluate a patient before discharge from a PACU? What should the evaluation include?

13. What criteria should be met before discharging a patient from the PACU to home?

14. What information should a PACU nurse provide a ward nurse before the transfer of a patient from the PACU to the ward?

EARLY POSTOPERATIVE PHYSIOLOGIC DISORDERS

15. What is the most common cause of upper airway obstruction in the PACU?

16. What is the clinical appearance of a patient with upper airway obstruction in the PACU?

17. What are some methods of relieving upper airway obstruction in the PACU?

18. How is laryngospasm in a patient in the PACU treated?

19. How might laryngeal edema after endotracheal intubation be treated? Why is it especially important to be vigilant about this possible complication in children?

20. How can prolonged upper airway obstruction lead to pulmonary edema?

21. How is arterial hypoxemia defined?

22. What is the incidence of arterial hypoxemia in the PACU?

23. What are some clinical signs of arterial hypoxemia?

24. What is the ventilatory response to arterial hypoxemia? Why might this be altered in the patient in the PACU?

25. What are some factors that place a patient at an increased risk of postoperative arterial hypoxemia?

26. Name at least eight possible causes of arterial hypoxemia that may present in the PACU.

27. What is the most common cause of postoperative arterial hypoxemia? What are some reasons why this might occur?

28. After which surgical procedures is arterial hypoxemia especially common?

29. How can a decrease in cardiac output result in arterial hypoxemia?

30. What are three ways in which the pulmonary aspiration of acidic gastric contents can result in arterial hypoxemia?

31. When should a pulmonary embolus be suspected in a patient in the PACU?

32. How does pulmonary edema present in the PACU?

33. How might arterial hypoxemia secondary to a pneumothorax present in the PACU? How should a postoperative pneumothorax be treated?

34. How can hyperventilation result in arterial hypoxemia?

35. Can diffusion hypoxia result in arterial hypoxemia in the PACU after the administration of nitrous oxide?

36. How can postoperative shivering result in arterial hypoxemia?

37. What is the treatment of arterial hypoxemia in the PACU?

38. How long should supplemental oxygen be continued in the PACU?

39. How is hypoventilation defined?

40. What are some clinical signs of hypoventilation?

41. What is the most likely cause of hypoventilation in the PACU?

42. Why might opioids produce a biphasic depression of ventilation?

43. What are three reasons why neuromuscular blocking drugs administered intraoperatively may have sufficient residual effects in the PACU to affect ventilation?

44. What are some ways to evaluate the patient for residual neuromuscular blockade in the PACU?

45. What are some reasons, other than pharmacologic, why a patient may have suboptimal ventilatory mechanics in the PACU leading to hypoventilation?

46. How should hypoventilation be treated in the PACU?

47. How should naloxone be administered in the PACU to treat hypoventilation due to the residual effects of opioids? What are some of the possible adverse effects of naloxone administration?

48. What are some of the criteria for extubation of a patient's trachea after surgery? How should extubation proceed under these circumstances?

49. Name some causes of hypotension in the PACU.

50. What is the most common cause of hypotension in the PACU?

51. How might the residual effects of anesthetics contribute to hypotension in the PACU?

52. What are some reasons why decreases in myocardial contractility may occur in the PACU and result in hypotension?

53. Which patients are most likely to have a perioperative myocardial infarction? What percent of patients who have had a myocardial infarction in the PACU experienced angina pectoris?

54. What clinical sign is a useful indicator that hypotension may be due to hypovolemia or a decreased cardiac output? How can hypotension from either of these two causes be distinguished from each other?

55. Which type of surgical procedure may be most likely to lead to sepsis postoperatively?

56. What clinical signs may be an indication of inadequate surgical hemostasis?

57. How should the hypotensive patient be managed in the PACU?

58. When might central venous pressure monitoring be considered in the hypotensive patient?

59. What pulmonary artery catheter values are indicative of hypovolemia?

60. What pulmonary artery catheter values are indicative of decreased myocardial contractility?

61. What pulmonary artery catheter values are indicative of sepsis?

62. Name some causes of hypertension that presents in the PACU. What is hypertension that develops in the PACU most frequently due to?

63. Approximately what percentage of patients with hypertension in the PACU had hypertension preoperatively? What can exaggerate this hypertensive response?

64. What adverse effects can result from sustained, excessive hypertension?

65. How should hypertension in the PACU be managed?

66. What is an adverse risk of nitroprusside administration? How can this risk be minimized?

67. Name some reasons why a patient may have cardiac dysrhythmias in the PACU.

68. What is the appropriate treatment of cardiac dysrhythmias occurring in the patient in the PACU?

69. Name some factors associated with postoperative renal dysfunction.

70. How is oliguria defined? What is oliguria that manifests in the PACU most likely due to? How should it be monitored?

71. What are some coagulation abnormalities that may present as postoperative bleeding in the PACU? What are some laboratory tests that should be ordered in the PACU when postoperative bleeding occurs?

72. What is a bedside whole-blood clotting test useful for the evaluation of?

73. What laboratory results are indicative of disseminated intravascular coagulation?

74. Why might platelet quality and function be impaired despite normal platelet counts?

75. What are some reasons for an elevated partial thromboplastin time in the PACU? What drug can be administered for the reversal of heparin-induced prolongation of the partial thromboplastin time?

76. What are some possible reasons for an elevated prothrombin time in the PACU? How can this be treated?

77. What are some reasons for hypothermia seen in the PACU? How can it be treated?

78. Name some reasons why a patient may awaken from anesthesia in an agitated state.

79. How can the emergence delirium in the PACU associated with scopolamine or atropine administration be treated?

80. Name some reasons why patients in the PACU may have delayed awakening from anesthesia. What is the most common cause of delayed awakening in the PACU after anesthesia?

81. After what time course postoperatively can patients be expected to respond to stimulation? How should delayed awakening from anesthesia in the PACU be evaluated?

82. What are some pharmacologic interventions that can be made to antagonize residual drug effects that can result in delayed awakening in the PACU?

83. Name some factors associated with an increased risk of postoperative nausea and vomiting. What is the incidence of nausea and vomiting in the PACU?

84. What are some medications that can be administered to patients at risk of postoperative nausea and vomiting preoperatively or that can be administered postoperatively to patients in the PACU with nausea and vomiting?

85. What are some examples of minor incidental trauma that may present in the PACU?

86. Name some factors that influence the incidence and severity of postoperative pain.

87. Which surgical procedures typically result in the most postoperative pain?

88. What is preemptive analgesia?

POSTOPERATIVE RESPIRATORY THERAPY

89. Name some factors that influence the risk of postoperative pulmonary complications.

90. Which surgical procedures typically result in the most postoperative pulmonary complications?

91. How does the choice of drugs used for anesthesia influence the incidence of postoperative pulmonary complications?

92. When is oxygen therapy indicated for a patient in the PACU? When is oxygen therapy indicated for patients with chronic obstructive pulmonary disease whose ventilatory drive may rely on arterial hypoxemia?

93. How frequently do patients require postoperative oxygen therapy?

94. What is an advantage of oxygen therapy by nasal cannula?

95. What factors are the inspired oxygen concentration achieved dependent on when oxygen is delivered via a nasal cannula?

96. For each 1 L/min of oxygen flow administered via a nasal cannula, what is the approximate increase in percent of oxygen delivered to the patient?

97. What is the maximum flow of oxygen that can be delivered via a nasal cannula? What might result from excessive flow rates?

98. How does mouth breathing affect the effectiveness of oxygen delivery to the patient via a nasal cannula?

99. What are some types of face masks used for oxygen delivery?

100. Describe a simple face mask. What inspired concentration of oxygen can be delivered to the patient with a simple face mask?

101. What should be the minimum amount of oxygen flow through a simple face mask?

102. How does a simple face mask compare with a nasal cannula with regard to the consistency in the oxygen concentration delivered to patients?

103. Describe a partial rebreathing face mask. What inspired concentration of oxygen can be delivered to the patient with a partial rebreathing face mask?

104. Describe a non-rebreathing face mask. What inspired concentration of oxygen can be delivered to the patient with a non-rebreathing face mask? What flow rates of oxygen should be used when administering oxygen therapy via a non-rebreathing face mask?

105. Describe an air-entrainment face mask. What is another name for this type of face mask? What inspired concentration of oxygen can be delivered to the patient with an air-entrainment face mask?

106. What is an advantage of the air-entrainment face mask over other methods of administering oxygen therapy?

107. How are inhaled gases normally warmed?

108. In what situations should an artificial humidifying device for inspired gases be considered? What are some potential consequences of not humidifying inspired gases in these patients?

109. Why should only sterile water be used as a suspension fluid for all humidifiers and nebulizers?

110. How do pass-over humidifiers work? On what does the relative humidity of the gases inspired by the patient depend?

111. What is the major limitation of a pass-over humidifier?

112. How do bubble-through humidifiers work? Why is heating the water important in bubble-through humidifiers?

113. What is the function of a jet nebulizer? How does it work?

114. What are some uses of a jet nebulizer?

115. What does bronchial hygiene refer to? What are some methods used for bronchial hygiene?

116. What is mucociliary clearance? What volume of secretions per day is cleared by mucociliary clearance?

117. What are some causes of the impairment of mucociliary clearance?

118. What are some problems that can result from routine tracheal suctioning?

119. How can arterial hypoxemia during tracheal suctioning be minimized?

120. What is the purpose of chest physiotherapy? What are the components of chest physiotherapy?

121. How does coughing clear secretions from large airways?

122. What might be some reasons for postoperative decreases in vital capacity and functional residual capacity? Why is the magnitude of postoperative decreases in vital capacity and functional residual capacity important?

123. Does the total relief of postoperative pain prevent postoperative decreases in functional residual capacity?

124. What are some specific therapies designed to increase a patient's functional residual capacity postoperatively?

125. How should voluntary deep breathing exercises be done to maximize their benefit? What is the benefit of voluntary deep breathing exercises?

126. What is incentive spirometry? How is it best utilized?

127. What is the major limitation of incentive spirometry?

128. Why is early postoperative ambulation thought to be beneficial for the prevention of postoperative pulmonary complications?

129. How effective is intermittent positive pressure breathing in decreasing the incidence of postoperative pulmonary complications?

130. Why are postoperative exhalation exercises not recommended?

ANSWERS*

1. The postanesthesia care unit (PACU) is the area in which patients recover immediately after surgery and anesthesia. This area, also known as the recovery room, is designed for the continuous monitoring and close observation of patients as the acute physiologic effects of anesthesia and surgery subside. The American Society of Anesthesiologists has endorsed standards for postanesthesia care. (408; **2302, 2306–2307**)

2. The PACU should be staffed with nurses who are specially trained in postanesthesia care. They should be able to promptly recognize postoperative complications. The medical director of the PACU should be a physician who is skilled and knowledgeable in anesthesia, postanesthesia, and postsurgical issues. Most often, the director of the PACU is an anesthesiologist. (408; **2305**)

3. There at least two obvious advantages to having a PACU in proximity to the operating rooms. First, the proximity lessens the distance the anesthesiologist must transport the patient after anesthesia, providing the anesthetic was not administered in a remote location. Second, the proximity to the operating rooms ensures that anesthesiologists and surgeons are also in proximity and readily available for consultation or assistance. (408; **2304**)

4. There should be about 1.5 beds in the recovery room per operating room. Equipment that should be available at every bedside includes supplemental oxygen; suction; monitors for vital signs including blood pressure, pulse oximetry, and electrocardiogram; and the capability for mechanical ventilation and the transduction of intravascular pressures. (408; **2304**)

LEVELS OF POSTOPERATIVE OBSERVATION

5. The type of surgery, duration of surgery, type of anesthesia, severity of underlying illness, and the potential for postanesthesia complications all influence what level of immediate postanesthesia care is needed in postoperative patients. For instance, a relatively healthy patient undergoing superficial surgery under local anesthesia with sedation may bypass the regular type of

*Numbers in parentheses: lightface numbers refer to pages, figures, or tables in Stoelting RK, Miller RD: Basics of Anesthesia, 4th ed. Philadelphia, Churchill Livingstone, 2000; **boldface numbers** refer to pages, figures, or tables in Miller RD: Anesthesia, 5th ed. Philadelphia, Churchill Livingstone, 2000.

PACU, instead going to a step-down unit where he or she can ambulate, drink and eat, read, and be reunited with family members. These phase II type PACUs allow for fewer PACU personnel and decrease PACU costs. (408; **2303**)

RECOVERY FROM ANESTHESIA

6. Extubation of the trachea usually occurs in the operating room at the conclusion of surgery. On occasion, however, the patient may be brought to the PACU with the trachea still intubated. (408; **2305**)

7. The rate of decrease in the alveolar concentration of an inhaled anesthetic is dependent on many factors, including the patient's alveolar ventilation and the duration of anesthesia. It is also dependent on properties specific to the inhaled anesthetic, such as its blood and lipid solubility and the magnitude of its metabolism. (408–409; **2305**)

8. The rate of recovery from injected anesthetic drugs is dependent on the dose of drug that was administered, the time that has passed since the last injection of drug, the drug's lipid solubility, and the rate and method of elimination of the drug by either hepatic metabolism and/or renal excretion. (408–409; **2305**)

ADMISSION TO THE PACU

9. The anesthesiologist should provide the nurse with information regarding the patient's medical history and condition. The nurse should also be provided with information regarding the surgical procedure, intraoperative events, and the type of anesthetic rendered to the patient. (409; **2305–2306**)

10. Patients recovering from anesthesia should have their oxygenation, ventilation, and circulation closely observed, monitored, and documented at regular intervals. The patient's oxygenation is reflected by pulse oximetry, the ventilation by breathing frequency and airway patency, and the circulation by blood pressure, heart rate, and heart rhythm. (409, Fig. 32–1; **2306**)

11. The patient's vital signs should be recorded every 15 minutes while in the PACU. (409; **2306**)

DISCHARGE CRITERIA FROM THE PACU

12. Evaluation of a patient before discharge from the PACU should be done by a physician knowledgeable about postanesthesia and postsurgical recovery, usually an anesthesiologist. The evaluation of a patient for discharge from the PACU should include an assessment of the patient's level of activity, response to commands, ease of breathing, stability of blood pressure, level of consciousness, and color. (409, Table 32–1; **2306**)

13. Before being discharged from a PACU to home the patient must have a responsible adult who will care for him or her at home. In addition, the patient must be able to ambulate without dizziness, stand without hypotension, be devoid of significant postoperative pain, and be able to tolerate liquids without nausea and vomiting. (410, Table 32–2; **2306**)

14. The PACU nurse should provide the ward nurse with information about the patient's medical history, medical condition, operative procedure, and postoperative course before being transferred to the ward. (410; **2306**)

EARLY POSTOPERATIVE PHYSIOLOGIC DISORDERS

15. The most common cause of upper airway obstruction in the PACU is occlusion of the pharynx by the tongue. Laryngeal obstruction in the PACU may

also occur secondary to laryngospasm, laryngeal edema, tumor, or a foreign body. Laryngeal edema can occur as a result of traumatic intubation, too large an endotracheal tube, excessive neck movements while the trachea is intubated during surgery, excessive coughing and bucking on the endotracheal tube on emergence, and the presence or recent history of upper airway respiratory tract infection. (411; **1447, 2308**)

16. Upper airway obstruction that presents in the PACU can be total or partial. It is important for the anesthesiologist to recognize airway obstruction when it occurs. These patients have a distinct clinical appearance. With each attempted breath the patient has flaring of the nares, retractions are apparent at both the suprasternal notch and at the intercostal spaces, and there are vigorous contractions by the diaphragm and abdomen. Inexperienced persons may wrongly interpret the tugging motions of the diaphragm as respiration. Partial upper airway obstruction may be accompanied by loud snoring or inspiratory stridor for obstruction near the larynx. Total obstruction leads to the lack of any air exchange or breath sounds. (412; **1415–1416**)

17. The most common cause of upper airway obstruction is soft tissue occlusion or reduction of the pharyngeal space at the base of the tongue. The most effective method of relieving this type of upper airway obstruction in the PACU is by extending the head while supporting the mandible in an anterior position. Often, extension of the head alone is enough to relieve the obstruction. This maneuver works by stretching muscles attached to the tongue. The stretch of these muscles pulls the tongue from the posterior pharynx where it occludes the airway. An alternative that may be tried if this method does not work is the placement of an oropharyngeal or nasopharyngeal airway once a foreign body has been excluded. If obstruction of the upper airway persists despite proper head position and the use of an airway, direct laryngoscopy and intubation of the trachea is indicated. Obstruction of the airway that occurs as a result of laryngeal edema may indicate that visualization of the vocal cords may be difficult, making tracheal intubation by direct laryngoscopy difficult. When intubation of the trachea is difficult under these conditions, the anesthesiologist must proceed with the algorithm for a difficult airway endorsed by the American Society of Anesthesiologists. Among the maneuvers that the anesthesiologist may attempt under these circumstances are transtracheal jet ventilation, a laryngeal mask airway, or cricothyrotomy. (412; **1415–1416, 2308–2309, Figs. 68–3, 68–4, 68–5**)

18. Laryngospasm in the PACU is treated by the manual management of the airway with the head tilt-jaw thrust and a well-fitted mask and the administration of continuous positive airway pressure with a bag and mask. The fraction of inspired oxygen during this maneuver should be 100%. Laryngospasm that is not complete will dissipate spontaneously, making this noninvasive form of management sufficient in most cases. Laryngospasm that is not reversed by this noninvasive maneuver must be managed by the intravenous administration of small doses of succinylcholine. (412; **1416, 2309**)

19. Laryngeal edema that follows endotracheal intubation might be treated by the administration of humidified inhaled gases and nebulized racemic epinephrine. Controversial with regard to its efficacy for the treatment of laryngeal edema is dexamethasone. It is important to be vigilant about postoperative laryngeal edema in children, because mild laryngeal edema may significantly reduce the size of the tracheal lumen. In this population of patients laryngeal edema can rapidly progress to complete airway obstruction. (412; **1447**)

20. Prolonged upper airway obstruction may lead to pulmonary edema as a result of a sustained reduction in interstitial hydrostatic pressure. Other terms for this type of pulmonary edema are noncardiogenic pulmonary edema and negative pressure pulmonary edema. (412; **2309**)

21. Arterial hypoxemia is defined as being a PaO_2 less than 60 mm Hg. It is usually recognized by the measurement of arterial hemoglobin oxygen saturation by pulse oximetry. The definitive diagnosis of arterial hypoxemia is made by the direct measurement of the PaO_2. (412; **2309, 2311**)

22. About 50% of postoperative patients are estimated to have an episode of arterial hypoxemia in the first 3 hours after surgery. (412; **2309**)

23. Clinical signs of arterial hypoxemia are nonspecific and can include hypertension, hypotension, tachycardia, bradycardia, cardiac dysrhythmias, and agitation. (413)

24. The normal ventilatory response to arterial hypoxemia is an increase in alveolar ventilation. In patients in the PACU the ventilatory response to arterial hypoxemia may be altered by the residual effects of anesthetics the patient had received intraoperatively. Alterations in the response to the hypoxia by peripheral chemoreceptors appears to be the mechanism by which volatile anesthetics exert this effect in postoperative patients. The synergistic effect of hypercapnia and hypoxia to stimulate ventilation is also affected. Indeed, this effect has been found to occur with volatile anesthetic concentrations equivalent to 0.1 minimum alveolar concentration (MAC). (413; **141–143, 641, 2311, Figs. 5–37, 5–38**)

25. Factors that place a patient at an increased risk of postoperative arterial hypoxemia include advanced age, obesity, a smoking history, and co-existing lung disease. Knowledge of these factors allows for the preoperative identification of patients at risk for postoperative arterial hypoxemia. (412; **963–964, 2309**)

26. The classic causes of arterial hypoxemia fall into one of four categories, which are hypoventilation, low inspired oxygen concentration, areas of low ventilation-to-perfusion matching, and an increase in intrapulmonary right-to-left shunt. Possible causes of postoperative arterial hypoxemia include atelectasis, decreased cardiac output, alveolar hypoventilation, the aspiration of gastric contents, pulmonary embolus, pulmonary edema, pneumothorax, post-hyperventilation hypoxia, increased oxygen consumption, advanced age, and obesity. (412; **2309–2311**)

27. The most common cause of postoperative arterial hypoxemia is an increase in right-to-left intrapulmonary shunting, as with atelectasis. Segmental atelectasis can result from bronchial obstruction due to secretions or blood. Diffuse atelectasis often occurs as a result of decreased lung volumes. (412; **2309**)

28. Arterial hypoxemia is especially common after upper abdominal or thoracic surgery. The PaO_2 decreases by about 20 mm Hg after upper abdominal or thoracic surgery. The PaO_2 decreases by about 10 mm Hg after abdominal surgery and by about 6 mm Hg after peripheral surgery. The decrease in the PaO_2 of patients after abdominal surgery occurs regardless of whether the procedure was done under general or regional anesthesia. Arterial hypoxemia after abdominal surgery is due in part to decreases in the patient's vital capacity. The vital capacity can decrease by as much as 60% in these patients. (412; **2311, 2313, Fig. 68–11**)

29. A decrease in cardiac output can contribute to arterial hypoxemia in patients who have existing intrapulmonary shunts. This occurs as a result of the effect of the lowered mixed-venous PO_2, which returns to the arterial circulation via a right-to-left intrapulmonary shunt. (412; **2311, Fig. 68–8**)

30. The pulmonary aspiration of acidic gastric contents can result in arterial hypoxemia in at least three ways. First, immediately after aspiration there may be reflexive airway closure. Second, the loss of surfactant in the affected

areas leads to atelectasis in those areas. Third, the loss of capillary integrity in the affected areas can result in noncardiogenic pulmonary edema. (412–413; **2310**)

31. A pulmonary embolus should be suspected in a postoperative patient who has an acute onset of pleuritic chest pain, dyspnea, and tachypnea that are coincident with acute decreases in the PaO_2. Patients with a pulmonary embolus may have right-sided heart strain on their electrocardiogram. A massive pulmonary embolus may be accompanied by pulmonary hypertension, elevated central venous pressures, and systemic hypotension. Patients who have been at bed rest for prolonged periods before surgery are especially at risk for a pulmonary embolus. (413; **2310**)

32. Pulmonary edema in the PACU usually presents in the first hour after surgery. It is often preceded by systemic hypertension and is frequently accompanied by wheezing. Pulmonary edema can occur as a result of high hydrostatic pressures in the pulmonary capillaries, increased capillary permeability, or decreased interstitial pressures that are sustained. Examples of a cause of each of these types of pulmonary edema include valvular heart disease, the adult respiratory distress syndrome, and prolonged airway obstruction with sustained intrathoracic negative pressures. (413; **2310, Fig. 68–6**)

33. A pneumothorax can result in arterial hypoxemia by causing atelectasis and an intrapulmonary shunt. It may present in the PACU as an increase in airway pressure, wheezing, decreased breath sounds, and labored breathing. Trauma or an attempt at central venous access can result in a pneumothorax. Surgical procedures that are most likely to be associated with a postoperative pneumothorax include a radical neck dissection, mastectomy, or nephrectomy. Treatment of a postoperative pneumothorax in a spontaneously ventilating patient with the insertion of a chest tube is recommended when the pneumothorax exceeds 20%. A pneumothorax of any size requires the insertion of a chest tube in mechanically ventilated patients. In the event of a tension pneumothorax and the associated circulatory compromise generated by compression of the mediastinum, the emergent placement of a 14-gauge catheter into the second intercostal space should proceed without delay. (413; **2309**)

34. Hyperventilation can result in arterial hypoxemia by the compensatory hypoventilation that follows. Hypoventilation follows hyperventilation in an effort to restore carbon dioxide levels to the baseline state. During this period of hypoventilation the patient may become hypoxemic. Arterial hypoxemia resulting from hyperventilation can be avoided by the administration of supplemental oxygen. (413; **604, 2310–2311, Fig. 68–7**)

35. It is unlikely that arterial hypoxemia in the PACU can be attributed to diffusion hypoxia after the administration of nitrous oxide. At the conclusion of an anesthetic only a few breaths of 100% oxygen are required to prevent the diffusion hypoxia that would otherwise result. In the vast majority of cases, the discontinuation of nitrous oxide and the administration of supplemental oxygen has taken place in the operating room before arrival to the PACU. (413; **92–93, 2310–2311, Figs. 4–23, 68–7**)

36. Postoperative shivering can result in arterial hypoxemia by increasing oxygen consumption. Oxygen consumption can increase by 300% to 500% in shivering patients. Postoperative shivering can be treated through skin surface warming or the administration of drugs such as meperidine, clonidine, and magnesium sulfate. (413; **1377–1378, 2311, 2319**)

37. The treatment of arterial hypoxemia in the PACU is with the administration of supplemental oxygen. It is important to realize that this is not actually a treatment for the hypoxemia but rather a temporizing procedure until a cause

can be determined and the appropriate treatment instituted. Treatment for arterial hypoxemia in the PACU depends on the cause of the hypoxemia and is aimed at reversing or treating the underlying cause. The persistence of arterial hypoxemia despite the administration of 100% oxygen is an indication for intubation of the patient's trachea and mechanical ventilation of the lungs. The application of positive end-expiratory pressure may be useful to increase the functional residual capacity in these patients. Likewise, hypercapnia after the administration of supplemental oxygen that does not resolve is an indication for intubation of the patient's trachea. (413; **2312–2313**)

38. There are no clear guidelines regarding how long supplemental oxygen should be administered in the postoperative period. In general, patients should have supplemental oxygen until they are able to maintain a reasonable oxygen saturation for 30 minutes after discontinuing the oxygen. The oxygen saturation that is considered reasonable varies for different individuals. (413; **2311–2312**)

39. Hypoventilation is considered present when the Pa_{CO_2} exceeds 45 mm Hg as a result of decreased alveolar ventilation. The diagnosis of hypoventilation in the PACU requires the direct measurement of the Pa_{CO_2}. (413; **2312–2313**)

40. Clinical signs of hypoventilation are related to the signs of acute carbon dioxide retention. These are nonspecific and include tachycardia, hypertension, and arrhythmias. Elderly patients may have an impaired response to increasing levels of carbon dioxide. (414; **613–614, 2312–2313**)

41. The most likely cause of hypoventilation in the PACU is the depression of ventilation secondary to the residual effects of inhaled and injected anesthetics. Hypercarbia results in the accumulation of carbon dioxide in the alveoli of the hypoventilatory patient. This results in a concomitant decrease in the Po_2 in the alveoli. Without supplemental oxygen, the patient may become hypoxemic. (413; **140–141, 613–614, 2312–2313, Fig. 5–36**)

42. Opioids administered intraoperatively may result in biphasic ventilatory depression. Biphasic ventilatory depression may occur based on the amount of external stimulation that a patient requires to stimulate ventilation. For instance, on extubation and transport to the PACU the patient may experience a sufficient amount of stimulation for ventilation to occur. After admission to the PACU the amount of external activity may diminish to the extent that the stimulation of ventilation does not take place, and the patient once again has depressed ventilation. (413, Fig. 32–3; **2312–2313, Fig. 68–10**)

43. Patients in the PACU may have residual neuromuscular blockade after the administration of neuromuscular blocking drugs intraoperatively for at least three reasons. First, the patient may have delayed excretion or metabolism of the neuromuscular blocking drug. Second, the neuromuscular blocking drug may be potentiated by hypermagnesemia, hypothermia, hypokalemia, respiratory acidosis, or the concomitant administration of aminoglycoside antibiotics. Third, the pharmacologic antagonism that was administered to the patient may have been inadequate. Any of these causes of residual neuromuscular blockade may affect ventilation in the PACU. These patients may also have double vision and difficulty swallowing. Patients who had received a long-acting neuromuscular blocking drug such as pancuronium are at a greater risk of residual neuromuscular blockade postoperatively. (414; **2313**)

44. There are several ways to evaluate the patient clinically for residual effects of neuromuscular blocking drugs in the PACU. The performance of a sustained head lift for 5 seconds, a vigorous hand grasp, and tongue protrusion for several seconds by the patient are each evidence for the recovery from the effects of neuromuscular blocking drugs. Likewise, the vital capacity can

also be used for the evaluation for the residual effects of neuromuscular blocking drugs. Finally, a peripheral nerve stimulator can be used to evaluate the patient's response to a train-of-four stimulus. (414; **417, 1361–1362**)

45. Hypoventilation may be seen in the PACU as a result of the suboptimal ventilatory mechanics. Examples of patients who may have this postoperative problem include patients who are obese, patients with gastric dilation, patients positioned poorly, patients with tight dressings or body casts, and patients experiencing pain from the surgical site. Patients with preoperative pulmonary disease and suboptimal ventilatory mechanics preoperatively are also at an increased risk postoperatively. (414; **2313**)

46. Hypoventilation that occurs in the PACU should be treated on an individual basis. If the cause of the hypoventilation is reversible, attempts to do so should be instituted. The provision of adequate pain control may allow for the patient to ventilate with greater tidal volumes when inhibited by postoperative pain. If hypoventilation occurs as a result of residual neuromuscular blockade, antagonism of the blockade should be administered. For hypoventilation that results from the residual effects of inhaled anesthetics, the reversal of the hypoventilation can only occur with the passage of time as the partial pressure of the anesthetic in the patient's tissues decreases. Under these circumstances, if the patient maintains a patent upper airway and appears alert, it may be permissible to allow for the spontaneous remission of the anesthetic while closely observing the patient. If, however, the patient is not alert or is not able to maintain a patent upper airway, intubation of the trachea and mechanical ventilation of the lungs may be indicated. (414–415; **2313**)

47. Hypoventilation in the PACU due to the residual effects of opioids can be treated by the administration of naloxone. Naloxone administration under these circumstances should be done incrementally in doses of 40 μg intravenously every 2 minutes. This allows for the titration of naloxone to the desired effect on ventilation without reversing all the beneficial analgesic effects of the opioid. Adverse effects associated with the administration of large doses of naloxone are related to the abrupt activation of the sympathetic nervous system. These adverse effects include nausea and vomiting, pulmonary edema, hypertension, and myocardial ischemia. Cardiac dysrhythmias and ventricular fibrillation have also resulted from the administration of a large dose of naloxone. (414–415; **348–350, 2313, Table 10–22**)

48. Readiness for extubation of the patient's trachea after surgery should be evaluated on an individual basis. Some useful criteria for patient readiness for an awake extubation include the patient's level of consciousness, a vital capacity greater than 15 mL/kg, an inspiratory force greater than −20 cm H_2O, and acceptable arterial blood gas values. Once the determination has been made to extubate the patient's trachea, the patient's oropharynx and trachea should be suctioned. The patient should inhale deeply or be assisted in doing so. The cuff of the endotracheal tube should then be deflated, and removal of the endotracheal tube should follow. Removal of the endotracheal tube must follow the patient's inhalation so as to ensure that the initial flow of gas is outward from the lungs, thus expelling instead of inhaling secretions. (415; **1446–1447, 2313**)

49. Hypotension postoperatively can be due to a decrease in ventricular preload, a decrease in myocardial contractility, or a decrease in systemic vascular resistance. Causes of hypotension in the PACU include hypovolemia, arterial hypoxemia, decreased myocardial contractility, decreased systemic vascular resistance, cardiac dysrhythmias, pulmonary embolus, pneumothorax, and cardiac tamponade. (415; **2313–2314**)

50. The most common cause of hypotension in the PACU is hypovolemia.

Hypovolemia and decreased ventricular preload may be due to intravascular fluid volume depletion from blood loss, excessive third space loss, or inadequate fluid replacement after fasting. Hypovolemia causes hypotension by the associated decreased venous return and subsequent decreased cardiac output. (415; **2313–2314**)

51. The residual effects of anesthetics can contribute to hypotension in the PACU by accentuating hypotension due to hypovolemia. The presence of residual anesthetics attenuates the peripheral vasoconstriction that would normally reflexively occur to compensate for hypovolemia. Residual anesthetics can also impair myocardial contractility. (415; **2314**)

52. Decreases in myocardial contractility may occur in the PACU for several reasons. First, the residual effects of anesthetics may have a direct myocardial depressant effect. Second, the patient may have co-existing cardiac dysfunction that is manifest as a decrease in myocardial contractility in the PACU. Finally, the patient may have myocardial ischemia or an acute myocardial infarction. Decreases in myocardial contractility from any of these causes can result in hypotension in the PACU. (415; **2314**)

53. Patients who are most likely to have a perioperative myocardial infarction include those with left ventricular hypertrophy, a history of hypertension, diabetes mellitus, or co-existing coronary artery disease. Of all the patients who are found to have had a myocardial infarction in the PACU, only about one fourth of them experienced any angina pectoris. Many of them did have a period of unexplained hypotension, some with concomitant ventricular premature contractions. (415)

54. Oliguria is a useful clinical indicator of hypovolemia or a decreased cardiac output. Oliguria under these conditions presumably corresponds to a decrease in renal perfusion. A urine output of less than 0.5 mL/kg per hour should alert the anesthesiologist that hypovolemia or a decrease in cardiac output may be present. In an attempt to determine which of these two is the cause of oliguria, a fluid challenge of lactated Ringer's solution in the amount of 3 to 6 mL/kg may be administered intravenously and the subsequent urine output monitored. For oliguria that results from hypovolemia, an increase in urine output may result. For oliguria that results from a decrease in myocardial contractility, the urine output probably would not change in response to a fluid challenge. (415; **1307–1308**)

55. Surgical procedures on the genitourinary tract are among the most likely to lead to sepsis postoperatively. Patients with postoperative sepsis may have fever, chills, tachycardia, and an elevated white blood cell count. (415; **1948**)

56. Evidence of bleeding at the operative site and/or a low hematocrit provide an indication of possible inadequate surgical hemostasis. A decreasing hematocrit on evaluation of serial blood samples postoperatively is indicative of ongoing losses and is more worrisome than one isolated low hematocrit value. (415)

57. Worrisome blood pressures, especially when they are a distinct change from baseline, should be confirmed before treatment is instituted. Artificially low readings from a mechanical blood pressure machine can occur secondary to the use of a blood pressure cuff that is too large. Artificially low readings from direct arterial blood pressure measurements can result from an inaccurately calibrated transducer or from a transducer that is positioned above the level of the right atrium. Once the presence of hypotension in the PACU has been confirmed it should be evaluated and treated. Conservative measures for increasing venous return and perhaps increasing cardiac output include positional changes, such as elevation of the legs or placing the patient in the Trendelenburg position if tolerated. Blood pressures that are not restored by

conservative measures may be supported by a sympathomimetic drug. This can serve as a temporizing measure until hypovolemia is corrected or an underlying cause is elucidated. (415–416; **2314–2315**)

58. Monitoring with a central venous catheter may be considered if hypotension persists despite resuscitation with intravenous fluids. If the patient has normal left ventricular function, the central venous pressure is a fairly accurate measure of the intravascular fluid volume. Central venous pressures are not as useful in patients with known left ventricular dysfunction. In these patients a pulmonary artery catheter may be able to provide the anesthesiologist with more precise information to evaluate the cause of the hypotension. (416; **2314–2315**)

59. Pulmonary artery catheter measurements that indicate hypovolemia is the cause of hypotension include a low pulmonary artery occlusion pressure, low cardiac index, and an increased calculated systemic vascular resistance. (416; **2314–2315**)

60. Pulmonary artery catheter measurements that indicate that decreased myocardial contractility is the cause of hypotension include a high pulmonary artery occlusion pressure and a low cardiac index. Hypotension secondary to decreased myocardial contractility can be treated with inotropic drugs. An electrocardiogram and laboratory analysis should be performed to exclude myocardial ischemia as a cause for the decrease in myocardial contractility. (416; **2314–2315**)

61. Pulmonary artery catheter measurements that indicate sepsis is the cause of hypotension include a low pulmonary artery occlusion pressure, high cardiac index, and a decreased calculated systemic vascular resistance. Hypotension that is due to sepsis should be treated with intravenous fluids and a vasopressor agent, such as an alpha agonist. (416; **2314–2315**)

62. Hypertension that presents in the PACU can be due to arterial hypoxemia, an increase in sympathetic nervous system activity, preexisting hypertension, or hypervolemia. Hypertension that develops in the PACU is most commonly due to increased sympathetic nervous system activity from pain. Hypertension in the PACU that results from pain usually occurs in the first 30 minutes after surgery as the patient recovers from the intraoperatively administered anesthetics. (416; **2315**)

63. More than 50% of patients who are hypertensive in the PACU had preoperative hypertension. Patients are at an increased risk of postoperative hypertension if their antihypertensive medications were withdrawn preoperatively. (416; **2315**)

64. There are several adverse effects that can result from sustained, excessive hypertension in the PACU. These include left ventricular failure with pulmonary edema, myocardial ischemia, cardiac dysrhythmias, and cerebral hemorrhage. (416; **2315**)

65. Hypertension in the PACU should be managed based on the underlying cause of the hypertension. For instance, if hypertension in the PACU occurs as a result of pain, relief of the pain should also lead to a decrease in the blood pressure. Among the antihypertensives that can be used to control elevated blood pressures in the PACU are nitroprusside, labetalol, and hydralazine. Nitroprusside should be administered by a continuous infusion and titrated to maintain the blood pressure in the desirable range. Labetalol can be administered at a dose of 5 to 10 mg IV, and hydralazine can be administered at a dose of 2.5 to 5 mg IV. (416; **2315–2316**)

66. An adverse risk of nitroprusside administration is the accumulation of cya-

nide, a metabolite of nitroprusside. The accumulation of cyanide can lead to tissue hypoxia. For this reason the total dose of nitroprusside should not exceed 1.5 mg/kg IV for 1 to 3 hours of administration of the drug. During the administration of nitroprusside the arterial pH should be measured periodically for the detection of metabolic acidosis suggestive of the accumulation of cyanide. (416; **1474–1476, 2315–2316**)

67. Reasons why a patient may have cardiac dysrhythmias in the PACU include arterial hypoxemia, hypovolemia, pain, hypothermia, anticholinesterases, myocardial ischemia, electrolyte abnormalities, respiratory acidosis, hypertension, digitalis intoxication, and preoperative cardiac dysrhythmias. (416–417; **2319**)

68. Cardiac dysrhythmias that occur in the PACU should be treated by confirming adequate arterial oxygenation and then seeking and treating the underlying cause of the dysrhythmias. The dysrhythmia itself may also be treated with the administration of medicines. Bradycardia in the PACU can be treated with the administration of atropine. Tachycardia in the PACU can be treated with the administration of a beta-adrenergic antagonist. Premature ventricular contractions occurring in the PACU can be treated with the administration of lidocaine. Patients who have atrial or ventricular tachydysrhythmias that result in hemodynamic instability should be treated by electrical cardioversion. (417; **1239–1245, 2319, 2550–2554**)

69. Factors associated with an increased risk of postoperative renal dysfunction include co-existing renal disease, major trauma, sepsis, advanced age, multiple intraoperative blood transfusions, prolonged intraoperative hypotension, and biliary tract surgery in the presence of obstructive jaundice. (417; **684–690**)

70. Oliguria is defined as a urine output that is less than 0.5 mL/kg in 1 hour. Oliguria that manifests in the PACU is most likely due to hypovolemia or a decreased cardiac output. Either of these can ultimately result in a decrease in renal blood flow and lead to oliguria. Oliguria in the PACU should be monitored by the placement of an indwelling Foley catheter for accurate measurements of urine output and for the evaluation of the efficacy of treatment interventions. (417; **1308–1309**)

71. Coagulation abnormalities can be a cause of postoperative bleeding in the PACU. Bleeding abnormalities that may present as bleeding in the recovery room include a dilutional thrombocytopenia, disseminated intravascular coagulation, factor V and/or factor VIII deficiencies, and dysfunctional platelets. Laboratory tests that may be ordered to determine if bleeding abnormalities may be a cause of otherwise unexplained bleeding in the recovery room are a platelet count, prothrombin time, partial thromboplastin time, fibrinogen levels, fibrin split product levels, bleeding time, and thromboelastography. Other causes of bleeding in the PACU, such as inadequate surgical hemostasis, must also be considered. (417, Table 32–3; **1621–1623**)

72. A bedside whole-blood clotting test is useful for the anesthesiologist because it provides early information about the patient's ability to clot blood. Clot formation should take place in less than 12 minutes. The time to clot, the blood clot size, clot stability, and the evaluation of the clot for lysis can all be observed at the bedside. In addition, retraction of the clot provides information about platelet function during a whole-blood clotting test. Although this bedside test can only provide the anesthesiologist with clinical indicators, it may be useful to determine if bleeding in the PACU is due to a bleeding abnormality or some other cause while the results of laboratory tests for platelet count, prothrombin time, partial thromboplastin time, fibrinogen, and fibrin split product levels are pending. (417; **1624**)

73. When disseminated intravascular coagulation occurs, the clotting system becomes deranged. Normally, the clotting of blood occurs to prevent excessive blood loss and fibrinolysis occurs to ensure blood flow within the microvasculature. In disseminated intravascular coagulation, fibrin deposition is disseminated. This leads to unclottable blood and poor perfusion in the microvasculature, which can result in ischemic necrosis of organs. Laboratory results indicative of disseminated intravascular coagulation include a low platelet count, a prolonged prothrombin time, a decreased serum concentration of fibrinogen, and an increased level of circulating fibrin split products. (417; **1622–1623**)

74. Platelet function can be impaired despite normal circulating levels of platelets in the serum. Reasons for platelet dysfunction include rare inherited genetic disorders, lupus, idiopathic thrombocytopenic purpura, hemolytic uremic syndrome, uremia, hypothermia, prolonged storage of platelets in the blood bank, and multiple different drugs. Some of the drugs that have been shown to affect platelet function include aspirin, vitamin E, indomethacin, dipyridamole, tricyclic antidepressants, furosemide, phenothiazines, and corticosteroids. Except for aspirin, these drugs usually only disturb platelet function for 24 to 48 hours after ingestion. The herb *Ginkgo Biloba* has also been implicated in impairing normal platelet function. (417; **988, 1621–1622**)

75. Reasons for an elevated partial thromboplastin time in the PACU include the inadequate reversal of heparin, a dilution of factors V and VIII by the massive transfusion of whole blood, and hemophilia. The reversal of heparin-induced prolongation of the partial thromboplastin time can be achieved with the administration of protamine. The administration of protamine must be done slowly with careful attention to the patient's blood pressure. The rapid administration of protamine places the patient at risk of hypotension, myocardial depression, histamine release, systemic vasodilation, pulmonary vasoconstriction, and anaphylactic reactions. (417; **1191, 1624**)

76. Reasons why a patient may have a prolonged prothrombin time include disseminated intravascular coagulation, a vitamin K deficiency, liver disease, and the ingestion of medicines that may prolong the prothrombin time, such as warfarin. An elevated prothrombin time can be treated by the administration of fresh frozen plasma. (417; **1622**)

77. Hypothermia is commonly seen in the PACU. The four mechanisms for heat loss from the patient in the operating room are radiation, evaporation, conduction, and convection. Hypothermia occurs mostly through radiation from the skin. The amount of heat lost in this manner depends on the temperature difference between the room and the patient and the amount of skin exposed. Evaporative heat losses occur from evaporation from exhaled gases and exposed viscera, whereas conductive losses occur from direct contact with cold surfaces, such as the operating room table or cold intravenous solutions. Convective heat losses occur by moving air flow around the patient. Anesthetized patients are less able to compensate for heat loss occurring in the operating room secondary to the attenuation of reflexive peripheral vasoconstriction and shivering responses. Heat losses intraoperatively can be minimized by warming the room, delivering warm inhaled gases at low flows, and using warming blankets for skin surface warming. Postoperative shivering in response to hypothermia can increase oxygen consumption by 300% to 500%. For hypothermia that presents in the PACU, warming can be instituted by forced air skin surface warming such as the Bair Huggar system. Postoperative shivering can be treated with the administration of drugs such as meperidine, clonidine, and magnesium sulfate. (417–418; **1377–1378, 2311, 2319**)

78. A patient may awaken from anesthesia in an agitated state secondary to arterial hypoxemia, hypercapnia, pain, gastric dilation, urinary retention, and drug effects. The incidence of awakening in an agitated state appears to be increased in young patients. (418; **2316–2317**)

79. Patients who have received scopolamine or atropine are at risk for emergence delirium on awakening from anesthesia secondary to the central nervous system side effects of these drugs. Scopolamine and atropine are muscarinic antagonists that have tertiary amine structures enabling these drugs to cross the blood-brain barrier. In the brain these drugs compete for acetylcholine receptors and prevent the muscarinic effects of acetylcholine. Emergence delirium from these causes can be treated by the administration of physostigmine at a dose of 15 to 45 μg/kg IV. Physostigmine inhibits the acetylcholinesterase enzyme, increasing the levels of acetylcholine in the brain. The increased levels of acetylcholine allow for increased competition by acetylcholine for acetylcholine receptor sites and reverses the effects of scopolamine and atropine. (418; **2316–2317**)

80. Reasons why a patient may be delayed in awakening from anesthesia include residual drug effects, hypothermia, hypoglycemia, electrolyte disturbances, arterial hypoxemia, increased intracranial pressure, air embolism, and hysteria. The most common cause of delayed awakening from anesthesia in the PACU is the residual effects of inhaled and injected anesthetic drugs. (418; **2316**)

81. Patients are typically responsive to stimuli within the first 60 to 90 minutes of their arrival to the PACU. The evaluation of delayed awakening in the PACU should include an evaluation of the patient's vital signs, the performance of a neurologic examination, analysis of arterial blood gases, and an evaluation for metabolic disturbances by measuring electrolytes and glucose levels in the serum. Radiographic procedures may also be indicated in given patients for the evaluation of possible intrathoracic or intracranial adverse processes. (418; **2316**)

82. When delayed awakening in the PACU may be due to opioids, naloxone may be administered in titrated doses in an attempt to reverse the opioid effect on the level of consciousness while still maintaining its beneficial analgesic effects. For delayed awakening in the PACU that may be due to anticholinergics such as atropine or scopolamine, the administration of physostigmine at a dose of 15 to 45 μg/kg intravenously may be useful as an attempt to reverse the anticholinergic effect. Delayed awakening in the PACU that may be due to benzodiazepines can be treated by the administration of flumazenil at a dose of 8 to 15 μg/kg IV to reverse the effect of the benzodiazepine. Hypoglycemia can be treated with the administration of 50% dextrose intravenously. (418–419; **2316**)

83. Factors associated with an increased risk of nausea and vomiting include a history of emesis with previous anesthetics, female gender, obesity, postoperative pain, the type of surgery, gastric distention, and anesthetic drugs administered such as opioids. Surgeries associated with an increased risk of postoperative nausea and vomiting include surgery on eye muscles, surgery on the middle ear, and laparoscopic procedures. The incidence of nausea and vomiting in the PACU may be as high as 20% to 30%. (419; **2318–2319**)

84. Among the medicines that can be administered to patients in the perioperative period for the prevention or treatment of nausea and vomiting are droperidol, ondansetron, metoclopramide, and transdermal scopolamine. Droperidol can be administered at a dose of 0.0625 to 1.25 mg IV. Larger doses of droperidol may result in increased levels of sedation. Ondansetron can be administered at a dose of 4 to 8 mg IV. The dose of metoclopramide is 10 to 20 mg IV,

although it is not believed to be as efficacious as the former two antiemetics. Transdermal scopolamine patches may lead to mental confusion and blurry vision, especially in elderly patients. (419; **2318–2319**)

85. Minor incidental trauma associated with surgery and anesthesia may present in the PACU. Examples include corneal injury; peripheral nerve injury; oral soft tissue trauma; pharyngitis and/or hoarse voice; loosened, damaged or missing teeth; and bruising or extravasation at intravenous sites. (419)

86. Factors that influence the incidence and severity of postoperative pain include the type of surgery, whether and when opioids were administered intraoperatively, preoperative personality traits, the quality of the preoperative visit by the anesthesiologist, and the age of the patient. Elderly patients and infants appear to experience a decreased amount of pain in comparison to patients of other ages. Patients who preoperatively received a detailed explanation of the events to follow, including a discussion of postoperative pain control, from their anesthesiologist have decreased postoperative pain medication requirements. (419, Fig. 32–4; **2317–2318, 2325, Fig. 68–14**)

87. Surgeries associated with the highest incidence and severity of postoperative pain include thoracic, upper abdominal, and orthopedic procedures. (420; **2317–2318**)

88. *Preemptive analgesia* is a term used to describe the theory that the intensity of pain that is subsequently perceived by patients after a painful stimulus can be decreased by the administration of an opioid preceding the stimulus. Preemptive analgesia has been defined as "antinociceptive treatment that prevents the establishment of altered central processing, which amplifies postoperative pain." It is believed that the inhibition of C-fiber stimulation prevents or attenuates the subsequent development of any "memory," sensitization, or "wind-up" of the painful stimulus in the nervous system when opioids have been administered before the painful stimulus. (420; **2317–2318, 2325**)

POSTOPERATIVE RESPIRATORY THERAPY

89. Factors that influence the risk of postoperative pulmonary complications include the site of surgery, co-existing pulmonary disease, cigarette smoking, obesity, and advanced age. (420; **963–965, Table 25–39**)

90. Surgical procedures that typically result in the most postoperative pulmonary complications include thoracic and upper abdominal procedures. These surgical procedures are also associated with the greatest decrease in arterial oxygenation postoperatively. Significant postoperative atelectasis occurs in 20% to 40% of patients having thoracic or upper abdominal procedures. A vertical versus transverse upper abdominal skin incision does not appear to influence the incidence of postoperative pulmonary complications. (420, Fig. 32–5; **963–965, 2311, Fig. 68–11, Table 25–39**)

91. The choice of drugs used for anesthesia does not appear to influence the incidence of postoperative pulmonary complications. (420)

92. Oxygen therapy should be instituted for any patient in the PACU who has a Pao_2 less than 60 mm Hg. For those patients with chronic obstructive pulmonary disease who preoperatively relied on arterial hypoxemia for their ventilatory drive, oxygen therapy should be instituted just as it is for other patients in the postoperative period. The institution of oxygen therapy can be done in graded doses to determine the optimum level of supplementary oxygen for these patients. (421; **2309, 2311**)

93. It is common practice to institute oxygen therapy in the recovery room for almost every postoperative patient because nearly every patient has some degree of arterial hypoxemia during the period of recovery from anesthesia and surgery. Oxygen therapy in the PACU is usually delivered via a face mask or nasal cannula. (421; **2309, 2311**)

94. The main advantage of delivering oxygen via a nasal cannula is how well tolerated it is by patients. Discomfort to the patient wearing a nasal cannula for oxygen therapy is minimal. (421; **2405**)

95. Oxygen concentrations that are inspired vary when oxygen is delivered via a nasal cannula. The factors that influence the inspired concentrations of oxygen include the flow rate of the oxygen, the volume of the patient's nasopharynx, the patient's tidal volume, breathing frequency, and inspiratory flow rate. (421; **2404**)

96. For each 1 L/min of oxygen flow administered to a patient via a nasal cannula, the inspired oxygen concentration increases by approximately 4%. (421; **2405, Table 72–1**)

97. The maximum flow of oxygen that can be delivered via a nasal cannula is about 6 L/min. When oxygen flow rates are increased above 6 L/min the inspired concentration of oxygen does not increase further. This is because the volume of the nasopharynx has been filled by the 6 L/min flow rate. Air swallowing and gastric distention may result from flow rates in excess of 6 L/min. (421; **2405**)

98. Mouth breathing does not affect the effectiveness of oxygen delivery to the patient via a nasal cannula. When a patient who has oxygen delivered by nasal cannula breathes through the mouth, the oxygen in the nasopharynx is entrained into the lungs with the inspiratory flow through the nasopharynx. (421)

99. Types of face masks that can be used for oxygen delivery include the simple face mask, the partial rebreathing face mask, the non-rebreathing face mask, and the air-entrainment or Venturi face mask. (421, Fig. 32–6)

100. A simple face mask for oxygen delivery is a mask that does not have any valves or reservoir bags. With a simple face mask the maximum inspired concentration of oxygen that can be delivered is between 35% and 60%. The flow rates that can be administered with this type of oxygen delivery system are 5 to 8 L/min. (421, Fig. 32–6A; **2405, Table 72–1**)

101. The minimum amount of oxygen flow through a simple face mask should be 5 L/min in adults. When oxygen flow through a simple face mask is less than 5 L/min there is a risk of rebreathing carbon dioxide. (421)

102. The constant fraction of the inspired concentration of oxygen achieved does not differ much when comparing a simple face mask with a nasal cannula. (421; **2405, Table 72–1**)

103. A partial rebreathing face mask does not have any valves but does contain a reservoir bag. The inspired concentration of oxygen that can be achieved by a patient with a partial rebreathing face mask is between 50% and 65%. The flow rates of oxygen required to achieve this are in excess of 10 L/min. (421, Fig. 32–6B; **2405, Fig. 72–3, Table 72–1**)

104. A non-rebreathing face mask has a valve ensuring the flow of gases is in one direction and a reservoir bag. The maximum inspired concentration of oxygen that can be achieved by a patient with a non-rebreathing face mask is nearly 100%. The limitation of achieving a 100% inspired oxygen concentration is the difficulty in obtaining a tight mask fit on the patient. The flow rates of

oxygen that should be administered to a patient with a non-rebreathing face mask are enough so that the reservoir bag remains inflated at the end of inspiration, thus ensuring that there is no rebreathing of gases. (421, Fig. 32–6C; **2405**)

105. An air-entrainment face mask is also referred to as a Venturi mask. Oxygen is delivered through an injector to the mask at flow rates of 2 to 12 L/min. Ports in the face mask allow the entrainment of room air into the mask as well. The fraction of inspired oxygen achieved depends on the size of the ports and, therefore, on the degree of mixing of the delivered oxygen with room air. High flows of gases fill the mask, and holes in the mask allow exhaled gases and excess gases to escape. The inspired concentration of oxygen that can be delivered to a patient with an air-entrainment face mask is between 24% and 40%. (421, Fig. 32–6D, Table 32–4; **2404, Fig. 72–2, Table 72–1**)

106. An air-entrainment face mask has as its advantage a consistent, reliable inspired concentration of oxygen delivered to the patient independent of the patient's breathing pattern. (421, Fig. 32–6D, Table 32–4; **2404, Fig. 72–2, Table 72–1**)

107. Inhaled gases are normally warmed and humidified mostly by the nose but also by the upper respiratory tract. (421, **2406**)

108. An artificial humidifying device should be considered in a patient whose trachea is intubated or who has a tracheostomy. In these patients the body's natural warming and humidifying systems are bypassed. When a humidifier is not used in these patients moisture from the mucus lining the tracheobronchial tree becomes exhausted. This can lead to drying of the tracheobronchial tree, ciliary dysfunction, impairment of the transport of mucus, inflammation and necrosis of the pulmonary epithelium, retention of dried secretions, atelectasis, bacterial infiltration of the pulmonary mucosa, and pneumonia. The use of a humidifier may prevent these consequences by increasing the water content of inspired gases. (421; **2405–2406**)

109. Only sterile water, free of pyrogens, should be used for all humidifiers and nebulizers. The reason for this is to prevent as much as possible the water reservoir becoming a source of hospital-acquired infections. (422; **2409**)

110. Pass-over humidifiers work by having gases pass over a water surface. Evaporation of the water adds water vapor to the gases. The relative humidity of the gases subsequently inspired by the patient depends on three things: the gas flow, the temperature of the water, and the temperature of the gases. (422; **2407**)

111. The major limitation of a pass-over humidifier is the inability to reliably deliver gases at 90% to 100% relative humidity. (422)

112. Bubble-through humidifiers are frequently used for patients who are mechanically ventilated. Bubble-through humidifiers work by having inspired gases pass through a heated water reservoir. As the gases pass through the heated water reservoir they are broken up into small bubbles. The temperature of the water reservoir in bubble-through humidifiers is important because it determines the capacity of the gases to hold moisture. The water reservoir in bubble-through humidifiers should be heated sufficiently to maintain the temperature of the inhaled gases entering the patient's airway ideally at, but no greater than, body temperature. A relative humidity of 100% is attained when inhaled gases are between 36°C and 37°C. The temperature of the water reservoir should be adjusted based on monitoring of the temperature of the inhaled gases at the patient's airway. (422; **2406–2407, Table 72–4**)

113. The function of a jet nebulizer is to aerosolize particles to a certain diameter for delivery to the patient's airways. Jet nebulizers work by placing the liquid for nebulization in a chamber containing a small-diameter vertically oriented tube. A jet stream of high-pressure gas is directed through a restricted orifice past the end of the top of the tube at a high velocity. The high velocity of the jet stream of gas pulls the liquid to the top of the tube and aerosolizes it. The gas exiting the jet nebulizer contains aerosolized particles with a diameter between 10 and 30 μm in diameter. Particles that are larger are not carried by the gas and fall back into the liquid reservoir chamber. (422; **2407, 2409**)

114. Uses of a jet nebulizer include the humidification of gases for inspiration, to decrease the viscosity of airway secretions, and the administration of nebulized medicines such as racemic epinephrine and albuterol. (422; **2407, 2409–2411, Table 72–5**)

115. Bronchial hygiene refers to the removal of secretions from the lungs. Methods used for bronchial hygiene include natural mucociliary clearance, tracheal suctioning, and chest physiotherapy. (422; **2405, Table 72–3**)

116. Mucociliary clearance is the clearance of respiratory secretions in the respiratory tract by the action of cilia. Cilia are located on epithelial cells that line the respiratory tract. Cilia move 10 to 100 mL of secretions per day from the respiratory tract toward the glottic opening. (422; **2405**)

117. Impairment of the activity and effectiveness of cilia occurs as a result of inhaled anesthetics, endotracheal tubes, the inhalation of gases that are cold and dry, high inhaled concentrations of oxygen, and pulmonary infections. (422; **2406**)

118. Problems that can result from routine tracheal suctioning include tracheal erosion and trauma, the colonization of the tracheal tree by bacteria, small airway closure and collapse due to the aspiration of pulmonary gases, and a vasovagal response due to stimulation of the trachea or carina by the suction catheter. Tracheal suctioning should be done when there are secretions heard on chest auscultation that do not clear with coughing. (422; **2408**)

119. Tracheal suctioning can result in arterial hypoxemia by the small airway closure and collapse that results from the aspiration of pulmonary gases. Arterial hypoxemia can be minimized under these circumstances by administering oxygen before suctioning, selecting a suction catheter of the appropriate size, limiting the duration of suctioning to less than 15 seconds, and manually inflating the lungs with oxygen after suctioning. The appropriate size of a suction catheter should be no more than one half of the internal diameter of the trachea. (422; **2408**)

120. The purpose of chest physiotherapy is the removal of airway secretions and the improvement of the inflation of poorly ventilated alveoli. Components of chest physiotherapy include postural drainage, percussion, vibration, deep breathing, and assisted coughing. (422; **957–959, 2407–2408, Fig. 72–4**)

121. Coughing is effective at clearing secretions from large airways due to the high air flow velocities that occur during a cough. The high air flow velocities generated during a cough propel secretions from the large airways outward. The high air flow velocity necessary to generate a cough requires that the patient can breathe with large lung volumes. Patients who are rapid, shallow breathers, such as postoperative patients in pain, are therefore not able to cough effectively. (422; **2405**)

122. Decreases in vital capacity and functional residual capacity postoperatively may occur as a result of an ineffective cough or shallow breathing due to pain, atelectasis that may result from the surgical procedure itself, and

decreases in the clearance of secretions in the airways. The magnitude of decreases in the vital capacity and functional residual capacity in postoperative patients has been shown to parallel the severity of postoperative pulmonary complications. (423; **605–609**)

123. The total relief of postoperative pain does not prevent postoperative decreases in functional residual capacity. This implies that surgical trauma itself may interfere with optimal chest wall and pulmonary function. (423)

124. Specific therapies designed to increase a patient's functional residual capacity postoperatively include voluntary deep breathing, ambulation, intermittent positive pressure breathing, and incentive spirometry. (423; **957–959**)

125. Voluntary deep breathing exercises should be done with maintenance of the peak inflation at end inspiration for 3 to 5 seconds to maximize their benefit. Restoration of preoperative lung volumes is the ultimate goal of voluntary deep breathing exercises. The benefit of voluntary deep breathing exercises comes as a result of the large transpulmonary pressure gradient facilitating reexpansion of collapsed alveoli. For voluntary deep breathing exercises to be effective the patient must be motivated and have adequate postoperative analgesia. (423; **2407**)

126. Incentive spirometry is another method by which the patient is encouraged to do voluntary deep breathing. The patient is given an incentive spirometer device that measures the inspired volume of gas. The patient should have an inspired volume as a goal to achieve and should attempt to sustain lung inflation at end inspiration to reexpand collapsed alveoli. The incentive spirometer is best utilized postoperatively by educating the patient preoperatively as to how to use the incentive spirometer and using the preoperative inspired volume as a goal to achieve postoperatively. (423; **957–959, 2407**)

127. The major limitation of incentive spirometry is that it requires an awake, motivated, cooperative, and pain-free patient to be beneficial. (424; **957–959, 2407**)

128. Early ambulation postoperatively is thought to increase lung volumes, in particular the functional residual capacity. It is believed that this may be the mechanism by which early ambulation has been shown to provide the patient with the benefit of a decreased risk of postoperative pulmonary complications. (423)

129. Intermittent positive pressure breathing has not been shown to decrease the incidence of postoperative pulmonary complications. When intermittent positive pressure breathing is prescribed to a patient postoperatively, the goal of the treatment should be the achievement of the optimal tidal volume for the patient. (423; **958–959, 2408**)

130. Exhalation exercises may include inflating balloons or the use of blow bottles. Postoperative exhalation exercises are not recommended because performing these exercises often causes the patient to exhale below the functional residual capacity. This could lead to atelectasis and increases in airway resistance. (423)

Chapter 32

Acute Postoperative Pain Management

1. What are some sources of acute postoperative pain?

2. What are some potential adverse physiologic effects of acute postoperative pain?

3. What are some potential benefits of the effective management of acute postoperative pain?

4. What are the goals of an acute pain management service?

NEUROPHYSIOLOGY OF PAIN

5. What is nociception?

6. What are nociceptors? How are they stimulated?

7. What is the neurologic pathway of afferent pain impulses?

8. Where along the neurologic pathway of afferent pain impulses can modulation of the painful stimulus occur?

9. How can the modulation of painful stimuli occur in the periphery? What pharmacologic agents may be particularly useful for modulation of painful stimuli in the periphery?

10. How can the modulation of painful stimuli occur at the level of the spinal cord?

11. How can the modulation of painful stimuli occur above the level of the spinal cord? What endogenous and exogenous agents may have a role in modulating painful stimuli above the spinal cord level?

12. Name some excitatory and inhibitory neurotransmitters believed to have a role in the modulation of painful stimuli.

ANALGESIA DELIVERY SYSTEMS

13. Name some routes for the administration of analgesic drugs.

14. What is the limitation of the oral administration of analgesic agents for the management of acute postoperative pain? When is this route of administration appropriate?

15. What benefit does the intramuscular administration of analgesic agents have over oral administration? What are some problems with this method of administration?

16. What is an advantage of intramuscular ketorolac over intramuscular opioids administered for acute postoperative pain management?

17. When is the intravenous administration of small, frequent doses of an analgesic agent by the nurse feasible? What is the benefit of the frequent administration of small doses of opioids intravenously for pain management?

18. Describe patient-controlled analgesia. What is the lockout interval?

19. What are some of the advantages of patient-controlled analgesia?

20. How do neuraxially administered opioids exert their effect?

512

21. What are some of the potential benefits of neuraxial opioids for postoperative analgesia?

22. What are some of the potential adverse effects of neuraxial opioids for postoperative analgesia?

23. What is the early depression of ventilation that may be seen with the neuraxial administration of opioid believed to be due to?

24. What is the delayed depression of ventilation that may be seen with the neuraxial administration of opioid believed to be due to? Why might this effect be more pronounced with morphine than with fentanyl?

25. Which patients may be most at risk for delayed depression of ventilation from the administration of neuraxial opioid?

26. What characteristic of the opioid administered intrathecally determines its time of onset and its duration of action?

27. What are the disadvantages of a single-dose administration of opioid in the intrathecal space for the management of acute postoperative pain?

28. What may be the reason for the clinical impression that the incidence of side effects associated with intrathecal opioid is higher than the incidence of side effects associated with the epidural administration of opioid for postoperative analgesia?

29. Why is the continuous administration of opioid via an intrathecal catheter controversial?

30. Why does the epidural administration of opioid require more drug than the intrathecal administration of the same opioid? What dose of epidural opioid is equipotent to the same opioid administered in the intrathecal space?

31. Why is it believed that fentanyl produces a more segmental band of anesthesia than morphine when administered in the epidural space?

32. How do the resulting plasma concentrations of fentanyl compare when the same dose of fentanyl is administered intravenously versus epidurally?

33. How can the delay in onset of analgesia be overcome when using epidural morphine for the management of postoperative pain?

34. What are some complications that can occur with the continuous administration of opioids in the epidural space for the management of postoperative pain?

35. How do the physiologic effects of the neuraxial placement of opioids compare with those associated with the neuraxial placement of local anesthetics?

36. Why might a local anesthetic be added to the opioid for administration in the epidural space for the management of postoperative pain?

37. What is the concern regarding the institution of regional anesthesia when the patient is to receive anticoagulants for thromboembolism prophylaxis?

ALTERNATIVE APPROACHES TO MANAGEMENT OF ACUTE POSTOPERATIVE PAIN

38. What is an advantage and a disadvantage of peripheral nerve blocks for the management of acute postoperative pain?

39. How is intrapleural regional analgesia achieved? What is an advantage and a disadvantage of this technique for the management of acute postoperative pain?

40. What is transcutaneous electrical nerve stimulation? How is it believed to achieve

analgesia? What is a limitation of this technique for the management of acute postoperative pain?

ANSWERS*

1. Sources of acute postoperative pain include tissue injury, visceral distention, and disease. (425; **2324**)

2. Potential adverse physiologic effects of acute postoperative pain include hypoventilation, atelectasis, ventilation-to-perfusion mismatching in the lungs, deep vein thrombosis, myocardial ischemia, ileus, nausea and vomiting, urinary retention, hyperglycemia, sodium and water retention, insomnia, fear, and anxiety. (425; **2324–2325**)

3. Some potential benefits of the effective management of acute postoperative pain include improvement in patient comfort, a decrease in perioperative morbidity, and a decrease in cost. The cost is decreased by decreasing the amount of time a patient spends in postanesthesia care units and in intensive care units and by shortening the time to patient discharge from the hospital. (425)

4. The goals of an acute pain management service are to evaluate and treat postoperative pain and to identify and manage the undesirable side effects associated with the postoperative pain relief medicines. (425; **2342–2343**)

NEUROPHYSIOLOGY OF PAIN

5. Nociception is a word used to describe the recognition and transmission of painful stimuli. (426; **2323–2324**)

6. Nociceptors are the free nerve endings of afferent myelinated A-delta and unmyelinated C nerve fibers. Nociceptors are stimulated by thermal, mechanical, or chemical tissue damage. (426)

7. Nociceptors, on stimulation, send axonal projections to the dorsal horn of the spinal cord and synapse on second order neurons there. The axonal projections of the second order neurons cross to the contralateral half of the spinal cord and ascend the spinothalamic tract to the thalamus in the brain. In the thalamus these second order neurons synapse with third order neurons that send axonal projections to the sensory cortex. Before reaching the thalamus, the second order neurons divide and also send axonal branches to the reticular formation and periaqueductal gray matter. (426; **2323–2324**)

8. Modulation of the painful stimulus can occur at almost every level along the afferent neurologic pain pathway. It can occur at the site of stimulation of the nociceptors or at any synapse. In addition, modulation of nociception can even occur by the inhibition of the afferent sensory pathways by descending inhibitory pathways originating at the level of the brain stem. (426, Figs. 33–1, 33–2; **2323–2324, Fig. 10–5**)

9. Modulation of painful stimuli can occur in the periphery by decreasing or eliminating the endogenous mediators of inflammation in the vicinity of the nociceptor. Examples of endogenous mediators of inflammation include prostaglandins, histamine, bradykinin, serotonin, acetylcholine, lactic acid, hydrogen ions, and potassium ions. These endogenous inflammatory mediators sensitize and excite nociceptors, leading to the conduction of the painful stimulus. Pharmacologic agents that are particularly useful for the modulation of painful stimuli in the periphery are aspirin and nonsteroidal anti-inflammatory agents

*Numbers in parentheses: lightface numbers refer to pages, figures, or tables in Stoelting RK, Miller RD: Basics of Anesthesia, 4th ed. Philadelphia, Churchill Livingstone, 2000; **boldface numbers** refer to pages, figures, or tables in Miller RD: Anesthesia, 5th ed. Philadelphia, Churchill Livingstone, 2000.

(NSAIDs). These agents modulate painful stimuli by decreasing the synthesis of prostaglandins. (426–427; **281–282, 2323–2324**)

10. The modulation of painful stimuli can occur at the level of the spinal cord through the effects of excitatory or inhibitory neurotransmitters in the dorsal horn of the spinal cord. (427; **2323–2324**)

11. The modulation of painful stimuli can occur above the level of the spinal cord through the effects of a descending inhibitory pathway that originates in the brain stem. The descending inhibitory pathway synapses in the substantia gelatinosa region of the spinal cord. There are at least two types of descending inhibitory pathways, the opioid and alpha-adrenergic pathways. The opioid descending pathway releases endorphins and enkephalins, whereas the alpha-adrenergic descending pathway releases norepinephrine. Both these pathways work by hyperpolarizing the nerve fibers of the ascending pain pathway and potentially negate the action potential that would otherwise have resulted from the stimulation of the nerve by the painful stimulus. Exogenous agents that may have a role in modulating painful stimuli above the level of the spinal cord include synthetic opioids and clonidine. Synthetic opioids act as agonists at receptors that are membrane bound and distributed throughout the spinal cord. Clonidine is thought to act via the alpha-adrenergic descending inhibitory pathway. (427–428; **281–285, 2325–2326, Fig. 10–5**)

12. Examples of excitatory neurotransmitters that are believed to modulate painful stimuli include glutamate, aspartate, vasoactive intestinal polypeptide, cholecystokinin, gastrin-releasing peptide, angiotensin, and substance P. Examples of inhibitory neurotransmitters that are believed to modulate painful stimuli include enkephalins, endorphins, substance P, and somatostatin. (428; **2324**)

ANALGESIC DELIVERY SYSTEMS

13. Routes for the administration of analgesic drugs include oral, transmucosal, transdermal, intramuscular, intrapleural, intravenous, neuraxial, and by injection to block a peripheral nerve. (428; **2326**)

14. The limitation of the oral administration of analgesic agents for the management of acute postoperative pain is the lack of titratability and the prolonged amount of time it takes to reach its peak effect. The oral route of administration for analgesic agents is appropriate when the pain the patient is experiencing has decreased and there is no longer a need for rapid adjustments in the level of analgesia. (428; **2326**)

15. The intramuscular injection of analgesic agents has a more rapid onset and more rapidly reaches its peak effect than the oral route of administration of analgesic agents. There are some problems with the intramuscular administration of analgesics. First, the plasma concentration of the drug can vary among patients by three to five times, making dosing of the drug difficult. Second, when intramuscular opioids are administered on a fixed time interval schedule, there is an associated cyclical period of sedation, adequate analgesia, and then inadequate analgesia. Only about 35% of the time will the patient have adequate pain management with this regimen. (428; **2326**)

16. An advantage of intramuscular ketorolac over intramuscular opioids administered for acute postoperative pain management is the lack of depression of ventilation and nausea and vomiting associated with its use. Its potency is less than that of opioids, however. In addition, ketorolac is a nonsteroidal anti-inflammatory agent that may have effects of increased postoperative bleeding and renal sequelae. (428; **2318, 2332–2333**)

17. The intravenous administration of small, frequent doses of an analgesic agent by the nurse is only feasible in the postanesthesia care unit or in an intensive

care unit where the nurse-to-patient ratio allows for continuous nursing observation and monitoring of the patient. This method of administration of an analgesic agent maintains a more stable plasma concentration of the drug in the analgesic range. This provides for more effective pain management with fewer negative side effects. (429; **2317**)

18. Patient-controlled analgesia is a method of delivering an opioid for analgesia to a patient. In this form of analgesic delivery the patient controls his or her own administration of the opioid by pressing a button connected to a pump. The pump is programmed to deliver a preset small intravenous dose of opioid when triggered by the patient. The lockout interval is the interval of time that must pass after the last self-administered dose before the patient can deliver another small dose of opioid to himself or herself. (429; **2317, 2326–2327**)

19. There are several advantages of patient-controlled analgesia. These include high patient acceptance and for patients a sense of control, improved titration of drug, and subsequent patient comfort with less total drug administered, less sedation, improved sleep at night, and a more rapid return to physical activity after surgery. (429; **2317, 2326–2327**)

20. Neuraxially administered opioids exert their effect by acting on a dense collection of opioid receptors in the substantia gelatinosa of the spinal cord. The neuraxial administration of opioids requires the opioids be placed in either the epidural or the intrathecal space. When in the epidural space, the opioid must diffuse across the dura to reach the receptors in the spinal cord. (429; **280–283**)

21. Potential benefits of the neuraxial administration of opioids for postoperative analgesia include superior pain control, improved postoperative pulmonary function, decreases in cardiovascular complications, decreases in infectious complications, and decreases in total hospital costs. (429; **2317–2318, 2328–2330**)

22. Potential adverse effects of the neuraxial administration of opioids for postoperative analgesia include pruritus, urinary retention, nausea and vomiting, sedation, and early and delayed depression of ventilation. (430; **2317, 2333**)

23. The early depression of ventilation that is seen with the neuraxial administration of opioids usually occurs in the first 2 hours after the administration of the opioid. Early respiratory depression is believed to occur as a result of vascular uptake and redistribution of the opioid. (430; **2331**)

24. The delayed depression of ventilation that is seen with the neuraxial administration of opioids usually occurs 6 to 24 hours after the administration of the opioid. It is believed to be due to the cephalad spread of the opioid in the cerebrospinal fluid to the medullary centers of the brain. The medullary centers are in the area of the fourth cerebral ventricle. This effect may be more pronounced with the less lipid-soluble opioids, such as morphine, than with the more lipid-soluble drugs, such as fentanyl. The more lipid soluble the opioid is, the more readily it will attach to opioid receptors on the spinal cord. This makes less drug available for diffusion to the brain. The opposite occurs with the less lipid soluble drug, leaving more drug available for diffusion to the medullary centers. (430; **2330–2333**)

25. Patient characteristics contribute to the risk of delayed depression of ventilation from the administration of neuraxial opioid. Patients at an increased risk for the delayed depression of ventilation include elderly patients, patients not tolerant to opioid medications, and patients receiving concomitant systemic opioids. (430; **2330–2333**)

26. The lipid solubility of the opioid administered intrathecally is the primary determinant of its time of onset and duration of action. The onset time is shorter

with more lipid-soluble drugs, and the duration of action is shorter. Conversely, less lipid-soluble drugs have a longer onset time and a prolonged duration of action. (430; **2330**)

27. Typically, the intrathecal administration of opioid is administered as a single dose in conjunction with a local anesthetic block for a surgical procedure. Disadvantages of a single dose intrathecal administration of opioid include the lack of titratability and the need for other analgesic options after the initial intrathecal opioid effect subsides. (430)

28. The clinical impression that intrathecal opioid results in a higher incidence of side effects when compared with the epidural administration of the same opioid probably comes as a result of the administration of excessive doses of opioid in the intrathecal space. The same receptors are being stimulated in both cases, so theoretically equipotent doses at the receptor should result in similar desired and undesired effects. (430; **2330**)

29. The continuous administration of opioid in the intrathecal space via a catheter is controversial for at least two reasons. First, there is the concern of the introduction of infection in the intrathecal space with a catheter that is left in place for a prolonged period of time. Second, small-diameter catheters that were introduced for the continuous intrathecal administration of local anesthetics have been associated with cauda equina syndrome, making anesthesiologists reconsider the administration of continuous medicines intrathecally via a catheter. (430)

30. The epidural administration of opioid requires more drug to be administered than if it were administered intrathecally because the drug must diffuse across the dura to reach the spinal cord and exert its effect. In addition, fat, connective tissue, and the epidural veins all take up opioid that is deposited in the epidural space. In contrast, the intrathecal administration of opioid places the opioid directly at its site of action. The dose of epidurally administered opioid is approximately ten times the dose of intrathecally administered opioid for resulting equipotent effects. (430; **2330, Table 69–4**)

31. Fentanyl administered in the epidural space is believed to produce a more segmental band of anesthesia than morphine because of its increased lipid solubility. The increased lipid solubility of fentanyl causes it to bind to opioid receptors in the spinal cord adjacent to the area in which they enter the intrathecal space. Morphine, being more hydrophilic, binds less readily and instead diffuses in the intrathecal space. This results in a wider distribution of anesthesia with morphine than with fentanyl when administered in the epidural space. (432; **2330**)

32. The plasma concentration of fentanyl when administered intravenously is similar to the plasma concentration of fentanyl when the same dose is administered epidurally. This is thought to occur from the systemic absorption of fentanyl from the epidural space by the vasculature in that space. This implies that at least part of the analgesic effect of fentanyl administered epidurally is through its systemic effects. (431, Fig. 33–3; **2331**)

33. When using epidural morphine for the management of postoperative pain there is a delay of 3 to 4 hours before the onset of effective analgesia. This can be overcome in a number of ways. First, the anesthesiologist may administer a bolus of local anesthetic through the epidural catheter to the patient before the patient awakens from anesthesia. Alternatively, a short-acting narcotic such as fentanyl can be administered through the epidural catheter in the interim until the epidural morphine takes its effect. The intravenous administration of analgesics may also provide pain relief in the interim. Finally, the anesthesiologist who plans in advance may actually begin the infusion with morphine intraopera-

tively such that the onset of effect of epidural morphine coincides with the patient's arrival to the postanesthesia care unit. (431; **2330**)

34. Complications that can occur with the continuous administration of opioids in the epidural space include, among others things, ventilatory depression, infection, and the accidental administration of opioid intrathecally. (432; **2334–2336**)

35. Local anesthetics administered neuraxially in dense concentrations block the conduction of all neural impulses. This results in sympathetic nervous system blockade, skeletal muscle weakness, and loss of proprioception as well as blockade of pain pathways. These effects prohibit the patient from ambulating. Opioids administered neuraxially specifically attach to opioid receptors and work to decrease the patient's pain. Neuraxial opioids lack all the other effects of local anesthetics, thus allowing for patient ambulation while neuraxial opioids are being administered. Of note, local anesthetics administered neuraxially in dilute concentrations may augment the beneficial effects of opioids without impairing ambulation or causing significant sympathetic nervous system blockade. (429; **2333–2334**)

36. Local anesthetic added to the opioid solution for administration in the epidural space results in a synergistic analgesic effect. This is believed to occur because of the blockade of painful stimuli at two different sites at the spinal cord. The opioid administered acts by binding to opioid receptors in the substantia gelatinosa. The local anesthetic administered acts at the nerve roots and in the dorsal root ganglia by blocking the transmission of afferent impulses. The synergistic effect of these two classes of drugs allows for a decreased dose of each to be administered to the patient. This has the added benefit of a decreased risk of the potential side effects of both drugs. (431; **2333–2334**)

37. There is a concern for the formation of an epidural or intrathecal hematoma associated with the institution of regional anesthesia when the patient is to receive anticoagulants for thromboembolism prophylaxis perioperatively. The American Society of Regional Anesthesia published a consensus statement regarding this issue in 1998. Among the recommendations is the timing of placement and withdrawal of epidural catheters in the presence of either heparin or low-molecular-weight heparin. Several large studies have verified that placing an epidural catheter in patients who are to receive heparin therapy has been safe when there was no detectable clinical bleeding for at least 1 hour after placement of the epidural catheter. Subsequent removal of the epidural catheter should be delayed until 10 to 12 hours have passed after the last dose of heparin. Re-dosing of heparin should again be delayed for 1 hour after removal of the catheter. The recommendations with regard to low-molecular-weight heparin are more stringent because it appears the risk of epidural hematoma in these patients is slightly greater. Patients who are receiving anticoagulants for thromboembolism prophylaxis and who also have received neuraxial anesthesia should be closely monitored for the prompt recognition of epidural or intrathecal hematoma formation. The diagnosis can be confirmed by computed tomography. Outcomes are best if diagnosis and operative decompression for treatment occur within 6 hours of the onset of hematoma formation. (432–433, Table 33–6; **2334–2336**)

ALTERNATIVE APPROACHES TO MANAGEMENT OF ACUTE POSTOPERATIVE PAIN

38. An advantage of peripheral nerve blocks for the management of acute postoperative pain is its ability to provide good management of postoperative pain while not affecting the patient systemically. Thus the patient is not at risk for any of the negative effects of systemic opioids. A disadvantage of peripheral nerve

blocks for postoperative pain is its relatively short duration of action. (434; **2228–2329**)

39. Intrapleural regional analgesia is most frequently used for the management of acute postoperative pain after a thoracotomy. It is achieved by the injection of a local anesthetic solution through a catheter placed in the intrapleural space. The catheter is often placed intraoperatively by the thoracic surgeon one interspace lower than that of the surgical incision. The local anesthetic diffuses to the intercostal nerves and produces a multilevel, unilateral intercostal nerve block. An advantage of this technique for postoperative pain management is the potential for effective pain relief for the patient, especially in the first 6 hours postoperatively. A disadvantage of this technique is that the local anesthetic may be lost through the pleural drainage tubes that are placed after a thoracotomy. Complications associated with this technique include pneumothorax and high plasma concentrations of local anesthetic. The efficacy of this technique for postoperative pain management is variable. (434; **1543–1545, 1724, 2318, 2328**)

40. Transcutaneous electrical nerve stimulation is the application of electrical stimulation to the skin to provide pain relief. Transcutaneous electrical nerve stimulation is thought to work by stimulating the release of endogenous endorphins by the electrical stimulation of cutaneous nerves. An advantage of this technique is its relative lack of side effects, its simplicity, and its noninvasiveness. A disadvantage of this technique is its variable efficacy, almost always being less efficacious than neuraxial opioid administration or patient-controlled analgesia for acute postoperative pain management. (434; **2339**)

Chapter 33

Critical Care Medicine and Management of the Trauma Patient

LIFE-THREATENING TRAUMA

1. What qualifies a trauma center as a level 1 trauma center?

2. What should be included in the initial evaluation of a person arriving to a trauma center? What is the first priority in this situation?

3. Name some indications for tracheal intubation after life-threatening trauma.

4. What approximate percent of all trauma victims sustain cervical spine injury? What types of trauma result in a high likelihood of cervical spine injury in the trauma patient?

5. By what percent of normal does a rigid collar decrease flexion of the neck? By what percent of normal does a rigid collar decrease lateral movement of the neck?

6. How must a patient's head be positioned for orotracheal intubation in a situation in which the airway must be secured but the cervical spine status is unknown?

7. What type of skull fracture is a contraindication to nasotracheal intubation?

8. In the event of airway obstruction and an inability to perform tracheal intubation, how should the airway be secured?

9. How can the anesthesiologist check nothing by mouth (NPO) status in the trauma patient?

10. What are some injuries that might result from thoracic trauma? How is the diagnosis of intravascular thoracic trauma made by chest radiography?

11. Describe the treatment of a pneumothorax or hemothorax.

12. What injuries might result from trauma to the abdomen? How is the diagnosis of intra-abdominal hemorrhage made in the trauma unit?

13. What may hematuria in the trauma unit indicate?

14. What drug might be used for the induction of general anesthesia in the trauma patient? How should anesthesia be maintained?

15. In the situation in which the dose of anesthesia hemodynamically tolerated by the patient is too small to prevent skeletal muscle movement intraoperatively, how should the patient be managed by the anesthesiologist?

16. How should hypovolemia be treated in the trauma patient? What are some signs of adequate intravascular fluid volume replacement in the trauma patient?

17. What laboratory tests can be ordered on a frequent basis during trauma surgery to assess continued blood loss and the adequacy of fluid volume replacement?

THERMAL BURN INJURY

18. What should be included in the initial evaluation of a patient with a burn injury arriving to the trauma unit?

19. What are some indications for endotracheal intubation in the trauma patient with a burn injury?

20. What are some pathophysiologic responses associated with thermal burn injury?

21. Why might burn injury victims have an inadequate oxygen-carrying capacity in their blood despite a normal PaO_2? How should it be treated?

22. What are some clinical signs of carbon monoxide toxicity? How is the diagnosis of carbon monoxide toxicity made?

23. What clinical information helps guide the anesthesiologist with regard to fluid volume resuscitation in the burn patient?

24. When is fluid loss in the patient greatest after a burn injury?

25. How does a patient's metabolism change after a burn injury?

26. What are some considerations for the anesthetic management of the burn injury patient with regard to intraoperative monitoring?

27. How should the induction and maintenance of anesthesia be accomplished in burn injury patients? Why might it be prudent to avoid halothane in these patients?

28. What are the recommendations regarding succinylcholine and nondepolarizing neuromuscular blocking drugs in the burn injury patient?

ACUTE RESPIRATORY FAILURE

29. What is the adult respiratory distress syndrome (ARDS)? What are some pulmonary physiologic derangements associated with ARDS?

30. What are some causes of ARDS?

31. How reversible is arterial hypoxemia in patients with ARDS when oxygen is administered?

32. What are some physiologic explanations for the arterial hypoxemia seen in patients with ARDS?

33. What is believed to be the reason for pulmonary edema seen in ARDS? What is the pulmonary artery occlusion pressure in these patients?

34. What is the utility of serial arterial blood gas analysis and pH measurements in the management of the patient with ARDS?

35. What is the aim of the treatment of ARDS? What are some treatment methods for ARDS?

36. How can acute respiratory failure be distinguished from chronic respiratory failure on the basis of arterial pH and $PaCO_2$?

37. What are some classifications of ventilators for mechanical ventilation of the lungs?

38. What is pressure-cycled ventilation? What physiologic factor of the patient will determine the tidal volume and inspiratory time in a patient being ventilated by pressure-cycled ventilation?

39. What are some problems with pressure-cycled mechanical ventilation of the lungs?

40. What is volume-cycled ventilation? How do changes in the patient's pulmonary compliance affect the tidal volume when mechanically ventilated with volume-cycled ventilation?

41. Explain what the compression volume of a ventilator circuit is. What is the approximate compression volume of the ventilator delivery circuit for every 1 cm H_2O of airway pressure?

42. In which patient population is it particularly important for the anesthesiologist to be aware of the compression volume of a circuit?

43. What is time-cycled ventilation? What factors determine the tidal volume delivered to a patient with time-cycled ventilation?

44. What is assist mode ventilation? What is the trigger for the ventilator to deliver a mechanical breath in assist mode ventilation?

45. What is control mode ventilation? What is the advantage of this mode of mechanical ventilation?

46. How do a patient's spontaneous breathing efforts affect control mode ventilation of the lungs? How might the anesthesiologist manage the patient in this regard?

47. What are some typical initial ventilator settings for the patient being mechanically ventilated with control mode ventilation? What might help guide the anesthesiologist in making changes to the initial ventilator settings?

48. What is pressure-control inverse-ratio ventilation? What is the principal advantage of this mode of mechanical ventilation? What is a risk of this mode of ventilation?

49. What is assist/control mode ventilation? When might this mode of mechanical ventilation be useful?

50. What is pressure support ventilation?

51. What is high-frequency ventilation?

52. What is positive end-expiratory pressure (PEEP)?

53. What are some potential benefits of PEEP?

54. When is the institution of PEEP recommended? What levels of PEEP should be used initially?

55. What are some potential negative effects of PEEP?

56. How does PEEP decrease cardiac output? In which patients is this effect most pronounced?

57. What level of PEEP begins to interfere with the interpretation of the pulmonary artery occlusion pressure as a monitor of left atrial pressure?

58. What are some adverse manifestations of pulmonary barotrauma that can result from PEEP?

59. How might PEEP lead to a redistribution of pulmonary blood flow?

60. What is noninvasive positive pressure ventilation? What are some advantages of this type of support of ventilation?

61. How can the adequacy of arterial oxygenation be monitored during the treatment of ARDS?

62. How can the adequacy of alveolar ventilation be monitored during the treatment of ARDS?

63. How can the adequacy of tissue oxygenation be monitored during the treatment of ARDS? What mixed venous P_{O_2} warrants a change in management?

64. How can the adequacy of acid-base equilibrium be monitored during the treatment of ARDS?

65. How can the adequacy of cardiac output be monitored during the treatment of ARDS?

66. When can the cessation of mechanical support of ventilation of the ARDS patient's

lungs be considered? What are some clinical guidelines that are used to predict successful cessation of mechanical ventilation of the lungs?

67. What are some methods used in weaning patients from mechanical ventilation of the lungs?

68. How is weaning accomplished using the T-tube method?

69. What is continuous positive airway pressure (CPAP)? Why is CPAP often delivered via the T-tube when this mode of weaning is selected?

70. What are some clinical indications in the patient breathing through a T-tube that weaning from mechanical ventilation of the lungs may be premature?

71. What is intermittent mandatory ventilation? What is the difference between synchronized intermittent mandatory ventilation and nonsynchronized intermittent mandatory ventilation?

72. How is weaning accomplished using intermittent mandatory ventilation?

CONGESTIVE HEART FAILURE

73. What is the goal of treatment for patients with congestive heart failure? What classes of drugs are used for this purpose?

74. What are some vasodilators used for congestive heart failure? What is the mechanism by which vasodilators increase cardiac output?

75. What are some limitations to vasodilator therapy for the treatment of congestive heart failure? How can the decrease in blood pressure that results from the administration of vasodilators be minimized?

76. What is the use of inotropic drugs in the treatment of congestive heart failure? What are some inotropic drugs administered in congestive heart failure?

77. How can the effectiveness of drugs used in congestive heart failure be measured?

78. In what patient is an intra-aortic balloon counterpulsation pump useful? How does it work?

SEPSIS

79. What are some common sources of infection in critically ill patients?

80. What are some clinical signs of septic shock? Is a positive blood culture necessary for the diagnosis of septic shock?

81. How is septic shock treated? When might dopamine be indicated?

82. When might surgical intervention be indicated for patients with sepsis? What induction agent might be useful under these circumstances?

HEAD INJURY

83. What are some mechanisms for the evaluation of a patient with a suspected closed-head injury?

84. How can intracranial pressure (ICP) be monitored? Which patients should have their ICP monitored?

85. What is a normal ICP? Is a normal ICP pulsatile or flat?

86. What is a plateau wave in the ICP wave tracing?

87. How can painful stimulation affect the ICP in an otherwise unresponsive patient?

88. At what ICP is treatment frequently recommended? Name some methods used to treat an increased ICP.

89. What posture should be maintained in a patient with an elevated ICP to facilitate postural drainage? How can flexion or extension of the head lead to an increase in ICP?

90. How does hyperventilation decrease ICP? What is the duration of efficacy of hyperventilation for decreasing ICP?

91. What Pa_{CO_2} should be maintained in adult patients to decrease the ICP? What Pa_{CO_2} should be maintained in children for this purpose? What is the danger of excessive hyperventilation?

92. What is the mechanism for the decrease in ICP seen with the administration of osmotic diuretics? What osmotic diuretic is frequently administered to patients to decrease elevated ICPs?

93. What are some physiologic effects, other than a decrease in ICP, seen with the administration of osmotic diuretics? What is the potential problem with administering glucose-containing intravenous solutions after the administration of an osmotic diuretic?

94. How does the administration of a tubular diuretic such as furosemide decrease the ICP?

95. Which corticosteroids are often administered to patients to decrease elevated ICP? How are they believed to exert their effect?

96. When might barbiturates be administered to patients for the treatment of elevated ICPs? What is their mechanism of action?

97. What is a potential hazard of barbiturate administration to patients with persistently elevated ICPs?

NEUROLOGIC COMPLICATIONS IN CRITICALLY ILL PATIENTS

98. What are some causes of failure to awaken in patients in the critical care unit?

99. What are some causes of skeletal muscle weakness in patients in the critical care unit?

100. What are some causes of seizures in patients in the critical care unit?

ACUTE RENAL FAILURE

101. What is the best method by which to avoid acute renal failure in a patient in an intensive care unit setting?

102. What is the treatment for acute renal tubular necrosis that may occur in a patient in the intensive care unit?

ACUTE HEPATIC FAILURE

103. Why do patients with early acute hepatic failure hyperventilate?

104. What physiologic dysfunctions are frequently associated with terminal hepatic failure?

105. What is the goal of treatment of acute hepatic failure? Which agents are used for this purpose?

MALNUTRITION

106. What are some reasons why critically ill patients often have increased caloric needs?

107. How is malnutrition in an intensive care unit setting usually managed?

108. Name some potential complications associated with total parental nutrition.

ANSWERS*

LIFE-THREATENING TRAUMA

1. A trauma center becomes qualified as a level 1 trauma center by the level of services it can provide on an immediate basis 24 hours a day. Immediately available at a level 1 trauma center are trauma surgeons, anesthesiologists, nurses, emergency rooms, operating rooms, ICU beds, radiologic services, stat laboratory analysis, and a blood bank. (436; **2157–2158, Table 62–1**)

2. The initial evaluation of any person arriving to the trauma center should always include an evaluation of the patient's airway, breathing, circulation, and neurologic status. The first priority in this situation is securing a patent airway and the administration of oxygen. The neurologic status is frequently assessed by using the Glasgow Coma Scale. (436–437, Table 34–1; **2163, Table 62–4**)

3. Indications for tracheal intubation after life-threatening trauma include head injury; protection against aspiration, airway obstruction, and unconsciousness; the provision of positive pressure ventilation; the need for sedation, general anesthesia, or skeletal muscle paralysis; and shock. (437; **2163, Table 62–5**)

4. The estimated number of trauma patients who have sustained cervical spine injury is 1.5% to 3%. Patients who are alert without neck pain or tenderness are not likely to have cervical spine injury. The mechanism of injury places some trauma patients at a high risk of cervical spine injury. Cervical spine injury is likely in patients who have been in a front-end motor vehicle accident without a seat belt, patients who have sustained a head-first fall, and patients with maxillofacial blunt trauma. (447; **2162–2163, 2169**)

5. A rigid collar can be placed on a patient for stabilization of the neck after trauma. A rigid collar acts by reducing neck motion. With a rigid collar, flexion and extension of the neck are reduced to about 30% of normal and rotation and lateral movements of the neck are reduced to about 50% of normal. (447)

6. In a situation in which the status of the patient's cervical spine is unknown, and the airway must be secured, orotracheal intubation should proceed only with the patient's head stabilized in the neutral position. This can be accomplished by manual immobilization of the head on a flat board surface. In-line stabilization of the head limits the amount of atlanto-occipital extension that occurs during direct laryngoscopy. (437, 447; **1918–1919, 2163–2164, Figs. 52–13, 62–2**)

7. Nasotracheal intubation is contraindicated in a patient with a basilar skull fracture. There is a risk of a nasally introduced endotracheal tube entering the cranium in these patients. (437; **1430, 1919**)

8. In the event of airway obstruction and an inability to perform endotracheal intubation, the airway must be secured immediately by emergency cricothyrotomy or tracheostomy. (437, Fig. 12–22; **2163–2164**)

---

*Numbers in parentheses: lightface numbers refer to pages, figures, or tables in Stoelting RK, Miller RD: Basics of Anesthesia, 4th ed. Philadelphia, Churchill Livingstone, 2000; **boldface numbers** refer to pages, figures, or tables in Miller RD: Anesthesia, 5th ed. Philadelphia, Churchill Livingstone, 2000.

9. The anesthesiologist must assume that all trauma patients are at risk for the aspiration of gastric contents, despite the time that has passed since their last ingestion. Therefore, in cases of an emergency and the need to secure the airway, cricoid pressure should be applied before the administration of induction agents in rapid sequence. Assessment of the patient's NPO status becomes irrelevant under these circumstances. (437, 447; **2163**)

10. Injuries that may be sustained in thoracic trauma include injury to the lungs or cardiovascular system or both. These injuries may include a pneumothorax, hemothorax, hemopericardium, pulmonary laceration, tracheobronchial laceration, rib fractures, flail chest, or vascular injury. The diagnosis of intravascular thoracic trauma is made by the presence of a widened mediastinum on a chest radiograph. (437; **2159–2162**)

11. The treatment of a pneumothorax or hemothorax is by the placement of a chest tube in the thorax to drain extrapulmonary air or blood. The chest tube is placed in the fourth or fifth interspace in the midaxillary line and directed posteriorly. After placement the chest tube should be attached to suction. (437; **2162**)

12. Injuries that may be sustained in abdominal trauma include soft tissue contusions or avulsions, rupture of visceral organs, or laceration of the spleen or liver. Injury to the spleen or liver can result in significant hemorrhage. The diagnosis of intra-abdominal hemorrhage is made by peritoneal lavage or by computed tomography. (437; **2159**)

13. Hematuria in the trauma unit may be an indication of bladder injury or injury to the genitourinary system. (437; **1305, 2167**)

14. General anesthesia is most often indicated in trauma surgery. The induction of general anesthesia in the trauma patient must be done with caution. The choice of induction agent must be made on an individual basis, because the extent of injuries, intravascular volume status, and level of consciousness can vary greatly among trauma patients. In general, drugs that minimize cardiovascular depression and intracranial hypertension may be chosen. Ketamine may be contraindicated in patients who have sustained head injury. Succinylcholine administration can result in a hyperkalemic response if administered to patients with spinal cord injury or burn injury after 24 hours after the injury. The maintenance of anesthesia can be achieved by the careful titration of drugs at a dose in which hemodynamic stability is maintained. Nitrous oxide is avoided in patients with a potential for pneumothorax or for abdominal procedures. (437; **2167–2168, Tables 62–6, 62–10**)

15. During trauma surgery the patient may be hemodynamically unstable such that anesthetics are not tolerated by the patient. When this occurs, skeletal muscle movement cannot be prevented by the anesthetics alone. A nondepolarizing neuromuscular blocking drug is then necessarily administered to prevent skeletal muscle movement and facilitate the surgical procedure. Under these conditions some patients experience some recall of the intraoperative events, making it important for the anesthesiologist to communicate with the patient during the procedure. Small doses of a benzodiazepine or scopolamine have been used under these circumstances in an attempt to prevent recall. (437; **2167–2168**)

16. Hypovolemia in the trauma patient must be treated sufficiently to regain intravascular fluid volume status near normal and to regain hemodynamic stability if possible. This may require pressurized infusion devices to deliver the fluids more rapidly. Warming the fluids before their administration also helps to decrease the risk of hypothermia in the patient. Signs of adequate intravascular fluid volume replacement include a heart rate <100 beats per

minute, a pulse pressure >30 mm Hg, a urine output >0.5 to 1 mL/kg per hour, the absence of metabolic acidosis, and minimal effects of positive pressure ventilation on systemic blood pressure. Fluid resuscitation may be initiated with crystalloid solutions. In situations in which there are massive or ongoing blood losses, the initial resuscitation may be with type O-negative or type-specific blood until blood can be typed and crossmatched with the patient's blood. Whole blood less than 6 hours old is preferable in this situation because it may also provide some factors for coagulation that may be deficient in the hemorrhaging trauma patient. Finally, if available, autotransfusion systems may also be used in the trauma patient. Clearly, the achievement of hemodynamic stability depends largely on the control of bleeding by the surgeons. (438; **2164–2168, Table 62–9**)

17. Laboratory tests that can be ordered on a frequent basis in trauma patients during trauma surgery include arterial blood gases, pH, and hematocrit. Electrolytes, glucose, and coagulation factors may also be measured on a less frequent basis as the situation allows. These laboratory analyses may facilitate the assessment of continued blood loss and adequate fluid volume replacement. (438; **2166–2167**)

THERMAL BURN INJURY

18. The initial evaluation of a patient with a burn injury arriving to the trauma unit, just as in all patients arriving to the trauma unit, should include an evaluation of the patient's airway, breathing, and circulation. (438; **2163, Table 62–4**)

19. For the burn injury patient arriving to the trauma unit, the presence of stridor or a hoarse voice is an indication for endotracheal intubation. The patient with stridor or hoarseness is likely to have subsequent facial and glottic edema that may lead to airway obstruction and may make future intubation of the trachea difficult. (438; **1610**)

20. Pathophysiologic responses associated with thermal burn injury include hypovolemia, upper airway edema, chemical pneumonitis, carbon monoxide toxicity, increased metabolism, impaired thermoregulation, ileus, oliguria, electrolyte abnormalities, hyperglycemia, and depressed immune function. After the first 24 hours the patient may have a hyperdynamic circulatory system, reflected by hypertension and tachycardia. (438–439)

21. Burn injury victims may have suffered from smoke inhalation injury with associated carbon monoxide inhalation, particularly if the patient had been exposed to smoke in a closed space. Carbon monoxide binds to hemoglobin with a higher affinity than oxygen by a factor of about 200 times. This can lead to an inadequate oxygen-carrying capacity despite the presence of a normal PaO_2, resulting in a functional anemia. In addition, the binding of carbon monoxide to hemoglobin shifts the oxyhemoglobin dissociation curve to the right, making the remaining oxygen bind more tightly to hemoglobin and decreasing the ability of hemoglobin to unload oxygen at the tissues. Carbon monoxide inhalation that compromises oxygen-carrying capacity should be treated with the administration of 100% oxygen. A high PaO_2 will lead to the removal of carbon monoxide from hemoglobin with greater rapidity. (438; **2276–2277, Table 67–6**)

22. Clinical signs of carbon monoxide toxicity include headache, nausea, restlessness, and confusion. A pulse oximeter will have normal readings despite carbon monoxide toxicity. Carbon monoxide toxicity is suspected by the presence of a decrease in arterial oxygen saturation in the presence of a normal PaO_2. A carboxyhemoglobin level confirms the diagnosis. A carboxyhemoglobin level of 40% is considered to be consistent with severe carbon

monoxide intoxication. Patients with this level of carboxyhemoglobin have a cherry-red appearance and are comatose. (438; **2276–2277**)

23. The burn injury patient often requires large volumes of fluid for volume resuscitation after his or her injury secondary to huge volume shifts into burned tissue and a subsequent decrease in plasma volume. The fluid shift occurs as a result of tissue injury, disruption of the capillary bed, local vasodilation, and increased permeability. In addition to fluid shifts, evaporative losses from the exposed wounded tissues and increases in the metabolic rate contribute to intravascular fluid losses. Several formulas exist to guide the anesthesiologist with respect to fluid resuscitation in the burn injury patient. Each of these formulas is dependent on the amount of body surface area that is burned. The Parkland formula calls for the administration of 4 mL/kg of lactated Ringer's solution in the first 24 hours for every 1% of the patient's body surface area that is burned. According to the Parkland formula, one half of the calculated volume should be administered in the first 8 hours and the remaining half administered in the subsequent 16 hours. Monitoring of the urine output and central venous pressures also facilitates volume resuscitation in these patients. (438; **1610**)

24. Fluid loss in the burn injury patient is greatest in the first 12 hours after the injury. Fluid loss subsides after 24 hours in these patients. (438)

25. The patient who has sustained a burn injury undergoes a dramatic change in metabolism after the injury. Within a few hours the patient becomes hypermetabolic, with increased oxygen consumption, tachycardia, and increased serum catecholamine concentrations. This has implications for increased oxygen and nutritive requirements. (438; **2510, Table 74–5**)

26. Considerations for the intraoperative monitoring of the burn injury patient include the potential difficulty for obtaining access for the placement of the monitoring equipment. In general, in large burns a blood pressure cuff may be placed over a burned area, but intra-arterial monitoring of blood pressure is recommended in these situations. Additionally, needle electrodes may be necessary for electrocardiographic and peripheral nerve stimulator monitors. The patient must also have the body temperature monitored closely and must be kept as close to normothermia as possible. (439; **2169**)

27. The induction and maintenance of anesthesia in burn injury patients should provide sufficient analgesia for the patient because both intraoperative and postoperative pain can be intense. Ketamine and opioids are often used for the induction and maintenance of anesthesia. If the burns are severe, the patient may be already intubated for airway patency and frequent excision and grafting procedures. It may be prudent to avoid halothane for maintenance anesthesia in burn injury patients because these patients may have epinephrine-soaked sponges applied to the burned surfaces to help control bleeding in areas to be excised and grafted. (439; **2169**)

28. Succinylcholine is not recommended for neuromuscular blockade in patients after 24 hours after the burn injury. The risk of administering succinylcholine after this time period is the potential for hyperkalemia. With regard to the administration of nondepolarizing neuromuscular blocking drugs in burn injury patients, it has been noted that these patients become resistant to the effects of these drugs. Burn injury patients often require higher doses of nondepolarizing neuromuscular blocking drugs to achieve a given effect. (439; **472, 2169, Table 62–10**)

ACUTE RESPIRATORY FAILURE

29. The adult respiratory distress syndrome (ARDS) is a term used to describe the patient with acute respiratory failure who has a combination of pathophys-

iologic pulmonary derangements that can result from a variety of causes. The pathophysiologic derangements include hypoxemia, decreased lung compliance, increased work of breathing, bilateral and diffuse pulmonary infiltrates on a chest radiograph, pulmonary hypertension, and pulmonary edema. (439; **2385, 2428, Fig. 72–23**)

30. ARDS can be caused by trauma, sepsis, acute pancreatitis, the aspiration of gastric contents, pneumonia, pulmonary disease, near-drowning, brain injury, high inspired concentrations of oxygen, high altitude, pulmonary embolus, the inhalation of toxic substances, massive blood transfusion, disseminated intravascular coagulation, uremia, prolonged cardiopulmonary bypass, and neuromuscular dysfunction as with myasthenia gravis, spinal cord transection, and Guillain-Barré syndrome. (439;**2385, 2428, Table 71–3**)

31. Arterial hypoxemia in patients with ARDS is not readily reversible with the administration of oxygen. Furthermore, a PaO_2 less than 60 mm Hg despite the administration of supplemental oxygen is a frequent accompaniment of ARDS. (440; **2385–2386, 2428–2429**)

32. Physiologic explanations for the arterial hypoxemia frequently seen in patients with ARDS include ventilation-to-perfusion mismatching, a decrease in functional residual capacity, decreased pulmonary compliance, and possible pulmonary edema. The most significant contributor to the arterial hypoxemia associated with ARDS is believed to be the ventilation-to-perfusion mismatch. (440; **2385–2386, 2428–2429**)

33. Pulmonary edema in patients with ARDS is thought to result from the loss of pulmonary capillary integrity. The pulmonary artery occlusion pressure is usually lower than 15 mm Hg in these patients. (440; **2428–2429**)

34. Serial arterial blood gas and pH measurements in the patient with ARDS are useful for the patient's management for several reasons. Serial arterial blood gas and pH measurements allow for the establishment of the diagnosis of ARDS, assist in the determination of the needs of mechanical ventilation, assist in assessing the effects of interventions and therapy, and help to confirm when the patient no longer requires the mechanical support of ventilation. (440)

35. The aim of the treatment of ARDS is the support of the function of the pulmonary system until the lungs recover from the injury that caused the pulmonary dysfunction. Treatment methods for ARDS include the supplementation of oxygen, improvement in gas exchange, and support of the intravascular fluid volume. The vast majority of patients with ARDS require mechanical ventilation of the lungs with positive end-expiratory pressure. The cause of death in most patients with ARDS is multiple system organ failure, sepsis, or the underlying pathology causing the ARDS. (440; **2385–2386, 2428–2429**)

36. Acute respiratory failure can be distinguished from chronic respiratory failure on the basis of arterial pH and $Paco_2$. In both these conditions the $Paco_2$ is elevated. If the elevation of $Paco_2$ is acute, as in acute respiratory failure, there has been inadequate time for the kidneys to compensate for the resulting acidosis and the arterial pH will be decreased. If the elevation of the $Paco_2$ is chronic, as in chronic respiratory failure, the kidneys have had adequate time to compensate for the acidosis by the renal tubular reabsorption of bicarbonate ions. This would lead to a near-normal pH in patients with chronic respiratory failure despite an elevated $Paco_2$. (440; **1404–1405**)

37. Ventilators used for mechanical ventilation of the lungs are classified by the mechanism by which the inspiratory cycle is terminated with each mechanical breath. Mechanical ventilators can be classified as pressure-cycled, volume-cycled, or time-cycled. (440; **2415, Tables 72–6, 72–7**)

38. Pressure-cycled ventilation of the lungs is the mechanical ventilation of the lungs in which the inspiratory phase of the ventilatory cycle is terminated when a selected pressure is achieved in the ventilatory circuit. The compliance or resistance of the patient's lungs will be the primary determinant of the tidal volume and inspiratory time achieved with the selected pressure. For instance, for a given selected pressure, a patient with poorly compliant lungs will achieve that pressure more quickly than another patient with more compliant lungs. Thus, the inspiratory cycle will be less in the patient with the poorly compliant lungs than in the patient with compliant lungs for a given selected pressure setting in pressure-cycled ventilation of the lungs. (440; **2417–2418**)

39. There are at least two significant problems with pressure-cycled mechanical ventilation of the lungs. First, in the event of a leak in the ventilatory circuit the pressure achieved in the ventilatory circuit may be insufficient to terminate the inspiratory phase and cycle the ventilator to exhalation. Second, significantly decreased pulmonary compliance or increased airway resistance of a patient's lungs may result in achievement of the selected pressure before the attainment of a breath with an adequate tidal volume. Finally, most mechanical ventilators that are pressure-cycled are not capable of providing a consistent tidal volume. (440; **2417–2418**)

40. Volume-cycled ventilation of the lungs is the mechanical ventilation of the lungs in which the inspiratory phase of the ventilatory cycle is terminated when a selected volume of gas has been delivered to the patient via the ventilatory circuit. Changes in the patient's pulmonary compliance or airway resistance do not have much of an effect on the tidal volume provided by the mechanical ventilator during volume-cycled ventilation of the lungs. This is true because the flow generator during volume-cycled mechanical ventilation of the lungs is uniform throughout the inspiratory phase independent of the patient's airway pressures. This allows for a more consistent tidal volume being delivered to the patient despite possible changes in the patient's airway pressures, as can occur with the administration of medicines such as albuterol. Most mechanical ventilators used in the critical care setting are volume-cycled. (440; **2415–2416**)

41. The compression volume of a ventilator circuit is the portion of the tidal volume that is generated by the mechanical ventilator that does not reach the patient but rather becomes lost to, or compressed within, the ventilator circuit. The compression volume of a ventilator circuit varies depending on the compliance of the entire patient-ventilator circuit system as well as the patient's peak inspiratory pressure. In general, however, most ventilator circuits have a compression volume of 3 to 5 mL for every 1 cm H_2O of airway pressure. (440; **196**)

42. It is particularly important for the anesthesiologist to be aware of the compression volume of a ventilator circuit when mechanically ventilating the lungs of a pediatric patient. The compression volume of a circuit during mechanical ventilation of a small child's lungs may actually exceed the tidal volume delivered to the patient. For example, if the patient weighs 10 kg and the ventilator has been set to ventilate the child's lungs at 10 mL/kg, the tidal volume to be delivered to the patient is 100 mL per mechanical breath. If the peak airway pressure of the lungs is 20 cm H_2O, and we assume the compression volume of the circuit to be 4 mL for every 1 cm H_2O of airway pressure, the compression volume of the circuit is 80 mL. This means that for every 100 mL tidal volume to be delivered to the patient, 80 mL will be lost to, or compressed within, the ventilator circuit. The effective tidal volume reaching the patient's lungs will thus be only 20 mL. For some patients it

may be prudent to monitor the exhaled tidal volume with a spirometer. (440–441; **196, 2107–2108**)

43. Time-cycled ventilation of the lungs is the mechanical ventilation of the lungs in which the inspiratory phase of the ventilatory cycle is terminated when a selected time interval of the inspiratory phase has elapsed. Factors that determine the tidal volume delivered to the patient with time-cycled ventilation include the inspiratory time selected and flow rate of the gases delivered during the inspiratory phase. (441)

44. Assist mode ventilation is the mechanical ventilation of a patient's lungs when the patient triggers the ventilator. The trigger for the ventilator to deliver a mechanical breath is the decrease in airway pressure that occurs when the patient makes a spontaneous breathing effort. The decrease in airway pressure that is necessary to trigger the ventilator to the inspiratory mode can be selected by the clinician caring for the patient. (441; **2415–2416, 2427, Table 72–9**)

45. Control mode ventilation is the mechanical ventilation of a patient's lungs at a selected rate independent of the patient's spontaneous effort to breathe. The advantage of this mode of ventilation is the guaranteed delivery of a selected minute ventilation independent of the patient's spontaneous breathing efforts. (441; **2415, 2427, Table 72–9**)

46. During control mode ventilation of the lungs the patient's spontaneous breathing efforts do not prevent the cycling of the mechanical ventilator. Negative pressure from a patient's spontaneous breathing efforts without the delivery of a breath can be stimulating to the patient's sympathetic nervous system, however. In this regard, it may be prudent for the anesthesiologist to depress the patient's own ventilatory drive while the patient's lungs are being mechanically ventilated with control mode ventilation. This can be achieved by administering sedative and opioid medicines to the patient or by deliberately hyperventilating the patient so that the $PaCO_2$ is below the apneic threshold. As a last result, neuromuscular blockade may be instituted to prevent patients from bucking and fighting mechanical ventilation. This may prevent the patient from harm and facilitate arterial oxygenation, particularly when small tidal volumes are being administered. Patients in whom neuromuscular blockade has been instituted should also have administered sedation, amnesia, and analgesia. (441; **2415–2416, 2423–2424, 2434**)

47. Typical ventilator settings for a patient whose lungs are being mechanically ventilated with control mode ventilation include a breathing rate of 6 to 10 breaths per minute, a tidal volume ranging between 10 and 15 mL/kg, and a fraction of inspired oxygen concentration of approximately 50%. The advantage of a slow breathing rate and a large tidal volume when a patient's lungs are being mechanically ventilated is better matching of ventilation to perfusion for the patient by decreasing the risk of atelectasis. Arterial blood gases and arterial pH can then be measured at serial intervals, depending on the patient's clinical condition, to adjust the ventilator settings accordingly. Typically, a PaO_2 between 60 and 100 mm Hg, a $PaCO_2$ between 36 and 44 mm Hg, and a pH between 7.36 and 7.44 are reflective of appropriate ventilator settings for control mode ventilation of the patient's lungs. Patients with ARDS may not tolerate large tidal volumes, however. In addition, there is a concern regarding large tidal volume trauma, or "volutrauma," in these patients resulting from alveolar hyperdistention. For this reason, smaller tidal volumes with a more rapid respiratory rate and possibly even permissive hypercapnia is frequently implemented in patients with ARDS. (441; **2424, 2428, 2430–2432**)

48. Pressure-control inverse-ratio ventilation is a form of mechanical ventilation

of a patient's lungs in which the inspiratory phase of the ventilatory cycle is longer than the exhalation phase of the cycle. The principal advantage of this form of ventilation is an improvement in oxygenation and ventilation for the patient by the recruitment of collapsed alveoli during the prolonged inspiratory phase cycle. With this mode of mechanical ventilation of a patient's lungs, however, there is the risk of having an inadequate exhalation time for the patient and subsequent overdistention of the patient's lungs. (441; **2432–2433**)

49. Assist/control mode ventilation is a form of mechanical ventilation of a patient's lungs in which the ventilatory cycle is set such that the control mode ventilatory cycle is less frequent than the patient's own spontaneous breathing efforts. If the patient should not breathe, the ventilator will then deliver a breath at the selected interval. The selected interval can be thought of as a back-up rate for ventilation should the patient not spontaneously ventilate adequately. This mode of mechanical ventilation is useful during weaning of the patient from mechanical ventilation of the lungs. Advantages to this mode of ventilation may include improved cardiac output in patients with normal left ventricular function, less hemodynamic compromise than when positive end-expiratory pressure is being applied, improved renal blood flow, and greater urine output. Patients with ventilatory fatigue or in cardiogenic shock may not tolerate the work of breathing associated with this mode of ventilation. (441; **2386, 2427**)

50. Pressure support ventilation is a mode of mechanical ventilation in which the patient's spontaneous inspiratory breathing effort leads to the delivery of high gas flow into the circuit of a preselected pressure. Pressure support ventilation decreases the patient's work of breathing by augmenting each inspiratory effort with positive pressure. The preselected pressure augmentation can be adjusted to achieve a given tidal volume. This mode of ventilation can be used to partially decrease the patient's work of breathing, known as partial unloading, or to entirely assume the patient's work of breathing by total unloading. (441; **2387, 2417, Figs. 72–11, 72–12**)

51. High-frequency ventilation is a mode of ventilation in which small tidal volumes are delivered at a rapid rate, usually between 30 and 60 breaths per minute. The tidal volume delivered is less than the volume of the anatomic deadspace. High-frequency ventilation may be used in patients with massive air leaks in whom conventional mechanical ventilation techniques have failed. This method of ventilation has also been used with some success in neonatal patients. Risks of high-frequency ventilation include barotrauma and alveolar hyperdistention that may occur if breaths become stacked and insufficient time or space is allowed for gases to escape. (441; **1285–1286, 1715, 2418–2419, 2464, Fig. 33–23**)

52. Positive end-expiratory pressure (PEEP) is the application of positive pressure to the patient's lungs at the conclusion of mechanical exhalation. (441, Figs. 34–1, 34–2; **2386, 2419–2420**)

53. The potential benefits of PEEP are the improved matching of ventilation-to-perfusion of the patient's lungs, as well as a decrease in the magnitude of right-to-left intrapulmonary shunting of blood. The mechanism by which PEEP is believed to achieve these benefits is through increasing the volume of patent alveoli and by the expansion of previously collapsed but perfused alveoli, thus improving pulmonary compliance and increasing the functional residual capacity of the lungs. The application of PEEP also results in the redistribution of extravascular lung water. This mechanism of action of PEEP is particularly beneficial to patients with pulmonary edema. In these patients, edema in the alveoli is mobilized from areas of gas exchange to the peribron-

chial and hilar regions. The benefits of PEEP are reflected by an increase in arterial oxygenation. When a patient's functional residual capacity of the lungs is normal or increased, or when the arterial hypoxemia seen in the patient is due to hypoventilation, the institution of PEEP does not improve the PaO_2. (441; **2386, 2419, Figs. 72–16, 72–17, 72–18**)

54. The institution of PEEP is recommended when a PaO_2 greater than 60 mm Hg cannot be maintained despite an inhaled concentration of oxygen greater than 50% in a patient whose lungs are being mechanically ventilated. Initially, the level of PEEP that is instituted should be 2.5 to 5.0 cm H_2O and an arterial blood gas sample taken to measure the PaO_2. The addition of PEEP should be done in 2.5 cm H_2O increments until arterial hypoxemia is minimized with the patient breathing 50% oxygen, without causing any of the potential negative effects of PEEP. Thus the minimal amount of PEEP that achieves these results is typically applied. (441–442; **2424–2425, Figs. 72–20, 72–21**)

55. Potential negative effects of PEEP include a decrease in cardiac output and pulmonary barotrauma. PEEP may also result in the redistribution of pulmonary blood flow. (442; **2386, 2419–2423, 2426**)

56. PEEP decreases cardiac output through three potential mechanisms. The primary mechanism appears to be due to an increase in intrathoracic positive pressure, which results in a decrease in venous return to the heart. The second mechanism by which PEEP can result in a decrease in cardiac output is by the leftward displacement of the cardiac ventricular septum that restricts left ventricular filling. A final potential mechanism is through the increase in right ventricular afterload produced by the increase in the intrathoracic pressure. The effect of PEEP on cardiac output appears to be the most pronounced in patients who are hypovolemic or in patients with normal lungs. Normal lungs allow for the maximal transmission of positive pressure to the thorax. The cardiovascular effects of PEEP may be minimized by ensuring adequate intravascular fluid volume status and adequate preload to the heart. (442; **2422–2423**)

57. The effects of PEEP on cardiac output can be monitored with the use of a pulmonary artery catheter. When PEEP is less than 10 cm H_2O, the pulmonary artery occlusion pressure measured by a pulmonary artery catheter is a fairly accurate representation of left atrial pressure. When the level of PEEP administered to a patient is greater than 10 cm H_2O, the pulmonary artery occlusion pressure measured by a pulmonary artery catheter is no longer an accurate representation of left atrial pressure. This occurs as a result of the transmission of positive pressure from the alveoli to the pulmonary capillaries, which is then measured as the pulmonary artery occlusion pressure. (442; **2422**)

58. Adverse manifestations of pulmonary barotrauma that can result from PEEP include pneumothorax, pneumomediastinum, pneumopericardium, pneumoperitoneum, and subcutaneous emphysema. These can occur as a result of overdistention of alveoli secondary to the positive pressure in the airways at end-exhalation. In retrospective studies the risk of barotrauma appeared to be increased in patients in whom peak inspiratory pressures were greater than 60 to 80 cm H_2O and when the level of PEEP was greater than 15 cm H_2O. The risk of barotrauma appeared to be most correlated with the nature and severity of lung disease. Pulmonary barotrauma significantly increases the risk of morbidity and mortality. The anesthesiologist should be immediately suspicious of possible pulmonary barotrauma when there is an abrupt deterioration of the PaO_2 and of cardiovascular function in a patient whose lungs are being mechanically ventilated with PEEP. (442; **2420–2422, 2425–2426, Fig. 72–22, Table 72–8**)

59. The administration of PEEP can lead to a redistribution of pulmonary blood flow. Although the exact mechanism for the redistribution of pulmonary blood flow is not clearly understood, it is believed to occur as a result of overdistention of alveoli. This causes compression of surrounding capillaries and an increased resistance to blood flow to these alveoli. Perfusion to these alveoli is thus decreased. This can result in an increase in ventilation-to-perfusion mismatch and a decrease in the Pa_{O_2}. The potential benefits of PEEP outweigh the detriments of the redistribution of pulmonary blood flow when the appropriate amount of PEEP is applied to diseased lungs. (442; **2422**)

60. Noninvasive positive pressure ventilation provides ventilatory support without tracheal intubation. It assists ventilation by providing positive airway pressure through either a nasal or an oral mask. This type of ventilatory support often involves continuous positive airway pressure (CPAP). Advantages of this type of support of ventilation include increased patient comfort, decreased length of stay in the intensive care unit, and the avoidance of tracheal intubation. Patient cooperation is required for noninvasive positive pressure ventilation to be effective. (442; **2312, 2386, 2419**)

61. The adequacy of arterial oxygenation during the treatment of ARDS can be monitored by evaluating the patient's Pa_{O_2}. The goal of treatment in ARDS is the reversal of arterial hypoxemia to a Pa_{O_2} between 60 and 100 mm Hg. When the ARDS patient's Pa_{O_2} is low, additional information can be gained with regard to arterial oxygenation by measuring the efficiency of gas exchange across the alveolar-to-capillary interface. This is reflected by the difference in the calculated PA_{O_2} in the alveolus and the measured Pa_{O_2}, or perhaps more efficiently by the ratio of these two values. This value provides the anesthesiologist with an estimate of the degree of right-to-left intrapulmonary shunting that is occurring and contributing to the arterial hypoxemia. (442–443; **2424–2425, 2434**)

62. The adequacy of alveolar ventilation in patients with ARDS can be monitored in two different ways. First, the Pa_{CO_2} can be directly measured. Normal values of Pa_{CO_2} range between 36 and 44 mm Hg, although hypercapnia may be permitted when attempting to minimize excessive airway pressures and the arterial pH is greater than 7.30. Alternatively, the efficiency of the exchange of carbon dioxide across the alveolar-to-capillary interface can also be measured as the ratio between volume of deadspace ventilation and volume of ventilation that leads to gas exchange (V_D/V_T). Normally, this number is less than 0.3, but in cases of ARDS, this ratio can more than double. (443; **2424–2425, 2432, 2434**)

63. The adequacy of tissue oxygenation in patients with ARDS can be monitored by the use of a pulmonary artery catheter. Blood obtained from the pulmonary artery can be evaluated for the partial pressure of oxygen. The partial pressure of oxygen in this sample is termed the *mixed venous partial pressure of oxygen* and serves as a reflection of the amount of oxygen that was extracted from the blood by the tissues for oxygenation. When the mixed venous partial pressure of oxygen is less than 30 mm Hg, it is thought that the delivery of oxygen to the tissues is inadequate. When oxygen delivery to the tissues is inadequate, attempts should be made to increase the cardiac output as well as the Pa_{O_2}. (443; **2424–2425**)

64. The adequacy of acid-base equilibrium in patients with ARDS can be monitored by the direct measurement of arterial pH. It is fairly common for patients with ARDS to be acidotic. Metabolic acidosis occurs as a result of arterial hypoxemia and the inadequate delivery of oxygen to the tissues that is frequently seen in these patients. Respiratory acidosis occurs as a result of alveolar hypoventilation and the concomitant increase in the Pa_{CO_2}. Potential

adverse effects of the acidosis frequently seen in ARDS patients include cardiac dysrhythmias, increased pulmonary vascular resistance, and a decreased responsiveness to catecholamines. (443; **2432, 2435**)

65. The adequacy of cardiac output in patients with ARDS can be monitored by its direct measurement with the use of a pulmonary artery catheter and the thermodilution technique. A cardiac output greater than 2.5 L/min per square meter of body surface area is desirable to maintain adequate oxygen delivery to tissues. (443)

66. During the treatment of ARDS the cessation of mechanical ventilation of the lungs can be considered when the patient is able to maintain normal arterial blood gases, pH, consciousness, and hemodynamic stability while spontaneously breathing through a T-tube or with a low mandatory ventilatory rate for 1 to 2 hours. In addition, the patient should have intact laryngeal and cough reflexes for airway protection, not be productive of copious secretions, have adequate nutrition, have normal electrolytes, and have favorable pulmonary mechanics. Some clinical guidelines that are used to predict successful cessation of mechanical ventilation of the lungs include a vital capacity greater than 15 mL/kg, an alveolar-to-arterial difference of oxygen less than 350 mm Hg while breathing 100% oxygen, an arterial-to-alveolar Po_2 ratio greater than 0.75, a maximum inspiratory pressure more negative than -20 cm H_2O, and a deadspace-to-tidal volume ratio less than 0.6. Of note, it is not necessary for the patient to be independent of oxygen requirements before extubation of the trachea. The patient may be weaned from mechanical ventilation of the lungs, have his or her trachea extubated, and subsequently be weaned gradually from oxygen while spontaneously breathing. The oxygen requirement of the patient should be sufficiently low such that it can be delivered reliably to the patient after extubation of the trachea. (443; **1285, 2434–2436, Table 33–4**)

67. There are several methods for weaning patients from mechanical ventilation of the lungs. Two methods that are commonly used include the use of a T-tube and intermittent mandatory ventilation (IMV). There are no data to indicate that the method used to wean patients from mechanical ventilation of the lungs has much influence on the success of weaning. (443–444; **1286–1287, 2434–2436**)

68. T-tube weaning involves the disconnection of the patient's endotracheal tube from the mechanical ventilator and its connection to a gas source through which oxygen-enriched humidified gases are delivered to the spontaneously breathing patient. Weaning via the T-tube is accomplished by having the patient breathe spontaneously via the T-tube for incrementally greater amounts of time while being closely observed for signs of premature weaning from mechanical ventilation of the lungs. (444; **1286–1287, 2434–2436**)

69. Continuous positive airway pressure (CPAP) is the continuous administration of airway pressure at 2.5 to 5 cm H_2O. CPAP is often delivered to the patient via the T-tube when this mode of weaning is selected for two reasons. First, it helps the patient overcome the resistance of the tracheal tube while breathing spontaneously. Second, it helps to prevent the decrease in functional residual capacity that can be associated with the cessation of positive pressure ventilation of the lungs. (444; **1286–1287, 2386, 2417, 2419, 2421–2423, Figs. 71–2, 72–15**)

70. Tachypnea, tachycardia, and a change in level of consciousness in a spontaneously breathing patient who is being weaned from mechanical ventilation may all be indications that weaning is premature. (444; **1286–1287, 2434–2436**)

71. Intermittent mandatory ventilation is the intermittent mechanical ventilation

of a patient's lungs while the patient spontaneously breathes. When intermittent mandatory ventilation is synchronized, the ventilatory breaths provided by the ventilator are triggered by, or synchronized with, the patient's efforts. Nonsynchronous intermittent mandatory ventilation is the delivery of an intermittent mechanical ventilatory breath by the ventilator that is not initiated by the patient but delivered at a preset interval independent of the patient's efforts. (444; **1286–1287, 2386, 2434–2436, Table 72–6**)

72. Weaning a patient from mechanical ventilation of the lungs using intermittent mandatory ventilation is usually accomplished by the incremental decrease in the number of ventilatory breaths per minute delivered by the ventilator. The goal of weaning from mechanical ventilation of the lungs through this method is that the spontaneously breathing patient will gradually rely less on the ventilator and be able to assume the work of breathing. When the ventilator is providing only 1 to 2 breaths/min, the patient is considered for the cessation of mechanical ventilation of the lungs. (444; **1286–1287, 2434–2436**)

CONGESTIVE HEART FAILURE

73. The goal of treatment for patients with congestive heart failure is to optimize their cardiac output. Classes of drugs that are used for this purpose include vasodilators and inotropic agents. (444)

74. Vasodilators that are commonly used to increase cardiac output include nitroprusside, nitroglycerin, hydralazine, and captopril. The mechanism by which vasodilators increase cardiac output is by decreasing the resistance the heart must pump against, thereby increasing the forward ejection of blood from the left ventricle. Nitroglycerin may be useful in patients with myocardial ischemia in that it redistributes coronary artery blood flow. (444; **1763**)

75. A limitation to vasodilator therapy for the treatment of cardiac output is the potential for decreasing the systemic blood pressure to the extent that the coronary perfusion pressure decreases, putting the patient at risk for myocardial ischemia. When using vasodilators for the treatment of congestive heart failure, maintaining the patient in the optimal fluid status may minimize the decrease in blood pressure that can result. (444; **1763**)

76. Inotropic drugs are used in the treatment of congestive heart failure as a means of increasing cardiac output. The mechanism by which inotropic drugs work to increase cardiac output is by increasing myocardial contractility. Examples of inotropic drugs that are used in congestive heart failure include dopamine, dobutamine, and epinephrine. (444)

77. The effectiveness of drugs that are used in congestive heart failure can be measured through the use of a pulmonary artery catheter. Information that can be gained by a pulmonary catheter that may reflect an increase in cardiac output secondary to pharmacologic interventions includes an improvement in the cardiac index, a decrease in atrial filling pressures, an increase in the mixed venous partial pressure of oxygen, and an associated improvement in arterial oxygenation. (444; **1776**)

78. An intra-aortic balloon counterpulsation pump may be useful in patients who are in cardiogenic shock after suffering from a myocardial infarction. The mechanism by which an intra-aortic balloon counterpulsation pump works is the inflation and deflation of a balloon in the proximal aorta timed with the electrocardiogram. Inflation of the balloon takes place during diastole, and the balloon deflates just before systole. Inflation of the balloon during diastole allows for an increase in diastolic blood pressure and possible improvement in coronary blood flow and myocardial oxygen delivery. Deflation of the balloon just before systole decreases the systemic blood pressure and de-

creases afterload, which leads to a decrease in myocardial work and myocardial oxygen requirements. (444–445; **1141–1142, 1764**)

SEPSIS

79. Common sources of infection in patients who are critically ill include pneumonia and infections of the urinary tract, surgical wounds, intravascular devices, and sinuses. Pneumonia is the most common infectious cause of death in the hospital. (445; **1948, 2484–2485, 2506**)

80. Clinical signs of septic shock include hypotension, peripheral vasodilation, and oliguria. If a pulmonary artery catheter were placed, the pulmonary artery occlusion pressure is usually low with a very high cardiac output. The patient may or may not have a fever and elevated white blood cell count. Blood cultures are useful when positive in diagnosing the source of the sepsis, but a positive blood culture is not necessary for the diagnosis of sepsis. (445; **688–689, 1305, 2315, 2484–2485, 2506**)

81. Septic shock is treated by the administration of intravascular fluids and antibiotics. The initial antibiotics chosen for this purpose usually cover a wide spectrum of bacteria. If a specific bacterial pathogen is cultured from the blood of the patient, the antibiotics can be modified to more specifically cover the pathogen. Patients with septic shock lose intravascular fluid secondary to capillary endothelial leak. The administration of intravascular fluids is often guided by monitoring right or left atrial pressures and urine output. Fluid replacement should be aggressive and instituted early to maintain systemic blood pressure. Dopamine and/or other vasopressors may be indicated for the maintenance of systemic blood pressure, cardiac output, and renal function. (445; **688–689, 1305, 2315, 2484–2485, 2506**)

82. Surgical intervention may become necessary for the treatment of the source of bacteremia. Ketamine may be a useful agent for the induction of anesthesia in these patients. (445; **2484–2485**)

HEAD INJURY

83. Patients suspected of having a closed-head injury can be evaluated by history, physical examination, and radiologic studies. The hallmark clinical sign of a closed-head injury is loss of consciousness. The Glasgow Coma Scale assigns a numerical score to patients based on eye opening and verbal and motor responses. A computed tomographic scan is diagnostic of a closed-head injury. Evidence of an increase in intracranial pressure (ICP), a subdural hematoma, or an epidural hematoma can be diagnosed by computed tomography. (445; **1918, 2158, 2395, 2468, Tables 62–3, 71–8, 73–12**)

84. ICP can be directly monitored by the use of a catheter placed through a bur hole into a cerebral ventricle. Alternatively, intracranial pressure can be monitored by the placement of a transducer on the surface of the brain. Patients who have sustained a closed-head injury and are at a high risk of complications should have their ICPs continually monitored. These patients include those who have cerebral edema, large brain tumors, cerebral aneurysms, or hydrocephalus or who are comatose. (445–446; **1922, 2393–2394, 2396, 2468**)

85. A normal ICP has a mean less than 15 mm Hg. The ICP is normally pulsatile and varies with the cardiac impulse and breathing. (446; **2393–2394**)

86. A plateau wave in the ICP wave tracing refers to an abrupt increase in the ICP observed during continuous monitoring. The plateau wave is usually sustained for 10 to 20 minutes, followed by a rapid decrease in the ICP. The

presence of plateau waves on an ICP wave tracing may indicate that the intracranial compliance is low. (446, Fig. 34–3)

87. Painful stimuli can elicit a plateau wave in an otherwise unresponsive patient. This implies that even unresponsive patients should be administered analgesics to avoid pain. (446)

88. Treatment of an elevated ICP is frequently recommended when the pressure exceeds 20 mm Hg for a sustained period of time. There are several methods by which elevations in ICP can be treated. These include the maintenance of an appropriate posture; the administration of osmotic diuretics, renal tubular diuretics, corticosteroids, and barbiturates; deliberate hyperventilation; and the institution of cerebrospinal fluid drainage. (446; **1916–1917, 2394, 2470–2471**)

89. The posture of a patient with an elevated ICP can significantly impact the patient's ICP. The head of the bed of the patient should be maintained in a 30-degree head-up position to facilitate venous drainage from the brain. In addition, the patient's head should not be extended or rotated in a manner that may obstruct jugular venous outflow from the brain. (446; **1902, 2470**)

90. Hyperventilation of the lungs results in a decrease in the patient's $PaCO_2$, subsequently leading to systemic alkalosis. This results in a decrease in cerebral blood flow and therefore a decrease in intracranial blood volume. The duration of efficacy of hyperventilation for decreasing a patient's ICP is estimated to be about 6 hours, after which cerebral blood flow returns to normal in healthy volunteers. The efficacy of hyperventilation for decreasing ICP is affected by the integrity of the cerebral blood vessels. For example, if cerebral blood vessels are damaged or diseased, as by trauma or tumor, the reactivity of the vessels in response to deliberate hyperventilation may be diminished. (446; **698, 1899–1900, 2470, Figs. 19–4, 52–5**)

91. The $PaCO_2$ that should be maintained in adults to decrease ICP by hyperventilation is between 25 and 30 mm Hg. Because of their higher cerebral blood flow relative to adults, the $PaCO_2$ that can be maintained in children to decrease ICP by hyperventilation is between 20 and 25 mm Hg. The danger of excessive hyperventilation in adults or children is the potential for cerebral ischemia that can result if the patient becomes too alkalotic. (446; **698, 1899–1900, 2470**)

92. Osmotic diuretics decrease ICP by drawing water out of tissues and into the intravascular space. Osmotic diuretics do so by transiently increasing the osmolarity of plasma. The osmotic diuretic that is most frequently administered for this purpose is mannitol. The dose of mannitol that is administered is 0.25 to 1 g/kg over 15 to 30 minutes. (446; **1901–1902, 2470**)

93. The administration of osmotic diuretics may have some adverse effects in addition to the desired effect of decreasing ICP. Osmotic diuretics may cause hypovolemia and electrolyte abnormalities. This effect can be minimized by replacing the urine output with equal volumes of crystalloid and colloid solutions. The administration of glucose-containing intravenous solutions after the administration of an osmotic diuretic is not recommended because these solutions rapidly become distributed throughout the total body water, including the brain. Furthermore, if the glucose concentration in the brain increases more rapidly than the serum glucose concentration, water enters the central nervous system and can further exacerbate existing cerebral edema. (446; **1901–1902, 2470**)

94. The administration of a tubular diuretic such as furosemide is useful in lowering increased ICPs that exist in the presence of an increased intravascu-

lar fluid volume. They work by decreasing the intravascular fluid volume and increasing urine output. (446; **1901–1902, 2470**)

95. Corticosteroids that are often administered to patients with elevated ICPs include dexamethasone and methylprednisolone. The exact mechanism by which corticosteroids decrease elevated ICPs is not known, but it may be through its effects on capillary membranes. Corticosteroids are most effective in decreasing elevated ICPs in the presence of focal edema, as opposed to global cerebral edema. (446; **1901, 2470**)

96. Patients with persistently elevated ICPs despite conventional interventions of positioning, deliberate hyperventilation, diuretics, and corticosteroids may benefit from the administration of barbiturates. Barbiturates are believed to decrease elevated ICPs by decreasing cerebral blood flow secondary to cerebral vasculature vasoconstriction. Barbiturates also decrease the cerebral metabolic oxygen requirements of the brain. Barbiturates that are administered to decrease elevated ICPs should be administered at a dose sufficient to maintain the ICP lower than 20 mm Hg, as well as to achieve the suppression of plateau waves. Barbiturates that are administered to decrease elevated ICPs should be discontinued when the ICP has been normal for 48 hours. (446–447; **223–224, 703, 719–720, 1917, 2471**)

97. The potential hazard of barbiturate administration to patients with persistently elevated ICP is that of hypotension. The hypotension that results may lead to an inadequate cerebral perfusion pressure. This risk can be minimized by the administration of an agent to support the mean arterial blood pressure. (447; **223–224, 703, 719–720, 1917, 2471**)

NEUROLOGIC COMPLICATIONS IN CRITICALLY ILL PATIENTS

98. Causes of failure to awaken patients in the critical care unit include septic encephalopathy, acute uremic encephalopathy, ischemic strokes, and persistent effects of residual sedative drugs. Patients who fail to awaken without explanation should be evaluated with laboratory and radiologic tests. (447; **2393**)

99. Causes of skeletal muscle weakness in patients in the critical care unit include polyneuropathy and generalized weakness related to the administration of nondepolarizing neuromuscular blocking drugs. Patients with polyneuropathy in the critical care unit may have areflexia and muscle wasting. Female patients with renal failure are at particular risk of generalized weakness related to the administration of nondepolarizing neuromuscular blocking drugs. The cause of generalized weakness in these patients may be persistent pharmacologic neuromuscular blockade. (447–448; **472–474**)

100. Causes of seizures in patients in the critical care unit include hyponatremia, hypocalcemia, hypoglycemia, and drug toxicity. (448)

ACUTE RENAL FAILURE

101. The best method by which to avoid acute renal failure in an intensive care unit setting is by the maintenance of the patient's intravascular fluid volume and cardiac output such that renal perfusion is maintained. (448; **1303–1304, 1945–1946, Fig. 34–5**)

102. The only treatment for acute tubular necrosis is hemodialysis. (448; **1945–1946**)

ACUTE HEPATIC FAILURE

103. Patients with early acute hepatic failure often hyperventilate. This is presumed to be as a result of the stimulation of ventilation by the accumulation of ammonia. (448)

104. Physiologic dysfunctions that are frequently associated with terminal hepatic failure include coagulopathy, renal failure, arterial hypoxemia, hypotension, hepatic encephalopathy, portal hypertension, varices, ascites, hypoglycemia, and an increased ICP. The cardiac output of a patient with acute hepatic failure is often increased. Cardiac output is believed to increase as a result of increased arteriovenous shunting and a decrease in systemic vasculature resistance. (448; **1966, 1984–1985, 2477–2478**)

105. The goal of treatment of acute hepatic failure is symptomatic and supportive. This frequently includes the administration of neomycin or lactulose to decrease the production of ammonia. (448; **1608, 1966, 2477–2478, 2526–2527**)

MALNUTRITION

106. Critically ill patients often have increased caloric needs as a result of being hypermetabolic. The hypermetabolic state of these patients can occur as a result of trauma, fever, sepsis, burns, and wound healing. (448; **2504–2505, Table 74–5**)

107. Malnutrition in an intensive care unit setting is usually managed by the administration of enteral nutrition directly to the stomach or intestines or by total parenteral nutrition. Total parenteral nutrition is usually delivered via central venous access. (448; **2519–2520**)

108. Some of the potential complications associated with total parenteral nutrition include hypoglycemia, hyperglycemia, hyperchloremic metabolic acidosis, increased carbon dioxide production, electrolyte abnormalities, and catheter-related sepsis. (448; **2520–2525, Tables 74–7, 74–8**)

Chapter 34

Chronic Pain Management

ROLE OF THE ANESTHESIOLOGIST IN THE DIAGNOSIS AND TREATMENT OF CHRONIC PAIN

1. What group of professionals are usually employed by a chronic pain clinic? How are patients usually referred to a pain clinic?

2. Who should evaluate a patient on his or her arrival to a chronic pain clinic? What kind of information about the patient should be gathered at that time? How is a treatment plan established for a patient at the chronic pain clinic?

3. Name some treatment modalities for the management of chronic pain.

4. What is the risk of performing diagnostic and therapeutic nerve blocks before the performance of a complete physical examination?

APPROACH TO THE PATIENT WITH CHRONIC PAIN

5. Name some psychological reactions to chronic pain. What is the potential value of the Minnesota Multiphasic Personality Inventory Test when evaluating patients with chronic pain?

6. What are some methods for the clinician to evaluate a patient's pain by history and physical examination?

DIAGNOSTIC NERVE BLOCKS

7. What is some of the information a diagnostic nerve block can provide the chronic pain clinician?

8. Describe how the graduated spinal technique is used to do a differential nerve block to determine whether the source of pain is a sympathetic nerve, a sensory nerve, a motor nerve, or psychogenic in a chronic pain patient.

9. How frequently will a placebo injection in lieu of local anesthetic during a diagnostic nerve block result in some relief of chronic pain? What does this imply regarding the basis of pain in the patient?

10. What are some disadvantages of a graduated spinal anesthetic technique as a diagnostic nerve block?

THERAPEUTIC NERVE BLOCKS

11. What types of chronic pain can be interrupted with the appropriately placed injection of local anesthetics? Is the pain relief achieved usually temporary or permanent?

12. How do sympathetic nerve blocks with local anesthetic affect vascular blood flow to areas supplied by the sympathetic nerve?

13. What are some agents that can be used as neurolytics for the destruction of nerves? Which is most efficacious?

14. Please complete the following table comparing alcohol and phenol:

	ALCOHOL	PHENOL
Pain with injection?		
Neurolysis prompt or delayed?		
Hypobaric or hyperbaric?		
Concentration used in somatic nerve blocks?		
Concentration used in sympathetic nerve blocks?		

15. Which patients are appropriate candidates for neurolysis of the nerves that are the source of chronic pain?

16. What is denervation hypersensitivity?

17. What are some disadvantages of neurolysis of the nerves that cause chronic pain?

18. Which opioid is used neuraxially most often for the treatment of chronic pain? What is the most common cause of pain in patients who are administered neuraxial opioids for chronic pain control?

19. What are some advantages of the neuraxial administration of opioids for the treatment of chronic pain?

20. What are some of the potential negative side effects of the neuraxial administration of opioids for chronic pain?

21. What are some potential advantages of the administration of neuraxial opioids via implantable infusion pumps? Approximately what percent of patients experience pain relief with this method?

22. What are some potential complications of the administration of neuraxial opioids via an implantable infusion pump?

23. Why should chronic neuraxial opioid infusions not be abruptly discontinued?

EVALUATION OF A NERVE BLOCK

24. How should the effectiveness of a nerve block be evaluated by the physician specializing in the treatment of chronic pain?

25. If a nerve block with local anesthetic results in excellent pain relief, how certain is it that surgical neurolysis will also result in excellent pain relief?

26. How permanent is the pain relief achieved by surgical neurolysis?

NEUROSTIMULATION THERAPY

27. What are some types of neurostimulation techniques?

28. What is transcutaneous electrical nerve stimulation (TENS)? What are some of its advantages for the treatment of pain?

29. How is TENS believed to work?

30. When is TENS most often used?

ORAL DRUG THERAPY

31. What dose of opioids should be given to the terminally ill patient with chronic pain?

32. What are some other drugs that are administered in combination with opioids in an effort to achieve the relief of chronic pain?

33. When might the administration of a nonsteroidal anti-inflammatory agent be useful in conjunction with opioids for the treatment of chronic pain?

34. When might the administration of an antidepressant drug be useful in conjunction with opioids for the treatment of chronic pain? How are antidepressants thought to exert their effects on pain?

35. When might the administration of an anticonvulsant drug be useful in conjunction with opioids for the treatment of chronic pain?

COMMON CHRONIC PAIN SYNDROMES

36. What is myofascial pain? What is a trigger point? What is the physiologic connection between a trigger point and myofascial pain?

37. What is the scapulocostal syndrome of myofascial pain? Where is the associated trigger point?

38. What is the treatment of myofascial pain?

39. What is lumbosacral radiculopathy? What are some characteristics of the pain associated with lumbosacral radiculopathy?

40. What are some other causes of chronic back pain that must be ruled out before the institution of treatment for lumbosacral radiculopathy?

41. What is the mechanism by which epidural corticosteroids are thought to decrease chronic back pain? Describe the procedure for an epidural corticosteroid injection.

42. What are some clinical circumstances in which repeated epidural corticosteroid injections will be unlikely to lead to any beneficial effect?

43. What are some potential complications of epidural corticosteroid injections?

44. How can the chronic low back pain associated with inflammation of the lumbar facet joint be distinguished from the chronic low back pain associated with lumbosacral radiculopathy?

45. What is the usual clinical presentation of intercostal neuralgia?

46. What is the most effective treatment plan for intercostal neuralgia? How effective is neurolysis with alcohol or phenol in these patients?

47. What is postherpetic neuralgia?

48. What treatment modalities have been used in the treatment of postherpetic neuralgia?

49. What are some of the side effects of tricyclic antidepressants that may limit their usefulness in elderly patients with postherpetic neuralgia?

50. What are the complex regional pain syndromes? What differentiates types I and II of these syndromes?

51. What are the clinical manifestations of the complex regional pain syndromes?

52. How is the diagnosis of complex regional pain syndrome of an upper or lower extremity made?

53. What is the treatment of complex regional pain syndrome? How does the time delay to diagnosis and treatment affect treatment outcome?

54. Why can't brachial plexus blockade be used for the treatment of a complex regional pain syndrome of the upper extremity?

55. What pharmacologic agents can be used for intravenous regional sympathetic nerve blockade? How is this technique believed to work? In which patients is this technique useful?

CANCER PAIN

56. What are some causes of pain in patients with cancer?

57. What are some oral medications that may be useful in the treatment of cancer pain?

58. What are some alternative routes of analgesic drug delivery for the cancer patient with chronic pain in whom the oral administration of medicines is not possible?

59. What are some neurosurgical procedures for the treatment of chronic pain that may be useful in cancer patients in whom less invasive procedures have been unsuccessful at pain control?

60. When might a neurolytic celiac plexus block be useful to treat cancer pain?

61. How is a neurolytic celiac plexus block achieved?

62. What are some potential complications of a celiac plexus block?

ANSWERS*

ROLE OF THE ANESTHESIOLOGIST IN THE DIAGNOSIS AND TREATMENT OF CHRONIC PAIN

1. Professionals employed by a chronic pain clinic include anesthesiologists, orthopedic surgeons, neurologists, psychologists, social workers, and behavioral and physical therapists. Patients are usually referred to a chronic pain clinic by their family physicians for a problem with chronic pain that has not responded to conventional medical interventions. The pain clinic professionals interact to solve the chronic pain problem from both a nociceptive and a psychological approach. (449; **2351–2352, 2355–2356**)

2. On their arrival to a chronic pain clinic, the patient should be evaluated by psychological and medical professionals, as well as by a social worker. During the initial evaluations the potential psychological, medical, and social contributions to the patient's pain should be evaluated. A multidisciplinary meeting is then scheduled to discuss the various aspects of the patient's case as well as the probable diagnosis. A treatment plan can then be established for the patient. (450; **2354–2355**)

3. Treatment modalities for the management of chronic pain include the oral administration of medicines, diagnostic and therapeutic nerve blocks, the neuraxial administration of opioids, neurostimulation, biofeedback, and physical therapy. (450; **2356–2372**)

4. The risk of performing diagnostic and therapeutic nerve blocks before the performance of a complete physical examination is that a disease process may be overlooked. (450; **2355**)

APPROACH TO THE PATIENT WITH CHRONIC PAIN

5. Psychological reactions to chronic pain vary. They may include mental depression, insomnia, avoidance of social and vocational obligations, dependence on analgesics, and visits to multiple physicians. Patients with chronic pain may be

*Numbers in parentheses: lightface numbers refer to pages, figures, or tables in Stoelting RK, Miller RD: Basics of Anesthesia, 4th ed. Philadelphia, Churchill Livingstone, 2000; **boldface numbers** refer to pages, figures, or tables in Miller RD: Anesthesia, 5th ed. Philadelphia, Churchill Livingstone, 2000.

demoralized and worried, sometimes even hostile and neurotic. It is important that patients with chronic pain who have a neurotic personality not be excluded from treatment. The Minnesota Multiphasic Personality Inventory test is a useful behavioral analysis test for the detection of any psychopathology existing within the patient that may be contributing to the chronic pain complaint. (450; **2354–2355, 2369–2370**)

6. The history elicited regarding the pain should include information about the onset of the pain, its location, radiation, characteristics, quality, constancy, attempted therapies, and responses to therapy. Aspects of the pain that should be evaluated by the anesthesiologist during the initial physical examination include the distribution of the pain, evidence of guarding or wasting of muscles and joints, any swelling of the painful area, temperature changes overlying the painful area, and maneuvers that alter the pain. The neurologic examination should be especially emphasized during the physical examination the patient receives on the initial visit to the chronic pain center. Also useful is documentation in a diary of daily activities and the level of associated pain. Medicines taken and their timing in relation to the pain should also be documented. A useful method of evaluating a patient's pain is by asking the patient to assign a number between 0 and 10 corresponding to the level of pain the patient is experiencing, where 0 would be no pain at all and 10 would be severe, extreme pain. The patient may be asked to assess the pain before and after an intervention in an attempt to quantify the success of the intervention. (450–451, Fig. 35–1; **2347–2348, 2353–2354, 2369–2370**)

DIAGNOSTIC NERVE BLOCKS

7. Diagnostic nerve blocks can provide the chronic pain clinician with several pieces of information regarding the pain. With a diagnostic nerve block the pain pathway may be identified, the size of the fibers that mediate the pain can be distinguished pharmacologically, and central pain may be differentiated from peripheral pain. Finally, a diagnostic nerve block may assist in determining if the performance of a neurolytic nerve block or surgical resection may provide the patient with relief from the pain. (451; **2359–2360**)

8. The size and fiber type of the nerve that is the source of chronic pain is important information for the clinician because it provides for a better understanding of the etiology of the pain. The different nerve fibers that may be the source for the pain include sympathetic nerves, sensory nerves, and motor nerves. Because different types of nerve fibers are different sizes, it is believed that a graduated spinal technique, or the application of different solutions to the nerve, will help the clinician to determine the fiber type and etiology of the pain. The graduated spinal technique for a differential nerve block is performed in a stepwise fashion. After the anesthesiologist performs a lumbar subarachnoid puncture, he or she first injects placebo into the intrathecal space. After that, incrementally increasing concentrations of a short-acting local anesthetic are injected. For example, a given volume of 0.2% procaine may be injected into the intrathecal space. This may be followed by the same volume of 0.5% procaine, and finally the same volume of 1.0% procaine is injected into the intrathecal space. The results of the differential nerve block are determined as follows: the cause of the pain is believed to be possibly psychogenic if relief of the pain occurs after the injection of placebo. The cause of the pain is believed to be primarily from the sympathetic nervous system if the first application of dilute procaine results in relief of the patient's pain. Likewise, the cause of the patient's pain is believed to be primarily sensory or motor if relief of the patient's pain occurred after the application of 0.5% and 1.0% procaine, respectively. If the patient's pain were to persist despite the application of 1.0% procaine in the subarachnoid space, the source of the pain may be central or psychogenic in origin. (451; **2359–2360**)

9. If a placebo is injected in lieu of local anesthetic during a diagnostic nerve block there will be some relief of the pain in 30% to 40% of patients. This does not imply that the basis for the pain experienced by the patient is not organic, however. (451; **2359–2360**)

10. There are several disadvantages of a graduated spinal technique as a diagnostic nerve block. First, if the patient requires some movement to elicit the pain, he or she may be unable to elicit the pain when a catheter is inserted in the lumbar subarachnoid space. Second, the administration of the placebo may result in some relief of pain in patients whose source for the pain is truly organic. Finally, although the various concentrations of the local anesthetic administered are believed to result in the selective blockade of various nerves, there is no certainty that this is in fact what is occurring. For example, with the administration of 0.5% procaine in the subarachnoid space, sensory nerves are being tested for conduction blockade as a possible source for the pain. It is possible that motor nerves are also inadvertently undergoing some degree of blockade as well and that relief of the patient's pain under these conditions may be due to motor nerve blockade and not sensory nerve blockade. This may make the results of the differential nerve block difficult to interpret. Indeed, critics of differential nerve blocks state that few studies have been done to demonstrate their value. (451–452; **2359–2360**)

THERAPEUTIC NERVE BLOCKS

11. Nerve blocks performed with the application of local anesthetics in chronic pain patients are usually done for diagnostic purposes and are usually of only temporary duration. In patients with complex regional pain syndrome the pain relief provided by the application of local anesthetics may result in sufficient pain relief to allow the patient to attend physical therapy sessions and possibly improve the patient's condition as a result. In patients with ischemic vascular disease in an extremity, the application of local anesthetics can result in improved blood flow to the extremity. Finally, although the application of local anesthetics usually provides only temporary relief of the pain, there are rare occasions when prolonged and even permanent pain relief has resulted from the application of local anesthetics. (452; **2360–2365**)

12. Patients undergoing a sympathetic nerve block of an extremity will have improved blood flow to the extremity as a result. Sympathetic nerve blocks are traditionally used for the diagnosis and treatment of patients with complex regional pain syndrome types I and II. (452; **2361–2362**)

13. Agents that may be administered to a nerve for permanent neurolysis of the nerve include alcohol and phenol. The effectiveness of alcohol and phenol when administered for neurolysis is similar. It is important to know whether a neurolytic is hypobaric or hyperbaric relative to cerebrospinal fluid because the way the neurolytic will settle in the subarachnoid space, and thus the nerves that are bathed by the neurolytic, is determined by the baricity of the neurolytic. (452; **2366–2367**)

14. (452, Table 35–1; **2366–2367**)

	ALCOHOL	PHENOL
Pain with injection?	Yes	No
Neurolysis prompt or delayed?	Prompt	Delayed
Hypobaric or hyperbaric?	Hypobaric	Hyperbaric
Concentration used in somatic nerve blocks?	100%	20%
Concentration used in sympathetic nerve blocks?	50%	5%

15. Patients with intractable pain are appropriate candidates for neurolysis of the nerves causing the pain. The patients chosen for neurolytic nerve blocks also usually have a short life expectancy, such as those patients with pain due to terminal cancer. Factors that should be considered in the decision to proceed with a neurolytic block include the patient's general medical condition, the location of the source of pain, the rapidity with which the pain source is growing, the type of pain, the patient's life expectancy, the risks of the procedure, the outcome of treatments with more conservative methods, the patient's tolerance of narcotics, the response to a diagnostic nerve block, and the patient's ability to tolerate any of the potential side effects of the neurolytic block. (452; **2366–2367**)

16. *Denervation hypersensitivity* is a term used to describe the pain that may immediately follow neurolysis of a nerve. This neuropathic pain that results can be worse than the original pain that the patient was seeking relief from. This occurs more commonly with the neurolysis of peripheral nerves, leading clinicians to administer neurolytics primarily in either the epidural or subarachnoid spaces. (452; **2366**)

17. There are several potential disadvantages of neurolysis of the nerves that are the source of chronic pain. First, the patient may experience denervation hypersensitivity of the nerve, which can result in pain worse than the original pain. Second, there may be unwanted spread of the neurolytic solutions, resulting in the destruction of nerves that were otherwise normal. This can lead to numbness, motor weakness, or incontinence. Third, neurolysis of the nerves that are the source of chronic pain may not lead to pain relief that is as profound as the pain relief the patient experienced with the diagnostic nerve block. The patient may therefore have had expectations for pain relief that were not met and be disappointed. Finally, neurolytic blockade is rarely permanent. Recovery of the sensation of pain often occurs within weeks to months. (452–453; **2366–2367**)

18. The opioid used neuraxially most often for the treatment of chronic pain is morphine. The most common cause of pain in patients who are administered neuraxial opioids for chronic pain control is cancer. (453; **2367**)

19. The principal advantage of the neuraxial administration of opioids for the treatment of chronic pain is its efficacy. Additional advantages include the potential for continuous delivery via indwelling catheters or implantable infusion pumps, the decreased amount of systemic side effects when administered neuraxially, the absence of sympathetic nervous system blockade, and the absence of skeletal muscle paralysis. (453; **2367–2369**)

20. Potential negative side effects of the neuraxial administration of opioids for chronic pain include delayed respiratory depression, pruritus, sedation, urinary retention, nausea, and vomiting. Unlike patients with acute postoperative pain, patients with chronic pain often have developed a tolerance to opioids such that these side effects occur rarely and are manageable. (453; **2367**)

21. Neuraxial opioids can be administered on a long-term basis via a subcutaneously or surgically implanted catheter. These long-term delivery systems deliver drug to the epidural or the subarachnoid space. There is typically an implanted infusion device that may be refilled percutaneously. The main advantage of this type of delivery system for the relief of chronic pain is that the patient often experiences pain relief with this modality. In fact, pain relief is excellent for more than 50% of patients who receive these catheters. Patients may also receive analgesia on an outpatient basis. Finally, only about 2% of patients will develop a tolerance to opioids with this method of drug delivery. (453; **2367–2369**)

22. Potential complications of the administration of neuraxial opioids via an implanted catheter include infection, leakage, and occlusion. When administered in the subarachnoid space, smaller doses of opioid may be used, but there are potential complications of cerebrospinal fluid leak and headache, meningitis, and arachnoiditis. (453; **2367–2369**)

23. Because approximately 2% of patients who receive epidural or subarachnoid opioid via a continuous infusion catheter develop a tolerance to the opioid, a withdrawal syndrome may accompany an abrupt discontinuation of the infusion. For this reason, the abrupt discontinuation of the infusion should be avoided. (453)

EVALUATION OF A NERVE BLOCK

24. The effectiveness of a nerve block should be evaluated by the chronic pain physician in an analytical manner. The initial evaluation of the pain should include a patient recording of various aspects of the pain and levels of activity at home. The intensity of the pain should be evaluated using patient activity as a marker for any changes. For instance, the patient should be asked to record hourly the intensity of the pain and how many hours were spent in bed versus reclining in a chair or standing. The patient should also record his or her ability to walk, bend, and work. Comparing the activities in number and difficulty before and after the intervention may be a useful tool for the clinician. Recreational and social activities should also be documented. Also useful is documentation of the number and type of medicines taken before and after the intervention. (453; **2360**)

25. Nerve blocks that are done for diagnostic purposes, and result in excellent pain relief, do not guarantee that surgical neurolysis of the nerve will also result in excellent pain relief. Local anesthetics will produce a more intense relief of pain than neurolysis. In addition, surgical neurolysis may result in denervation hypersensitivity. Finally, regeneration of the nerve may occur after neurolysis with a return of the pain that may be even more severe than the original pain. (453; **2360, 2366**)

26. Pain relief achieved by surgical neurolysis is not always permanent. For instance, regeneration of the nerve may occur after neurolysis with a return of the pain that may be even more severe than the original pain. (453; **2360, 2366**)

NEUROSTIMULATION THERAPY

27. Types of neurostimulation techniques include transcutaneous electrical nerve stimulation (TENS), spinal cord stimulation, and peripheral nerve stimulation. TENS is a noninvasive technique beneficial in some pain syndromes. Spinal cord stimulation is generally reserved for patients who have failed all other treatment modalities. Peripheral nerve stimulation is typically reserved for patients with a peripheral mononeuropathy who had a favorable response to a diagnostic nerve block and stimulation trial. (453; **2370–2372**)

28. TENS is the delivery of a pulsed electric current to skin overlying a painful area. The delivery of the electrical current is patient activated via a small, battery-powered, portable unit. It can be a continuously applied stimulation or may be intermittent for periods of about 30 minutes. The maximal paresthesia that can be tolerated by the patient appears to achieve the best results for that patient. The advantages of TENS are that it is patient controlled, noninvasive, and portable and has very few side effects. (454; **2370–2371, Fig. 70–4**)

29. The delivery of an electric current by TENS is believed to work through the activation of large afferent fibers and the descending inhibitory system for the

transmission of pain. This activation of the larger afferent fibers may result in the stimulation of inhibitory dorsal horn neurons and/or the release of endorphins. TENS has also been noted to increase cerebrospinal fluid levels of substance P and 5-hydroxytryptamine. (454; **2370–2371**)

30. TENS is most often used in patients with pain caused by myofascial syndromes and peripheral nerve injury and with phantom limb pain after the amputation of an extremity. TENS has also been used for the pain that is associated with postherpetic neuralgia. (454; **2370–2371**)

ORAL DRUG THERAPY

31. Opioids that are administered to a terminally ill patient for the control of chronic pain should be in doses sufficient to achieve that end. The drug should be administered in a manner in which sufficient blood levels of the drug are sustained so that the effect of the drug does not wane. It is likely that the drug will need to be administered at regular intervals. (454; **2357–2358**)

32. Other drugs that can be administered in combination with opioids to achieve the relief of chronic pain include nonsteroidal anti-inflammatory agents, antidepressants, benzodiazepines, antipsychotics, and anticonvulsants. (454; **2357–2359**)

33. The administration of nonsteroidal anti-inflammatory agents may be useful in conjunction with opioids for the treatment of chronic pain in patients with pain that involves an inflammatory process or in patients with bone pain such as arthritis. (454; **2357**)

34. The administration of an antidepressant drug may be useful in conjunction with opioids for the treatment of chronic pain for some patients. Antidepressants are thought to exert their effect by normalizing sleep patterns, decreasing anxiety, and decreasing the patient's perception of the pain. Antidepressants may enhance neurotransmitters acting on descending efferent inhibitory pain pathways, thus augmenting the analgesia achieved with the opioids. (454; **2359**)

35. The administration of anticonvulsant agents may be useful in conjunction with opioids for the treatment of chronic pain in patients who have neuropathic pain or neuralgias such as trigeminal neuralgia, postherpetic neuralgia, phantom limb pain, or denervation dysesthesias. (454; **2359**)

COMMON CHRONIC PAIN SYNDROMES

36. Myofascial pain is pain located within skeletal muscles and supporting tissues. Myofascial pain may occur after injury to muscles, bones, or joints, or it may occur secondary to pain from a distant site that leads to alterations in position and repeated stress and strain of muscles over time. Discrete tender points in muscle or surrounding tissue are termed *trigger points* when pressure applied to that area reproduces the patient's pain. Trigger points can be caused by a specific traumatic event or chronic repeated stress. The muscles that are affected by trigger points are tight and ropy. There is no physiologic connection between a trigger point and myofascial pain. (455; **2361**)

37. The scapulocostal syndrome is a myofascial pain syndrome whose pain is associated with a trigger point located just medial to and superior to the scapula. The pain commonly radiates to the occiput, shoulder, and anterior chest. (455)

38. The treatment of myofascial pain is through physical therapy with the goal of restoring muscle strength and elasticity. Trigger point injections may be performed at the site of maximal tenderness. Successful trigger point injections have been performed with local anesthetic, saline, and dry needling. This

suggests that it is the mechanical stimulation of the trigger point that provides the benefit. The diagnosis of myofascial trigger points is confirmed by the relief of pain after injection. The onset of analgesia in that area also allows for the patient to participate in physical therapy. (455–456; **2361**)

39. The usual cause of pain in patients with chronic back pain is lumbosacral radiculopathy. Often patients have sought relief with conservative and/or surgical methods before coming to the chronic pain clinic. Lumbosacral radiculopathy usually occurs as a result of inflammation of the nerve root or compression of the dorsal root ganglion. Persistence of the acute inflammatory reaction can lead to intraneural ischemia and degeneration. Patients may experience low back pain, pain radiating down the lower extremity, and motor or sensory nerve loss in the distribution of the affected nerve root in more severe cases. Patients may have chronic pain, decreased productivity, and/or disability as a result of their symptoms. Lumbosacral radiculopathy can be treated with epidural steroid injections when other treatment methods have failed. (455; **2365–2366**)

40. A careful diagnostic examination should be done before administering treatment of the pain associated with lumbosacral radiculopathy in an effort to rule out chronic pain due to infection or space-occupying lesions. This might include a neurologic examination and/or a CT scan. (455, Table 35–2; **2354–2355, 2365–2366**)

41. Epidural corticosteroids are thought to decrease chronic back pain by decreasing the inflammation surrounding the nerve root. The procedure for the administration of epidural corticosteroids begins in a similar fashion to the procedure for the placement of an epidural catheter. The patient is positioned appropriately, and local anesthetic is used to infiltrate the subcutaneous tissues. The epidural space is identified via the loss of resistance technique. A solution containing 3 to 4 mL of a local anesthetic is administered into the epidural space, followed by 80 mg methylprednisolone or 50 mg triamcinolone. An attempt should be made to inject into the epidural space as close to the affected nerve root as possible. The purpose of the injection of local anesthetic is to confirm proper needle placement and to provide the patient with some acute, temporary pain relief. Repeated injections of epidural corticosteroids may follow if the patient has experienced some relief from symptoms for 1 to 2 weeks. (455; **2365–2366**)

42. Repeated epidural corticosteroid injections are unlikely to lead to any beneficial effect if the first injection provided no benefit, if the radicular pain has been present for 6 months or more, or if a laminectomy had been previously performed. This may be due to the formation of thick scar and fibrous tissue around the damaged tissue surrounding the nerve root. (455; **2365–2366**)

43. There are several potential complications of epidural steroid injections, although the risks of these are low. Patients may have backache, postdural puncture headache, or a vasovagal reaction associated with the injection. Case reports of nausea, dizziness, nerve root injury, durocutaneous fistula, and meningitis are also in the literature. Symptoms of aseptic meningitis have occurred in some patients after the administration of corticosteroids in the intrathecal space, although studies have not demonstrated any risk of the intrathecal administration of corticosteroids. There is also concern regarding the systemic absorption of corticosteroids. There are potential risks of acute and chronic adrenal suppression and Cushing's syndrome in these patients. It has been recommended that repeated doses of epidural corticosteroid injections should not be given more frequently than every 6 weeks, owing to the risk of developing Cushing's syndrome from excessive corticosteroid administration. (455; **2365–2366**)

44. Degeneration and inflammation of the lumbar facet and sacroiliac joints can usually be seen by computed tomography. The chronic low back pain associated with this pathology can radiate to the lower extremity, making it difficult to

distinguish from pain due to lumbar radiculopathy. Chronic low back pain from inflammation of the lumbar facet and sacroiliac joints can usually be distinguished from radicular back pain by the injection of 1 mL of local anesthetic into the facet joint. This is often done under fluoroscopy to guide needle placement. If the injection of local anesthetic results in prolonged pain relief, it is then believed that the pain is due to inflammation of the lumbar facet and is not radicular in origin. (455–456)

45. Intercostal neuralgia usually occurs as a result of nerve injury after a thoracotomy or rib fracture. Clinically it presents as paresthesias and pain in response to touch or movement of the thorax. Intercostal neuralgia usually subsides within 2 weeks, but on occasion it can persist for several months or years. It is these patients who usually seek some form of treatment. (456)

46. The most effective treatment plan for intercostal neuralgia is the repeated administration of local anesthetic intercostal or paravertebral nerve blocks. After each injection, the patient should undergo physical therapy while free of pain. Neurolysis with alcohol or phenol in these patients is associated with a high incidence of post-block neuritis and pain that is worse than the original pain. (456)

47. Postherpetic neuralgia refers to the pain that can persist for extended periods of time in patients after they have had an acute infection of herpes zoster. Postherpetic neuralgia usually occurs in elderly or immunocompromised patients. (456)

48. Postherpetic neuralgia has been treated with occasional success with sympathetic nerve blocks in patients who have sought early treatment, with TENS, with the administration of phenothiazines and tricyclic antidepressants as combination therapy, or with the subcutaneous injection of a local anesthetic and triamcinolone under the painful skin area. Local anesthetic, alcohol, and phenol intercostal nerve blocks for postherpetic neuralgia have not been shown to be very effective in relieving the pain. (456; **2359**)

49. Side effects of tricyclic antidepressants include orthostatic hypotension, sedation, and a decrease in appetite. These side effects may limit the usefulness of tricyclic antidepressant medication therapy in elderly patients suffering from postherpetic neuralgia. (456; **2359**)

50. The complex regional pain syndromes refer to the effects on a given extremity that are mediated by sympathetic nervous system dysfunction after trauma, infections, or surgery. These syndromes also result in sympathetically mediated pain. The degree of inciting injury does not correlate with the severity of symptoms. The pathophysiology of these syndromes is poorly understood. Traditionally, these syndromes were referred to as reflex sympathetic dystrophy and causalgia. The complex regional pain syndrome types I and II can be differentiated from each other by the history of the injury. Complex regional pain syndrome type I (reflex sympathetic dystrophy) exists when the history of nerve injury is not specifically known, although there may be a history of tissue injury. Complex regional pain syndrome type II (causalgia) exists when there was at least partial nerve damage inciting the syndrome. (456; **2361–2362**)

51. Clinical manifestations of the complex regional pain syndromes include chronic, severe burning pain, hyperalgesia, bone demineralization, joint stiffness, and atrophic changes. The patient typically has localized sympathetic nervous system dysfunction, which is manifest as warm, erythematous, dry and swollen skin early in the disease process, followed by vasoconstriction, cool, pale and edematous skin later in the course. Patients usually characterize the pain in these syndromes as aching, intense, and/or agonizing. The pain appears to be enhanced by mechanical stimulation, movement, and the application of heat or cold. (456–457; **2361–2362**)

52. The diagnosis of complex regional pain syndrome is made by performing sympathetic blocks in the affected extremity and evaluating the patient for relief of the pain. For the upper extremity a stellate ganglion block may be performed, while for the lower extremity a lumbar sympathetic block may be performed. If sympathetic nerve blockade results in relief of the pain, the diagnosis of complex regional pain syndrome is made. (456; **2361–2362**)

53. The treatment of complex regional pain syndrome is the administration of a series of sympathetic blocks until the symptoms are minimized. After each sympathetic block the patient should participate in physical therapy and possibly TENS to improve muscular strength and function. A delay in the diagnosis and treatment of complex regional pain syndrome results in poorer outcome from interventions and treatments. For example, if the delay of treatment is longer than 6 months, the success rate becomes 50% or less. This is in contrast to a success rate of about 90% in patients whose treatment with sympathetic blocks began within 1 month of the onset of symptoms. (456–457; **2361–2362**)

54. Brachial plexus blockade produces unnecessary blockade of sensory and motor nerve fibers in addition to the nerves of the sympathetic nervous system. The blockade will result in relief of the pain associated with complex regional pain syndrome but is in excess of what is necessary. (456; **2361–2362**)

55. Pharmacologic agents that can be used for intravenous regional sympathetic nerve blockade include guanethidine and phentolamine. These agents are believed to work by blocking alpha receptors that may be present in injured nerves, resulting in a decrease in sympathetic nervous system input to these receptors. This technique appears to be most useful in patients who have undergone stellate ganglion or lumbar sympathetic blockade that has been unsuccessful in alleviating the patient's pain or in patients who have undergone surgical excision of sympathetic ganglia but are experiencing a return of sympathetic nervous system function. (456; **2361–2362**)

CANCER PAIN

56. Patients with cancer may experience pain from local tumor infiltration or metastases. Tumor or metastases to bone or infiltrating nerves are especially painful. Patients may also experience pain as a side effect of chemotherapy, irradiation, or surgical treatment. Examples include phantom limb pain, peripheral neuropathy, and radiation fibrosis. Approximately 40% of patients with cancer experience chronic pain. (457; **2353**)

57. The mainstay of treatment of chronic pain for cancer patients is opioid drug therapy. The patient should be made as comfortable as possible. Addiction to drugs is not an issue in these patients given that their illness is terminal. A stable dosing regimen is usually able to be achieved in the absence of the progression of symptoms associated with progressing disease. Tricyclic antidepressants may be useful in patients with cancer for the treatment of depression that is associated with their illness, to potentiate the effects of opioids, to facilitate nocturnal sleep, and to improve mood. Anticonvulsant medications may be useful in patients with cancer for the treatment of pain that is neuropathic in origin. Corticosteroid medications may be useful in patients with cancer to decrease the sensation of pain, to improve mood, and to increase appetite. (457; **2357–2359**)

58. Intravenous, neuraxial, transdermal, and transmucosal routes of administration are alternative routes of analgesic drug delivery for the cancer patient with chronic pain in whom the oral administration of medicines is not possible. (458; **2358**)

59. Patients with chronic pain secondary to cancer who have not had success with

pain control with less invasive procedures may benefit from some neurosurgical procedures for the treatment of the pain. Neurosurgical procedures that may be useful in these cancer patients include a cordotomy or dorsal rhizotomy. A cordotomy is the open or percutaneous interruption of the spinothalamic tract. A dorsal rhizotomy is the interruption of the sensory nerve root. (458; **2367–2368**)

60. A neurolytic celiac plexus block may be useful to treat pain associated with cancer of the pancreas or upper abdominal organs. Except for the left colon and pelvic organs, the sensory and autonomic nervous system fibers from the abdominal viscera are carried by the celiac plexus. In one study, blockade of the celiac plexus results in partial to complete analgesia in 90% of patients who were alive 3 months after the procedure. (458; **1545, 2364–2365**)

61. A neurolytic celiac plexus block can be performed with 30 to 50 mL of either 50% alcohol or 6% phenol. The injection of these medicines may result in some pain, so premedication of the patient with analgesics is recommended. The position of the needle is usually verified by radiography or computed tomography. (458; **1545, 2364–2365**)

62. The complication rate of celiac plexus blocks is about 2%. Complications include intravascular injection, epidural or subarachnoid injection resulting in paraplegia, or needle trauma to the kidney, lung, or intestine. Postblock orthostatic hypotension can occur after the performance of a celiac plexus block as a result of the splanchnic vasodilation that occurs after the nerves supplying those organs are blocked. The risk of orthostatic hypotension can be decreased by the prophylactic infusion of intravenous fluids. A potential side effect of celiac plexus blockade is diarrhea. (458; **1545, 2364–2365**)

Chapter 35

Cardiopulmonary Resuscitation

1. What is cardiopulmonary resuscitation (CPR)? What is basic life support (BLS)? What is advanced cardiac life support (ACLS)?

2. What are the responsibilities of the team leader during CPR?

3. What are some determinants of survival after CPR?

PROVISION OF A PATENT UPPER AIRWAY

4. What is the head tilt/jaw thrust? What is its goal? How can it be modified in a patient with a suggested neck injury?

EXHALED AIR VENTILATION

5. What inspired concentration of oxygen is delivered during mouth-to-mouth ventilation? Why is arterial hypoxemia predictable during mouth-to-mouth ventilation?

6. How can gastric distention be prevented during mouth-to-mouth ventilation?

CLOSED-CHEST (EXTERNAL) CARDIAC COMPRESSION

7. Where should the rescuer's hands be placed on the adult patient to maximize blood flow during closed-chest cardiac compression? What are some risks to the patient when the rescuer's hands are erroneously placed during closed-chest cardiac compression?

8. How should the rescuer be positioned relative to the patient during closed-chest cardiac compression? How much should the sternum of an adult patient be depressed during closed-chest cardiac compression?

9. What is the minimum number of recommended compressions per minute for adult closed-chest cardiac compression? What is the ratio of cardiac compressions to mouth-to-mouth ventilation during one-rescuer CPR? What is the ratio of cardiac compressions to mouth-to-mouth ventilation during two-rescuer CPR?

10. What are the two proposed mechanisms for blood flow during closed-chest cardiac compression? Which of these is thought to predominate?

11. How can the effectiveness of closed-chest cardiac compression be verified? If end-tidal CO_2 monitors are available, what end-tidal CO_2 during CPR is suggestive of a grave prognosis?

12. What systolic blood pressure can be produced by closed-chest cardiac compression? What systolic blood pressure is palpable? What diastolic blood pressure can be produced by closed-chest cardiac compression?

13. Which organ is most vulnerable to hypoxemic damage from cardiac arrest?

SPECIALIZED EQUIPMENT TO MAINTAIN THE AIRWAY

14. What is the advantage to the rescuer of a portable pocket face mask for mouth-to-mouth ventilation?

15. What are some advantages of reservoir bags attached to a pocket face mask for mouth-to-mouth ventilation?

16. What is a potential risk of placing an oropharyngeal airway in a conscious or semi-conscious patient for the maintenance of a patent airway?

17. What are the advantages of the placement of a cuffed endotracheal tube for ventilation of the lungs of the patient during CPR?

18. How effective are mechanical ventilators during CPR?

EXTERNAL DEFIBRILLATION AND TREATMENT OF VENTRICULAR FIBRILLATION

19. What is the definitive treatment of ventricular fibrillation? What is the most important determinant of the success of external defibrillation for the patient's survival?

20. How many joules of electrical shock should be delivered for the initial attempt at external defibrillation of the adult patient's heart? How many joules should be delivered in subsequent defibrillation attempts, provided they are necessary?

21. What is the appropriate paddle size and placement on the chest for external defibrillation?

22. What is the risk of external defibrillation in the patient with an artificial cardiac pacemaker?

DRUG THERAPY

23. What is the goal of initial drug therapy during CPR? What are the mainstays of treatment for the patient in cardiac arrest?

24. What actions of epinephrine are thought to be responsible for its beneficial effects during cardiac arrest?

25. What actions of vasopressin are thought to be responsible for its beneficial effects during cardiac arrest?

26. When might amiodarone be administered during cardiac arrest?

27. What is the advantage of the delivery of drugs by a centrally placed catheter during CPR? How long should the rescuers wait for drug administered via a peripheral vein to reach the central circulation?

28. What are two alternatives for drug delivery when vascular access is not available?

CARDIAC ASYSTOLE

29. What are some causes of cardiac asystole?

30. What is the survival rate to hospital discharge for patients who have had cardiac asystole and have undergone resuscitative efforts? What treatment modality should be considered in patients with cardiac asystole?

PULSELESS ELECTRICAL ACTIVITY

31. What are some causes of pulseless electrical activity?

32. What is pulseless electrical activity? How should it be treated?

VENTRICULAR TACHYCARDIA

33. What are some causes of ventricular tachycardia?

34. What is the appropriate treatment of ventricular tachycardia?

35. What is the risk of cardioversion that is not synchronized?

36. What is torsades de pointes? What are some causes of torsades de pointes?

37. What is the treatment of torsades de pointes?

PAROXYSMAL SUPRAVENTRICULAR TACHYCARDIA

38. What is the appropriate treatment of paroxysmal supraventricular tachycardia?

39. What are some side effects of the administration of adenosine?

MANAGEMENT OF THE OBSTRUCTED AIRWAY

40. What is the recommended method of treating a foreign body in the glottic opening obstructing the airway in both conscious and unconscious patients? What are some complications of this maneuver?

41. What is the recommended method of treating a foreign body in the glottic opening obstructing the airway in a morbidly obese patient or near-term parturient?

42. When should a blind finger examination of the pharynx be performed in an adult? When should a blind finger examination of the pharynx be performed in a child? What is the risk of a blind finger examination of the pharynx?

PRECORDIAL THUMP

43. What is a precordial thump? When is a precordial thump recommended in adult patients? When is a precordial thump recommended in pediatric patients?

RESUSCITATION OF INFANTS AND CHILDREN

44. Where is the most palpable pulse in infants up to 1 year of age? Where is the most palpable pulse in children?

45. How should the head tilt/jaw thrust be modified in infants and children?

46. How should mouth-to-mouth ventilation be modified in infants?

47. How should closed-chest cardiac compression be performed in infants?

48. How should closed-chest cardiac compression be performed in children?

49. What energy setting in joules should be applied for optimal success of shock delivery for external defibrillation in children? If the initial attempt at defibrillation is unsuccessful, what energy setting should be used for the subsequent attempt?

POSTRESUSCITATION LIFE SUPPORT

50. How should a cardiac arrest patient be managed after the establishment of a spontaneous cardiac output?

51. After what length of time of global cerebral ischemia produced by cardiac arrest is irreversible brain injury thought to result? What is the controversy regarding the administration of calcium during and after CPR with regard to cerebral ischemia?

52. What are some monitors and supportive measures specific for the central nervous system in the cardiac arrest patient with residual neurologic dysfunction? What is the goal of treatment in these patients?

53. What is the potential benefit of barbiturates during the postresuscitation period?

54. Does the postresuscitation administration of corticosteroids or hypothermia improve patient survival or outcome?

55. Why are patients with hyperglycemia at the time of cardiac arrest believed to have a less favorable outcome than patients who are normoglycemic?

56. What are some of the criteria for brain death in an adult?

DO NOT RESUSCITATE ORDERS

57. When should Do Not Resuscitate orders be considered? Who should make this decision for a patient if the patient is incapable?

58. What are some treatment modalities relatively common in the practice of anesthesia that may require discussion before the delivery of anesthesia to the patient who has Do Not Resuscitate orders?

ANSWERS*

1. Cardiopulmonary resuscitation (CPR) is the institution of artificial circulation and ventilation until advanced cardiac life support can be rendered or until spontaneous cardiopulmonary function returns. Basic life support (BLS) is the evaluation of and provision for a patent upper airway, mouth-to-mouth ventilation, and circulation through closed-chest cardiac compressions. BLS can be instituted by any lay person who has been trained to provide BLS, because no specialized equipment is necessary. Advanced cardiac life support (ACLS) provides for the same things as BLS, that is, ventilation and circulation, but also utilizes specialized equipment, drugs, and training to achieve those ends. (459, Table 36–1; **2533**)

2. Responsibilities of the team leader during CPR include ensuring the quality of BLS, facilitating the early use of electrical defibrillation, directing and monitoring the adequacy of drug therapy, and making the decision to end resuscitative efforts when in vain. (459)

3. Patients with an unwitnessed cardiac arrest, asystole, or pulseless electrical activity, and patients in the hospital with preexisting oliguria, metastatic cancer, sepsis, pneumonia, cardiogenic shock, or acute stroke have all been shown to have very poor outcomes with CPR. The most critical factors in outcome for patients with ventricular fibrillation or ventricular tachycardia are whether it was witnessed and the time elapsed before defibrillation. Patients who have had CPR initiated in the hospital appear to have a 10% to 20% rate of survival to hospital discharge. (459; **2548**)

PROVISION OF A PATENT UPPER AIRWAY

4. The head tilt/jaw thrust is a maneuver that is used to provide the patient with a patent upper airway. Because most upper airway obstruction in unconscious patients occurs because of the tongue falling against the posterior pharynx, the maneuver involves extension of the head and displacement of the mandible to an anterior position to stretch the muscles attached to the tongue. When done appropriately, the head tilt/jaw thrust pulls the tongue off the posterior pharynx and may provide the patient with a patent upper airway. For patients with a suspected neck injury the rescuer should modify the head tilt/jaw thrust maneuver to avoid exacerbating potential spinal cord trauma. The head tilt should be

*Numbers in parentheses: lightface numbers refer to pages, figures, or tables in Stoelting RK, Miller RD: Basics of Anesthesia, 4th ed. Philadelphia, Churchill Livingstone, 2000; **boldface numbers** refer to pages, figures, or tables in Miller RD: Anesthesia, 5th ed. Philadelphia, Churchill Livingstone, 2000.

excluded from the maneuver and only the jaw thrust performed in these patients. (459–460, Fig. 36–1; **1415–1416, 2533–2534**)

EXHALED AIR VENTILATION

5. Mouth-to-mouth ventilation, when performed properly, delivers an inspired concentration of oxygen of 16% to 17%. The alveolar Po_2 that is maximally obtainable from mouth-to-mouth ventilation is about 80 mm Hg, such that the arterial Po_2 that is usually achieved under these circumstances is even lower. This means that arterial hypoxemia is predictable during mouth-to-mouth ventilation even when properly performed. Interestingly, in the absence of airway obstruction substantial air exchange occurs with closed-chest cardiac compressions, leading some to question the need for mouth-to-mouth ventilation during initial BLS. (460)

6. Gastric distention is likely to occur during mouth-to-mouth ventilation. It can be prevented by using inflation pressures that are less than 15 cm H_2O. It is not recommended to place manual pressure over the patient's epigastrium to prevent air entering the stomach, because this may increase the likelihood of regurgitation in the patient. (460; **2533–2534**)

CLOSED-CHEST (EXTERNAL) CARDIAC COMPRESSION

7. For closed-chest cardiac compression in the adult patient, the rescuer's hands should be placed over and parallel to the lower one third of the patient's sternum. This provides for maximum compression to the underlying cardiac ventricles and optimizes blood flow produced by the compressions. If the rescuer's hands are erroneously placed during closed-chest cardiac compression, not only is blood flow not optimized but the patient may suffer from damage as well. For example, pressure over the xiphoid process or rib cage can result in damage to abdominal organs, especially the liver, or cause rib fractures. Rib fractures can result in damage to the heart and lungs. (460–461; **2491**)

8. During closed-chest cardiac compression the rescuer should be positioned in a kneeling position next to the patient. The rescuer's upper body should be directly over the patient's chest, the rescuer's shoulders positioned directly over his or her hands, and his or her elbows kept straight. This position enables the rescuer to use the weight of his or her upper body for compression and may prevent early tiring. The sternum of an adult patient should be depressed 3.8 to 5 cm (1.5 to 2 inches) during closed-chest cardiac compression. (461, Fig. 35–2; **2534**)

9. The minimum number of compressions per minute for adult closed-chest cardiac compression is 80. The ratio of cardiac compressions to mouth-to-mouth ventilation during one-rescuer CPR is 15:2. The ratio of cardiac compressions to mouth-to-mouth ventilation during two-rescuer CPR is 5:1. (461; **2534**)

10. There are two proposed mechanisms for blood flow during closed-chest cardiac compression. The one traditionally thought of is that of direct compression of the cardiac ventricles between the sternum and the spine, resulting in an increase in intra-cardiac pressures, closure of the tricuspid and mitral valves, and the forward flow of blood into the pulmonary arteries and aorta. This is referred to as the *cardiac pump* mechanism. The second proposed mechanism for blood flow is the facilitation of forward blood flow secondary to the increase in intrathoracic pressure that accompanies closed-chest compressions. This mechanism is commonly referred to as the *thoracic pump* mechanism. Evidence for the thoracic pump mechanism is that increases in the intrathoracic pressure produced by repeated, forceful coughing can sustain consciousness for as long as 1.5 minutes. The predominant mechanism for blood flow achieved during

closed-chest compression is unclear. Patient-related factors such as heart size, the anterior-to-posterior chest distance, and thoracic compliance are believed to influence which of these predominate. In addition, rescuer technique may also have an influence. For example, manual versus mechanical compression and the duration and depth of the compression may also be factors. (461, Fig. 36–3; **2534–2536, Figs. 75–1, 75–2**)

11. Verification of the effectiveness of closed-chest cardiac compression can be estimated by the palpation of peripheral pulses and by observation of pupillary size. A capnogram may also be used to guide the effectiveness of closed-chest cardiac compression. When ventilation and CO_2 production are constant, alterations in the end-tidal CO_2 are reflective of alterations in pulmonary blood flow and cardiac output. When end-tidal CO_2 monitors are available during closed-chest cardiac compression, an end-tidal CO_2 of 20 mm Hg or more suggests effective CPR. Conversely, an end-tidal CO_2 of 10 mm Hg or less is suggestive of a grave prognosis. (462; **2536–2537**)

12. A systolic blood pressure in excess of 100 mm Hg can be produced by closed-chest cardiac compression. A pulse becomes palpable when the systolic blood pressure is 70 mm Hg or greater. Diastolic blood pressures produced by closed-chest cardiac compression are usually between 10 and 40 mm Hg. (461–462)

13. The organ most vulnerable to hypoxemic damage from cardiac arrest is the heart. This is because of the poor coronary artery blood flow that is achievable by closed-chest cardiac compression. Coronary artery blood flow during closed-chest cardiac compression is usually only 5% to 10% of normal coronary artery blood flow. The discrepancy between normal coronary artery blood flow and coronary artery blood flow achieved during closed-chest cardiac compression is accounted for by the poor diastolic blood pressure achievable by closed-chest cardiac compression. (461–462)

SPECIALIZED EQUIPMENT TO MAINTAIN THE AIRWAY

14. A portable pocket face mask for mouth-to-mouth ventilation offers the rescuer the advantage of isolation from the patient's saliva and potentially from viral diseases and vomitus. (462)

15. Advantages of a reservoir bag that attaches to a pocket face mask for mouth-to-mouth ventilation are that, in addition to the protection conferred by the pocket face mask, the reservoir bag has a one-way valve that allows for the manual ventilation of the patient's lungs. It also offers the ability to deliver supplemental oxygen while ventilating the lungs. (463)

16. Coughing, vomiting, laryngospasm, and bronchospasm are potential risks of placing an oropharyngeal airway in a conscious or semi-conscious patient. (463; **1421**)

17. There are several advantages of the placement of a cuffed endotracheal tube for ventilation of the lungs of the patient during CPR. First, it allows for the adjustment of tidal volume and frequency of breathing. Patients requiring high inspiratory pressures for ventilation and oxygenation may require endotracheal intubation. Endotracheal intubation also allows for the addition of supplemental oxygen in a reliable manner. Finally, it provides the lungs with some protection against the aspiration of gastric contents when the endotracheal tube cuff is inflated with air. Endotracheal intubation is the standard of care for airway control in patients during CPR in critical care settings. (463; **2354**)

18. Mechanical ventilators are not effective during CPR with any reliability. Pressure-cycled ventilation may lead to a prematurely terminated inspiratory cycle when intrathoracic pressures increase associated with closed-chest cardiac com-

pression. Volume-cycled ventilation is also unable to deliver reliable tidal volumes during closed-chest cardiac compression. Ventilation of the lungs may be done manually or with a manually triggered oxygen-powered breathing device. (463)

EXTERNAL DEFIBRILLATION AND TREATMENT OF VENTRICULAR FIBRILLATION

19. The definitive treatment of ventricular fibrillation is external defibrillation. The most important determinant of the success of external defibrillation for ventricular fibrillation is the duration of the time lapse between cardiopulmonary arrest and external defibrillation. For this reason the current recommendation is to apply external defibrillation as soon as possible in these patients. (463, Fig. 36–4; **2545**)

20. The initial attempt at external defibrillation requires a shock of 200 joules for adult patients. A second defibrillation attempt, if necessary, involves the delivery of a shock of 200 to 300 joules. A third attempt should not exceed a setting of 360 joules. (463–464; **2545–2546**)

21. External defibrillation of an adult's heart should be with paddles that are 8 to 10 cm in diameter. External defibrillation of an infant's or child's heart should be with paddles that are about 4.5 cm in diameter. The paddles should be applied to the chest with firm pressure in positions that will maximize the flow of electrical current through the myocardium. The standard for placement is with one electrode below the clavicle and to the right of the sternum, whereas the second electrode is usually placed at the level of the apex of the heart in the midaxillary line. Poor technique can lead to an increase in the resistance to current flow during shock delivery. (464, Fig. 36–5; **2545**)

22. The risk of external defibrillation in the patient with an artificial cardiac pacemaker is malfunction of the pacemaker if the electrodes are placed too near the pacemaker. It is therefore recommended that the paddles be placed 10 to 12 cm away from the pacemaker generator. (464)

DRUG THERAPY

23. The goal of initial drug therapy during CPR is the correction of arterial hypoxemia and the increasing of coronary and cerebral perfusion pressures. The mainstay for treatment of the patient in cardiopulmonary arrest is the administration of oxygen and epinephrine. (464, Table 35–2; **2546–2547**)

24. The effects of epinephrine that are thought to be primarily responsible for its beneficial effects during cardiac arrest occur as a result of its action on alpha-1 receptors. These effects include increased cerebral and coronary perfusion pressures, intense arterial vasoconstriction in other vascular beds, and a selective redistribution of cardiac output. There is evidence that epinephrine administered early in the resuscitative effort after cardiac arrest is correlated with improved outcome. The dose of epinephrine during cardiac arrest that provides optimal outcome has not been determined, but maintenance of a diastolic pressure of 40 mm Hg as measured by direct arterial pressure monitoring is desirable. (464; **2546**)

25. Newly revised ACLS guidelines have recently been issued by the American Heart Association. One change is the addition of vasopressin (antidiuretic hormone) to the algorithm for pulseless ventricular fibrillation and/or ventricular tachycardia. Vasopressin, if administered, is in lieu of epinephrine after the three initial defibrillation attempts by electric shock have failed. Under these conditions, the dose of vasopressin administered should be a single dose of 40

units intravenously. Subsequent dosing should be with epinephrine. The potent vasoconstrictor action of vasopressin is thought to be primarily responsible for its beneficial effects during cardiac arrest. Vasopressin administration also results in the tubular concentration of water, increased urine osmolality, and negative free water clearance by the kidneys. **(679–680)**

26. Amiodarone has also been added to the algorithm for pulseless ventricular fibrillation and/or ventricular tachycardia in the newly revised ACLS guidelines issued by the American Heart Association. Amiodarone is considered an alternative to lidocaine for shock-refractory ventricular fibrillation and ventricular tachycardia. Amiodarone has a broad antiarrhythmic spectrum with little inotropic effect. (**1245**)

27. The advantage of the delivery of drugs by a centrally placed catheter during CPR is the rapid delivery of drugs to the heart. When a peripheral intravenous site is used for the administration of drugs during cardiopulmonary arrest, a period of 1 to 2 minutes should be allowed for drugs to reach the central circulation. CPR should not be interrupted for placement of central venous access, however. (464; **2546**)

28. Two alternatives for drug delivery when vascular access is not available include drug delivery via an endotracheal tube to be absorbed across the tracheal and bronchial mucosa and the interosseous infusion of drugs. Drugs that can be absorbed across the tracheal mucosa include epinephrine, lidocaine, and atropine. The interosseous infusion of drugs is most useful in pediatric patients when intravenous access is not readily available. (464–465; **2546, 2552, Fig. 75–19**)

CARDIAC ASYSTOLE

29. Causes of cardiac asystole include persistent hypoxia, severe hyperkalemia, massive drug overdose, myocardial infarction, and hypothermia. (465; **2547**)

30. The survival rate to hospital discharge for patients who have had cardiac asystole and have undergone resuscitative efforts is less than 2%. CPR, epinephrine, atropine, and transcutaneous pacing are all treatment modalities that should be considered for the patient in cardiac asystole. (465, Fig. 36–6; **2547**)

PULSELESS ELECTRICAL ACTIVITY

31. Causes of pulseless electrical activity include hypoxia, hypovolemia, cardiac tamponade, tension pneumothorax, pulmonary embolus, hypothermia, hyperkalemia, acidosis, myocardial infarction, or overdose with digitalis, beta blockers, calcium channel blockers, and tricyclic antidepressants. (466; **2547**)

32. *Pulseless electrical activity* is a term used to describe the presence of a cardiac rhythm on the electrocardiogram while an inadequate stroke volume is being generated. In patients with pulseless electrical activity there will be a disappearance of peripheral pulses or systemic blood pressure. Cardiac rhythms that may be present include organized electrical activity, idioventricular rhythms, ventricular escape rhythms, and bradyasystole. Electromechanical dissociation is a type of pulseless electrical activity in which the cardiac rhythm appears to have organized electrical activity. Pulseless electrical activity should be treated with the rapid administration of epinephrine, as well as with a search for, and correction of, possible causes. (466, Fig. 36–7; **2547**)

VENTRICULAR TACHYCARDIA

33. Causes of ventricular tachycardia include hypoxemia, hypercarbia, hypokalemia, hypomagnesemia, digitalis toxicity, and derangements in the arterial pH. (467; **2542**)

34. The appropriate treatment of ventricular tachycardia is determined by the stability of the patient. Patients who are hemodynamically unstable, show evidence of acute myocardial ischemia or infarction, or have acute pulmonary edema should undergo immediate synchronized cardioversion. Cardioversion is initially with a shock of 100 joules, with the energy setting incrementally increased as needed. Patients whose condition is stable can undergo drug treatment of ventricular tachycardia. Medicines that may be used include amiodarone, lidocaine, procainamide, or bretylium. In the newly revised ACLS guidelines, amiodarone dominates the management of ventricular tachycardia because of its antiarrhythmic potential and minimal inotropic effect. Amiodarone exerts its effect within one hour of its intravenous administration. Underlying causes of ventricular tachycardia should be sought and treated. Although the administration of verapamil to patients with a paroxysmal supraventricular tachycardia is an acceptable treatment option, the administration of verapamil to patients with ventricular tachycardia can be lethal. (467, Fig. 36–8; **2542–2545**)

35. The risk of cardioversion that is not synchronized is ventricular fibrillation. Ventricular fibrillation results if the cardioversion shock occurs on the relative refractory period of the cardiac cycle. (467)

36. Torsades de pointes is an atypical form of ventricular tachycardia with a characteristic twisting of the QRS around the baseline such that it appears as a sine wave. Causes of torsades de pointes include drugs such as quinidine, procainamide, disopyramide, phenothiazines, and tricyclic antidepressants; bradycardia; hypokalemia; hypomagnesemia; and acute myocardial ischemia or infarction. (**2543**)

37. The treatment of torsades de pointes may include overdrive pacing of the cardiac atria or ventricles and/or treatment with magnesium sulfate for stable patients. Isoproterenol may also be used to break the arrhythmia. Patients whose condition is unstable should undergo defibrillation. (**2543–2544**)

PAROXYSMAL SUPRAVENTRICULAR TACHYCARDIA

38. The factor that determines the appropriate method of treatment of paroxysmal supraventricular tachycardia is the amount of hemodynamic compromise that occurs as a result of the cardiac dysrhythmia. Patients who are hemodynamically unstable should undergo immediate synchronized cardioversion. The treatment of patients with paroxysmal ventricular tachycardia whose condition is stable includes vagal maneuvers, adenosine, and amiodarone. (467, Fig. 36–9; **2539–2541**)

39. Side effects of the administration of adenosine include flushing, dyspnea, chest pain, and bronchospasm. (467; **2540**)

MANAGEMENT OF THE OBSTRUCTED AIRWAY

40. The recommended method of treatment for both conscious and unconscious patients with a foreign body in the glottic opening is the rapid, manual delivery of pressure in an inward and upward direction overlying the patient's epigastrium. This maneuver has been termed *abdominal thrust, external subdiaphragmatic compression,* or the *Heimlich maneuver.* With the maneuver the diaphragm is forced cephalad, the lungs become compressed, and an outward force of air occurs as a result of the increased airway pressures. Complications of the maneuver include rib fractures or the rupture or laceration of thoracic or abdominal viscera. (468, Fig. 36–10, Table 36–1; **2467**)

41. The recommended method of treating a morbidly obese patient or near-term parturient with a foreign body in the glottic opening is the chest thrust. The chest thrust is manual compression over the middle or lower sternum. Alternatively, in the adult patient a precordial thump may be delivered because it creates airway pressures that are similar to those achieved with a chest thrust. (468, Fig. 36–10)

42. A blind finger examination of the pharynx of an unconscious adult patient who has an obstruction of the glottic opening should only be performed when the other appropriate maneuvers have been attempted without success. A blind finger examination of the pharynx of an unconscious child who has an obstruction of the glottic opening is not recommended unless the object of obstruction is visualized. The risk of a blind finger examination of the pharynx is impaction of the object deeper into the airway. This risk is greatest in children. (469)

PRECORDIAL THUMP

43. A precordial thump is the delivery of a single, forceful blow by the rescuer with a closed fist to the middle portion of the patient's sternum. A precordial thump is recommended in adult patients for the initial treatment of ventricular fibrillation or tachycardia or for cardiac asystole due to complete heart block when a defibrillator is not immediately available. Immediate external defibrillation should not be delayed for a precordial thump. A precordial thump is not recommended in pediatric patients. (469; **2546**)

RESUSCITATION OF INFANTS AND CHILDREN

44. The most palpable pulse in infants up to 1 year of age is the brachial artery pulse in the mid-upper arm. The most palpable pulse in children older than 1 year of age is the carotid artery pulse. (467; **2549, Table 75–3**)

45. The head tilt/jaw thrust maneuver should be modified when applied to infants. In infants, care must be taken to avoid excessive extension of the head, because this may result in obstruction of the upper airway. Moderate extension of the head may be useful in pediatric patients for opening the upper airway. (467; **2076–2077**)

46. Mouth-to-mouth ventilation of the infant patient should be modified from that of adults given their smaller body size and smaller tidal volumes. The rescuer should use his or her mouth to cover and seal the entire nose and mouth of the infant. The cephalad position of the infant's larynx and the proximity of the epiglottis to the palate actually make ventilation of the infant's lungs easier via the nose than the mouth. (467)

47. The heart in infants and children has been confirmed to be positioned below the lower sternum, as in adults. Hand placement during closed-chest cardiac compression in infants can be accomplished two ways. The rescuer's hands can encircle the infant's chest, with the thumbs used to depress the lower sternum. Alternatively, the rescuer's one hand can be used to support the back while the compressions are performed with two fingers of the other hand. Closed-chest cardiac compression in the infant should be performed at a rate of at least 100 per minute. The sternum of the infant patient during closed-chest cardiac compression should be depressed by 1.25 to 2.5 cm (0.5 to 1 inch) per compression. (467; **2490–2491, 2549, Table 75–3**)

48. Closed-chest cardiac compression in children can be accomplished with the heel of one hand directed over the lower sternum. The recommended rate of closed-chest cardiac compression in children is 100 per minute as in infants, whereas depression of the sternum should be by 2.5 to 4 cm (1.0 to 1.5 inches) per compression. (467; **2490–2491, 2549, Table 75–3**)

49. The energy setting that should be used for the optimal success of external defibrillation of children is directly related to their body weight. The recommended energy setting is 2 joules/kg. If the initial attempt at defibrillation is unsuccessful, the subsequent attempt should be made with double the initial energy setting. (469; **2553–2554, Fig. 75–20**)

POSTRESUSCITATION LIFE SUPPORT

50. The management of the cardiac arrest patient after the establishment of a spontaneous cardiac output is termed *postresuscitation life support*. Postresuscitation life support should include close monitoring, supplemental oxygen, and radiography of the chest; drug therapy as needed to maintain organ function; and optimal adjustment of the intravascular fluid volume. Hemodialysis may also be required if the patient suffers from renal failure. (469)

51. Irreversible brain injury was once thought to occur after 4 to 6 minutes of global cerebral ischemia produced by cardiac arrest. More recent evidence suggests that the central nervous system neurons may actually tolerate 20 to 60 minutes of complete anoxia without always sustaining irreversible injury. Calcium is believed to play a role in small vessel vasoconstriction in the cerebral vessels, making its administration controversial during periods of cerebral hypoperfusion or ischemia as during cardiac arrest. (469–470; **721, 2392–2393**)

52. Monitoring of the central nervous system of cardiac arrest patients who may have suffered from central nervous system damage includes the monitoring of intracranial pressures, an electroencephalogram, computed tomography of the brain, determination of cortical evoked potentials, the measurement of total and/ or regional cerebral blood flow, and frequent neurologic examinations. Supportive measures for these patients include the control of the intracranial pressure, maintenance of cerebral oxygen delivery, and decreasing the cerebral metabolic oxygen requirement. The goal of treatment in these patients is the minimization of the degree of secondary injury that can occur with postresuscitation cerebral hypoperfusion. (470; **721, 2392–2393**)

53. There was some belief that barbiturates may have potential benefit during the postresuscitation period owing to the ability of barbiturates to decrease intracranial pressures, suppress seizure activity, and produce dose-dependent decreases in cerebral metabolic oxygen requirements to a maximum of about 50%. Barbiturates may be titrated to achieve a maximum decrease in cerebral metabolic oxygen requirements by the use of an electroencephalogram. The maximum decrease in cerebral metabolic oxygen requirements attainable corresponds to an isoelectric electroencephalogram. The isoelectric point on the electroencephalogram reflects the point at which there is maximal depression of mentation without a change in the amount of oxygen needed to maintain cell viability. There has been no evidence of any derived benefit from the administration of barbiturates after cardiac arrest, however. (470; **223–224, 719–721, 1329, 2392–2393**)

54. The postresuscitation administration of corticosteroids or hypothermia has not been shown to improve patient survival or outcome. (470)

55. Patients with hyperglycemia at the time of cardiac arrest are believed to have a less favorable outcome than normoglycemic patients, possibly because the hyperglycemia reflects the production of lactate and intracellular acidosis due to anaerobic glycolysis. Solutions containing glucose should not be administered during cardiac arrest because glucose is associated with worsened survivor neurologic outcomes. (470; **2546, 2553**)

56. Criteria for brain death include a coma persisting more than 12 hours in the

presence of a known cause, angiographic evidence of absent cerebral circulation, absent cortical function as reflected by a flat electroencephalogram for 60 minutes, and absent brain stem function as reflected by either fixed and unreactive pupils or apnea despite a normal to increased $Paco_2$. These criteria must hold true in the absence of hypothermia or drug overdose. (470; **2396, 2560–2570, Table 76–2**)

DO NOT RESUSCITATE ORDERS

57. Do Not Resuscitate (DNR) orders should be considered when it is believed that efforts at CPR would be futile, when CPR is not in the best interest for the patient, or when CPR is not desired by the patient. If the patient is incapable of making the decision for the application of DNR orders, a third party should be solicited to make the decision. Often, the surrogate decision maker is a member of the patient's immediate family or is appointed by the courts. All decisions regarding the resuscitation status of the patient should be documented clearly in the patient's chart and discussed with the patient's health care team. (470; **2392, 2548, 2721–2722**)

58. There are several treatment modalities that are relatively common in the practice of anesthesia that may require discussion with the patient or the patient's surrogate before the delivery of anesthesia to patients with DNR orders. Some of the treatments are blood product transfusion, the maintenance of intravascular volume with nonblood products, the administration of supplemental oxygen, tracheal intubation, external cardiac chest compression, electrical defibrillation and artificial cardiac pacing, vasoactive drug administration, and postoperative support of ventilation of the lungs. (470–471; **2392, 2548, 2721–2722**)

Index

Note: Page numbers followed by t refer to tables.